Chronic Kidney Disease: An Evidence-Based Approach

Chronic Kidney Disease: An Evidence-Based Approach

Edited by Felicity Darko

hayle
medical

New York

Hayle Medical,
750 Third Avenue, 9th Floor,
New York, NY 10017, USA

Visit us on the World Wide Web at:
www.haylemedical.com

ISBN: 978-1-63241-663-6

Cataloging-in-Publication Data

Chronic kidney disease : an evidence-based approach / edited by Felicity Darko.
    p. cm.
Includes bibliographical references and index.
ISBN 978-1-63241-663-6
1. Kidneys--Diseases. 2. Chronic diseases. 3. Nephrology. I. Darko, Felicity.
RC902 .C47 2019
616.61--dc23

Contents

Preface

Chronic kidney disease is a form of kidney disease, in which the loss of kidney's function or failure takes place gradually over a period of months or years. High blood pressure, leg swelling, anemia and loss of appetite are some of its symptoms. The main causes which lead to the loss of kidney function include diabetes, high blood pressure and glomerular nephritis. Urine dipstick, nuclear medicine MAG3 scan and renal ultrasonography are some of the most commonly used techniques to assess the functioning of kidneys. Renal dialysis and kidney transplant are two of the most effective ways to treat chronic kidney disease. This book discusses the fundamentals as well as modern approaches of chronic kidney disease. It presents researches and studies performed by experts across the globe. This book will help new researchers by foregrounding their knowledge in this branch.

The information shared in this book is based on empirical researches made by veterans in this field of study. The elaborative information provided in this book will help the readers further their scope of knowledge leading to advancements in this field.

Finally, I would like to thank my fellow researchers who gave constructive feedback and my family members who supported me at every step of my research.

Editor

The Use of Surrogate Endpoints in Regulating Medicines for Cardio-Renal Disease: Opinions of Stakeholders

Bauke Schievink[1], Hiddo Lambers Heerspink[1]*, Hubert Leufkens[2,3], Dick De Zeeuw[1], Jarno Hoekman[2]

1 Department of Clinical Pharmacy and Pharmacology, University of Groningen, University Medical Center Groningen, Groningen, The Netherlands, 2 Utrecht Institute for Pharmaceutical Sciences, Division of Pharmacoepidemiology and Clinical Pharmacology, Utrecht University, Utrecht, The Netherlands, 3 Medicines Evaluation Board, Utrecht, The Netherlands

Abstract

Aim: There is discussion whether medicines can be authorized on the market based on evidence from surrogate endpoints. We assessed opinions of different stakeholders on this topic.

Methods: We conducted an online questionnaire that targeted various stakeholder groups (regulatory agencies, pharmaceutical industry, academia, relevant public sector organisations) and medical specialties (cardiology or nephrology vs. other). Participants were enrolled through purposeful sampling. We inquired for conditions under which surrogate endpoints can be used, the validity of various cardio-renal biomarkers and new approaches for biomarker use.

Results: Participants agreed that surrogate endpoints can be used when the surrogate is scientifically valid (5-point Likert response format, mean score: 4.3, SD: 0.9) or when there is an unmet clinical need (mean score: 3.8, SD: 1.2). Industry participants agreed to a greater extent than regulators and academics. However, out of four proposed surrogates (blood pressure (BP), HbA1c, albuminuria, CRP) for cardiovascular outcomes or end-stage renal disease, only use of BP for cardiovascular outcomes was deemed moderately accurate (mean: 3.6, SD: 1.1). Specialists in cardiology or nephrology tended to be more positive about the use of surrogate endpoints.

Conclusion: Stakeholders in drug development do not oppose to the use of surrogate endpoints in drug marketing authorization, but most surrogates are not considered valid. To solve this impasse, increased efforts are required to validate surrogate endpoints and to explore alternative ways to use them.

Editor: John Matthew Koomen, Moffitt Cancer Center, United States of America

Funding: The research was funded by TI Pharma (project number T6-503) http://www.tipharma.com/. Hiddo Lambers Heerspink is supported by a VENI-Grant from the Netherlands Organization for Scientific Research. The funders had no role in study design, data collection and analysis, decision to publish, or preparation of the manuscript.

Competing Interests: HLH has consultancy agreements with the following companies: AbbVie, Astellas, Johnson & Johnson, Reata, and Vitae. All honoraria are paid to his employer/institution University of Groningen. DDZ is a consultant for and received honoraria (to employer/institution) from AbbVie, Astellas, AstraZeneca, Chemocentryx, J&J, Hemocue, Novartis, Reata, Takeda, and Vitae. HL is chairman of the Dutch Medicines Evaluation Board; the views in this paper are not necessarily the views of the MEB. This study was funded by TI Pharma.

* Email: h.j.lambers.heerspink@umcg.nl

Introduction

Cardiovascular and renal disease place an increasing burden on the healthcare system because of a growing incidence of diabetes and a high unmet need in useful protective therapies. The use of surrogate endpoints in clinical trials reduces the time to marketing authorization, which provides patients with earlier access to new medicines and lowers drug development costs [1–4]. However, there is a long-standing debate whether surrogate endpoints are valid proxies of clinically meaningful outcomes, especially in the prevention of cardiovascular and renal disease [5–9]. The debate has recently been reinvigorated by results from clinical trials that showed promising effects of medicines on surrogate endpoints without any effect on clinically meaningful outcomes [9–11]. For example, the anti-diabetic medicine rosiglitazone reduces the surrogate HbA1c, yet increases the risk of myocardial infarction [12,13]; the antihypertensive medicine aliskiren increased the risk of stroke in the ALTITUDE trial despite reducing blood pressure and albuminuria [14,15], and sibutramine increases risk of myocardial infarction and stroke despite lowering body weight [16].

Despite the debate, it remains unclear how stakeholders in drug development perceive the current use of surrogate endpoints in the marketing authorization of medicines. Therefore, we conducted a survey to assess opinions on the utility and validity of surrogate endpoints, with a focus on surrogates used for cardio-renal disease.

Methods

Ethics statement

We did not require IRB approval for conducting the presented survey, which is in compliance with the Dutch regulations on research with human participants. All gathered data was handled anonymously.

Survey design

An online survey (see Survey Form S1) was designed with software from SurveyMonkey (www.surveymonkey.com, Palo Alto, CA, USA). The survey was checked for content validity by a pilot panel consisting of regulators from the Dutch Medicines Evaluation Board (MEB) and academic employees working at the University Medical Center Groningen. We targeted regulatory agencies (e.g. FDA, EMA), representatives from the pharmaceutical industry, relevant public sector organizations (e.g. Critical Path Institute (C-path), National Institute for Health and Care Excellence (NICE), National Institutes of Health (NIH)) and academic clinicians, including specialists in cardiology or nephrology as well as other specialists. The survey contained questions on the general use of surrogate endpoints, and on the validity of currently used surrogate endpoints for cardio-renal disease, and biomarkers that have been proposed as surrogates. We included blood pressure, HbA1c, albuminuria and CRP as surrogate endpoints for end-stage renal disease or cardiovascular (CV) disease (composite of myocardial infarction, stroke and CV death), while weight, carotid intima thickness and left ventricular hypertrophy were only included as surrogates for CV disease. We also included a medicine case scenario with questions on the use and validity of a composite score capturing the effect on multiple biomarkers as surrogate endpoint for clinically meaningful outcomes. Answers were provided on a 5-point Likert response format (i.e. strongly disagree, disagree, neutral, agree, strongly agree corresponding to a score of 1 to 5), ranking format or multiple choice format. We pre-specified to analyze differences in opinions between stakeholder groups and medical specialties.

Sampling and population

Due to the relatively small and specialized population, we used purposeful sampling at stakeholder level to include participants. We did not perform a formal sample size calculation but strived to create equally sized stakeholder groups. The sample consisted of all participants from two international conferences on the topic of regulatory science and clinical trial design, where the use of surrogate endpoints was discussed. We observed a low participation rate of regulators and therefore invited additional participants from the European Medicines Agency (EMA) and assessors from the Dutch MEB. Participants were targeted by e-mail and a maximum of two reminders were sent in a time span of two months.

Statistical analysis

Means and standard deviations (SD) were computed for questions based on a 5-point Likert response format. All reported p values were calculated by ANCOVA adjusted for age, gender, cardio-renal profession, stakeholder group and years of experience. Tukey HSD post-hoc tests were used for pairwise comparison between industry participants, regulators and academics. All other questions were analyzed non-parametrically. Participants from public sector organizations were excluded from comparisons between stakeholders due to small sample size. Background characteristics of participants that partially and completely filled out the survey were similar. Question answers were therefore analyzed with all available data. Analyses were conducted with R version 3.0.1 (R Foundation for Statistical Computing, Vienna, Austria. http://www.r-project.org).

Results

Survey and background characteristics

Background characteristics of surveyed participants are listed in Table 1. The population consisted of 193 individuals. A total of 74 persons participated (38% response): 18 representing the pharmaceutical industry, 18 from regulatory agencies, 34 from academia and 4 with other backgrounds, including public sector organizations (e.g. C-path, NICE, NIH). A total of 55 respondents (70%) were medical specialists in cardiology or nephrology. Median years of professional experience of all participants was 10 to 15 years. Most respondents were from the United States or Europe (91%), with a ratio of approximately 1:1. No statistical differences between respondents and non-responders in the distribution of geographical location and gender were found.

Stakeholders

As shown in Figure 1A, there was consensus among stakeholder groups that surrogate endpoints can be used in drug marketing authorization under certain conditions. Specifically, all stakeholder groups agreed that a scientifically valid surrogate endpoint (pooled mean: 4.3, SD: 0.9) or an unmet clinical need are valid conditions for surrogate endpoint use, provided that a post-marketing study with hard outcomes is conducted (pooled mean: 3.8, SD: 1.2).

Industry participants were more positive towards the use of surrogate endpoints than both regulators and academic clinicians (Table 2). Industry participants were also more positive towards the statement that surrogate endpoints can be used when hard clinical outcome studies are perceived as too costly (mean 3.4, SD: 0.9). Academic clinicians and regulators ranked surrogate endpoints as the most beneficial for the pharmaceutical industry, while industry participants ranked surrogate endpoints as the most beneficial for patients (P<0.001 for difference).

Despite the positive attitude towards the use of surrogate endpoints among all stakeholders, they did not consider most currently used surrogates such as blood pressure, HbA1c, albuminuria and CRP valid substitutes for end-stage renal disease and cardiovascular (CV) outcomes. Only blood pressure for CV outcomes was considered a moderately accurate surrogate endpoint (pooled mean: 3.6 SD: 1.1; Figure 1B). Industry valued the accuracy of biomarkers consistently higher (exception: HbA1c for CV outcomes, Table 3). Additionally, all stakeholder groups indicated that weight, carotid intima thickness and left ventricular hypertrophy are not valid and should not be qualified by regulators as surrogate endpoints for CV outcomes in drug marketing authorization (data not shown).

Cardio-renal specialty

Specialists in cardiology or nephrology tended to agree more to the proposed statements regarding valid conditions for surrogate endpoint use compared to participants that are active in other fields. However, none of these differences were statistically significant (Table 2). Respondents with a specialty in cardiology or nephrology perceived blood pressure (mean: 3.8 vs 3.1, P<0.05) for CV outcomes as more accurate than those in other fields. Significant differences for the validity of other biomarkers were not observed (Table 3).

Use of a risk score based on multiple biomarkers

We presented a hypothetical case of an antihypertensive medicine that fulfilled all the regulatory requirements for marketing authorization, including a significant reduction in blood pressure compared to placebo (Textbox S1). We found that 41 respondents were willing to accept this particular medicine for

Table 1. Characteristics of respondents.

Characteristic	Number (%)
Respondents	74 (38%*)
Males	53 (72.6%)
Age group (years)	
18–24	1 (1.4%)
25–34	2 (2.7%)
35–44	21 (28.4%)
45–54	26 (35.1%)
55–64	19 (25.7%)
64–75	5 (6.8%)
75+	0 (0%)
Experience	
0–5 years	9 (12.2%)
5–10 years	11 (14.9%)
10–15 years	21 (28.4%)
15+ years	33 (44.6%)
Stakeholders	
regulator	18 (24.3%)
industry	18 (24.3%)
academia	34 (46.0%)
other	4 (5.4%)
Specializations	
cardio-renal	55 (74.3%)
other	19 (25.7%)

*Percentage compared to surveyed population.

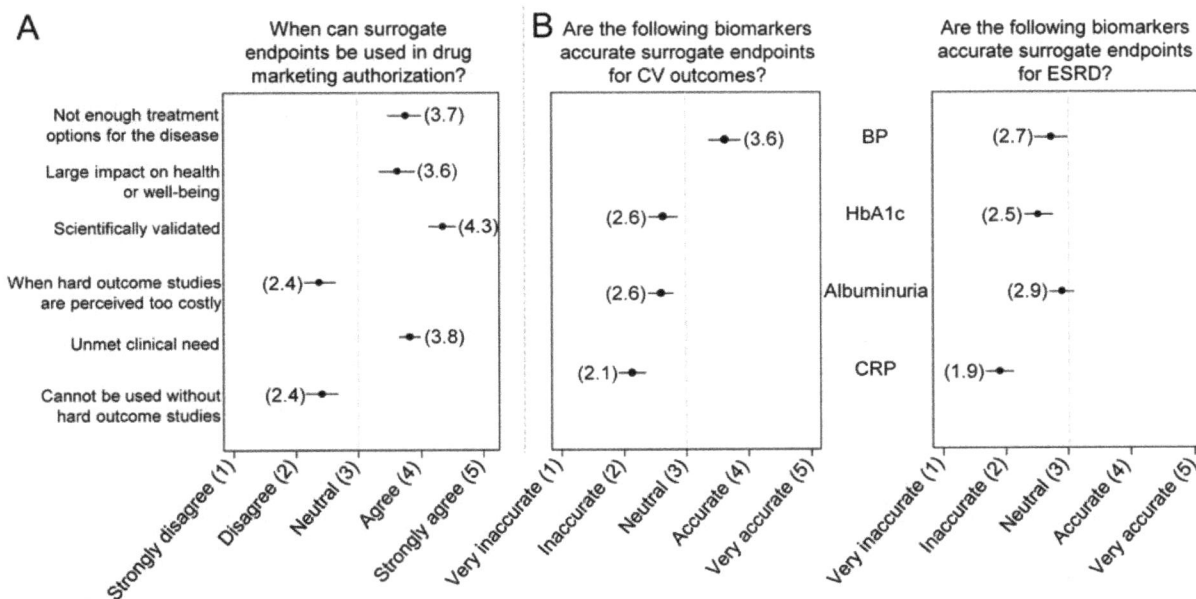

Figure 1. Pooled responses to survey questions. A: pooled responses (mean+95% CI) of all stakeholders on when surrogate endpoints can be used in drug marketing authorization, provided that a post-marketing study with hard outcomes is conducted. B: pooled answers on which biomarkers are perceived as accurate surrogate endpoints for either cardiovascular outcomes or end-stage renal disease. Absolute mean values are provided in brackets. Abbreviations: CV, cardiovascular; ESRD, end-stage renal disease; BP, blood pressure; CRP, C-reactive protein.

Table 2. Question: When can surrogate endpoints be used?

	Stakeholder groups				Medical specialty			Pooled mean
	Regulator	Academia	Industry	P	CR	Other	P	
Not enough treatment options	3.5 (1.2)	3.6 (1.2)	4.5 (0.6)	0.012	3.9 (1.1)	3.4 (1.3)	0.24	3.7 (1.2)
Large impact on health and well-being	3.3 (1.4)	3.4 (1.2)	4.6 (0.5)	0.001	3.8 (1.2)	3.2 (1.3)	0.08	3.6 (1.2)
Scientifically validated	4.3 (0.7)	4.3 (1.0)	4.8 (0.4)	0.058	4.4 (0.9)	4.2 (1.0)	0.63	4.3 (1.0)
Hard outcome studies are too costly	2.1 (0.7)	2.1 (1.0)	3.4 (0.9)	<0.001	2.4 (1.1)	2.4 (1.1)	0.86	2.4 (1.1)
Unmet clinical need	3.9 (1.1)	3.4 (1.1)	4.7 (0.6)	<0.001	3.8 (1.2)	3.7 (1.2)	0.96	3.8 (1.2)
Cannot be used without hard outcome studies	2.4 (1.0)	2.9 (1.1)	1.6 (0.6)	<0.001	2.4 (1.1)	2.5 (1.1)	0.55	2.4 (1.1)

Statements on when surrogate endpoints can be used in drug marketing authorization, provided that a post-marketing study with hard outcomes will be conducted. Results from a 5-point Likert response format (strongly disagree – strongly agree) are presented in mean (SD) according to stakeholder group or medical specialty group (cardio-renal vs. no cardio-renal). Statistical differences between groups are mainly driven by differences of industry respondents vs. regulators and academia. Abbreviations: CR, cardiorenal background; P, P value.

Table 3. Question: are these biomarkers accurate surrogates?

	Stakeholder groups				Medical specialty			Pooled mean
	Regulator	Academia	Industry	P	CR	Other	P	
BP for CV outcomes	3.3 (1.1)	3.7 (1.0)	4.1 (0.7)	0.07	3.8 (1.0)	3.1 (1.0)	0.03	3.6 (1.1)
BP for ESRD	2.6 (0.7)	2.8 (0.9)	2.9 (0.9)	0.67	2.8 (0.9)	2.6 (0.7)	0.79	2.7 (0.9)
HbA1c for CV outcomes	2.8 (0.9)	2.6 (1.0)	2.7 (0.8)	0.87	2.7 (1.0)	2.3 (0.6)	0.28	2.6 (0.9)
HbA1c for ESRD	2.5 (1.0)	2.5 (1.1)	2.7 (0.7)	0.78	2.6 (1.0)	2.1 (0.7)	0.13	2.5 (1.0)
Albuminuria for CV outcomes	2.3 (0.7)	2.7 (0.8)	2.8 (0.8)	0.18	3.1 (0.8)	2.7 (0.8)	0.07	2.6 (0.8)
Albuminuria for ESRD	2.9 (0.9)	2.8 (1.0)	3.4 (0.7)	0.07	3.0 (1.0)	2.7 (1.0)	0.48	2.9 (1.0)
CRP for CV outcomes	1.8 (0.7)	2.2 (0.9)	2.5 (0.9)	0.06	2.1 (0.9)	2.3 (0.9)	0.17	2.1 (0.9)
CRP for ESRD	1.9 (0.7)	1.9 (0.9)	2.1 (0.8)	0.70	1.8 (0.8)	2.1 (0.7)	0.11	1.9 (0.8)

Qualification of four biomarkers as accurate surrogate endpoints for CV outcomes or ESRD. Results from a 5-point Likert response format (strongly disagree – strongly agree) are shown in mean+SD according to professional background or medical specialty. Abbreviations: BP, blood pressure; CV, cardiovascular; ESRD, end-stage renal disease; CRP, C-reactive protein; CR, cardio-renal background; P, P value.

marketing authorization, while 18 respondents indicated that the medicine could not be marketed before conducting studies with clinically meaningful outcomes. Willingness to accept the medicine decreased significantly after showing that a risk score incorporating medicine-induced changes in multiple biomarkers predicted no CV protective effect of the medicine. Respondents indicated that such predictions incorporating medicine-induced changes in multiple biomarkers may be particularly useful for the selection of promising medicine candidates by pharmaceutical companies in phase II studies (mean: 3.9, SD: 0.9). Industry respondents tended to be more positive towards the use of predictions based on multiple biomarkers than other respondents (Table 4).

Discussion

We conducted an online survey to assess the opinions of stakeholders on the use of surrogate endpoints in marketing authorization of medicines. Although respondents generally agreed that there are valid reasons for use of surrogate endpoints, they did not perceive currently accepted surrogates as well as novel surrogates for cardiovascular and renal endpoints as valid.

Our results indicate an impasse in the perception and use of surrogate endpoints. In the past, surrogate endpoints such as blood pressure, cholesterol and glucose metabolism have been endorsed by regulators and used to allow medicines on the market, after which the effect on clinically meaningful outcomes was established in the post-marketing phase. However in recent years, many medicines authorized on the base of surrogate endpoints were shown to be harmful after results from trials with clinical meaningful outcomes became available. As a result, there is fierce debate among stakeholders about the use and purpose of current surrogate endpoints in the marketing authorization of medicines. Against this background, we foresee three ways along which the future use of surrogate endpoints in regulating medicines may evolve.

Firstly, reducing reliance on surrogate endpoints in marketing authorization of medicines may be a desired approach in light of recent experiences. Indeed, a call for less reliance on surrogate endpoints has been regularly expressed in the academic community [5,8,9,17]. Use of surrogate endpoints could be restricted to situations where measuring clinically meaningful outcomes is not feasible, either due to practical or ethical concerns. For example, surrogates could be used in situations where it takes too long to measure a clinically meaningful endpoint due to slow disease progression [17]. This approach does not necessarily imply that the use of surrogate endpoints should be completely abandoned as evidence from biomarkers may provide important ancillary information in the regulatory assessment of the benefit and risks of medicines.

Less reliance on surrogate endpoints may also be achieved by requesting the conduct of hard clinical outcome trials. These trials could already be ongoing upon marketing authorization or be initiated shortly after medicines have been authorized based on surrogate endpoints. For instance, the FDA recently revised its guidelines on HbA1c-lowering medicines after the rosiglitazone incident by requiring hard clinical outcome studies to rule out harmful cardiovascular effects [18], thereby reducing reliance on HbA1c. Additionally, there is discussion whether regulatory authorities will require evidence on hard clinical outcomes for marketing authorization of upcoming PCSK9 inhibitors; novel medicine candidates that lower LDL cholesterol. As a result, several pharmaceutical companies have already initiated long-term hard outcome studies for PCSK9 inhibitors before marketing authorization [19,20,21], while other companies seem to base their

Table 4. Statements on use of multiple biomarkers.

	Stakeholder groups				Profession			Pooled mean
	industry	regulator	academia	P	CR	other	P	
more accurate predictions on hard outcomes than a single biomarker	4.0 (0.6)	3.9 (0.6)	3.3 (0.8)	0.01	3.6 (0.8)	3.3 (1.1)	0.39	3.5 (0.8)
select promising drug candidates during phase II clinical trials	4.5 (0.7)	3.8 (1.0)	3.9 (0.6)	0.01	4.0 (0.7)	3.5 (1.3)	0.16	3.9 (0.9)
substitute for hard clinical outcome studies, post-marketing studies required	3.5 (1.3)	3.1 (0.9)	2.7 (1.1)	0.11	2.9 (1.2)	2.8 (1.2)	0.90	2.9 (1.2)
substitute for hard clinical outcome studies, no post-marketing studies	2.2 (1.1)	2.3 (0.9)	1.6 (0.6)	0.02	1.9 (0.8)	1.8 (0.8)	0.93	1.9 (0.8)
no benefit for current registration practice	2.1 (0.9)	2.5 (0.9)	2.8 (0.9)	0.09	2.6 (1.0)	2.3 (0.8)	0.51	2.5 (0.9)
if multiple markers affect risk, approval cannot be based on a single marker	4.0 (0.8)	3.8 (0.7)	3.9 (0.8)	0.76	3.8 (0.9)	3.7 (0.6)	0.50	3.8 (0.8)
regulators should stimulate development of tools using multiple biomarkers	4.2 (0.6)	3.5 (1.0)	3.7 (1.0)	0.16	3.8 (1.0)	3.6 (0.8)	0.33	3.8 (1.0)

Statements on use of multiple biomarkers instead of single biomarkers to assess drug effects. Results from a 5-point Likert response format (strongly disagree – strongly agree) are shown in mean±SD according to professional background or medical specialty. Significant P values are driven by industry vs. academia (statement 1 and 2) and regulators vs. academia (statement 4). Abbreviations: CR, cardiorenal background.

drug development programs on the premise that LDL cholesterol is still considered a valid surrogate endpoint, knowing that a hard-clinical outcome study may be requested by regulatory authorities as a post-marketing commitment [22].

Secondly, further validation efforts may be conducted to rigorously evaluate currently used and proposed surrogate endpoints. Several criteria for formal scientific validation of surrogate endpoints have been proposed. Most of them require that there is thorough scientific understanding of the mechanistic relation between the surrogate and the hard clinical outcome as well as extensive preclinical (including animal studies) and clinical evidence confirming a quantifiable relationship between (treatment-induced) change in the surrogate outcome and change in the true clinical outcome [23]. One of the most well-known criteria for validation of surrogate endpoints was given by Prentice, who provided four operational criteria for the use of surrogates in clinical trials to 'capture any relationship between the treatment and the true endpoint' [24]. While the Prentice criteria are widely regarded as principles to scientifically validate a biomarker as surrogate endpoint, there is discussion whether they can reasonably be implemented in practice. In response, some scientists have proposed to validate surrogate endpoints based on the proportion of treatment effect explained or the strength of the relationship with the outcome of interest, as a quantifiable and less stringent measure [25,26]. However, there is no golden rule on how much treatment effect needs to be explained before a biomarker qualifies.

Although currently no single accepted framework for the scientific validation of surrogate endpoints exists, there is widespread agreement that the conduct of prospective studies on clinically meaningful outcomes as well as retrospective analysis on data from already conducted clinical trials are key to further evaluate used and proposed surrogate endpoints. Prospective validation can be done in clinical trials by stratifying and randomizing a patient population based on their response on a surrogate marker [27]. This approach is currently used in the SONAR trial (Clinical Trial identifier NCT01858532) in which approximately 4,000 patients with type 2 diabetes and nephropathy are randomized to the investigational medicine or placebo as either responders or non-responders based on medicine-induced responses to the biomarker albuminuria. The biomarker-outcome association will be confirmed when the patient population randomized as responders also experience more benefit on clinically meaningful outcomes compared to non-responders.

Retrospective validation may rely on large scale meta-analyses of clinical trials and post-hoc analysis of individual patient data by measuring the relationship between short-term medicine-induced changes in biomarkers and medicine effects on clinically meaningful outcomes. In order to perform these analyses, incentives to make clinical trial data or clinical study reports accessible to academic investigators are needed [28]. Moreover, when relying on published data one should be aware of publication bias which may inflate the perceived association between biomarker and outcome [29,30].

Thirdly, alternative ways of using biomarkers in the regulatory assessment of medicines are currently considered. The FDA and EMA recently introduced a procedural framework for the qualification of novel biomarkers [31,32]. The qualification procedure facilitates early dialogue between regulatory authorities, scientists and companies to delineate a specific fit-for-purpose use and to objectively evaluate whether performance standards are met and claims on fit-for-purpose are supported [33,34,35]. It seems that these efforts mainly focus on the use of biomarkers for safety rather than efficacy purposes. For example, a consortium of stakeholders including scientists and representatives from the pharmaceutical industry under the umbrella of the Critical Path Institute focuses exclusively on the development of biomarkers for early prediction of nephrotoxicity or hepatotoxicity [36], while in Europe, several initiatives for safety markers are currently ongoing as part of the Innovative Medicines Initiative [37].

Another new approach is to use medicine-induced changes in multiple biomarkers to predict effects on clinically meaningful outcomes in early stages. The rationale for this approach is that many medicines have effects on multiple biomarkers, with each of these biomarkers being associated with changes in clinically meaningful outcomes, either positively or negatively. A score that integrates medicine-induced responses to multiple biomarkers may therefore better capture the medicine effect on clinically meaningful outcomes than changes in single biomarkers alone. Indeed, we recently developed a risk score that accurately predicted the efficacy of angiotensin receptor blockers on cardiovascular and renal endpoints in a post-hoc analysis [38]. Moreover, the score was prospectively validated by predicting the treatment effect of aliskiren on hard clinical outcomes in the ALTITUDE trial before the trial was completed [39]. A similar model has been developed by Archimedes, which uses multiple parameters from existing clinical trial data to predict cardiovascular risk [40]. In our survey, respondents valued the use of these scores to provide early insights in medicine efficacy, although it was not considered a replacement for conducting studies on clinically meaningful outcomes.

Our study has limitations. Firstly, we used a non-random sample for enrolment. Gathering a random sample was not feasible due to the relatively small and specialized population. Secondly, 38% of the targeted population responded to our survey. However, internet-based surveys traditionally have a low response rate [41–43]. Thirdly, the contribution of the regulatory community is mainly based on European input, not necessarily representing other authorities. Fourthly, we did not include community physicians, payers or patient groups as stakeholder. These parties mainly play a role in the post-marketing domain but also increasingly contribute to the decision-making process before and during marketing authorization.

In conclusion, stakeholders in drug development do not oppose to the use of surrogate endpoints although they consider most surrogates inaccurate substitutes for clinically meaningful outcomes. To solve this impasse, increased efforts are required to validate surrogate endpoints and to explore alternative ways to use them.

Acknowledgments

We express our gratitude to the participants in our survey and the MEB for helping us develop the survey.

Author Contributions

Conceived and designed the experiments: BS HLH HL DDZ JH. Performed the experiments: BS JH. Analyzed the data: BS JH. Contributed reagents/materials/analysis tools: JH. Wrote the paper: BS JH HLH. Reviewed manuscript: BS HLH HL DDZ JH.

References

1. Lonn E (2001) The use of surrogate endpoints in clinical trials: focus on clinical trials in cardiovascular diseases. Pharmacoepidemiol Drug Saf 10: 497–508.
2. Aronson JK (2005) Biomarkers and surrogate endpoints. Br J Clin Pharmacol 59: 491–494.
3. Aronson JK (2012) An agenda for UK clinical pharmacology: Research priorities in biomarkers and surrogate end-points. Br J Clin Pharmacol 73: 900–907.
4. Domanski M, Pocock S, Bernaud C, Borer J, Geller N, et al (2011) Surrogate endpoints in randomized cardiovascular clinical trials. Fundam Clin Pharmacol 25: 411–413.
5. Fleming TRDD (1996) Surrogate End Points in Clinical Trials: Are We Being Misled? Ann Intern Med 125: 605–613.
6. Temple R (1999) Are surrogate markers adequate to assess cardiovascular disease drugs? JAMA 282: 790–795.
7. Psaty BM, Weiss NS, Furberg CD, Koepsell TD, Siscovick DS, et al (1999) Surrogate end points, health outcomes, and the drug-approval process for the treatment of risk factors for cardiovascular disease. JAMA 282: 786–790.
8. D'Agostino R (2000) Debate: The slippery slope of surrogate outcomes. Curr Control Trials Cardiovasc Med 1: 76–78.
9. Moynihan R (2011) Surrogates under scrutiny: fallible correlations, fatal consequences. BMJ 343: d5160.
10. Halimi J, Sautenet B, Gatault P, Roland M, Giraudeau B (2012) Renal endpoints in renal and cardiovascular randomized clinical trials: time for a consensus? Fundam Clin Pharmacol 26: 771–782.
11. Messerli FH, Staessen JA, Zannad F (2010) Of fads, fashion, surrogate endpoints and dual RAS blockade. Eur Heart J 31: 2205–2208.
12. Nissen SE, Wolski K (2007) Effect of Rosiglitazone on the Risk of Myocardial Infarction and Death from Cardiovascular Causes. N Engl J Med 356: 2457–2471.
13. Psaty BM, Furberg CD (2007) The Record on Rosiglitazone and the Risk of Myocardial Infarction. N Engl J Med 357: 67–69.
14. Parving H, Brenner BM, McMurray JJV, de Zeeuw D, Haffner SM, et al (2012) Cardiorenal End Points in a Trial of Aliskiren for Type 2 Diabetes. N Engl J Med 367: 2204–2213.
15. Messerli FH, Bangalore S (2013) ALTITUDE Trial and Dual RAS Blockade: The Alluring but Soft Science of the Surrogate End Point. Am J Med 126: e1–e3.
16. James WP, Caterson ID, Coutinho W, Finer N, Van Gaal LF, et al Effect of Sibutramine on Cardiovascular Outcomes in Overweight and Obese Subjects (2010) N Engl J Med 363: 905–917.
17. Svensson S, Menkes DB, Lexchin J (2013) Surrogate outcomes in clinical trials: A cautionary tale. JAMA Intern Med 173: 611–612.
18. Joffe HV, Parks MH, Temple R (2010) Impact of cardiovascular outcomes on the development and approval of medications for the treatment of diabetes mellitus. Rev Endocr Metab Disord 11: 21–30.
19. Amgen (2013) Further Cardiovascular Outcomes Research With PCSK9 Inhibition in Subjects With Elevated Risk (FOURIER). Available: http://clinicaltrials.gov/show/NCT01764633. Accessed 2014, April 7.
20. Pfizer (2013) The Evaluation Of PF-04950615 (RN316), In Reducing The Occurrence Of Major Cardiovascular Events In High Risk Subjects (SPIRE-1). Available: http://clinicaltrials.gov/show/NCT01975376. Accessed 2014, April 7.
21. Pfizer (2013) The Evaluation Of PF-04950615 (RN316) In Reducing The Occurrence Of Major Cardiovascular Events In High Risk Subjects (SPIRE-2). Available: http://clinicaltrials.gov/show/NCT01975389. Accessed 2014, April 7.
22. Mullard A (2012) Cholesterol-lowering blockbuster candidates speed into Phase III trials. Nat. Rev Drug Discov 11: 817–819.
23. Lesko LJ, Atkinson AJ (2001) Use of Biomarkers and Surrogate Endpoints in Drug Development and Regulatory Decision Making: Criteria, Validation, Strategies. Annu Rev Toxicol 41: 347–366.
24. Prentice RL (1989) Surrogate endpoints in clinical trials: definition and operational criteria. Stat Med 8: 431–440.
25. O'Quigley J (2006) Quantification of the Prentice Criteria for Surrogate Endpoints. Biometrics 62: 297–300.
26. Domanski M, Pocock S, Bernaud C, Borer J, Geller N, et al (2011) Surrogate endpoints in randomized cardiovascular clinical trials. Fundam Clin Pharmacol 25: 411–413.
27. Boessen R (2012) Methods to improve the efficiency of confirmatory clinical trials. PhD thesis. Utrecht University. Available: http://www.tipharma.com/fileadmin/user_upload/Theses/PDF/Ruud_Boessen_T6-202.pdf. Accessed 2014, September 5.
28. Eichler HG, Abadie E, Breckenridge A, Leufkens H, Rasi G (2012) Open Clinical Trial Data for All? A View from Regulators. PLOS Med DOI: 10.1371/journal.pmed.1001202.
29. Doshi P, Dickersin K, Healy D, Vedula S, Jefferson T (2013) Restoring invisible and abandoned trials: a call for people to publish the findings. BMJ 346: f2865.
30. Tzoulaki I, Siontis KC, Evangelou E, Ioannidis JA (2013) Bias in associations of emerging biomarkers with cardiovascular disease. JAMA Intern Med 173: 664–671.
31. European Medicines Agency (2008) EMA/CHMP/SAWP/72894/2008: Qualification of novel methodologies for drug development: guidance to applicants. Available: http://www.ema.europa.eu/docs/en_GB/document_library/Regulatory_and_procedural_guideline/2009/10/WC500004201.pdf. Accessed 2014, January 27.
32. Food and Drug Administration (2013) Biomarker Qualification Program. Available: http://www.fda.gov/Drugs/DevelopmentApprovalProcess/DrugDevelopmentToolsQualificationProgram/ucm284076.htm. Accessed 2014, January 27.
33. Goldman M, Compton C, Mittleman B (2013) Public-private partnerships as driving forces in the quest for innovative medicines. Clin Trans Med 2: 1–3.
34. Sistare FD, Dieterle F, Troth S, Holder DJ, Gerhold D, et al (2010). Towards consensus practices to qualify safety biomarkers for use in early drug development. Nat Biotechnol 28: 446–454.
35. Dieterle F, Sistare F, Goodsaid F, Papaluca M, Ozer JS (2010) Renal biomarker qualification submission: a dialog between the FDA-EMEA and Predictive Safety Testing Consortium. Nat Biotechnol 28: 455–462.
36. Mattes WB, Walker EG (2009) Translational Toxicology and the Work of the Predictive Safety Testing Consortium. Clin Pharmacol Ther 85: 327–330.
37. Goldman M (2012) The Innovative Medicines Initiative: A European Response to the Innovation Challenge. Clin Pharmacol Ther 91: 418–425.
38. Smink PA, Miao Y, Eijkemans MJC, Bakker SJL, Raz I, et al (2014) The Importance of Short-Term Off-Target Effects in Estimating the Long-Term Renal and Cardiovascular Protection of Angiotensin Receptor Blockers. Clin Pharmacol Ther 95: 208–215.
39. Smink P, Hoekman J, Grobbee D, Eijkemans M, Parving HH, et al (2013) A prediction of the renal and cardiovascular efficacy of aliskiren in ALTITUDE using short-term changes in multiple risk markers. Eur J Prev Cardiol DOI: 10.1177/2047487313481754.
40. Krishna R (2009) Model-Based Benefit-Risk Assessment: Can Archimedes Help? Clin Pharmacol Ther 85: 239–240.
41. Kroth PJ, McPherson L, Leverence R, Pace W, Daniels E, et al (2009) Combining Web-Based and Mail Surveys Improves Response Rates: A PBRN Study From PRIME Net. Ann Fam Med 7: 245–248.
42. Yarger JB, James TA, Ashikaga T, Hayanga AJ, Takyi V, et al (2013) Characteristics in response rates for surveys administered to surgery residents. Surgery 154: 38–45.
43. Leece P, Bhandari M, Sprague S, Swiontkowski M, Schemitsch E, et al (2004) Internet Versus Mailed Questionnaires: A Controlled Comparison. J Med Internet Res 6: e39.

2

Adverse Outcomes of Anticoagulant Use among Hospitalized Patients with Chronic Kidney Disease: A Comparison of the Rates of Major Bleeding Events between Unfractionated Heparin and Enoxaparin

Fatemeh Saheb Sharif-Askari[1]*, Syed Azhar Syed Sulaiman[1], Narjes Saheb Sharif-Askari[1], Ali Al Sayed Hussain[2], Mohammad Jaffar Railey[3]

1 School of Pharmacy, Universiti Sains Malaysia, Penang, Malaysia, 2 Pharmacy Department, Dubai Health Authority, Dubai, United Arab Emirates, 3 Nephrology Unit, Dubai Hospital, Dubai, United Arab Emirates

Abstract

Background: Anticoagulation therapy is usually required in patients with chronic kidney disease (CKD) for treatment or prevention of thromboembolic diseases. However, this benefit could easily be offset by the risk of bleeding.

Objectives: To determine the incidence of adverse outcomes of anticoagulants in hospitalized patients with CKD, and to compare the rates of major bleeding events between the unfractionated heparin (UFH) and enoxaparin users.

Methods: One year prospective observational study was conducted in patients with CKD stages 3 to 5 (estimated GFR, 10–59 ml/min/1.73 m^2) who were admitted to the renal unit of Dubai Hospital. Propensity scores for the use of anticoagulants, estimated for each of the 488 patients, were used to identify a cohort of 117 pairs of patients. Cox regression method was used to estimate association between anticoagulant use and adverse outcomes.

Results: Major bleeding occurred in 1 in 3 patients who received anticoagulation during hospitalization (hazard ratio [HR], 4.61 [95% confidence interval [CI], 2.05–10.35]). Compared with enoxaparin users, patients who received anticoagulation with unfractionated heparin had a lower mean [SD] serum level of platelet counts (139.95 [113]×10^3/µL vs 205.56 [123]×10^3/µL; P<0.001), and had a higher risk of major bleeding (HR, 4.79 [95% CI, 1.85–12.36]). Furthermore, compared with those who did not receive anticoagulants, patients who did had a higher in-hospital mortality (HR, 2.54 [95% CI, 1.03–6.25]); longer length of hospitalization (HR, 1.04 [95% CI, 1.01–1.06]); and higher hospital readmission at 30 days (HR, 1.79 [95% CI, 1.10–2.91]).

Conclusions: Anticoagulation among hospitalized patients with CKD was significantly associated with an increased risk of bleeding and in-hospital mortality. Hence, intensive monitoring and preventive measures such as laboratory monitoring and/or dose adjustment are warranted.

Editor: Cordula M. Stover, University of Leicester, United Kingdom

Funding: The authors have no support or funding to report.

Competing Interests: The authors have declared that no competing interests exist.

* Email: dr.fatemeh.askari@gmail.com

Introduction

Chronic kidney disease (CKD) affects 10% to 15% of the adult population in United States, Europe, and Asia [1–3]. Patients with CKD display a wide range of abnormalities in the homeostatic pathway that may account for their increased risk for both thrombotic events and bleeding [4]. The early stages of CKD are mainly associated with the prothrombotic tendency [4], whereas in its more advanced stages, beside the procoagulant state, platelets can become dysfunctional due to uremic-related toxin exposure leading to an increased bleeding tendency [4,5].

The increased risk of thromboembolic diseases among CKD patients commonly requires anticoagulation therapy [6]. However, many randomized trials have demonstrated the greater safety and clinical efficacy of low molecular weight heparin (enoxaparin) compared to unfractionated heparin (UFH) in non CKD patients [7]. The ease of use, and the predictable anticoagulant effect of enoxaparin eliminates the need for routine laboratory monitoring [8]. A disadvantage of enoxaparin is its dependence on kidney function for excretion and accumulation of its anticoagulant effect in patients with decreased kidney function [9]; therefore dosage reduction is recommended in patients with severe CKD, defined as creatinine clearance of less than 30 ml/min [10]. To date, it is unknown whether enoxaparin in adjusted therapeutic doses is as safe to prescribe in CKD patients as UFH whose elimination does not depend on the kidney.

In support of these matters, ensuring an accurate enoxaparin dose may have a significant impact on thromboembolic disease outcomes. Therefore, an appropriate therapeutic dose would appear essential in order to maintain a proper balance of efficacy and safety in patients with reduced kidney function. Data from large clinical trials regarding the approval of current enoxaparin dosing have excluded patients with CKD [7], and smaller observational studies [11] have used full therapeutic doses without dose adjustment.

Thus, we conducted a one year prospective study to examine whether the use of anticoagulants (UFH or enoxaparin) for the treatment of thrombotic events in hospitalized patients with CKD was associated with adverse outcomes. Using these data, we first explored the relationship between anticoagulant use and major bleeding events, in-hospital mortality, length of hospital stay, and readmission at 30 days. To limit the potential for confounding by indication, we then examined the association among the subgroup of patients with anticoagulant use and the occurrence of major bleeding events. Finally, we compared the risk of major bleeding in the use of UFH versus adjusted therapeutic doses of enoxaparin.

Materials and Methods

Study Design and Participants

This prospective, observational study was conducted at the renal unit of Dubai Hospital, a 625-bed general hospital in Dubai, the United Arab Emirates. Consecutive patients with CKD stages 3 to 5 (estimated glomerular filtration rate [eGFR], 10–59 ml/min/1.73 m^2) who were admitted to the renal unit, between December 1, 2011, and December 31, 2012 were included. This study was approved by the Medical Research Committee of Dubai Health Authority. The Medical Research Committee did not require a written informed consent from each study participant. However, in case further information was needed, a verbal consent was taken from the respective patient and was documented in the patient data collection form. This consent procedure was approved by the Medical Research Committee.

Data Collection

For each patient who met the study criteria baseline data was collected on admission and was updated daily by the researcher in charge using a standardized form. Data collected covered demographic characteristics, including age and sex; physical examination results, including blood pressure and weight; comorbid conditions, including diabetes, hypertension, vascular disease, heart failure, and anaemia; laboratory tests, including serum and biochemical parameters; and coadministration of medications taken before admission or during hospital stay that might affect patients bleeding tendencies. The baseline laboratory data was defined as the first test result before the anticoagulant administration. Furthermore, patients risk factors for bleeding such as history of uncontrolled hypertension, cerebrovascular accidents, cancer, falls, or recent surgery were also collected [12].

Anticoagulant Exposure

In our study, systemic anticoagulants (UFH or enoxaparin) that were administrated for the treatment of deep-vein thrombosis, pulmonary embolism, atrial fibrillation, ischemic stroke, myocar-

dial infarction, unstable coronary artery disease, and acute peripheral arterial occlusion, were included. We defined anticoagulant exposure on the basis of a patient receiving at least 1 course of either UFH or enoxaparin for the treatment of a new thrombotic indication during hospitalization, thus, excluding patients who received only prophylactic doses of either UFH or enoxaparin. We also excluded patients who received concurrent anticoagulation therapy or oral anticoagulants (warfarin sodium) during hospital stay.

In this study, all the anticoagulant drug orders were physician based. Patients baseline laboratory results and body weight were documented before the administration of anticoagulants, and the data was used to calculate the dose according to the British National Formulary [10] and other evidence based guidelines [8]. The doses of enoxaparin were adjusted based on the degree of kidney function. The dosages used were either 1 mg/kg body weight administered subcutaneously every 24 hours or 0.75 mg/kg every 12 hours. The doses of UFH were up to 30,000 units of heparin over 2–3 times per day. The anticoagulation activity of UFH was monitored by measuring the activated partial thromboplastin time (APTT) for all patients daily, and the doses were then adjusted accordingly.

Adverse Outcomes

The main outcome measures studied were the effect of anticoagulation therapy on, major bleeding events, in-hospital mortality, length of hospital stay, and readmission at 30 days. A major bleeding was defined as overt bleeding resulting in death, transfusion of two or more units of packed blood cells, a fall in haemoglobin level to ≥ 3 g/dL, the need for corrective surgery intervention, or the occurrence of intracranial, retroperitoneal, or intraocular bleeding [13,14]. Anticoagulant-related bleeding was defined as bleeding that occurred (1) during UFH or enoxaparin therapy (2) following the discontinuation of UFH or enoxaparin therapy within 24 hours prior to the bleeding events. In-hospital mortality was defined as all cause death occurring during the hospital stay. Readmission was detected by screening for a patient revisit within the specific period.

Statistical Analysis

Baseline characteristics of patients with and those without anticoagulation treatment were compared by using either a chi-square test for categorical variables and t-test or Mann-Whitney test, depending on skewness of data, for continuously distributed variables.

Propensity-Based Matching. Because anticoagulant users may differ in key baseline characteristics from those of non-users, and to allow for an unbiased comparison between these two groups, a propensity score-matching was performed [15,16]. The propensity scores were estimated using logistic regression with the dependent variable of anticoagulant use and the independent variables selected from baseline characteristics of study cohort. To remove confounding bias, patient variables that were considered as confounders of the association between anticoagulation therapy and major bleeding events were used to create the propensity score [17,18]. Variables used in the propensity score included: age, sex, estimated GFR, serum albumin, serum platelet counts, Charlson Comorbidity Index score [19], diabetes, hypertension, vascular disease, anaemia, history of gastrointestinal bleeding, history of stroke, and use of aspirin and clopidogrel. Matching was performed using the 'psmatching' custom dialogue in conjunction with SPSS version 21 [16]. Study cohorts were matched using nearest neighbour one-to-one matching, without replacement, and a caliber width of 0.2 of the standard deviation. Adequacy of

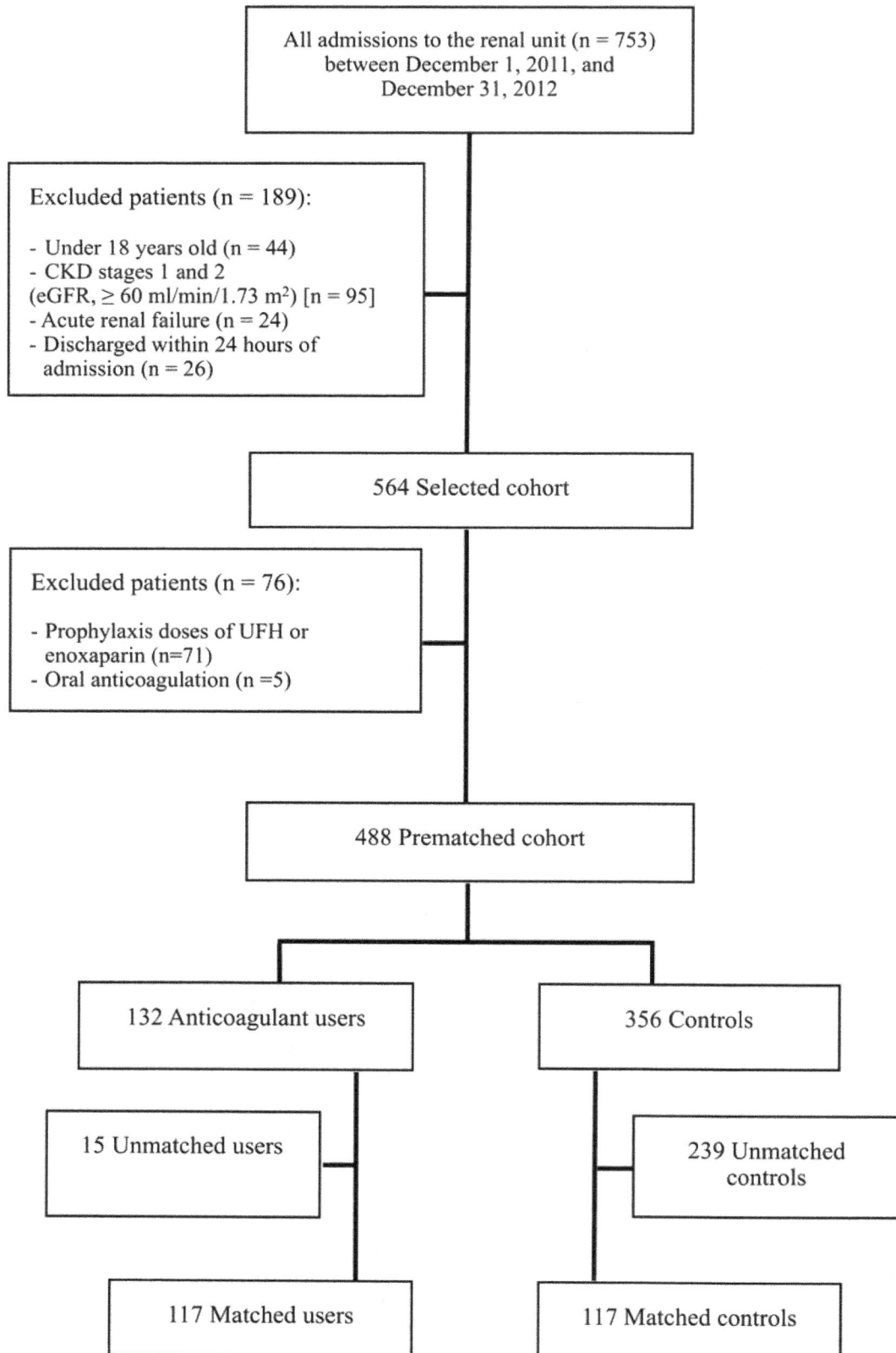

Figure 1. Cohort creation.

Table 1. Baseline characteristics of patients with and without anticoagulant use.

Characteristics	No. (%) of Participants		
	Anticoagulant Use		
	Treated (n = 132)	Untreated (n = 356)	P Value
Demographics			
Age, mean (SD), y	67 (13)	58 (16)	<0.001
Female sex	56 (42)	152 (43)	0.957
Male sex	76 (58)	204 (57)	0.957
Comorbid conditions			
Diabetes	104 (79)	256 (72)	0.133
Hypertension	128 (97)	322 (90)	0.021
Vascular disease[a]	77 (58)	146 (41)	0.001
Ischemic stroke	18 (14)	44 (12)	0.760
Anaemia	66 (50)	164 (46)	0.475
History of gastrointestinal bleeding	27 (20)	44 (12)	0.030
Liver cirrhosis	8 (6)	28 (8)	0.564
Charlson Comorbidity Index score, mean (SD)	3.87 (1.21)	3.14 (1.21)	<0.001
Laboratory data			
GFR, mL/min/1.73 m^2			
Baseline, mean (SD)	17.83 (14)	12.16 (11)	<0.001
30–59	26 (20)	35 (10)	0.005
15–29	30 (23)	56 (16)	0.082
<15	76 (58)	265 (74)	0.001
Serum creatinine, mean (SD), mg/dL	4.48 (3.29)	7.05 (4.59)	<0.001
Serum albumin, mean (SD), g/dL	3.25 (0.70)	3.60 (0.62)	<0.001
Serum platelet count, mean (SD), 10^3/μL	185.61 (123)	225.99 (106)	<0.001
Medication Use			
Aspirin	62 (47)	136 (38)	0.097
Clopidogrel	51 (39)	80 (22)	0.001
Aspirin and clopidogrel	36 (27)	50 (14)	0.001
NSAID	3 (2)	4 (1)	0.395

Abbreviations: GFR, glomerular filtration rate; NSAID, non-steroidal anti-inflammatory drug; SD, standard deviation.
SI conversions: To convert serum creatinine to μmol/L, multiply by 88.4.
[a]Vascular disease is defined as presence of coronary artery disease or peripheral vascular disease.

balance for the covariates in the matched samples was assessed using a standardized mean difference between the prematch and postmatch groups, considering differences less than 10% as good balance [20].

Outcome Analyses. The outcome analysis was performed comparing these propensity-matched anticoagulant users and nonusers. The risk of in-hospital mortality, the occurrence of major bleeding, length of hospital stay, and readmission at 30 days in relation with the anticoagulation therapy, was estimated separately using a Cox proportional hazard regression model that stratified on the matched pairs. The hazard ratio of major bleeding in relation with the use of UFH and enoxaparin was reported graphically using Kaplan-Meier estimates, plotting the log-minus-log survival function over time. The log-rank test was used to investigate the crude association with the use of UFH and enoxaparin and risk of major bleeding.

Sensitivity Analyses. The association of anticoagulation therapy with major bleeding events was further explored by stratifying the cohorts by age, sex, history of diabetes, hypertension, vascular disease, estimated GFR, serum level of platelet counts, and treatment with aspirin and clopidogrel. For these (subgroup) analyses, the risk of major bleeding in relation to anticoagulants exposure was estimated separately using proportional Cox regression models that incorporated propensity scores.

All tests were 2 tailed and a P value of less than 0.05 was considered statistically significant.

Results

During the study period, a total of 488 patients with CKD stages 3 to 5 (estimated glomerular filtration rate [GFR], 10–59 ml/min/1.73 m^2) fulfilled the inclusion criteria of the study. (Figure 1) Of these, 132 (27%) received anticoagulation therapy during hospital stay. The mean (SD) duration of anticoagulation therapy was 3.5 (0.2) days for UFH, and 4.2 (0.3) days for enoxaparin (P = 0.410).

Table 2. Characteristics of patients with and without anticoagulant use after propensity matched analysis.

| | No. (%) of Participants | | |
| | Anticoagulant Use After Matching | | |
Characteristics	Treated (n = 117)	Untreated (n = 117)	P Value
Demographics			
Age, mean (SD), y	66 (14)	66 (14)	0.969
Female sex	52 (44)	50 (43)	0.895
Comorbid conditions			
Diabetes	91 (78)	90 (77)	0.876
Hypertension	113 (97)	112 (96)	0.734
Vascular disease[a]	65 (56)	67 (57)	0.895
Ischemic stroke	15 (13)	17 (14)	0.849
Anaemia	60 (51)	53 (45)	0.475
History of gastrointestinal bleeding	23 (20)	16 (14)	0.293
Charlson Comorbidity Index score, mean (SD)	3.79 (1.3)	3.76 (1.3)	0.838
Laboratory data			
GFR, mean (SD), mL/min/1.73 m^2	15.73 (13)	16.55 (13)	0.616
Serum albumin, mean (SD), g/dL	3.30 (0.7)	3.36 (0.7)	0.535
Serum platelet count, mean (SD), 10^3/µL	188 (85)	188 (85)	0.977
Medication Use			
Aspirin and clopidogrel	28 (24)	28 (24)	1.000

Abbreviations: GFR, glomerular filtration rate; SD, standard deviation.
[a]Vascular disease is defined as presence of coronary artery disease or peripheral vascular disease.

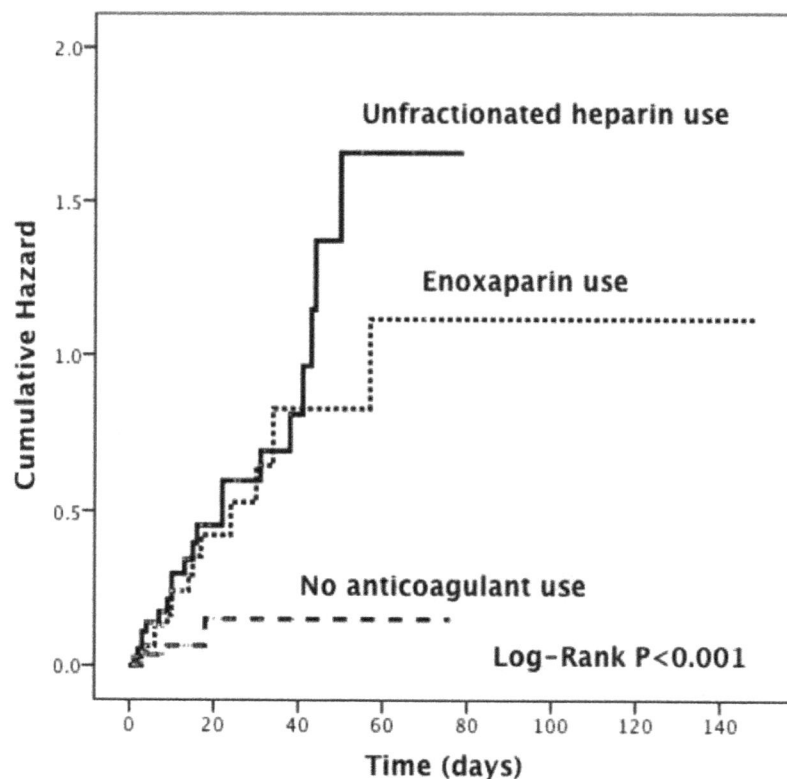

Figure 2. Kaplan-Meier estimates of cumulative hazard of major bleeding events with the use of unfractionated heparin or enoxaparin use.

Table 3. Crude and propensity adjusted hazard ratios of anticoagulant-related adverse outcomes.

	Major bleeding events		
	No. of Events/No. of Patients		
	No Anticoagulant	Anticoagulant Use	HR (95% CI)
Crude analysis	9/356	42/132	5.48 (2.61–11.51)
Propensity analysis	5/117	37/117	4.61 (2.05–10.35)
	In-hospital mortality		
	No. of Events/No. of Patients		
	No Anticoagulant	Anticoagulant Use	HR (95% CI)
Crude analysis	8/356	23/132	2.96 (1.27–6.91)
Propensity analysis	3/117	21/117	2.54 (1.03–6.25)
	Length of hospital stay		
	Median (IQR), days		
	No Anticoagulant	Anticoagulant Use	HR (95% CI)
Crude analysis	4 (6)	8 (15)	1.05 (1.03–1.07)
Propensity analysis	5 (6)	8 (14)	1.04 (1.01–1.06)
	Readmission at 30 days		
	No. of Events/No. of Patients		
	No Anticoagulant	Anticoagulant Use	HR (95% CI)
Crude analysis	44/356	50/132	1.72 (1.13–2.62)
Propensity analysis	15/117	44/117	1.79 (1.10–2.91)

Abbreviations: CI, confidence interval; HR, hazard ratio; IQR, interquartile range; SD, standard deviation.

Baseline Characteristics

Baseline characteristics for patients with and those without anticoagulant use are reported in Table 1. Patients who received anticoagulants were older with the mean (SD) age of 67 (13) years, versus 58 (16) years in the non anticoagulant use group (P<0.001); were more likely to have a history of vascular disease (58% vs 41%; P = 0.001), and a history of gastrointestinal bleeding (20% vs 12%; P = 0.030). Moreover, patients who received anticoagulants had lower serum level of albumin, with the mean (SD) serum level of albumin of 3.25 (0.70) g/dL, versus 3.60 (0.62) g/dL in the non anticoagulant use group (P<0.001); and had lower serum level of platelet counts, with the mean (SD) serum level of platelet counts of 185.61 (123)×10^3/μL, versus 225.99 (106) ×10^3/μL in the non anticoagulant use group (P<0.001).

Propensity-Based Matching

From the initial cohort of 132 patients with anticoagulant use, 117 were selected using propensity score matching. In the propensity score matched analysis, 15 patients remained unmatched and were thus excluded from the analysis. Prematching characteristics widely differed between those with anticoagulant use and those without anticoagulant use but propensity score matching led to an adequate balance for all characteristics considered (Table 2). The absolute standardized differences for all variables were less than 10%, indicating an adequate postmatch balance.

Outcome Analyses

In this study, 51 major bleeding events were identified. The rate of major bleeding was higher in anticoagulants treated patients than in matched controls (37 vs 5 events, respectively). The hazard

Table 4. Propensity adjusted hazard ratio of major bleeding events with the use of unfractionated heparin or enoxaparin.

Anticoagulant	No. of Events (% of Patients)	HR (95% CI)	P Value
UFH	20 (51)	4.79 (1.85–12.36)	0.001
Enoxaparin	17 (22)	2.10 (1.36–3.24)	0.001

Abbreviations: CI, confidence interval, HR, hazard ratio; UFH, unfractionated heparin.

Table 5. Hazard ratios of major bleeding events with anticoagulant use stratified by cohort characteristics.

Subgroups	No. of Events/No. Of Patients	HR (95% CI)	P value for Interaction
All patients	37/117	4.61 (2.05–10.35)	
sAged ≥65 y	22/64	2.99 (1.70–5.28)	<0.001
Aged 18–65 y	15/53	0.96 (0.49–1.89)	
Male sex	20/65	1.87 (1.05–3.31)	0.028
Female sex	17/52	1.69 (0.92–3.10)	
Diabetes	34/91	3.64 (1.80–7.35)	<0.001
No diabetes	3/26	1.10 (0.39–3.13)	
Hypertension	35/113	3.88 (1.86–8.09)	<0.001
No hypertension	2/4	0.87 (0.20–3.72)	
Vascular disease[a]	27/65	3.91 (2.18–7.02)	<0.001
No vascular disease	10/52	0.66 (0.32–1.34)	
Anaemia	24/60	2.01 (1.11–3.64)	0.018
No anaemia	13/57	1.64 (0.89–3.02)	
GFR ≤30 mL/min/1.73 m^2	36/102	3.41 (1.62–7.16)	0.001
GFR 30–59 mL/min/1.73 m^2	1/15	1.96 (0.69–5.59)	
Platelet count ≤150×10^3/µL	29/52	4.52 (2.44–8.39)	<0.001
Platelet count >150×10^3/µL	8/65	0.61 (0.29–1.27)	
Dual antiplatelets[b]	9/28	2.32 (1.21–4.46)	0.009
No dual antiplatelets	28/89	1.83 (0.98–3.43)	

Abbreviations: CI, confidence interval; GFR, glomerular filtration rate; HR, hazard ratio; UFH, unfractionated heparin.
[a]Vascular disease is defined as presence of coronary artery disease or peripheral vascular disease.
[b]Dual antiplatelets is defined as dual use of aspirin and clopidogrel.

ratio for anticoagulants exposure was 4.61 (95% confidence interval [CI], 2.05–10.35) (Table 3). Compared with enoxaparin users, patients who received anticoagulation therapy with UFH had a higher risk of major bleeding (hazard ratio [HR], 4.79 [95% CI, 1.85–12.36]; Figure 2, and Table 4). Furthermore, compared with those who did not receive anticoagulants, patients who did had higher in-hospital mortality (HR, 2.54 [95% CI, 1.03–6.25]; Table 3); longer length of hospital stay (HR, 1.04 [95% CI, 1.01–

1.06]; Table 3); and higher hospital readmission at 30 days (HR, 1.79 [95% CI, 1.10–2.91]; Table 3).

Sensitivity Analyses

As presented in Table 5, significant interactions were detected between anticoagulant use and age, sex, presence of diabetes, hypertension, vascular disease, anaemia, estimated GFR, serum level of platelet counts, and use of dual antiplatelet agents. The risk

Table 6. Frequency of risk factors for major bleeding between unfractionated heparin and enoxaparin users.

	No. (%) of Participants		
	Anticoagulant Use		
Variable	UFH (n = 39)	Enoxaparin (n = 78)	P Value
Aged ≥65 y	19 (49)	45 (58)	0.432
Male sex	21 (54)	44 (46)	0.845
Diabetes	30 (77)	61 (78)	0.875
Hypertension	37 (95)	76 (97)	0.600
Vascular diseasea	24 (61)	41 (53)	0.431
Anaemia	23 (59)	37 (47)	0.327
GFR ≤30 mL/min/1.73 m^2	36 (92)	66 (85)	0.380
Platelet count ≤150×103/µL	22 (56)	30 (38)	0.078
Dual antiplateletsb	6 (15)	22 (28)	0.169

Abbreviations: UFH, unfractionated heparin.
[a]Vascular disease is defined as presence of coronary artery disease or peripheral vascular disease.
[b]Dual antiplatelets is defined as dual use of aspirin and clopidogrel.

of bleeding associated with the use of anticoagulants was high in individuals older than 65 years (HR, 2.99; 95% CI, 1.70–5.28); in male sex (HR, 1.87; 95% CI, 1.05–3.31); presence of diabetes mellitus (HR, 3.64; 95% CI, 1.80–7.35); hypertension (HR, 3.88; 95% CI, 1.86–8.09); vascular disease (HR, 3.91; 95% CI, 2.18–7.02); anaemia (HR, 2.01; 95% CI, 1.11–3.64); estimated GFR less than or equal to 30 mL/min/1.73 m^2 (HR, 3.41; 95% CI, 1.62–7.16); serum platelet counts less than or equal to 150×10^3/µL (HR, 4.52; 95% CI, 2.44–8.39); and use of dual antiplatelet agents (HR, 2.32; 95% CI, 1.21–4.46).

The Risk Factors for Major Bleeding Events

The frequency of risk factors for bleeding between UFH and enoxaparin was statistically equivalence in all of subgroup evaluated (Table 6). However, after receiving anticoagulants, patients who received UFH had a lower serum level of platelet counts, with the mean (SD) serum level of platelet counts of 139.95 $(113) \times 10^3$/µL in the UFH use group, versus 205.56 (123) $\times 10^3$/µL in the enoxaparin use group (P<0.001).

Discussion

In this prospective observational study of hospitalized patients with moderate to severe CKD, exposure to anticoagulants in recommended doses was associated with a range of adverse outcomes. Major bleeding occurred in 1 in 3 patients who received anticoagulation therapy during their hospital stay. This rate of major bleeding is higher than that of the large trials of anticoagulants [13,21–26]. Noticeably, these large trials excluded CKD patients and renal function of randomized subjects was not reported. Results from this study are consistent with the previous observational study that showed a similar rate of bleeding in patients with severe CKD [11].

In this study, the risk of major bleeding was higher with UFH compared to enoxaparin. Despite the fact that enoxaparin is dependent on the kidney for its elimination and that it can bioaccumulate with reduced kidney function; this did not result into higher bleeding rates according to our findings. The increased rate of bleeding observed with UFH may be attributed to the inhibition of platelet function and increase in vascular permeability; properties that are independent to anticoagulant effects [8]. Unlike UFH, enoxaparin binds less to platelets because of its smaller molecular size and hence has fewer incidences of heparin-induced thrombocytopenia and bleeding events. This is of particular concern because patients with advanced CKD are already more susceptible to bleeding from uraemia-related platelet dysfunction [8].

In a study by Thorevska and colleagues [11], a retrospective medical record review of 620 patients with an estimated GFR of < 60 ml/min/1.73 m^2, which compared the rates of bleeding in patients who received anticoagulation therapy with full-therapeutic dose of UFH, or with enoxaparin, authors reported that the rates of major bleeding increased for both UFH and enoxaparin therapy at each stage of CKD, suggesting that factors other than drug clearance is responsible for anticoagulant bleeding complications. More recently, another retrospective observational study

of 7721 dialysis patients who received thrombophylaxis therapy with either UFH or enoxaparin, was able to confirm Thorevska and colleagues [11] results that enoxaparin was not associated with higher bleeding risk in comparison with UFH (risk ratio, 0.98; 95% CI 0.78–1.23), concluding that thrombophylaxis doses of enoxaparin appeared to be safe and could be used as an alternative to UFH in dialysis patients [27]. Of note in the studies mentioned above [11,27], enoxaparin doses were not reduced to account for kidney function that resulted in bleeding events compared to UFH, whilst in our study, enoxaparin was administrated in adjusted therapeutic doses to CKD patients, who were associated with lower bleeding events compared to UFH. The results of our study highlight the safety of enoxaparin if administered in therapeutic doses with dose adjustment to patients with advanced CKD.

In our study, in-hospital mortality occurred in 1 in 5 patients who received anticoagulation therapy during their hospital stay. This result is comparable with those of Koo and colleagues [28], who in a prospective cohort study investigated the association between anticoagulant usage and mortality in 101 patients admitted with major bleeding during anticoagulation with warfarin, unfractionated heparin or low molecular weight heparin. They reported that at 60 days, the overall mortality was 18%; 6 patients (21%) with excessive warfarin therapy, 5 patients (39%) with UFH or LMWH alone therapy, and 7 patients (60%) UFH or LMWH as a bridge to warfarin therapy. Moreover, the length of hospital stay was longer among anticoagulant users compared with those with no anticoagulation therapy. This fact, in part, can be related to in-hospital bleeding-related complications. At least two-thirds of anticoagulant users had 30 days readmission. This rate of readmission was higher compared with those with no anticoagulation therapy.

Similar to any observational study, this investigation has a number of limitations. Although, through propensity and sensitivity analysis, the effect of observed cofounders were adjusted, there might be a number of unobservable factors that could only be controlled with a randomized controlled trial. In addition, the limited sample size of this study could have resulted in some bias in the results produced. Finally, this study was performed in one hospital, which may also limit the generalizability of the results.

In conclusion, anticoagulation therapy in hospitalized patients with CKD is significantly associated with an increased risk of major bleeding and in-hospital mortality. Higher risk was observed in a range of patient groups and was not reduced after adjusting for the common cofounders. These results suggest that to reduce the risk of bleeding associated with anticoagulation therapy further preventive measures such as laboratory monitoring and/or dose adjustment are warranted.

Author Contributions

Conceived and designed the experiments: FSSA SASS AASH MJR. Performed the experiments: FSSA NSSA MJR. Analyzed the data: FSSA SASS AASH. Contributed reagents/materials/analysis tools: FSSA SASS AASH MJR. Contributed to the writing of the manuscript: FSSA SASS.

References

1. Coresh J, Selvin E, Stevens LA, Manzi J, Kusek JW, et al. (2007) Prevalence of Chronic Kidney Disease in the United States. JAMA 298: 2038–2047.
2. Hallan SI, Coresh J, Astor BC, Åsberg A, Powe NR, et al. (2006) International comparison of the relationship of chronic kidney disease prevalence and ESRD risk. J Am Soc Nephrol 17: 2275–2284.
3. Zhang L, Zhang P, Wang F, Zuo L, Zhou Y, et al. (2008) Prevalence and factors associated with CKD: a population study from Beijing. Am J Kidney Dis 51: 373–384.
4. Jalal DI, Chonchol M, Targher G (2010) Disorders of hemostasis associated with chronic kidney disease. Semin Thromb Hemost 36: 34–40.
5. Boccardo P, Remuzzi G, Galbusera M (2004) Platelet dysfunction in renal failure. Semin Thromb Hemost 30: 579–589.

6. Dager WE, Kiser TH (2010) Systemic anticoagulation considerations in chronic kidney disease. Adv Chronic Kidney Dis 17: 420–427.

7. Sherman DG, Albers GW, Bladin C, Fieschi C, Gabbai AA, et al. (2007) The efficacy and safety of enoxaparin versus unfractionated heparin for the prevention of venous thromboembolism after acute ischaemic stroke (PREVAIL Study): an open-label randomised comparison. The Lancet 369: 1347–1355.

8. Hirsh J, Bauer KA, Donati MB, Gould M, Samama MM, et al. (2008) Parenteral AnticoagulantsAmerican College of Chest Physicians Evidence-Based Clinical Practice Guidelines. Chest Journal 133: 141S–159S.

9. Verbeeck R, Musuamba F (2009) Pharmacokinetics and dosage adjustment in patients with renal dysfunction. Eur J Clin Pharmacol 65: 757–773.

10. British Medical Association, Royal Pharmaceutical Society of Great Britain(2012) British National Formulary. London: BMA, RPS, (No 64).

11. Thorevska N, Amoateng-Adjepong Y, Sabahi R, Schiopescu I, Salloum A, et al. (2004) Anticoagulation in hospitalized patients with renal insufficiency: a comparison of bleeding rates with unfractionated heparin vs enoxaparin. Chest Journal 125: 856–863.

12. Schulman S, Beyth RJ, Kearon C, Levine MN (2008) Hemorrhagic Complications of Anticoagulant and Thrombolytic Treatment. American College of Chest Physicians Evidence-Based Clinical Practice Guidelines. Chest Journal 133: 257S–298S.

13. Cohen M, Demers C, Gurfinkel EP, Turpie AG, Fromell GJ, et al. (1997) A comparison of low-molecular-weight heparin with unfractionated heparin for unstable coronary artery disease. Efficacy and Safety of Subcutaneous Enoxaparin in Non-Q-Wave Coronary Events Study Group. N Engl J Med 337: 447–452.

14. Prism P (1998) Study Investigators. Inhibition of the platelet glycoprotein IIb/IIIa receptor with tirofiban in unstable angina and non-Q-wave myocardial infarction. N Engl J Med 338: 1488–1497.

15. Rubin DB (2001) Using propensity scores to help design observational studies: application to the tobacco litigation. Health Serv Outcomes Res Methodol 2: 169–188.

16. Thoemmes F (2012) Propensity score matching in SPSS. http://arxivorg/abs/12016385 Accessed March 18, 2013.

17. Brookhart MA, Schneeweiss S, Rothman KJ, Glynn RJ, Avorn J, et al. (2006) Variable selection for propensity score models. Am J Epidemiol 163: 1149–1156.

18. Pisters R, Lane DA, Nieuwlaat R, de Vos CB, Crijns HJGM, et al. (2010) A Novel User-Friendly Score (HAS-BLED) To Assess 1-Year Risk of Major Bleeding in Patients With Atrial Fibrillation The Euro Heart Survey. Chest Journal 138: 1093–1100.

19. Deyo RA, Cherkin DC, Ciol MA (1992) Adapting a clinical comorbidity index for use with ICD-9-CM administrative databases. J Clin Epidemiol 45: 613–619.

20. Austin PC, Grootendorst P, Anderson GM (2007) A comparison of the ability of different propensity score models to balance measured variables between treated and untreated subjects: a Monte Carlo study. Stat Med 26: 734–753.

21. Levine M, Gent M, Hirsh J, Leclerc J, Anderson D, et al. (1996) A comparison of low-molecular-weight heparin administered primarily at home with unfractionated heparin administered in the hospital for proximal deep-vein thrombosis. N Engl J Med 334: 677–681.

22. Merli G, Spiro TE, Olsson C-G, Abildgaard U, Davidson BL, et al. (2001) Subcutaneous enoxaparin once or twice daily compared with intravenous unfractionated heparin for treatment of venous thromboembolic disease. Ann Intern Med 134: 191–202.

23. Blazing MA, de Lemos JA, White HD, Fox KAA, Verheugt FWA, et al. (2004) Safety and Efficacy of Enoxaparin vs Unfractionated Heparin in Patients With Non–ST-Segment Elevation Acute Coronary Syndromes Who Receive Tirofiban and Aspirin. JAMA 292: 55–64.

24. Antman EM, McCabe CH, Gurfinkel EP, Turpie AGG, Bernink PJLM, et al. (1999) Enoxaparin Prevents Death and Cardiac Ischemic Events in Unstable Angina/Non–Q-Wave Myocardial Infarction Results of the Thrombolysis In Myocardial Infarction (TIMI) 11B Trial. Circulation 100: 1593–1601.

25. Decousus H, Leizorovicz A, Parent F, Page Y, Tardy B, et al. (1998) A clinical trial of vena caval filters in the prevention of pulmonary embolism in patients with proximal deep-vein thrombosis. N Engl J Med 338: 409–416.

26. Antman EM, Morrow DA, McCabe CH, Murphy SA, Ruda M, et al. (2006) Enoxaparin versus Unfractionated Heparin with Fibrinolysis for ST-Elevation Myocardial Infarction. N Engl J Med 354: 1477–1488.

27. Chan KE, Thadhani RI, Maddux FW (2013) No difference in bleeding risk between subcutaneous enoxaparin and heparin for thromboprophylaxis in end-stage renal disease. Kidney Int 84: 555–561.

28. Koo S, Kucher N, Nguyen PL, Fanikos J, Marks PW, et al. (2004) The effect of excessive anticoagulation on mortality and morbidity in hospitalized patients with anticoagulant-related major hemorrhage. Archives of internal medicine 164: 1557.

3

The Clinical Characteristics and Pathological Patterns of Postinfectious Glomerulonephritis in HIV-Infected Patients

Christine A. Murakami[1,⌙], Doaa Attia[2,⌙], Naima Carter-Monroe[3], Gregory M. Lucas[1], Michelle M. Estrella[1], Derek M. Fine[1], Mohamed G. Atta[1]*

1 Department of Medicine, Johns Hopkins University School of Medicine, Baltimore, Maryland, United States of America, 2 Faculty of Medicine, Alexandria, Egypt, 3 Department of Pathology, Johns Hopkins University School of Medicine, Baltimore, Maryland, United States of America

Abstract

Background: Postinfectious glomerulonephritis (PIGN), a form of immune complex GN, is not well-defined in HIV-infected patients. This study characterizes PIGN in this patients' population and determine the impact of histopathological patterns on renal outcome and mortality.

Methods: HIV-infected patients with PIGN from September 1998 to July 2013 were identified. Archived slides were reviewed by a blinded renal pathologist, classified into acute, persistent and healed PIGN. Groups were compared using Wilcoxon rank-sum and Fisher's exact test. Survival analyses were performed to determine association of histopathological pattern with renal outcome and mortality.

Results: Seventy-two HIV-infected predominantly African American males were identified with PIGN. Median (interquartile range) age and creatinine at the time of renal biopsy was 48 years (41, 53) and 2.5 mg/dl (1.5, 4.9) respectively. Only 2 (3%) had acute PIGN, 42 (58%) had persistent PIGN and 28 (39%) had healed PIGN. Three patients (4%) had IgA-dominant PIGN. Only 46% of the patients had confirmed positive cultures with *Staphylococcus* the most common infectious agent. During a median follow up of 17 months, the pathological pattern had no impact on renal outcome ($P = 0.95$). Overall mortality was high occurring in 14 patients (19%); patients with healed PIGN had significantly increased mortality ($P = 0.05$).

Conclusion: In HIV-infected patients, *Staphylococcus* is the most common cause of PIGN. Renal outcome was not influenced by the histopathological pattern but those with healed PIGN had greater mortality which was potentially due to a confounder not accounted for in the study.

Editor: Antonio C. Seguro, University of São Paulo School of Medicine, Brazil

Funding: Mohamed G. Atta is supported by the National Institute of Diabetes and Digestive and Kidney Diseases grant P01DK056492. Dr. Lucas was supported by the National Institute on Drug Abuse (K24 DA035684 and R01 DA026770) and by the Johns Hopkins University Center for AIDS Research (P30 AI094189). The funders had no role in study design, data collection and analysis, decision to publish, or preparation of the manuscript.

Competing Interests: The authors have declared that no competing interests exist.

* Email: matta1@jhmi.edu

⌙ These authors contributed equally to this work.

Introduction

Renal diseases in patients infected with HIV cover a wide array of renal pathologies [1–3]. These pathologies could be the direct effect of the HIV-1 virus, such as HIV-1 associated nephropathy (HIVAN), or the consequence of coexisting conditions such as diabetes, hypertension, intravenous drug use, or exposure to antiretroviral medications [4]. The incidence of HIVAN, the most aggressive histologic lesion in the HIV population, has substantially declined in recent years due to the introduction of highly-active antiretroviral therapy (HAART) [5,6]. However, HIV-immune complex-mediated kidney disease (HIVICK) continues to be a pervasive histologic finding [7]. HIVICK refers to a spectrum of pathological entities consisting of post-infectious glomerulonephritis (PIGN), "lupus-like" glomerulonephritis, IgA nephropathy, membranoproliferative glomerulonephritis (MPGN), and membranous nephropathy [4]. In a study by Foy *et al*, PIGN was identified as the most common immune-complex glomerulonephritis in HIV patients [4].

In recent years, the disease pattern and epidemiology of PIGN has markedly evolved [8,9]. Infections with *Staphylococcal* and gram-negative bacteria have now been identified as increasingly common antecedent of PIGN. Studies have also reported a more unfavorable prognosis than two to three decades ago; this has been attributed to changes in the disease profile as well as delayed diagnosis and treatment [8,10]. Complete remission has been reported in some studies to occur in 26% to 69% of adults with PIGN [8,11,12]. While there have been several studies describing the clinicopathologic spectrum of PIGN in the adult population, data on the prevalence and prognosis of PIGN among adults HIV patients are lacking [8,10,13]. Histologically, PIGN is characterized by diffuse endocapillary proliferative and exudative glomerulonephritis on light microscopy with granular deposits of complement 3 (C3) and immunoglobulin G (IgG) in the mesangium and glomerular basement membranes on immunofluorescence (IF). On electron microscopy, large subepithelial electron-dense deposits or "humps" are characteristic findings [14]. Although, classic cases of PIGN are diagnosed histologically without difficulty, a large number of patients have PIGN with atypical histological features [10]. In 2003, Haas reviewed 1012 renal biopsies and classified PIGN as acute or subacute glomerulonephritis (GN), persistent or progressive glomerulonephritis and healed or latent glomerulonephritis [15]. In this classification, acute or subacute GN pertains to cases with diffuse mesangial and endocapillary hypercellularity on light microscopy, multiple subepithelial humps on electron microscopy (EM), characteristic granular glomerular basement membrane staining for IgG and or C3 on IF, and clinical findings consistent with acute or subacute kidney injury. Persistent or progressive GN lacks the intense degree of diffuse mesangial and endocapillary hypercellularity seen in acute PIGN, and has variable granular mesangial C3 and or IgG deposits with some capillary wall deposits. On EM, patients with persistent PIGN have fewer subepithelial humps compared to acute PIGN. Healed or latent GN refers to cases with mild mesangial hypercellularity and immunofluorescence (IF) similar to persistent GN, with partially or markedly resorbed subepithelial deposits on EM. Although this classification may be helpful, it is not known whether it has clinical implications, particularly in HIV-infected patients.

In this study, the clinical features of PIGN in HIV-infected patients and their correlation with the different aforementioned pathological patterns are explored. In addition, the impact of these pathological findings on renal outcome and mortality is determined.

Materials and Methods

Study Design and Patient Selection

Patients with the diagnosis of PIGN on renal biopsy from September 1998 to July 2013 were identified through linkage with the institutional pathology database. Patients who met all the following criteria were included: 18 years of age and older, diagnosis of HIV-1 infection, hospital admission at Johns Hopkins University from September 1998 to July 2013. Pediatric patients, patients who received any type of organ transplantation as well as those who received care at other institutions were excluded. We initially identified 90 adult HIV-infected patients who met these criteria (Figure 1) but only 72 patients were eventually included in the study due to uncertain pathological diagnoses in 18 cases. The Institutional Review Board of Johns Hopkins University approved the study. Patient records and information were de-identified prior to analysis.

Data Collection and Definitions

The diagnosis of PIGN was established from the pathological report generated by the renal pathologist at the time of the renal biopsy. A renal pathologist, who was blinded to clinical characteristics, reviewed the slides of the 90 patients screened for this study. All renal biopsies were processed by light microscopy and EM. All but 4 slides were also examined by IF. The patients

with PIGN were further subclassified into acute, persistent, or healed PIGN based on the system proposed by Haas et al summarized in Table 1 [15]. Demographic, clinical, laboratory and pharmaceutical data collected at the time of renal biopsy and at 2 months before and after the biopsy, were abstracted from electronic patient records. The following clinical definitions were used: HIV-1 infection based on documented diagnosis from medical records and or use of antiretroviral medications; diabetes and hypertension were defined by prescription of anti-diabetic or anti-hypertensive medications, respectively; hepatitis C virus (HCV) infection was based on presence of hepatitis C viral antibodies and/or detection of hepatitis C viral load by polymerase chain reaction. Cirrhosis was based on patient medical history and/or liver biopsy findings and end-stage renal disease (ESRD) was defined as initiation of renal replacement therapy. Nephrotic-range proteinuria was defined by >3.0 g/d (if 24 hour urine collected) or >3.0 g/g creatinine (by random urine protein-to-creatinine ratio).

Statistical Analyses

Stata statistical software version 10 (Stata Corp, College Station, TX) was used for the statistical analysis. Continuous variables were reported as median and interquartile range (IQR). Continuous and categorical variables were compared using Wilcoxon rank-sum and the Fisher's exact test, respectively. A P-value <0.05 was considered statistically significant. We used Kaplan-Meier plots and log-rank test to compare time to ESRD or death in groups with different kidney pathology features. Finally, we used Cox proportional hazards models to determine hazard ratios (HR) and 95% confidence intervals (CI).

Results

Pathological Findings

There were 1250 patients with a diagnosis of PIGN on renal biopsies performed from September 1998 to July 2013. After excluding 156 pediatric patients, 946 HIV-uninfected patients, 45 transplant recipients, 13 patients admitted at other institutions, there were 90 patients for evaluation. The blinded pathological review excluded 18 cases that were classified as immune-complex GN where there was no solid histologic evidence of PIGN. This resulted in 72 adult patients with confirmed PIGN and HIV-1 infection in the analysis (Figure 1). In the blinded pathological review of the archived renal tissues, 2 (3%) were designated as having acute PIGN, 42 (58%) persistent PIGN, and 28 (39%) healed PIGN. Three of the 72 PIGN cases (4%) were IgA-dominant PIGN. Twenty-six patients (36%) had PIGN as the sole diagnosis on their renal biopsy while 31 (43%) had PIGN with either concurrent classic FSGS or HIVAN and 15 (21%) have other pathological findings on renal biopsy.

Clinical Characteristics of Participants with Different Histological Classification of PIGN

The majority of patients were African American (89%) and male in gender (64%). The median (interquartile range [IQR]) age at the time of the renal biopsy was 48 years (41, 53). The median (IQR) CD4 count and viral load at the time of biopsy were 322 cells/mm^3 (156, 498) and 13,346 copies/mL (504, 100,566), respectively. The median (IQR) creatinine at the time of biopsy was 2.5 mg/dl (1.5, 4.9). Fifty-nine patients (82%) had hypertension and 17 (24%) had underlying diabetes mellitus. Forty out of 72 patients (56%) were coinfected with Hepatitis C. Only 12 patients (17%) exhibited a low C3 or C4. Bacterial infection was

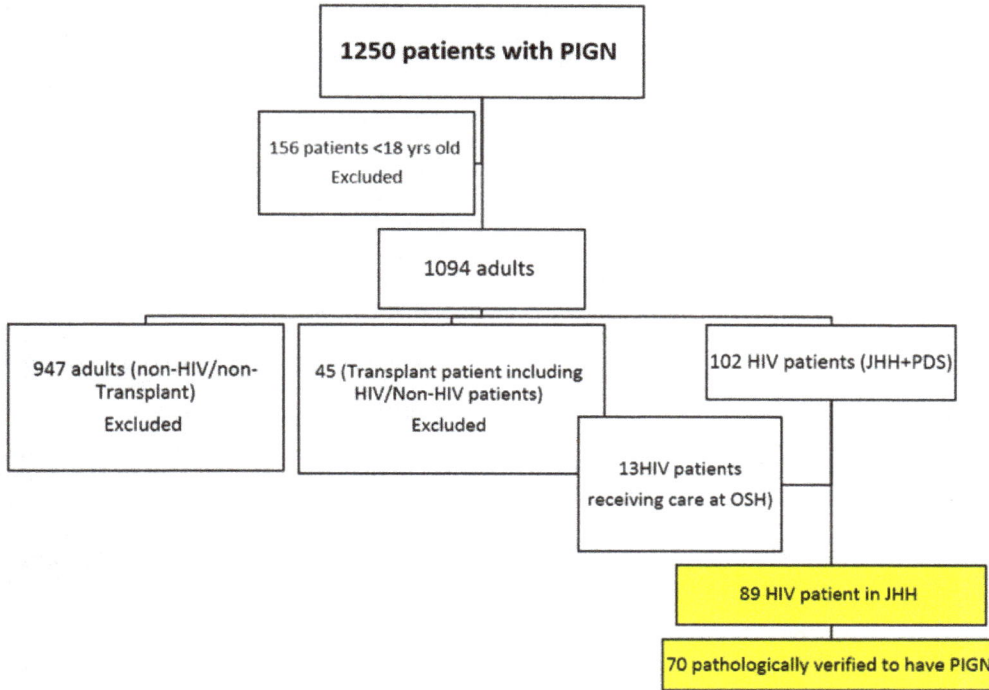

Figure 1. Screening of patients: Out of 1250 patients screened, 72 HIV infected individuals with Post infectious glomerulonephritis were included in the final analysis.

Table 1. Histopathological classification of postinfectious glomerulonephritis.

	Acute PIGN	Persistent PIGN	Healed PIGN
Light microscopy (H&E, PAS, Masson's trichrome and PAS -Methenimine silver stained slides)	• Diffuse, moderate to marked, segmental to global endocapillary hypercellularity (mostly neutrophilic)	• Focal, mild to moderate, segmental endocapillary hypercellularity (mostly mononuclear)	• Focal, absent to mild segmental endocapillary hypercellularity (mostly mononuclear)
	• ± Moderate to marked mesangial hypercellularity	• ± Mild to marked mesangial hypercellularity	• ± Absent to moderate mesangial hypercellularity
Immunofluorescence	• Granular capillary wall (GBM), with ± mesangial IgG and/or C3 deposits	• Variable granular mesangial C3± IgG with ± capillary wall (GBM) deposits	• Variable granular mesangial C3± IgG with ± capillary wall (GBM) deposits
	• Mesangial IgA in IgA -dominant PIGN	• ± IgA, IgM, C1q, kappa or lambda	• ± IgA, IgM, C1q, kappa or lambda
	• ± IgA, IgM, C1q, Kappa or lambda		
Electron microscopy	• Numerous irregularly-spaced subepithelial electron dense deposits, frequently in mesangial "notch", rare "humps", undergoing minimal to mild resorption	• Occasional to numerous subepithelial electron dense deposits, a few "humps", a few (at least 1) in mesangial "notch", undergoing variable (mild to marked) resorption	• Few subepithelial electron dense deposits, rare "humps" (up to 2), a few in mesangial "notch", undergoing moderate to marked resorption
	• ±Rare intramembranous, mesangial, subendothelial	• ± Variable numbers of subendothelial, intramembranous, mesangial	• Numerous subendothelial, intramembranous, mesangial, undergoing moderate to marked resorption

Adapted from Haas, M., Hum Pathol, 2003. 34(1): p. 3–10.

confirmed by positive blood culture in less than half of the patients (46%).

The two patients with acute PIGN were both African American males with HCV coinfection, hypertension, and history of intravenous drug use. Both presented with low C3 and normal C4 levels. At the time of renal biopsy, both were on antiretroviral therapy although one had a higher CD4 count and lower HIV-1 viral load (VL) compared to the other (CD4 657 vs. 50 and VL 400 vs. 939,000 respectively). However, the patient with better immunological status had underlying chronic kidney disease and ultimately required renal replacement therapy. The one with poor immune status had histological findings consistent with IgA-dominant PIGN. No preceding infection was identified in either patient.

The demographics and clinical characteristics of the remaining 70 patients with persistent and healed PIGN are summarized in Table 2. Hypertension and diabetes mellitus occurred in similar frequencies in the patients with persistent PIGN and healed PIGN (88% and 28% persistent PIGN vs. 79% and 23% healed, respectively). HCV coinfection was similar between the two groups, comprising 63% of patients with persistent PIGN and 56% of those with healed PIGN.

Most of the patients with persistent and healed PIGN were on antiretroviral therapy at the time of renal biopsy (66% persistent and 78% healed PIGN). The CD4 counts were also similar between the two groups. More patients with persistent PIGN (62%) exhibited statistically significant hematuria compared to those with healed PIGN ($P = 0.02$). In contrast, nephrotic-range proteinuria occurred more frequently in those with healed PIGN but these were not noted to be statistically significant ($P = 0.16$). The degree of renal dysfunction at the time of the renal biopsy was also similar between the 2 groups (median creatinine of 2.2 and 2.6 mg/dl). When identified, the heart or endocardium was the most common source of infection among patients with persistent PIGN while other infections were more frequently associated with healed PIGN (17%). However, the association between the source of infection and histopathological pattern was not statistically significant. In those with an isolated organism, *Staphylococcus* was identified as the most common infectious agent isolated in 42% of patients with persistent PIGN and 56% of those with healed PIGN.

Use of antimicrobials, angiotensin-converting enzyme inhibitor (ACE-I) and corticosteroid were similar between those with persistent PIGN and healed PIGN ($P = 0.92$, $P = 0.80$ and $P = 0.51$, respectively).

Pathological Findings

The two patients with acute PIGN have very similar pathological findings. Neither patient had crescents. Both of their renal biopsies showed subepithelial humps, subendothelial deposits and mesangial deposits. One of them had a positive C3 with trace IgM and intense IgA staining on IF while the other one was C3 negative. Both patients exhibited significant interstitial fibrosis, one with moderate interstitial fibrosis and the other with marked interstitial fibrosis. The pathological characteristics of the 70 HIV patients with persistent and healed PIGN are summarized in Table 3.

Only 3 patients out of 70 were found to have crescents on renal biopsy, all of whom had persistent PIGN. One had a fibrocellular crescent while the two others had cellular crescents. IF was positive for C3 and Ig (either IgA, IgM or IgG) on 55% of patients with persistent PIGN and 36% of patients with healed PIGN. Among the patients with positive C3 and Ig on IF, majority of the patients, both in the persistent and healed PIGN, had IgM positive deposits

along with C3 (26% persistent PIGN group and 25% healed PIGN group). A small proportion of patients on both groups (19% persistent PIGN and 11% with healed PIGN) had IF that was positive for C3 only. Subepithelial humps were identified in in the majority of patients with persistent and healed PIGN. In contrast, subendothelial deposits were significantly predominant in patients with persistent PIGN compared to those with healed PIGN (57% vs 7%, $P = <0.0001$). The majority of the patients with persistent PIGN (76%) had interstitial fibrosis, mostly mild and moderate interstitial fibrosis (33% and 26% respectively). The same percentage of patients with healed PIGN (76%), had interstitial fibrosis which were mostly moderate (31%) and mild (28%). Similarly, interstitial inflammation was noted in 76% of patients with persistent PIGN and 86% of patients with healed PIGN.

Mortality and Incidence of CKD

The patients were followed up for a median (IQR) of 17 months (1–45 months). Mortality occurred in 14 out of 72 patients (19%) during the follow-up period. Among those who died, 6 patients had a sole diagnosis of PIGN, 5 with PIGN and other pathologies and 3 have PIGN with FSGS or HIVAN. Two of the patients with PIGN who died exhibited histopathological features of IgA-dominant PIGN.

Fourteen patients (19%), including one with acute PIGN, required renal replacement. None of the patients with IgA dominant PIGN required renal replacement therapy. We found no significant association between the histopathological classification of PIGN and ESRD. The cumulative progression to ESRD was similar in patients with persistent PIGN and healed PIGN (19% and 18%, respectively; $P = 0.95$ log-rank test). Individuals with healed PIGN had a similar risk of progressing to ESRD as those with persistent PIGN (HR, 0.96; 95% CI, 0.31 to 3.00). Similarly, the cumulative incidence of ESRD in patients with an exclusive diagnosis of PIGN was similar to patients with PIGN in combination with HIVAN or FSGS, and PIGN with other pathologies (15%, 25% and 14%, respectively; $P = 0.72$ log-rank test) (Table 4). Compared to those with a sole diagnosis of PIGN, the risk of progressing to ESRD was similar in those with PIGN plus HIVAN or FSGS (1.09; 95% CI 0.28–4.18) and those with PIGN plus other pathologies (0.66; 95% CI 0.11–4.06).

Mortality rates, on the other hand, showed differences based on the histopathological pattern of PIGN. The cumulative incidence of mortality in individuals with healed PIGN was higher compared to those with persistent PIGN (36% and 10%; *P = 0.05 log-rank test*) (Figure 2). This significant difference was eliminated in a separate analysis where cases with co-existing histopathological diagnoses were excluded. Including only those with pure PIGN, there were 15 patients with persistent PIGN and 10 patients with healed PIGN. Of these, 2 and 4 patients died respectively and the log-rank P value for this comparison was 0.41 (data not shown). However, the significant drop in the sample size may limit the interpretation of this result. Patients with IgA-dominant PIGN did not show increased mortality (*P = 0.69*) or increased need for renal replacement ($P = 0.16$).

Discussion

This is the first study to explore the clinical and pathological characteristics of PIGN in HIV- infected individuals. In this study *Staphylococcus* was the most common etiology of an identified infection prior to diagnosis of PIGN. Interestingly, renal outcome was not influenced by the histopathological pattern, but mortality was relatively high (19%) in this cohort during the follow-up period, with patients with healed PIGN having greater mortality.

Table 2. Demographics, clinical characteristics and source of Infection of 71 patients at the time of diagnosis.

	Persistent PIGN (n = 42)	Healed PIGN (n = 28)	*P*-value
Sex			
Male (%)	27 (64)	17 (61)	0.8
Female (%)	15 (36)	11 (39)	
Age (median, IQR)	45 (41, 52)	48.5 (42, 54.5)	0.47
Race - no. of patients (%)			
Black	38 (91)	24 (86)	0.41
White	2 (5)	4 (14)	
Asian	1 (2)	0 (0.00)	
Others	1 (2)	0 (0.00)	
Serum creatinine (Median, IQR)	2.2 (1.1, 4.9)	2.6 (1.9, 5.1)	0.31
CD4 count (Median, IQR)	327 (199, 506)	238 (77, 459)	0.26
Comorbidities - no. of patients (%)			
Diabetes	11 (28)	6 (23)	0.8
Hypertension	35 (88)	22 (79)	0.34
Hepatitis C	24 (63)	14 (56)	0.61
Cirrhosis	1 (3)	2 (7)	0.57
Malignancy	8 (21)	3 (11)	0.34
Other systemic diseases	5 (13)	5 (20)	0.5
Intravenous drug use	19 (50)	10 (42)	0.61
Low C3	8 (25)	2 (10)	0.28
Low C4	8 (25)	2 (10)	0.28
Site of Infection –no. of patients (%)			
Endocardium	12 (29)	4 (14)	0.59
Bone/Joint	1 (2)	2 (7)	
Pleura	1 (2)	0 (0)	
Skin	4 (10)	4 (14)	
Lung/URTI	6 (14)	5 (18)	
Others	2 (5)	0 (0.00)	
None identified	16 (38)	14 (50)	
Infectious Agent - no. of patients (%)	N = 26	N = 25	
Staphylococcus	11 (42)	14 (56)	0.31
Streptococcus	7 (27)	8 (32)	
Others	8 (31)	3 (12)	
HIV medications - no. of patients (%)			
NRTI	21 (66)	11 (78)	0.5
NNRTI	7 (22)	2 (14)	0.7
PI	19 (59)	8 (57)	1
Other medications - no. of patients (%)			
ACE Inhibitors	19 (50)	12 (46)	0.8
ARB	1 (3)	1 (4)	1
Corticosteroid	9 (23)	3 (11)	0.51
Antibiotic use	24 (62)	16 (62)	0.92
Nephrotic Proteinuria	8 (26)	11 (46)	0.16
Hematuria	23 (62)	8 (30)	0.02

PIGN has been traditionally linked to Streptococcal pharyngitis or skin infection [13]. In our HIV-infected cohort with PIGN, *Staphylococcus* was the most common causative agent identified. This supports the findings of various authors, who described a shift in the epidemiologic features of PIGN over the past decades [8,9]. Nasr *et al* described *Staphylococcus* as the most common causative

Table 3. Summary of pathological findings on 70 patients with persistent and healed PIGN.

Pathological Finding – no of patients (%)	Persistent PIGN (n = 42)	Healed (n = 28)	p- value
Interstitial inflammation			
Mild/Minimal	13 (31)	13 (45)	0.22
Moderate	14 (33)	8 (28)	0.80
Marked	5 (12)	3 (10)	1.00
No inflammation	10 (24)	4 (14)	0.38
Crescents			
Fibrocellular	1 (2)	0 (0)	1.00
Cellular	2 (5)	0 (0)	0.51
Subepithelial humps	31 (74)	17 (59)	0.30
Subendothelial deposits	24 (57)	2 (7)	<0.0001
Mesangial deposits	34 (81)	15 (52)	0.02
Immunofluorescence			
C3+ Ig	23 (55)	10 (34)	0.15
C3+ IgM	11 (26)	7 (24)	1.00
C3+ IgG	2 (5)	0 (0)	0.51
C3+ IgM+ IgG	10 (24)	3 (10)	0.22
C3 only	8 (19)	3 (10)	0.51
C3 negative	8 (19)	13 (45)	0.02
Interstitial fibrosis			
Mild	14 (33)	8 (28)	0.79
Moderate	11 (26)	9 (31)	0.60
Marked	7 (17)	5 (17)	1.00
No fibrosis	10 (24)	7 (24)	1.00

agent in the elderly population [16] and in IgA dominant PIGN [17]. Our study showed that this is true even in younger patients with HIV-1 infection with no pathological features of IgA-dominant PIGN.

In our HIV-infected cohort, bacterial infection was only confirmed in 46% of the patients, which is consistent with a study which revealed that in as much as 24% to 59% of patients with PIGN, the causative organism cannot be identified [13]. The low yield of bacterial culture in identifying the causative organism could be due to the diversity of organisms that can cause PIGN which include viruses and parasites. Furthermore, the role of HIV and HCV infection in the development of PIGN in this cohort is not clear although one can argue that antigens of these viruses may be playing a role in this process. Hepatitis C infection was noted in more than 50% of our HIV-infected cohort. However, the presence of HCV coinfection did not increase predisposition for a specific histological pattern of PIGN. Previous studies reported

that HCV coinfection with HIV-1 increases predisposition to immune-complex glomerulonephritis [18]. HIV-1 itself may promote an increase in circulating immune complexes by promoting polyclonal hypergammaglobulinemia [19]. One study also suggested that formation of anti-HIV antibodies might play a role in forming immune complexes in some HIV patients [20] Whether HIVICK is caused by passive trapping of the circulating immune complex, or in situ deposition of antibody-antigen complex, is still not completely understood.

The lack of clinical signs of infection may explain the lower frequency of acute pattern of PIGN in our cohort. The majority of our patients with PIGN had healed and persistent PIGN on renal biopsy, and only 2 had acute PIGN. One study reported that as much as 16% of adult patients may not have any clinical manifestation of infection [13]. The absence of overt signs of acute infection is believed to be one of the reasons for delayed diagnosis [10]. Although, the patients with PIGN had comparable degrees of

Table 4. Estimated rates of mortality and ESRD 12 months following kidney biopsy, according to pathologic findings.

No. of patients (%)	PIGN only (n = 26)	PIGN+FSGS/HIVAN (n = 31)	PIGN + other* (n = 15)	P-value**
Mortality	6 (23)	3 (9)	5 (36)	0.09
ESRD	4 (15)	8 (25)	2 (14)	0.74

*Others: MPGN, lupus-like, membranous, diabetic glomerulosclerosis.
**Log-rank test.

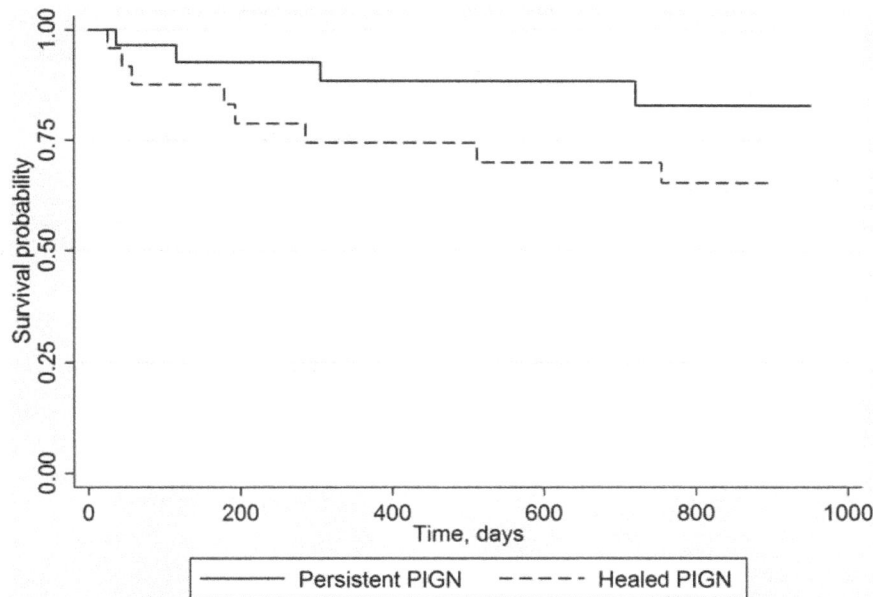

Figure 2. Mortality according to histopathological pattern of PIGN: Patients with healed PIGN had significantly worse survival compared to those of persistent PIGN, log-rank test.

renal dysfunction regardless of the histopathological pattern, early diagnosis in the HIV population may be important since patients with healed PIGN tend to have a higher mortality. Hence, PIGN should always be entertained as a differential diagnosis in HIV patients with renal dysfunction, even in the absence of a source of infection. Given the heterogeneity of renal pathologies in HIV as well as the absence of a reliable clinical indicator of PIGN in HIV patients, a timely renal biopsy is very valuable in this population.

Our study comprising of predominantly male African American HIV-infected patients, a large proportion (82%) of the patients were hypertensive. This is slightly higher than what has been previously reported [13]. However, the occurrence of hypertension did not differ between the patients with different histologic pattern of PIGN. Conversely, diabetes mellitus, which has been identified as the most frequent risk factor in a study of adults with acute PIGN [13], was only documented in 17 patients (24%) in our HIV-infected cohort. This finding may be partially explained by the demographic differences with other studies and suggests that diabetes mellitus is not a major risk factor for PIGN among young African American patients with HIV-infected patients.

Our study showed that individuals with persistent PIGN had a similar risk of progressing to ESRD as those with healed PIGN. Two prior PIGN studies identified the absence of interstitial inflammation as one of the pathological findings which correlates with renal recovery [11,13]. Interstitial fibrosis was identified by *Montseny* et al as one of the predictors of persistent renal dysfunction [8]. In our cohort of patients, the proportion of patients with interstitial inflammation and interstitial fibrosis were very similar between the persistent PIGN and healed PIGN groups. Perhaps, this explains why the mean creatinine at the time of renal biopsy and progression to ESRD during the follow-up period were similar between the two groups were similar. The association between the presence of crescents and renal outcome seems to be less straightforward in PIGN. While *Nasr* et al [13] did not find a correlation between crescents and renal outcome, another study reported poorer renal outcomes with crescentic PIGN [21]. In our patient population, only 3 patients exhibited

crescents on renal biopsy. Owing to the low number of patients with crescentic GN, we cannot determine if there is a correlation between renal outcome and crescentic glomerulonephritis in HIV-infected patients. It might be worthwhile to look into this on future studies involving a larger number of HIV patients with PIGN.

Studies on HIV-infected population have suggested that HIVAN progresses more rapidly than non-HIVAN renal diseases [1,22,23]. In our study, some of the patients with PIGN had concomitant findings consistent with HIVAN. However, these patients did not show an increased progression to ESRD compared to those patients with the sole diagnosis of PIGN or with PIGN in conjunction with other pathologies. The short follow-up period of our study may not have limited our ability to distinguish differences. Perhaps and more importantly, a substantial proportion of our patients were on antiretroviral therapy at the time of diagnosis, which could have delayed the progression of HIVAN in this cohort to ESRD.

Although renal outcome did not differ between the persistent and healed PIGN groups, healed PIGN appears to correlate with higher mortality during the follow-up period. Although this may be counterintuitive and there is real possibility of a chance finding, there is evidence that at the time of biopsy more patients with healed PIGN exhibiting more nephrotic-range proteinuria which may have been associated with worse outcome in this group of patients. Alternatively, since we did not account for the timing of institution of antibiotic and HAART use, this could have played a crucial role in the different mortality between the 2 groups.

Our study has several limitations. It is a single-center study with patients mostly coming from an inner city urban hospital. Our patient population consisted mostly of African American patients; hence the results may not apply to other populations. Only patients who had renal biopsies were included, which potentially excluded the HIV patients who are coagulopathic or with severe illness. We also did not account for the duration of HIV-1 infection or timing of initiation of HAART or antibiotic therapy, which could have an impact on the renal outcome or mortality. Although the histological pattern proposed by Haas is not widely utilized in practice, our study was an attempt at using some form of standardization for the study.

In conclusion, PIGN is a common histopathologic diagnosis in HIV patients. *Staphylococcus* is the most commonly identified organism in a preceding infection in HIV-associated PIGN. The histopathological classification of PIGN has no bearing on the renal outcome but this group of patients incur overall high mortality rate. Patients with healed PIGN have the highest mortality suggesting that delayed diagnosis may have a negative impact on overall outcome.

Acknowledgments

All authors abide by the Association for Medical Ethics (AME) ethical rules of disclosure.

Author Contributions

Conceived and designed the experiments: MGA GML DMF. Performed the experiments: NCM DA CM. Analyzed the data: MGA GML. Contributed reagents/materials/analysis tools: MGA GML. Contributed to the writing of the manuscript: CM DA MGA MME.

References

1. Berliner AR, Fine DM, Lucas GM, Rahman MH, Racusen LC, et al. (2008) Observations on a cohort of HIV-infected patients undergoing native renal biopsy. Am J Nephrol 28: 478–486.
2. Nebuloni M, Barbiano di Belgiojoso G, Genderini A, Tosoni A, L N, et al. (2009) Glomerular lesions in HIV-positive patients: a 20-year biopsy experience from Northern Italy. Clin Nephrol 72: 38–45.
3. Gerntholtz TE, Goetsch SJ, Katz I (2006) HIV-related nephropathy: a South African perspective. Kidney Int 69: 1885–1891.
4. Foy MC, Estrella MM, Lucas GM, Tahir F, Fine DM, et al. (2013) Comparison of risk factors and outcomes in HIV immune complex kidney disease and HIV-associated nephropathy. Clin J Am Soc Nephrol 8: 1524–1532.
5. Lucas GM, Eustace JA, Sozio S, Mentari EK, Appiah KA, et al. (2004) Highly active antiretroviral therapy and the incidence of HIV-1-associated nephropathy: a 12-year cohort study. Aids 18: 541–546.
6. Atta MG, Gallant JE, Rahman MH, Nagajothi N, Racusen LC, et al. (2006) Antiretroviral therapy in the treatment of HIV-associated nephropathy. Nephrol Dial Transplant 21: 2809–2813.
7. Estrella MM, Fine DM, Atta MG (2010) Recent developments in HIV-related kidney disease. HIV Ther 4: 589–603.
8. Montseny JJ, Meyrier A, Kleinknecht D, Callard P (1995) The current spectrum of infectious glomerulonephritis. Experience with 76 patients and review of the literature. Medicine (Baltimore) 74: 63–73.
9. Nast CC (2012) Infection-related glomerulonephritis: changing demographics and outcomes. Adv Chronic Kidney Dis 19: 68–75.
10. Wen YK (2009) The spectrum of adult postinfectious glomerulonephritis in the new millennium. Ren Fail 31: 676–682.
11. Moroni G, Pozzi C, Quaglini S, Segagni S, Banfi G, et al. (2002) Long-term prognosis of diffuse proliferative glomerulonephritis associated with infection in adults. Nephrol Dial Transplant 17: 1204–1211.
12. Vogl W, Renke M, Mayer-Eichberger D, Schmitt H, Bohle A (1986) Long-term prognosis for endocapillary glomerulonephritis of poststreptococcal type in children and adults. Nephron 44: 58–65.
13. Nasr SH, Markowitz GS, Stokes MB, Said SM, Valeri AM, et al. (2008) Acute postinfectious glomerulonephritis in the modern era: experience with 86 adults and review of the literature. Medicine (Baltimore) 87: 21–32.
14. Haas M, Racusen LC, Bagnasco SM (2008) IgA-dominant postinfectious glomerulonephritis: a report of 13 cases with common ultrastructural features. Hum Pathol 39: 1309–1316.
15. Haas M (2003) Incidental healed postinfectious glomerulonephritis: a study of 1012 renal biopsy specimens examined by electron microscopy. Hum Pathol 34: 3–10.
16. Nasr SH, Fidler ME, Valeri AM, Cornell LD, Sethi S, et al. (2011) Postinfectious glomerulonephritis in the elderly. J Am Soc Nephrol 22: 187–195.
17. Nasr SH, D'Agati VD (2011) IgA-dominant postinfectious glomerulonephritis: a new twist on an old disease. Nephron Clin Pract 119: c18–25; discussion c26.
18. George E, Nadkarni GN, Estrella MM, Lucas GM, Sperati CJ, et al. (2011) The impact of hepatitis C coinfection on kidney disease related to human immunodeficiency virus (HIV): a biopsy study. Medicine (Baltimore) 90: 289–295.
19. Cohen SD, Kimmel PL (2008) Immune complex renal disease and human immunodeficiency virus infection. Semin Nephrol 28: 535–544.
20. Kimmel PL, Phillips TM, Ferreira-Centeno A, Farkas-Szallasi T, Abraham AA, et al. (1993) HIV-associated immune-mediated renal disease. Kidney Int 44: 1327–1340.
21. Zent R, Van Zyl Smit R, Duffield M, Cassidy MJ (1994) Crescentic nephritis at Groote Schuur Hospital, South Africa–not a benign disease. Clin Nephrol 42: 22–29.
22. Wearne N, Swanepoel CR, Boulle A, Duffield MS, Rayner BL (2012) The spectrum of renal histologies seen in HIV with outcomes, prognostic indicators and clinical correlations. Nephrol Dial Transplant 27: 4109–4118.
23. Szczech LA, Gupta SK, Habash R, Guasch A, Kalayjian R, et al. (2004) The clinical epidemiology and course of the spectrum of renal diseases associated with HIV infection. Kidney Int 66: 1145–1152.

4

Increased Risk of Urinary Tract Cancer in ESRD Patients Associated with Usage of Chinese Herbal Products Suspected of Containing Aristolochic Acid

Shuo-Meng Wang[1,4], Ming-Nan Lai[2], Alan Wei[3], Ya-Yin Chen[1,2], Yeong-Shiau Pu[1], Pau-Chung Chen[4], Jung-Der Wang[5,6]*

1 Department of Urology, National Taiwan University Hospital, Taipei, Taiwan, 2 Department of Statistics, Feng Chia University, Taichung, Taiwan, 3 School of Medicine, Stony Brook University, Stony Brook, New York, United States of America, 4 Institute of Occupational Medicine and Industrial Hygiene, College of Public Health, National Taiwan University, Taipei, Taiwan, 5 Department of Public Health, National Cheng Kung University Medical College, Tainan City, Taiwan, 6 Departments of Internal Medicine and Occupational and Environmental Medicine, National Cheng Kung University Hospital, Tainan City, Taiwan

Abstract

Introduction: Both end-stage renal disease (ESRD) and urothelial cancer (UC) are associated with the consumption of Chinese herbal products containing aristolochic acid (AA) by the general population. The objective of this study was to determine the risk of UC associated with AA-related Chinese herbal products among ESRD patients.

Methods: We conducted a cohort study using the National Health Insurance reimbursement database to enroll all ESRD patients in Taiwan from 1998–2002. Cox regression models were constructed and hazard ratios and confidence intervals were estimated after controlling for potential confounders, including age, sex, residence in region with endemic black foot disease, urinary tract infection, and use of non-steroidal anti-inflammatory drugs and acetaminophen.

Results: A total of 38,995 ESRD patients were included in the final analysis, and 320 patients developed UC after ESRD. Having been prescribed Mu Tong that was adulterated with Guan Mu Tong (*Aristolochia manshuriensis*) before 2004, or an estimated consumption of more than 1–100 mg of aristolochic acid, were both associated with an increased risk of UC in the multivariable analyses. Analgesic consumption of more than 150 pills was also associated with an increased risk of UC, although there was little correlation between the two risk factors.

Conclusion: Consumption of aristolochic acid-related Chinese herbal products was associated with an increased risk of developing UC in ESRD patients. Regular follow-up screening for UC in ESRD patients who have consumed Chinese herbal products is thus necessary.

Editor: Francisco X. Real, Centro Nacional de Investigaciones Oncológicas (CNIO), Spain

Funding: This study was supported by the National Health Research Institutes of Taiwan (intramural project EO-100-EO-PP04), and a grant from the Headquarters of University Advancement at the National Cheng Kung University. The funders had no role in study design, data collection and analysis, decision to publish, or preparation of the manuscript.

Competing Interests: The authors have declared that no competing interests exist.

* Email: jdwang121@gmail.com

Introduction

Aristolochic acid nephropathy—a progressive form of renal interstitial fibrosis—was first reported in a group of young Belgian patients with end-stage renal disease in 1993, and was thought to be caused by the use of Chinese herbal medicines that contained aristolochic acid [1–3]. Aristolochic acid has been shown to be associated with urothelial cancer (UC) in many studies of clinical cases around the world, in animal models, and by the detection of aristolochic acid–DNA adducts in the kidney and ureteral tissues [4][5,6]. Prior studies observed increased risks of developing UC and ESRD in the general population in association with the consumption of Chinese herbal products [7][8], and patients with ESRD have a higher incidence of malignancies than the general population [9–12]. We have noticed an extraordinarily high incidence of UC in uremic or ESRD patients in the past decade in

Taiwan [13–16], but the reason for this remains unknown. Some researchers suggest that chronic bladder irritation, a decreased urinary washout effect, atrophic involution of the bladder, compound analgesic abuse [17–19], use of Chinese herbs [4,5,20], groundwater intake (arsenic exposure) [21,22], and uremia per se [15,16] may play roles in the development of UC. A report published by the International Agency in Research on Cancer (IARC) [23] stated that the risk factors associated with UC include analgesics (phenacetin), herbal usage (aristolochic acid), heavy metals (arsenic) and tobacco smoking.

Although the IARC classifies aristolochic acid as a group 1 carcinogen, to the best of our knowledge there have been no cohort studies that examine the association between urinary tract cancer and the use of herbs or herbal products containing aristolochic acid in ESRD patients. In March of 1995, Taiwan established the National Health Insurance (NHI) program, which covers more than 99% of the population [24]. The NHI routinely reimburses enrollees for the cost of prescribed medicines, including Chinese herbal products containing aristolochic acid, which were widely prescribed before being banned in December 2003. We thus used the NHI reimbursement database to conduct an ESRD population-based cohort study to examine the association between having been prescribed Chinese herbal products that contain substantial amounts of aristolochic acid, including Guan Mu Tong and Guang Fangchi, and the risk of urinary tract cancer, as well as the possibility of a dose–response relationship between the two.

Materials and Methods

Study Population

Established in Taiwan in March 1995, the National Health Insurance program (NHI) covers over 99% of the population residents [24]. Standard mixtures of Chinese herbal products (CHP) are included in the regular schedule of reimbursement. The National Health Research Institutes (NHRI) transformed the NHI reimbursement data into files suitable for use by researchers, and which contain detailed information about the usage of conventional drugs and CHP [25]. This study was conducted using ESRD patient data obtained from the database of approximately more than 22 million people enrolled in the NHI. The data collection period began in 1996, but became more comprehensive after January 1997. As noted above, the NHRI anonymized and converted the reimbursement data into research-ready files, called the National Health Insurance Research Database (NHIRD) [25]. The identification numbers of all the individuals in the database were doubly encrypted to ensure their privacy.

The dataset to which we had access provided detailed demographic data (including birth date and sex) and information regarding the health-care services provided for each patient, including all payments for outpatient visits, hospitalizations, and prescriptions, as well as where each patient lived. The data for each hospitalization contained up to five diagnoses that were coded according to the International Classification of Diseases, Ninth Revision (ICD-9) [26], all drugs prescribed and the doses (i.e., conventional medicines, including generic and commercial brands of acetaminophen and non-steroidal anti-inflammatory drugs, as well as Chinese herbal products), and the date of each prescription. During the study period (i.e., from January 1, 1998, to December 31, 2002), all prescribed medications were covered under the NHI of Taiwan, and no drug could be dispensed at a pharmacy without a doctor's prescription.

To select potential case subjects for this study, we first obtained the NHI catastrophic illness registry files for all patients who were diagnosed with end-stage renal disease from January 1, 1998, to December 31, 2002. Because all patients who are registered as having a catastrophic illness are exempt from all copayments, their data is very comprehensive and has been carefully validated. A diagnosis of urinary tract cancer or end-stage renal disease made by doctors and officials of the NHI is usually accurate: urinary tract cancer must be proven by tissue pathology, and is classified as cancer of the upper urinary tract, which includes the renal pelvis and ureter (ICD-9 codes 189.1 and 189.2, respectively) or bladder cancer (ICD-9 code 188). The database contains 38,675 Non-UTC and 839 UTC prevalent cases of end-stage renal disease that were diagnosed from January 1, 1998, to December 31, 2002.Within this population, we identified 320 patients who were newly diagnosed with urinary tract cancer from January 1, 2001, to December 31, 2002, to allow at least four years between January 1, 1997, and the date of diagnosis to give sufficient time

for the case subjects to accumulate sufficient doses of herbal products to induce UTC.

Exposure Assessment

The reimbursement database contained all the details of the prescribed conventional medicines, which included acetaminophen and the commercial names of 45 kinds of non-steroidal anti-inflammatory drugs (NSAIDs), shown in the File S1.

As phenacetin has been totally banned by the Department of Health since 1986, it was not included. Doses of each drug were determined according to the number of pills prescribed and cumulative doses were calculated before ESRD. The use of 600–1000 pills of acetaminophen, NSAIDs, or mixed analgesics has been associated with an increased risk of renal damage or renal cancer in previous studies [27,28]. We thus accumulated the total number of analgesics pills for each subject before dialysis during 1998–2002.

According to the standard prescription recommended by the Committee on Chinese Medicine and Pharmacy (CCMP) in Taiwan, the following Chinese herbal products may contain AA: Xi-Xin (Asarum heterotoppoides), Guan-Mu-Tong (Aristolochia manshuriensis), and Guang-Fangchi (A. fangchi). However, Guan-Mu-Tong and Guang-Fangchi were once offered under the names Mu-Tong (Akebia sp.) and Fangchi (Stephania sp.), respectively, in Taiwan before 2003, because of similarities of gross morphology and common practices [29]. In addition, according to an investigation by the Bureau of Food and Drug Analysis in Taiwan, as well as some studies, approximately 89.2–100% of Fangchi preparations were actually Guang-Fangchi [30–32] and 84% of Mu-Tong were actually Guan-Mu-Tong [33]. These three herbs were prescribed as single products or included as components of some mixed CHP. Each pharmaceutical company has published and submitted the detailed composition of every product it produces, and data on this can be retrieved from the website of the Committee on Chinese Medicine and Pharmacy of the Department of Health [29]. With this information, the original amounts of herbs, in grams, could be determined for each mixture of CHP, and the cumulative dose for each herb prescribed to an individual before developing ESRD could thus be calculated. We also calculated the estimated cumulative dose of aristolochic acid for each subject by using the following estimates obtained in previous studies: the estimated average doses of aristolochic acid per 1 g of Guan Mu Tong, Guang Fangchi, and Xi Xin are 2.59 mg, 2.04 mg, and 0.042 mg, respectively [30,32–35].

The reimbursement database also has data on where all the subjects lived. We identified subjects who lived in the four townships in Taiwan that have been reported to be areas endemic for black foot disease—Pu-Tai and Yi-Chu in Chiayi County, and Hsueh-Chia and Pei-Men in Tainan County [36,37]. Black foot disease is a peripheral vascular disease that has been endemic to the coastal region of Taiwan for the past 60 years, and is associated with drinking water from artesian wells containing arsenic, and has been documented to be associated with an increased incidence of bladder cancer [36,37]. We controlled for this factor (townships) as a surrogate for arsenic exposure.

According to the Committee on Chinese Medicine and Pharmacy [29], Mu Tong is usually prescribed for the treatment of hepatitis, urinary tract infection, rhinitis, dysmenorrhea, and eczema. Recurrent or chronic urinary tract infection, associated with Schistosomiasis or prolonged indwelling catheters in patients with spinal cord injury, is associated with an increase risk of bladder cancer [38,39], whereas urinary tract infection from other causes does not show any consistent association with bladder cancer risk [38,40]. We thus defined patients with chronic urinary tract infection (UTI) as those who had such a diagnosis at least 12 times up to one year before the diagnosis of UC, and we controlled for the above potential confounders during the risk-estimate analysis. The patients with diabetes or hypertension were also ascertained based on the related diagnosis numbers in ICD-9 before ESRD diagnosis.

Statistical Analyses

To assess the independent association of various risk factors with new occurrences of UC, univariate and multivariable Cox regression models were used to analyze the population of ESRD patients and those cases that developed UC subsequent to ESRD diagnosis. Potential risk factors, including age, sex, hypertension, diabetes mellitus, chronic UTI, and prescriptions of NSAIDs, acetaminophen or any of the aforementioned Chinese herbs suspected to contain AA, were assessed for independent association with new occurrences of UC. We constructed models for two different types of exposure assessment: prescribed dosages of Chinese herbs (model 1) and different estimated dosages of AA as risk factors (model 2). The dose–response association between cumulative dose of Chinese herbs, analgesics and occurrence of UC was tested by the Mantel–Haenszel extension for the trend. For each potential risk factor, multivariate Cox proportional hazards models were constructed to estimate the relative risk and its 95% confidence interval (CI) for UC incidence. An estimate with the 95% CI that did not contain the number 1 was considered statistically significant. We also ran a correlation analysis between the total numbers of analgesics pills and cumulative doses (in mg) of AA. All the above analyses were conducted using the SAS ver. 9.2 software package (SAS Institute, Cary, NC, USA).

Results

After excluding people with incomplete data or aged over 100 years, a total of 39,514 prevalent cases of end-stage renal disease were included in the data, with 839 of these developing UTC between January 1, 1998 and December 31, 2002. Among these patients, there were 38,675 cases without UTC and 320 UTC cases who were newly diagnosed with urinary tract cancer between January 1, 2001 and December 31, 2002. A total of 38,995 ESRD patients were thus included in the final analysis, with 18,522 (47.5%) men and 20,473 (52.5%) women. There were high prevalence rates of hypertension (88.5%) and diabetes mellitus (55.7%). The average crude incidence rate of UTC for these ESRD patients was 1,368 per million person-years.

Table 1 summarizes the frequency data of the ESRD patient population with respect to different potential risk factors, including sex, age, follow-up time after ESRD diagnosis, residence in township with endemic black foot disease, hypertension, diabetes, chronic UTI, and analgesics (NSAID and acetaminophen) consumption. The patient population was also characterized in terms of Chinese herb consumption for individual herbs (Mu-Tong, Fangchi, and Xi-Xin), as well as total estimated consumption of AA calculated based on total consumption of Chinese herbs containing this substance. The incidence rate of UTC appears to increase with the time after diagnosis of ESRD (Table 1).

Because only one UTC patient and 254 non-UTC controls had lived in area with endemic black foot disease (Table 1), we decided to exclude subjects with this characteristic in the final analysis for both cases and controls.

The number of new UTC cases and adjusted hazard ratios (aHR) calculated from the Cox regression models for multiple risk factors (sex, age, diabetes, hypertension, chronic UTI, analgesics

and cumulative doses for different herbs) are summarized in Table 2. The crude and adjusted HR (aHR) for development of UTC increased significantly for older patients, whereas the crude and adjusted HR for development of UTC was not significantly related to either hypertension or diabetes. Crude HR's also increased for prescribed cumulative doses of Mu-Tong greater than 1 g, Fangchi 1–30 g, >100 g, as well as for prescribed Xi-Xin and for estimated AA consumptions of 1–100 mg, 101–200 g, and >300 mg. Prescription of analgesics also increased the crude HR. After control of potential confounding by other risk factors, we found that the aHR for development of UTC increased for ESRD patients prescribed Mu Tong, and that the various estimated consumptions of AA were each associated with an increased risk of UTC in the multivariable analyses (Mu Tong: at 1–30 g, aHR = 1.8, 95% CI = 1.3 to 2.6, and each 30 g increase, aHR = 1.3, 95% CI = 1.2 to 1.5; AA: at 1–100 mg, aHR = 2.1, 95% CI = 1.6 to 2.6, and each 100 g increase, aHR = 1.6, 95% CI = 1.4 to 1.8). Prescription of analgesics is associated with a greater risk of urothelial cancer, with an increased aHR of 1.3 (95% CI = 1.2 to 1.4) for each increment of 150 pills, as summarized in models 1 and 2 of Table 2. However, there is little association between the prescribed numbers of analgesic pills and cumulative doses of AA, as shown in Figure 1.

Discussion

To the best of our knowledge, this is the first population-based study to document a linear dose–response relationship between prescription of Chinese herbal products containing AA and the risk of UTC in ESRD patients after controlling for confounding by age, sex, living in a township endemic for black foot disease (a surrogate of arsenic contamination in the water supply), analgesic consumption, and history of chronic urinary tract infection. In fact, because the NHI reimbursement database collects all prescription information prospectively, we can rule out the possibility of recall bias for the intake doses of various Chinese herbal products. Since we included all ESRD patients newly diagnosed in Taiwan from 1998 to 2002, and the diagnosis of urinary tract cancer or end-stage renal disease made by doctors and officials of the NHI is usually accurate, we can also rule out the possibility of selection bias. Moreover, we excluded all subjects who had lived in townships endemic for black foot disease (a surrogate of high arsenic exposure) to prevent confounding the results due to the carcinogenic effects of arsenic exposure. Although increased prescription of analgesics was also associated with UTC (Table 2), the effect has been controlled in the multivariable regression model, and Figure 1 also shows no association between the number of analgesics pills and cumulative dose of AA. Finally, this study has documented a dose-dependent association between the cumulative estimated prescribed dose of AA and urinary tract cancer, as well as a dose-dependent association between the cumulative prescribed dose of Mu-Tong and UTC. We thus tentatively conclude that the urothelial cancers developed by ESRD patients are associated with prescription of AA-associated Chinese herbal products.

This study found a consistent dose-response relationship between the estimated intake of AA (or prescribed dose of AA-containing CHP) and urinary tract cancer in ESRD patients, suggesting that AA may be responsible for increased cancer risk of these patients. Fangchi and Xi-Xin both showed increased hazard ratios at higher doses, but these results did not reach statistical significance after adjustment for risk factors, likely due to the small number of case subjects. However, the increased hazard ratios for the occurrence of UC were found to be significantly higher in

Table 1. Frequency distributions of various risk factors for the occurrence of urinary tract cancers (UTC) stratified by different inclusion criteria in 38,995 patients with end-stage renal disease (ESRD).

Risk Factors	All ESRD Patients	
	UTC Cases (n = 320)	Non-UTC Cases (n = 38675)
Sex		
Men	131 (40.94%)	18391 (47.55%)
Women	189 (59.06%)	20284 (52.45%)
Age (year)		
<50	67 (20.94%)	9804 (25.35%)
50–59	80 (25.00%)	7790 (20.14%)
60–69	99 (30.94%)	10572 (27.34%)
70–99	74 (23.13%)	10509 (27.17%)
Residence in township where black foot disease was endemic		
No	319 (99.69%)	38421 (99.34%)
Yes	1 (0.31%)	254 (0.66%)
Hypertension		
No	68 (21.25%)	4297 (11.11%)
Yes	252 (78.75%)	34378 (88.89%)
Diabetes		
No	219 (68.44%)	17045 (44.07%)
Yes	101 (31.56%)	21630 (55.93%)
Chronic UTI		
No	312 (97.50%)	38511 (99.58%)
Yes	8 (2.50%)	164 (0.42%)
Analgesics *(pills) NSAID & acetaminophen		
0–150	123 (38.44%)	16116 (41.65%)
151–300	74 (23.13%)	8187 (21.16%)
351–450	32 (10.00%)	4405 (11.40%)
451–600	25 (7.81%)	2665 (6.90%)
>600	66 (20.63%)	7306 (18.88%)
Mu-Tong (g) total amount prescribed		
0	286 (89.38%)	35968 (93.00%)
1–30	20 (6.25%)	1845 (4.77%)
30–60	3 (0.94%)	348 (0.90%)
61–100	3 (0.94%)	179 (0.46%)
101–200	4 (1.25%)	164 (0.42%)
>200	4 (1.25%)	171 (0.44%)
Fangchi (g) total amount prescribed		
0	295 (92.19%)	35731 (92.39%)
1–30	19 (5.94%)	2417 (6.25%)
31–60 (31–100)	4 (1.25%)	271 (0.70%)
61–100	0 (0%)	121 (0.31%)
101–200 (>100)	2 (0.63%)	86 (0.22%)
>200	0 (0%)	49 (0.13%)
Xi-Xin (g) total amount prescribed		
0	283 (88.44%)	34679 (89.67%)
1–30	22 (6.88%)	2995 (7.74%)
31–60	5 (1.56%)	465 (1.20%)
61–100	5 (1.56%)	231 (0.60%)
101–200	3 (0.94%)	185 (0.48%)
>200	2 (0.63%)	120 (0.32%)
Aristolochic acid (mg) estimated total consumption		

Table 1. Cont.

Risk Factors	All ESRD Patients	
	UTC Cases (n = 320)	Non-UTC Cases (n = 38675)
0	270 (84.38%)	32550 (84.16%)
1–100	33 (10.31%)	5363 (13.09%)
101–200	4 (1.25%)	464 (1.20%)
201–300	4 (1.25%)	197 (0.51%)
>300	9 (2.81%)	.04%)

Analgesics *, sum of acetaminophen and non-steroidal anti-inflammatory drugs (NSAIDs).

ESRD patients when over 1–30 g of Mu-Tong or over 1–100 mg cumulative AA were prescribed. Because these doses are much smaller than those reported by Belgian scholars [4] and our previous report [7], it suggests that patients with ESRD might be more vulnerable to the carcinogenic effects of AA. Although these subgroups do not correlate with a cumulative dose of higher than 147-mg AA, as reported in the Belgian report [4], the observation of increased hazard ratios at lower cumulative levels of AA-containing Chinese herbal products in ESRD patients who consume these products suggests potential pathogenic effects at lower doses, and this is an issue that deserves further investigation, with more long-term follow-up of these patients.

Forty-five percent of the UTC cases in this study were upper urinary tract cancer, which is similar to the rates seen in the general population, as reported by the National Cancer Registry and in a previous clinical report examining pathology-confirmed urinary tract cancer cases in Taiwan [41]. However, these rates are much higher than those in other countries, in which less than 10% of all UTC cases are upper urinary tract cancer. In this study, prescription of Chinese herbal products was associated with urothelial cancers that occurred in all parts of the urinary tract, similar to what was reported in a recent case study of Belgian women who received kidney transplants for end-stage AA nephropathy, in which 44.7% had upper urinary tract cancer

and 39.5% had bladder cancer [42]. We thus hypothesize that AA induces urothelial cancers in the upper urinary tract and bladder with approximately equal tendency.

We also found a dose-dependent association between analgesics and occurrence of UTC among patients with ESRD, corroborating previous reports [17–19]. Unfortunately, we did not have a sufficiently large sample size to further explore this issue. Future studies are thus recommended to collect more UTC cases among patients with ESRD, and determine if the effect is associated with acetaminophen, aspirin, or any other NSAID.

There are some limitations to this study, as follows. First, because patient identities were not obtainable from the NHI reimbursement database, histopathology reports were unavailable to confirm the diagnoses. However, accurate diagnosis of UTC in the NHI database is based on pathology and/or cytology evidence and made after serious consideration with histopathologic proof in 95% of bladder cancers and 91%–92% of upper urinary tract cancers [43]. Second, we were unable to contact patients directly about their use of herbs due to anonymization of the database; therefore, we were unable to rule out the possibility that subjects may have taken additional nephrotoxic herbs or agents that were not prescribed. However, the comprehensive coverage and copayment for prescriptions is universally 50 NT$ (approximately equal to US $1.5), which is generally less than the cost of herbs

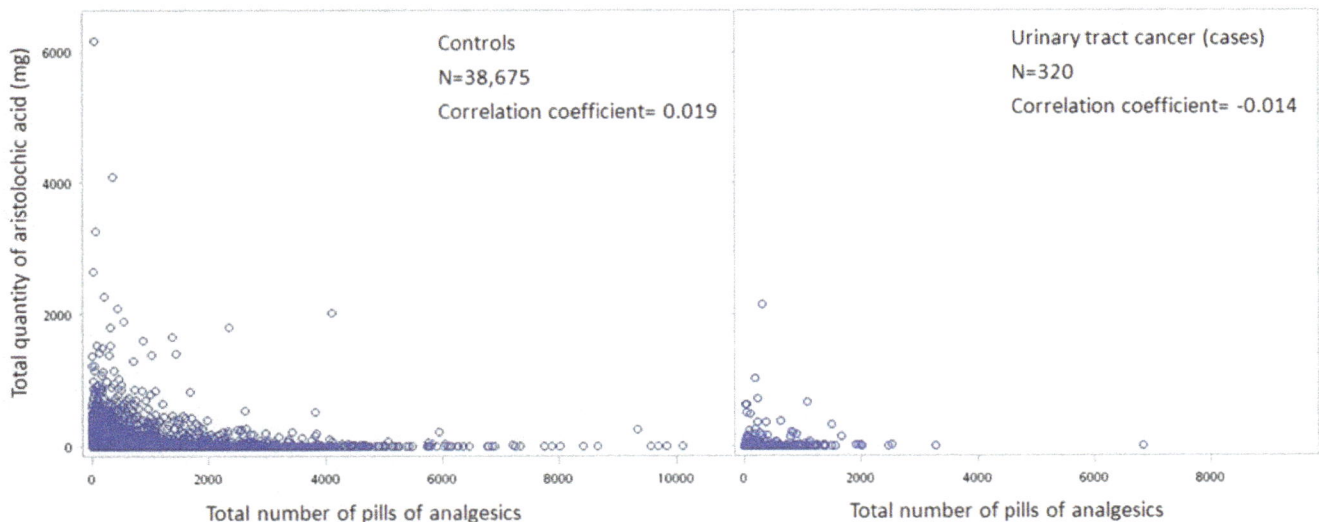

Figure 1. Correlation analysis between prescription of analgesics (number of pills) and cumulative dose of aristolochic acid for both cases and controls.

Table 2. Crude and adjusted hazards ratios (HR), and 95% confidence intervals (CI) estimated from multivariate Cox regression models for urinary tract cancer developed in patients with ESRD.

Risk Factors	Crude HR (95% CI)	Model 1 Adjusted HR (95% CI)†	Model 2 Adjusted HR (95% CI)†
Sex			
Men	1	1	1
Women	1.02 (0.82 to 1.27)	0.89 (0.71 to 1.12)	0.91 (0.73 to 1.14)
Age (years)			
<50	1	1	1
50–59	1.38 (1.04 to 1.85)*	1.43 (1.06 to 1.93)*	1.44 (1.07 to 1.92)*
60–69	1.77 (1.34 to 2.35)**	1.75 (1.30 to 2.36)**	1.73 (1.29 to 2.32)**
70–99	1.93 (1.39 to 2.66)**	1.90 (1.35 to 2.67)**	1.83 (1.31 to 2.56)**
Diabetes			
No	1	1	1
Yes	1.12 (0.90 to 1.40)	0.95 (0.76 to 1.20)	0.94 (0.75 to 1.19)
Hypertension			
No	1	1	1
Yes	1.00 (0.78 to 1.29)	0.74 (0.57 to 0.97)*	0.78 (0.60 to 1.01)
Chronic UTI			
No	1	1	1
Yes	4.77 (2.46 to 9.26)**	6.85 (3.52 to 13.34)**	6.68 (3.43 to 12.99)**
Analgesics (pills)			
0–150	1	1	1
151–300	2.03 (1.54 to 2.67)**	1.91 (1.44 to 2.53)**	1.93 (1.46 to 2.55)**
301–450	2.26 (1.55 to 3.28)**	1.97 (1.35 to 2.89)**	2.02 (1.39 to 2.95)**
451–600	2.92 (1.93 to 4.43)**	2.70 (1.75 to 4.15)**	2.72 (1.78 to 4.16)**
>600	3.36 (2.51 to 4.49)**	2.98 (2.19 to 4.06)**	2.83 (2.09 to 3.83)**
Each 150 pills increase	1.35 (1.26 to 1.44)**	1.32 (1.23 to 1.41)**	1.31 (1.22 to 1.40)**
Mu-Tong (g) total amount prescribed			
0	1	1	-
1–30	2.38 (1.79 to 3.16)**	1.83 (1.30 to 2.57)**	-
31–60	2.21 (1.29 to 3.82)‡	1.98 (1.07 to 3.69)*	-
61–100	3.08 (1.58 to 6.02)**	2.51 (1.19 to 5.28)*	-
101–200	2.73 (1.61 to 4.63)**	3.16 (1.63 to 6.14)**	-
>200	3.45 (1.88 to 6.36)**	3.46 (1.70 to 7.03)**	-
Each 30 g increase	1.33 (1.23 to 1.44)**	1.31 (1.17 to 1.48)**	-
Fangchi (g) total amount prescribed			
0	1	1	-
1–30	2.24 (1.73 to 2.92)**	1.23 (0.91 to 1.67)	-
31–100	1.41 (0.75 to 2.66)	0.84 (0.43 to 1.62)	-
>100	3.18 (1.31 to 7.70)*	1.89 (0.76 to 4.68)	-
Each 30 g increase	1.56 (1.33 to 1.84)**	1.22 (1.00 to 1.48)	-
Xi-Xin (g) total amount prescribed			
0	1	1	-
1–30	2.02 (1.55 to 2.63)**	1.27 (0.91 to 1.78)	-
31–60	2.40 (1.44 to 3.99)**	1.50 (0.84 to 2.70)	-
61–100	2.90 (1.62 to 5.20)**	1.34 (0.69 to 2.60)	-
101–200	2.47 (1.26 to 4.83)‡	1.17 (0.53 to 2.59)	-
>200	2.25 (1.15 to 4.21)*	0.78 (0.34 to 1.81)	-
Each 30 g increase	1.28 (1.18 to 1.39)**	1.02 (0.89 to 1.16)	-
Aristolochic acid (mg) estimated total consumption			
0	1	-	1

Table 2. Cont.

Risk Factors	Crude HR (95% CI)	Model 1 Adjusted HR (95% CI)†	Model 2 Adjusted HR (95% CI)†
1–100	1.21 (0.83 to 1.78)	-	2.05 (1.61 to 2.60)**
101–200	2.16 (0.80 to 5.80)	-	2.84 (1.66 to 4.86)**
201–300	4.80 (1.79 to 12.91)‡	-	2.42 (0.89 to 6.55)
>300	6.29 (3.23 to 12.26)**	-	5.18 (2.86 to 9.40)**
Each 100 mg increase	1.56 (1.40 to 1.74)**	-	1.57 (1.40 to 1.75)**

†Logistic regression models for different dosages of Chinese herbs (model 1) and different estimated dosages of aristolochic acid as risk factors (model 2) were adjusted for age, sex, residence in township with endemic black foot disease, and history of chronic UTI.
*$P<0.05$.
‡$P<0.01$.
**$P<0.001$.

sold in Taiwan's markets. It is thus unlikely that the subjects purchased AA-containing herbs or nephrotoxic drugs without a prescription. Third, we also could not validate the actual intake of prescribed herbal product by the patients. Because 95% of the dosing frequenciesfor Chinese herbal products last for only one week [44], a large cumulative dose indicates that patients on long-term prescriptions actually consumed the prescribed medication. However, if the patients did not take all of the prescribed medication, our findings would underestimate the effects of AA-related Chinese herbal consumption. Fourth, because the NHI data did not include smoking history, we could not control for this variable in our models. However, because smoking rates in Taiwan in the last two decades have ranged from 47% to 62% and from 2.3% to 5.3%, for males and females, respectively, male patients with ESRD would be expected to have a higher risk of developing UTC if smoking were a major contributing risk factor [45]. As we did not find any increased risk of UTC in males compared to females, our results do not seem to be confounded by smoking.

Conclusions

This study finds that AA from Chinese herbal products and analgesics is associated with increased risk of developing UTC in ESRD patients, due to these having been prescribed low doses of Mu-Tong. The linear dose-response relationships found in this work may be useful in consideration of a total ban or establishment of limits on the consumption of such herbal products among patients with ESRD and/or chronic kidney disease. More studies are needed to examine the potential carcinogenic effects of analgesics on patients with ESRD and/or chronic renal failure. In addition, regular follow-up screening for UC in ESRD patients who have consumed AA-related Chinese herbal products is also necessary.

Author Contributions

Conceived and designed the experiments: SMW JD. Performed the experiments: JDW PC. Analyzed the data: SMW. Contributed reagents/materials/analysis tools: PCC. Wrote the paper: SMW. Contributed to the idea and design in this work: MNL AW YYC YSP.

References

1. Vanherweghem JL, Depierreux M, Tielemans C, Abramowicz D, Dratwa M, et al. (1993) Rapidly progressive interstitial renal fibrosis in young women: association with slimming regimen including Chinese herbs. Lancet 341: 387–391.
2. Vanhaelen M, Vanhaelen-Fastre R, But P, Vanherweghem JL (1994) Identification of aristolochic acid in Chinese herbs. Lancet 343: 174.
3. Cosyns JP (2003) Aristolochic acid and 'Chinese herbs nephropathy': a review of the evidence to date. Drug safety : an international journal of medical toxicology and drug experience 26: 33–48.
4. Nortier JL, Martinez MC, Schmeiser HH, Arlt VM, Bieler CA, et al. (2000) Urothelial carcinoma associated with the use of a Chinese herb (Aristolochia fangchi). N Engl J Med 342: 1686–1692.
5. Cosyns JP, Jadoul M, Squifflet JP, Wese FX, van Ypersele de Strihou C (1999) Urothelial lesions in Chinese-herb nephropathy. American journal of kidney diseases : the official journal of the National Kidney Foundation 33: 1011–1017.
6. Arlt VM, Stiborova M, Schmeiser HH (2002) Aristolochic acid as a probable human cancer hazard in herbal remedies: a review. Mutagenesis 17: 265–277.
7. Lai MN, Wang SM, Chen PC, Chen YY, Wang JD (2010) Population-based case-control study of Chinese herbal products containing aristolochic acid and urinary tract cancer risk. J Natl Cancer Inst 102: 179–186.
8. Lai MN, Wang SM, Chen PC, Chen YY, Wang JD (2009) Population-based case-control study of Chinese herbal products containing aristolochic acid and urinary tract cancer risk. J Natl Cancer Inst 102: 179–186.

9. Matas AJ, Simmons RL, Kjellstrand CM, Buselmeier TJ, Najarian JS (1975) Increased incidence of malignancy during chronic renal failure. Lancet 1: 883–886.
10. Port FK, Ragheb NE, Schwartz AG, Hawthorne VM (1989) Neoplasms in dialysis patients: a population-based study. American journal of kidney diseases : the official journal of the National Kidney Foundation 14: 119–123.
11. Kjellstrand CM (1979) Are malignancies increased in uremia? Nephron 23: 159–161.
12. Maisonneuve P, Agodoa L, Gellert R, Stewart JH, Buccianti G, et al. (1999) Cancer in patients on dialysis for end-stage renal disease: an international collaborative study. Lancet 354: 93–99.
13. Chuang CH, Lee CT, Tsai TL, Chen JB, Hsu KT, et al. (2002) Urological malignancy in chronic dialysis patients. Acta Nephrologica 16: 19–24.
14. Chang CH, Yang CM, Yang AH (2007) Renal diagnosis of chronic hemodialysis patients with urinary tract transitional cell carcinoma in Taiwan. Cancer 109: 1487–1492.
15. Ou JH, Pan CC, Lin JS, Tzai TS, Yang WH, et al. (2000) Transitional cell carcinoma in dialysis patients. European urology 37: 90–94.
16. Chen KS, Lai MK, Huang CC, Chu SH, Leu ML (1995) Urologic cancers in uremic patients. American journal of kidney diseases : the official journal of the National Kidney Foundation 25: 694–700.
17. Gonwa TA, Corbett WT, Schey HM, Buckalew VM, Jr. (1980) Analgesic-associated nephropathy and transitional cell carcinoma of the urinary tract. Annals of internal medicine 93: 249–252.

18. Swindle P, Falk M, Rigby R, Petrie J, Hawley C, et al. (1998) Transitional cell carcinoma in renal transplant recipients: the influence of compound analgesics. British journal of urology 81: 229–233.

19. Kliem V, Thon W, Krautzig S, Kolditz M, Behrend M, et al. (1996) High mortality from urothelial carcinoma despite regular tumor screening in patients with analgesic nephropathy after renal transplantation. Transplant international : official journal of the European Society for Organ Transplantation 9: 231–235.

20. Vanherweghem LJ (1998) Misuse of herbal remedies: the case of an outbreak of terminal renal failure in Belgium (Chinese herbs nephropathy). Journal of alternative and complementary medicine 4: 9–13.

21. Chiang HS, Guo HR, Hong CL, Lin SM, Lee EF (1993) The incidence of bladder cancer in the black foot disease endemic area in Taiwan. British journal of urology 71: 274–278.

22. Chiou HY, Chiou ST, Hsu YH, Chou YL, Tseng CH, et al. (2001) Incidence of transitional cell carcinoma and arsenic in drinking water: a follow-up study of 8,102 residents in an arseniasis-endemic area in northeastern Taiwan. American journal of epidemiology 153: 411–418.

23. Wiessler M (1994) DNA adducts of pyrrolizidine alkaloids, nitroimidazoles and aristolochic acid. IARC Sci Publ: 165–177.

24. TaiwanYearbook2009 Public Health: Health Insurance.

25. NHRI-Taiwan (2003) National Health Research Database.

26. Centers_for_Disease_Control_and_Prevention (2009) International Classification of Diseases, Ninth Revision (ICD-9). Atlanta, Georgia.

27. Perneger TV, Whelton PK, Klag MJ (1994) Risk of kidney failure associated with the use of acetaminophen, aspirin, and nonsteroidal antiinflammatory drugs. N Engl J Med 331: 1675–1679.

28. Gago-Dominguez M, Yuan JM, Castelao JE, Ross RK, Yu MC (1999) Regular use of analgesics is a risk factor for renal cell carcinoma. Br J Cancer 81: 542–548.

29. Committee Chinese Medicine and Pharmacy DOH-T (2002) Unified Formulas.

30. Hsu Y, Tseng H, Wen K (1997) Determination of aristolochic acid in Fangchi radix. Ann Rept NLFD Taiwan ROC: 136–142 (In Chinese).

31. Tung C, Ho Y, Tsai H, Chong Y (1999) Studies on the commonly musused and adulterated Chinese crude drug species in Taiwan. Chin Med Coll J: 35–46.

32. Deng J (2002) Quality evaluation of Fang-Ji and analysis of marker constituents [dissertation]. Taiwan: Institute of Chiense Pharmaceutical Sciences, China Medical University: 75–77.

33. Chuang M, Hsu Y, Chang H, Lin J, Liao C (2002) Studies on adulteration and misusage of marketed Akebiae caulisn. Ann Rept NLFD Taiwan ROC: 104–119 (In Chinese).

34. Jong TT, Lee MR, Hsiao SS, Hsai JL, Wu TS, et al. (2003) Analysis of aristolochic acid in nine sources of Xixin, a traditional Chinese medicine, by liquid chromatography/atmospheric pressure chemical ionization/tandem mass spectrometry. J Pharm Biomed Anal 33: 831–837.

35. Hsu Y, Lo C, Chang H, Lin J (2003) Studies on adulteration and misusage of Asari radi in the market. Ann Rept NLFD Taiwan ROC: 153–167 (In Chinese).

36. Chen CJ, Chuang YC, Lin TM, Wu HY (1985) Malignant neoplasms among residents of a blackfoot disease-endemic area in Taiwan: high-arsenic artesian well water and cancers. Cancer research 45: 5895–5899.

37. Chen CJ, Chuang YC, You SL, Lin TM, Wu HY (1986) A retrospective study on malignant neoplasms of bladder, lung and liver in blackfoot disease endemic area in Taiwan. British journal of cancer 53: 399–405.

38. Johansson SL, Cohen SM (1997) Epidemiology and etiology of bladder cancer. Seminars in surgical oncology 13: 291–298.

39. Groah SL, Weitzenkamp DA, Lammertse DP, Whiteneck GG, Lezotte DC, et al. (2002) Excess risk of bladder cancer in spinal cord injury: Evidence for an association between indwelling catheter use and bladder cancer. Archives of Physical Medicine and Rehabilitation 83: 346–351.

40. Jiang X, Castelao JE, Groshen S, Cortessis VK, Shibata D, et al. (2009) Urinary tract infections and reduced risk of bladder cancer in Los Angeles. British journal of cancer 100: 834–839.

41. (2008) Cancer Incidence Rate in Taiwan, 1998–2002 & 2003–2007 http://tcr. cph.ntu.edu.tw/main.php?Page = N2: Taiwan cancer registry.

42. Achenbach H, Fischer A (1997) 6-O-beta-D-glucoside of aristolochic acid IIIa and other components from the roots of Aristolochia baetica. Planta Med 63: 579.

43. TaiwanCancerRegistry (2009) Cancer incidence rate in Taiwan, 1998–2002.

44. Hsieh SC, Lai JN, Lee CF, Hu FC, Tseng WL, et al. (2008) The prescribing of Chinese herbal products in Taiwan: a cross-sectional analysis of the national health insurance reimbursement database. Pharmacoepidemiology and drug safety 17: 609–619.

45. (2013) Adult Smoking Behavior Surveillance System,ASBS. Taipei, Taiwan.

5

Association of Angiopoietin-2 with Renal Outcome in Chronic Kidney Disease

Yi-Chun Tsai[1,2,3], Yi-Wen Chiu[2,3], Jer-Chia Tsai[2,3], Hung-Tien Kuo[2,3], Su-Chu Lee[2], Chi-Chih Hung[2,3], Ming-Yen Lin[3], Shang-Jyh Hwang[1,2,3,4], Mei-Chuan Kuo[1,2,3*], Hung-Chun Chen[2,3]

1 Graduate Institute of Clinical Medicine, Kaohsiung Medical University, Kaohsiung, Taiwan, 2 Division of Nephrology, Department of Internal Medicine, Kaohsiung Medical University Hospital, Kaohsiung, Taiwan, 3 Faculty of Renal Care, College of Medicine, Kaohsiung Medical University, Kaohsiung, Taiwan, 4 Institute of Population Sciences, National Health Research Institutes, Miaoli, Taiwan

Abstract

Background: The pathophysiological mechanisms of renal function progression in chronic kidney disease (CKD) have still not been completely explored. In addition to well-known traditional risk factors, non-traditional risk factors, such as endothelial dysfunction, have gradually attracted physicians' attention. Angiopoietin-2 (Ang-2) impairs endothelial function through preventing angiopoietin-1 from binding to Tie2 receptor. Whether Ang-2 is associated with renal function progression in CKD is unknown.

Methods: This study enrolled 621 patients with stages 3–5 CKD to assess the association of circulating Ang-2 with commencing dialysis, doubling creatinine and rapid decline in renal function (the slope of estimated glomerular filtration rate (eGFR) greater than 5 ml/min per 1.73 m^2/y) over follow-up of more than 3 years.

Results: Of all patients, 224 patients (36.1%) progressed to commencing dialysis and 165 (26.6%) reached doubling creatinine. 85 subjects (13.9%) had rapid decline in renal function. Ang-2 quartile was divided at 1494.1, 1948.8, and 2593.1 pg/ml. The adjusted HR of composite outcomes, either commencing dialysis or doubling creatinine was 1.53 (95% CI: 1.06–2.23) for subjects of quartile 4 compared with those of quartile 1. The adjusted OR for rapid decline in renal function was 2.96 (95% CI: 1.13–7.76) for subjects of quartile 4 compared with those of quartile 1. The linear mixed-effects model shows a more rapid decrease in eGFR over time in patients with quartile 3 or more of Ang-2 than those with the lowest quartile of Ang-2.

Conclusions: Ang-2 is an independent predictor of adverse renal outcome in CKD. Further study is needed to identify the pathogenic role of Ang-2 in CKD progression.

Editor: Effie C. Tsilibary, National Center for Scientific Research Demokritos, Greece

Funding: These authors have no support or funding to report.

Competing Interests: The authors have declared that no competing interests exist.

* Email: mechku@cc.kmu.edu.tw

Introduction

Chronic kidney disease (CKD) has been recognized as a worldwide health issue [1]. The pathophysiological mechanisms of renal function progression in CKD have still not been completely explored. In addition to well-known traditional risk factors, non-traditional risk factors, such as endothelial dysfunction, which might lead to cell apoptosis, vascular regression and renal fibrosis, have gradually attracted physicians' attention [2].

The angiopoietin (Ang)/Tie ligand-receptor system tightly controls the endothelial phenotype during angiogenesis and vascular inflammation [3]. Among the members of Ang family, Ang-1 and Ang-2 have attracted much attention [4]. Ang-1-driven Tie2 phosphorylation maintains structure integrity of vasculature, and protects the endothelium from excessive activation by cytokines and growth factors [5]. On the other hand, Ang-2 is

expressed in endothelial cells, and stored in Weibel-Palade bodies (WPB) [6]. The rapid release of Ang-2 from endothelial cells upon activation of the endothelium by hypoxia, histamine, and thrombin would disrupt the protective, constitutive Ang-1/Tie2 signaling by preventing Ang-1 from binding to the receptor [5,7]. Consequently, the loss of Tie2 signaling destabilizes the endothelium and contributes to angiogenic or inflammatory response to cytokines and growth factors [8].

Increased circulating Ang-2 has been found in diabetes mellitus [9], arterial hypertension [10], congestive heart failure [11], peripheral artery disease [12], coronary artery disease [13], sepsis [14], critical illness [15], and acute kidney injury [16]. Additionally, accumulating evidence shows that circulating Ang-2 is also markedly elevated in CKD and dialysis patients [17]. Elevated Ang-2 levels are also correlated with long-term mortality in patients with CKD stage 4 and on dialysis [18]. Although Ang-2 is associated with microalbuminuria [19], a clinical marker of renal injury, the relationship between Ang-2 and renal progression has not been well-explored in CKD patients not on dialysis. This study tries to analyze whether Ang-2 is associated with renal outcome, including reaching commencing dialysis and rapid decline in renal function (estimated glomerular filtration rate (eGFR) decline per year), in patients with CKD stages 3–5.

Materials and Methods

Study Participants

This observational study was conducted at a tertiary hospital in Southern Taiwan. Six hundred and twenty-one patients with CKD stages 3–5, who had follow-up for one year at least in our integrated CKD program, were enrolled in the study from January 2006 to December 2011. CKD was staged according to K/DOQI definitions and the eGFR was calculated using the equation of the 4-variable Modification of Diet in Renal Disease (MDRD) Study (CKD stage 3, eGFR: 30–59 ml/min/1.73 m^2; CKD stage 4, eGFR: 15–29 ml/min/1.73 m^2; CKD stage 5, eGFR <15 ml/min/1.73 m^2) [20].

Ethics Statement

The study protocol was approved by the Institutional Review Board of the Kaohsiung Medical University Hospital (KMUH-IRB-990198). Informed consents were obtained in written form from patients and all clinical investigations were conducted according to the principles expressed in the Declaration of Helsinki.

Data Collection

Demographic and clinical data were obtained from medical records and interviews with patients at enrollment. The participant was asked to fast for at least 12 hours before blood sample collection for the biochemistry study and protein in urine was measured using urine protein-creatinine ratio. Patients were classified as diabetic by history and blood glucose values using the American Diabetes Association criteria, oral hypoglycemia agent use, or insulin use. Hypertension was defined as those with a history, or antihypertensive drugs use. Heart disease was defined as a history of heart failure, acute or chronic ischemic heart disease, or myocardial infarction. Cerebrovascular disease was defined as a history of cerebral infarction or hemorrhage. Information regarding patient medications including β-blocker, calcium channel blockers, angiotensin converting enzyme inhibitors (ACEI), and angiotensin II receptor blockers (ARB) before and after enrollment was obtained from medical records.

Quantification of circulating Angiopoietin-2

Plasma Angiopoietin-2 was measured in duplicate using commercial enzyme-linked immunosorbent assays (R&D Systems Inc, Minneapolis, MN) according to the instructions of the manufacturer. The sensitivity of Ang-2 assay was 1.20 pg/ml. Intraassay and interassay coefficients of variation of Ang-2 were 1.8% and 1.2%, respectively.

Renal Outcomes

Patients were contacted at outpatient clinics at 3-month intervals to ascertain the clinical status. Renal outcomes included commencing dialysis, doubling creatinine and rapid decline in renal function. Commencing dialysis was defined as requiring maintenance hemodialysis and peritoneal dialysis and confirmed by reviewing medical charts or catastrophic illness certificate (issued by the Bureau of National Health Insurance in Taiwan).

The timing for commencing dialysis was considered according to the regulations of the Bureau of the National Health Insurance of Taiwan regarding eGFR, uremic status, nutritional status, and the laboratory data. The timing for doubling creatinine was considered based on all creatinine values from enrollment to the end of the observation period. The decline in renal function was assessed by the eGFR slope, defined as the regression coefficient between eGFR and time in units of ml/min per 1.73 m^2 per year. All eGFR values available from enrollment to the end of the observation period were included for calculation. At least three eGFR values were required to estimate the eGFR slope. Rapid decline in renal function was defined as the eGFR slope greater than 5 ml/min/1.73 m^2 per year based on Kidney Disease: Improving Global Outcomes (KDIGO) suggestion [21]. Patients were censored at death, last contact, or the end of observation in October 2013.

Statistical Analysis

Baseline characteristics of all subjects were stratified by quartiles of Ang-2, cut at 1494.1, 1948.8, and 2593.1 pg/ml. Continuous variables were expressed as mean ±SD or median (25th, 75th percentile), as appropriate, and categorical variables were expressed as percentages. Skewed distribution continuous variables were log-transformed to approximate normal distribution. The significance of differences in continuous variables between groups was tested using one-way analysis of variance (ANOVA) or the Kruskal-Wallis H test, as appropriate. The difference in the distribution of categorical variables was tested using the Chi-square test. Kaplan-Meier survival analysis was used to test Ang-2 as a predictor of the risk of composite outcomes either commencing dialysis or doubling creatinine. Cox regression models were applied to examine the relationship between Ang-2 and composite outcomes either commencing dialysis or doubling creatinine. Multivariable logistic regression models were also used to evaluate the association of Ang-2 with rapid decline in renal function. A linear mixed-effects model analysis was used to identify the factors associated with a change of eGFR, with control for internal correlations and other covariates. All the variables in Table 1 were tested by univariate analysis and those variables with P-value less than 0.05, including diabetes, heart disease, eGFR, urine protein-creatinine ratio cut at 1 g/g, serum albumin, phosphate, calcium, hemoglobin and cholesterol levels, and age, gender, and ACEI/ARB use were selected for multivariate cox and logistic analyses and linear mixed-effects model analysis. Statistical analyses were conducted using SPSS 18.0 for Windows (SPSS Inc., Chicago, Illinois). Statistical significance was set at a two-sided p-value of less than 0.05.

Results

Characteristics of Entire Cohort

A total of 621 participants with CKD stages 3 to 5 were analyzed (mean eGFR 21.8 ml/min/1.73 m^2, 146 in stage 3, 243 in stage 4, 232 in stage 5). The mean age was 65.3±12.7 years and 55.4% were male. Table 1 shows the baseline clinical characteristics stratified by quartiles of Ang-2, divided at 1494.1, 1948.8, and 2593.1 pg/ml. Of all patients, 532 (85.7%) were hypertensive and 239(38.5%)were diabetic mellitus. Pre-existing and documented heart disease and cerebral vascular disease were noted in 111(17.9%) and 55(8.9%) of patients respectively. The proportion of diabetes and β-blocker, serum blood urea nitrogen, phosphate and high-sensitivity C-reactive protein levels, and urine protein-creatinine ratio increased and eGFR, serum hemoglobin, calcium, and albumin levels decreased with Ang-2 quartiles.

Table 1. The clinical characteristics of study subjects stratified by angiopoietin-2 quartile.

		Angiopoietin-2[a]				
	Entire Cohort N = 621	Quartile 1 N = 151	Quartile 2 N = 157	Quartile 3 N = 157	Quartile 4 N = 156	P-trend
Demographics						
Age (year)	65.3±12.7	62.2±13.6[#]	67.1±11.0*	65.9±12.2	66.0±13.2	0.005
Sex (male), n(%)	344(55.4)	98(64.9)	89(56.7)	83(52.9)	74(47.4)*	0.01
Smoke, n(%)	120(19.4)	36(23.8)	22(14.0)	26(17.0)	36(23.1)	0.1
Alcohol,n(%)	49(7.9)	20(13.2)[†]	13(8.3)	7(4.6)*	9(5.8)	0.03
Cardiovascular disease, n(%)	111(17.9)	27(17.9)	20(12.7)	33(21.0)	31(19.9)	0.2
Cerebral vascular disease,n(%)	55(8.9)	11(7.3)	19(12.1)	15(9.6)	10(6.4)	0.2
Hypertension, n(%)	532(85.7)	133(88.1)	138(87.9)	129(82.2)	132(84.6)	0.3
Diabetes mellitus, n(%)	239(38.5)	48(31.8)	57(36.3)	60(38.2)	74(47.4)	0.03
Hyperlipidemia, n(%)	272(43.8)	66(43.7)[†]	77(49.0)	65(41.4)	64(41.0)	0.4
CKD cause, n(%)						
Chronic glomerulonephritis	232(37.4)	57(37.7)	55(35.0)	61(38.9)	59(37.8)	0.6
Diabetic nephropathy	180(29)	41(27.2)	41(26.1)	47(29.9)	51(32.7)*	
Others	209(33.7)	53(35.1)	61(38.9)	49(31.2)	46(29.5)	
CKD stage 3 n(%)	146(23.5)	45(29.8)	37(23.6)	37(23.6)	27(17.3)	0.003
4 n(%)	243(39.1)	62(41.1)	72(45.9)	57(36.3)	52(33.3)	
5 n(%)	232(37.4)	44(29.1)	48(30.6)	63(40.1)	77(49.4)	
Medications						
Calcium channel blocker, n (%)	341(54.9)	80(53.0)	89(56.7)	78(49.7)	94(60.3)	0.3
β-blocker, n (%)	147(23.7)	26(17.2)	28(17.8)	45(28.7)	48(30.8)*[#]	0.005
ACEI/ARB, n (%)	353(56.8)	89(58.9)	90(57.3)	85(54.1)	89(57.1)	0.8
Statin, n(%)	170(27.4)	40(26.5)	47(29.9)	40(25.5)	43(27.6)	0.8
Laboratory parameters						
Blood urea nitrogen (mg/dl)	41.1(30.0,60.0)	34.9(26.9,52.8)	38.7(29.5,55.1)	41.5(30.9,60.1)	50.6(35.5,66.1)*[#]	<0.001
Creatinine (mg/dl)	2.9(2.1,5.0)	2.8(1.9,4.4)	2.8(2.0,4.6)	3.0(2.2,5.6)	3.6(2.3,5.6)	0.005
eGFR (ml/min/1.73 m^2)	21.8±12.6	24.7±13.9[†]	22.7±11.8	20.7±12.3*	18.9±11.9*[#]	<0.001
Fasting sugar (g/dl)	101(92,117)	99(91,111)	100(94,119)	100(91,117)	102(92,126)* [†]	0.3
Glycated hemoglobin (%)	5.8(5.5,6.7)	5.7(5.4,6.4)	5.9(5.6,6.8)	5.7(5.4,6.4)	6.1(5.5,7.2)*[†]	0.01
Hemoglobin (g/dl)	10.9±2.1	11.7±2.1[#†]	11.0±2.1*	10.7±2.1*	10.4±1.9*[#]	<0.001
Albumin (g/dl)	4.1(3.9,4.3)	4.2(4.0,4.4)[†]	4.2(3.9,4.3)[†]	4.0(3.8,4.3)*[#]	4.0(3.7,4.2)*[#]	<0.001
Phosphate (mg/dl)	4.1(3.6,4.8)	4.0(3.5,4.6)	4.0(3.6,4.6)	4.1(3.7,4.8)	4.3(3.8,5.1)	0.02
Calcium (mg/dl)	8.9±0.6	9.1±0.6[†]	9.0±0.6	8.8±0.6*	8.8±0.8*	<0.001
Uric acid (mg/dl)	7.6±1.9	7.5±1.9	7.6±1.8	7.4±1.5	7.8±2.1	0.2
Cholesterol (mg/dl)	187±45	192±47	190±40	182±45	188±46	0.2
Triglyceride (mg/dl)	115(78,173)	115(78,181)	112(82,172)	108(76,162)	126(79,181)	0.6
hsCRP (mg/L)	1.6(0.6,4.2)	1.4(0.7,3.5)	1.5(0.5,3.7)	1.5(0.6,3.5)	2.2(0.8,6.5)*[#] [†]	0.03
Parathyroid hormone (pg/ml)	72(37,157)	62(36,142)	63(35,120)	76(40,190)	106(33,191)	0.2
Urine protein-creatinine ratio >1 g/g n (%)	275(49.3)	57(41.0)	66(46.8)	70(49.6)	82(59.9)*[#]	0.01

Data are expressed as number (percentage) for categorical variables and mean±SD or median (25th, 75th percentile) for continuous variables, as appropriate.
Conversion factors for units: eGFR in mL/min/1.73 m^2 to mL/s/1.73 m^2, ×0.01667 ; hemoglobin in g/dL to g/L, ×10; albumin in g/dL to g/L, ×10; calcium-phosphate product in mg^2/dL^2 to mmol^2/L^2, ×0.0806; cholesterol in mg/dL to mmol/L, ×0.02586; triglyceride in mg/dL to mmol/L, ×0.01129; uric acid in mg/dL toμmol/L, ×59.48.
Abbreviations: CKD, chronic kidney disease; ECW, extracellular water; ICW, intracellular water; TBW, total body water; ACEI, angiotensin converting enzyme inhibitors; ARB, angiotensin II receptor blockers; eGFR, estimated glomerular filtration rate; hsCRP, high-sensitivity C-reactive protein.
*P<0.05 compared with quartile 1; [#]P<0.05 compared with quartile 2; [†]P<0.05 compared with quartile 3.
[a]Angiopoietin-2 quartile cut at 1494.1, 1948.8, and 2593.1 pg/ml.

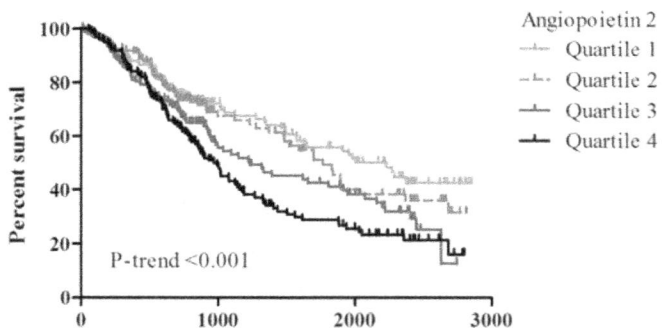

(A) Composite outcomes

Quartile 1	151	64	37	(No. Patients at Risk)
Quartile 2	157	43	22	
Quartile 3	157	43	26	
Quartile 4	156	50	22	

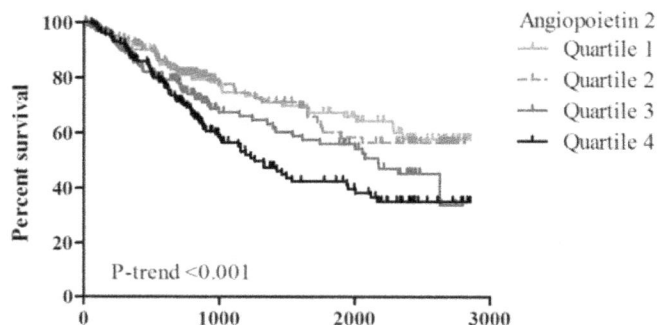

(B) Commencing dialysis

Quartile 1	151	66	42	(No. Patients at Risk)
Quartile 2	157	48	31	
Quartile 3	157	49	34	
Quartile 4	156	56	27	

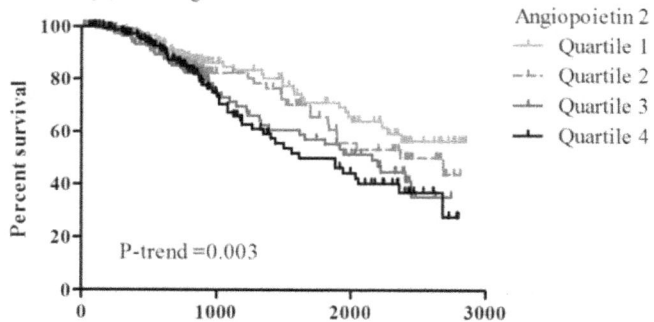

(C) Doubing creatinine

Quartile 1	151	64	37	(No. Patients at Risk)
Quartile 2	157	43	22	
Quartile 3	157	43	26	
Quartile 4	156	50	22	

Figure 1. Kaplan-Meier survival curve for composite outcomes, either commencing dialysis or doubling creatinine of all subjects stratified by angiopoietin-2 quartile.

Ang-2 and composite outcomes, either commencing dialysis or doubling creatinine

Over a mean follow-up period of 38.2 ± 26.3 months, 224 patients (36.1%) progressed to commencing dialysis (198 hemodialysis and 26 peritoneal dialysis, Table 2). Seventy-one (11.4%) had mortality before reaching commencing dialysis. 18 (2.9%) were lost to follow-up (the mean follow-up period: 19.7 ± 10.9 months), and no significant difference of proportion from quartile 1 to quartile 4 was found. A stepwise increase in the proportion of commencing dialysis from quartile 1 to quartile 4 was found (P-trend <0.001). Of all subjects, 165 (26.6%) reached doubling creatinine during follow-up period, but there was no significant difference among Ang-2 quartiles. Kaplan-Meier survival curve showed a significant correlation between quartiles of Ang-2 and composite outcomes, either commencing dialysis or doubling creatinine (Figure 1). Table 3 presents the longitudinal associations between stepwise increases in Ang-2 levels and composite outcomes, either commencing dialysis or doubling creatinine. The unadjusted hazard ratio (HR) of composite outcomes was 1.96 (95% Confidence interval (CI): 1.43–2.69) for subjects of quartile 4 compared with those of quartile 1. The adjusted HR of composite outcomes was 1.53 (95% CI: 1.06–2.23) for subjects of quartile 4 compared with those of quartile 1. The longitudinal association between composite outcomes and stepwise increases in Ang-2 levels (P-trend = 0.03).

The unadjusted risk for commencing dialysis increased 2 fold (HR: 2.01, 95% CI: 1.39–2.90) for subjects of quartile 4 compared with those of quartile 1. The adjusted risk for commencing dialysis increased 85% (HR: 1.85, 95% CI: 1.20–2.85) for subjects of quartile 4 compared with those of quartile 1. The longitudinal association between commencing dialysis and stepwise increases in Ang-2 levels (P-trend = 0.005). The unadjusted risk for doubling creatinine increased 89% (HR: 1.89, 95% CI: 1.21–2.93) for subjects of quartile 4 compared with those of quartile 1. However, there was no significant association of doubling creatinine with Ang-2 quartiles in adjusted model.

Ang-2, rapid decline in renal function and change in eGFR

Eighty-five subjects (13.9%) had rapid decline in renal function. Patients of progressive decline in renal function (eGFR slope greater than 5 ml/min/1.73 m^2/yr) were more likely to have higher level of Ang-2 than those of non-progressive decline in renal function (eGFR slope less than 5 ml/min/1.73 m^2/yr) (median: 1944.9 $v.s.$ 2066.0 pg/ml, P=0.01). No significant different in baseline eGFR was found between the two groups. The adjusted risk for rapid decline in renal function increased 2.9 folds (OR: 2.96, 95% CI: 1.13–7.76) for subjects of quartile 4 compared with those of quartile 1 (Table 4). Table 4 also shows the effect of study group on the change in eGFR in the linear mixed-effects model. The highest quartile of Ang-2 was associated with a significant decrease in eGFR over time as compared with the lowest quartile of Ang-2 (unstandardized coefficient $\beta = -1.73$, 95% CI: $-3.34, -0.11$, P = 0.03).

Discussion

To our knowledge, this study is the first to evaluate the association of Ang-2 with adverse renal outcome in patients with stages 3–5 CKD over an observation period of 3 years. Ang-2 is associated with composite renal outcomes, either commencing dialysis or doubling creatinine after adjustment of baseline renal function and associated risk factors. Patients with quartile 3 or more of Ang-2 have more than 1.7 and 3.0-fold increase in risk for commencing dialysis and rapid decline in renal function respectively. Additionally, the linear mixed-effects model shows a more rapid decrease in eGFR over time in patients with quartile 3 or more of Ang-2 than those with quartile 1 of Ang-2. CKD patients with quartile 3(1948.8 pg/ml) or more of Ang-2 are more likely to reach the plateau of adverse renal outcome.

With regard to glomerular diseases, studies by Belinda et al. [22] pointed out that increased glomerular expression of Ang-2 would tend to antagonize Ang-1-induced Tie-2 activation and destabilize capillaries and glomerular endothelia in podocin/Ang-2 transgene mice. There were significant increases in albuminuria and glomerular endothelial apoptosis, with significant decreases of both nephrin proteins and vascular endothelial growth factor A (VEGF-A), which were critical for maintenance of glomerular endothelia and glomerular filtration barrier integrity [23–25]. Besides, Seron et al. [26] indicated a chronic loss of renal interstitial capillaries in human nephropathy, and Futrakul et al. [27] suggested that an "anti-angiogenic environment" may exist in long-standing nephropathies. In clinical views, accumulating evidence shows that circulating Ang-2 is inversely related to eGFR and increases with advanced CKD and Ang-2 level is still increasing even after entering maintenance of dialysis [17]. However, little is known about a clinical relationship between Ang-2 and adverse renal outcome. The present study identifies that increased circulating Ang-2 is associated with risks for commencing dialysis and rapid decline in renal function in patients not on dialysis, and Ang-2 is an independent predictor of adverse renal outcome in CKD cohort.

Consistent with reports by Chang et al. [19], our results also showed a significant association of circulating Ang-2 with hypoalbuminemia and high-sensitivity C-reactive protein (hs-CRP), as indicators of malnutrition-inflammation. Fiedler et al. identified Ang-2 as an autocrine regulator of endothelial cell inflammatory responses and Ang-2 acts as a switch of vascular responsiveness exerting a permissive role for the activities of proinflammatory cytokines [11]. Ang-2 serves the link between angiogenic and inflammatory pathway, Ang-2 signaling between cellular elements in renal fibrosis, including endothelial cells, pericytes, myofibroblasts, and macrophages [23]. Meanwhile, CKD has been regarded as a disease with persistent and low-grade inflammation, and our previous study indicated that inflammation is an independent predictor of rapid decline in renal function in CKD cohort [28]. Hence, there might be an interaction among Ang-2, inflammation and rapid decline in renal function. The findings of our subgroup analysis show that elevated Ang-2 is independently associated with risk for maintenance dialysis in subjects of less than the median of hsCRP (1.56 mg/l; HR for log Ang-2: 4.80, 95%CI: 1.68–13.76). In addition, there is a significant association between Ang-2 and maintenance dialysis in subjects of serum albumin above 3.5 g/dl (HR for log Ang-2: 2.15, 95%CI: 1.05–4.38). Thus, circulating Ang-2 is possibly a significant risk factor for adverse renal outcome independent of malnutrition-inflammation.

Increased endothelial Ang-2 secretion is stimulated by exogenous stimuli such as angiotensin II, tumor necrosis factor-α, hypoxia, and reactive oxygen species, which are characteristics in

Table 2. Renal outcome of all subjects stratified by Angiopoietin-2 quartile.

| | Entire Cohort N = 621 | Angiopoietin-2[a] | | | | |
		Quartile 1 N = 151	Quartile 2 N = 157	Quartile 3 N = 157	Quartile 4 N = 156	P-trend
Follow-up time (month)	38.2±26.3	43.8±28.1	38.0±25.9	35.7±26.0	35.5±24.6	0.02
No. of SCr measurement	17 (9,27)	18(8, 27)	15(9,23)	15(9,24)	20(12,28)	0.01
Doubling creatinine (n,%)	165(26.6)	35(23.2)	37(23.6)	45(28.7)	48(30.8)	0.3
eGFR decline (mL/min/1.73 m²/year)	−1.6(−3.3,−0.4)	−1.3(−2.8,0.1)	−1.8(−3.6,−0.9)	−1.8(−3.8,−0.6)	−1.5(−3.1,−0.2)	0.01
Commencing dialysis (n,%)	224(36.1)	45(29.8)	43(27.4)	59(37.6)	77(49.4)	<0.001

Data are expressed as number (percentage) for categorical variables and median (25th, 75th percentile) for continuous variables, as appropriate.
Conversion factors for units: eGFR in mL/min/1.73 m² to mL/s/1.73 m², ×0.01667.
Abbreviations: eGFR, estimated glomerular filtration rate.
[a]Angiopoietin-2 quartile cut at 1494.1, 1948.8, and 2593.1 pg/ml.

CKD progression [5]. Endothelial injury in glomerular vasculature may induce endothelial Ang-2 secretion, and meanwhile, increased Ang-2 may lead to glomerular albuminuria through endothelial injury. It is difficult to evaluate whether increased Ang-2 is a cause or consequence of CKD progression [5]. Because of this complicated interaction among Ang-2, traditional risk factors, and CKD, we adjusted associated risk factors for rapid decline in renal function in multivariate analysis. We also performed subgroup analysis in different CKD stages, but the results did not consistent at all (Figure S1–S3). It is probably related to relative small number of subgroup and short observation period. We need further study to evaluate whether these risk factors are modifiers or confounders in association of Ang-2 and commencing dialysis. Besides, to consider the influence of competing risk of death on commencing dialysis, we performed further analysis, and the results are consistent (HR for quartile 4 compared with quartile 1: 1.85 (95% CI: 1.20–2.86). Our findings show a strong association of Ang-2 and adverse renal outcome and emphasize its importance as a predictor in CKD cohort.

Despite exogenous stimuli, Ang-2 was excreted by factors influencing the exocytosis of Weibel-Palade body, including thrombin, histamine, serotonin, vascular endothelial growth factor (VEGF) and epinephrine [29]. Therefore, it could be influenced by medication. In this study, no significant difference of medication was found among Ang-2 quartiles except for β-blocker. In post hoc multiple comparisons, subjects of Ang-2 quartile 4 had higher proportion of using β-blocker than those of

Ang-2 quartile 1 and 2. The reason might be related to blood pressure control or arrhythmia. The present study has a limitation that we did not record blood pressure and arrhythmia at enrollment. In late CKD, patients usually need three or more kinds of anti-hypertension medicines to keep adequate blood pressure and use β-blocker for arrhythmia. It is probably the reason for the different proportion of β-blocker usage. Contrarily, β-blocker promotes cardiac angiogenesis in heart failure via activation of VEGF signaling pathway [30]. Hence, higher level of Ang-2 in late CKD patients may be partially related to long term usage of β-blocker. We also add β-blocker usage into multivariate analysis, and Ang-2 is still associated with adverse renal outcome. Further study is needed to investigate the relationship of ang-2 and β-blocker.

Ang-2 is usually elevated in diabetes and associated with endothelial dysfunction, which leads to microvascular and macrovascular complications [9,31,32]. The pathophysiological mechanisms by which Ang-2 participates in rapid decline in renal function are complicated and include various pathways, such as arterial stiffness or oxidative stress [17,19]. Our results show an association of Ang-2 quartiles with the proportion of diabetes, but no correlation between Ang-2 quartiles and glycated hemoglobin in patients with integrated CKD care program. Although average sugar level is under strict control, some patients still reach adverse renal outcome. Accumulating evidence indicates that strict glycemic control might not be enough to prevent rapid decline in renal function in late CKD [33]. It is probably that Ang-2 is

Table 3. The adjusted risks for composite outcomes, either commencing dialysis or doubling creatinine according to Angiopoietin-2 quartile.

| Angiopoietin-2[a] | Composite outcomes | | Commencing dialysis | | Double creatinine | |
	Hazard ratio (95% CI)	P-value	Hazard ratio (95% CI)	P-value	Hazard ratio (95% CI)	P-value
Quartile 1	Reference		Reference		Reference	
Quartile 2	1.42(0.95–2.13)	0.08	1.50(0.92–2.44)	0.01	1.43(0.83–2.47)	0.1
Quartile 3	1.54(1.05–2.27)	0.02	1.73(1.10–2.71)	0.02	1.47(0.87–2.48)	0.1
Quartile 4	1.53(1.06–2.23)	0.02	1.85(1.20–2.85)	0.02	1.47(0.87–2.45)	0.1

Abbreviations: CI, Confidence Interval; eGFR, estimated glomerular filtration rate.
Adjusted model: age, sex, cardiovascular disease, diabetes mellitus, angiotensin converting enzyme inhibitors/angiotensin II receptor blockers use, estimated glomerular filtration rate, hemoglobin, serum calcium and cholesterol levels, log serum albumin and phosphate, and urine protein-creatinine ratio cut at 1 g/g.
[a]Angiopoietin-2 quartile cut at 1494.1, 1948.8, and 2593.1 pg/ml.

Table 4. The adjusted risks for rapid decline in renal function and change of eGFR according to Angiopoietin-2 quartile.

Angiopoietin-2[a]	Rapid decline in renal function		Change of eGFR	
	Odds ratio (95% CI)	P-value	Unstandardized coefficient β[b] (95% CI)	P-value
Quartile 1	Reference		Reference	
Quartile 2	3.40(1.32–8.75)	0.01	−1.03(−2.63,0.57)	0.1
Quartile 3	3.04(1.18–7.82)	0.02	−1.66(−3.25,−0.07)	0.03
Quartile 4	2.96(1.13–7.76)	0.02	−1.73(−3.33,−0.11)	0.03

Abbreviations: CI, Confidence Interval; eGFR, estimated glomerular filtration rate.
Adjusted model: age, sex, cardiovascular disease, diabetes mellitus, angiotensin converting enzyme inhibitors/angiotensin II receptor blockers use, estimated glomerular filtration rate, hemoglobin, serum calcium and cholesterol levels, log serum albumin and phosphate, , and urine protein-creatinine ratio cut at 1 g/g.
[a]Angiopoietin-2 quartile cut at 1494.1, 1948.8, and 2593.1 pg/ml.
[b]β expressed as ml/min/1.73 m^2/year in eGFR.

associated with adverse renal outcome beyond the effects of diabetes. Additionally, patients with cardiovascular disease, cerebrovascular disease or hypertension are more likely to have higher circulating Ang-2 level [10,11,13,34]. Ang-2 has been associated with cardiovascular markers, such as cell adhesion molecules and inflammation [35], and increases endothelial apoptosis, enhances myocardial microvascular inflammation, and promotes cardiac fibrosis [31]. Although there was no different proportion of cardiovascular disease, cerebrovascular disease and hypertension in Ang-2 quartiles at baseline in our cohort, Ang-2 might be probably associated with cardiovascular events in the future. Thus, further study is needed to evaluate the relationship between Ang-2 and cardiovascular outcome.

On the other hand, previous study reported a significant correlation between Ang-2 and asymmetric dimethylarginine (ADMA), as the nitric oxide (NO) synthase inhibitor [17]. CKD has been regarded as a NO-deficient state, and the oxidative stress leads to not only renal function decline, but also adverse cardiovascular sequelae [36,37]. Thus, ADMA is not only a uremic toxin, but also a strong marker of endothelial dysfunction and atherosclerosis [38]. Sascha et al. speculated that the increased Ang-2 levels might reveal excess Weibel-Palade body exocytosis as a consequence of decreased NO bioavailability in the presence of high ADMA levels [17]. Although further in vivo and in vitro studies are needed to evaluate the interaction between Ang-2 and NO bioavailability, it could possibly explain one of the potential mechanisms responsible for the association between Ang-2 and adverse renal outcome.

This study has some limitations that must be considered. The major uncertainty is whether circulating Ang-2 is biologically active in CKD patients. The biological implication of Ang-2 changes in the range observed in our patients is still unknown. Besides, Ang-2 was measured once at enrollment. The effect of the time-varying Ang-2 levels might be underestimated. Additionally, the mechanism contributing to the association between increased circulating Ang-2 and rapid decline in renal function has not been well-explored. Further study is needed to investigate the pathogenic link between Ang-2 and rapid decline in renal function.

In conclusion, our study demonstrates that elevated circulating Ang-2 is associated with increased risks for adverse renal outcome in stages 3–5 CKD patients. Future studies will be necessary to evaluate the pathogenic role of Ang-2 in renal progression, and to establish the beneficial renal function by targeting Ang-2.

Supporting Information

Figure S1   Adjusted hazard ratios (HRs) of commencing dialysis for Angiopoietin-2 (Ang-2) quartile 4 compared with Ang-2 quartile 1 in CKD stages 3–5 subjects stratified by proteinuria, high sensitivity c-reactive protein (hsCRP), serum albumin and angiotensin converting enzyme inhibitors (ACEI)/angiotensin II receptor blockers (ARB) usage. Ratios were adjusted for age, sex, cardiovascular disease, diabetes mellitus, ACEI/ARB usage, estimated glomerular filtration rate, hemoglobin, serum calcium and cholesterol levels, log serum albumin and phosphate, and urine protein-creatinine ratio cut at 1 g/g. The median values of serum albumin and hsCRP are 3.8 g/dl and 1.5 mg/l respectively.

Figure S2   Adjusted hazard ratios (HRs) of commencing dialysis for Angiopoietin-2 (Ang-2) quartile 4 compared with Ang-2 quartile 1 in CKD stages 3–4 subjects stratified by proteinuria, high sensitivity c-reactive protein (hsCRP), serum albumin and angiotensin converting enzyme inhibitors (ACEI)/angiotensin II receptor blockers (ARB) usage. Ratios were adjusted for age, sex, cardiovascular disease, diabetes mellitus, ACEI/ARB usage, estimated glomerular filtration rate, hemoglobin, serum calcium and cholesterol levels, log serum albumin and phosphate, and urine protein-creatinine ratio cut at 1 g/g. The median values of serum albumin and hsCRP are 3.8 g/dl and 1.5 mg/l respectively.

Figure S3   Adjusted hazard ratios (HRs) of commencing dialysis for Angiopoietin-2 (Ang-2) quartile 4 compared with Ang-2 quartile 1 in CKD stage 5 subjects stratified by proteinuria, high sensitivity c-reactive protein (hsCRP), serum albumin and angiotensin converting enzyme inhibitors (ACEI)/angiotensin II receptor blockers (ARB) usage. Ratios were adjusted for age, sex, cardiovascular disease, diabetes mellitus, ACEI/ARB usage, estimated glomerular filtration rate, hemoglobin, serum calcium and cholesterol levels, log serum albumin and phosphate, and urine protein-creatinine ratio cut at 1 g/g. The median values of serum albumin and hsCRP are 3.8 g/dl and 1.5 mg/l respectively.

Acknowledgments

The authors thank the help from the Statistical Analysis Laboratory, Department of Medical Research, Kaohsiung Medical University Hospital, Kaohsiung Medical University. **Support**: Dr. Tsai's research was supported by the Kaohsiung Medical University Faculty of Renal Care.

Author Contributions

Conceived and designed the experiments: Y-CT M-CK. Performed the experiments: S-CL M-CK. Analyzed the data: Y-CT C-CH M-YL. Contributed reagents/materials/analysis tools: Y-WC J-CT H-TK S-JH M-CK H-CC. Wrote the paper: Y-CT M-CK.

Reference

1. Nugent RA, Fathima SF, Feigl AB, Chyung D (2011) The burden of chronic kidney disease on developing nations: a 21st century challenge in global health. Nephron Clin Pract 118: 269–277.
2. Chang FC, Lin SL (2013) The role of angiopoietin-2 in progressive renal fibrosis. J Formos Med Assoc 112: 175–176.
3. Brindle NP, Saharinen P, Alitalo K (2006) Signaling and functions of angiopoietin-1 in vascular protection. Circ Res 98: 1014–1023.
4. Fam NP, Verma S, Kutryk M, Stewart DJ (2003) Clinician guide to angiogenesis. Circulation 108: 2613–2618.
5. Fiedler U, Augustin HG (2006) Angiopoietins: a link between angiogenesis and inflammation. Trends Immuno 27: 552–558.
6. Fiedler U, Scharpfenecker M, Koidl S, Hegen A, Grunow V, et al. (2004) The Tie-2 ligand angiopoietin-2 is stored in and rapidly released upon stimulation from endothelial cell Weibel-Palade bodies. Blood 103: 4150–4156.
7. Huang YQ, Li JJ, Hu L, Lee M, Karpatkin S (2002) Thrombin induces increased expression and secretion of angiopoietin-2 from human umbilical vein endothelial cells. Blood 99: 1646–1650.
8. Fiedler U, Reiss Y, Scharpfenecker M, Grunow V, Koidl S, et al. (2006) Angiopoietin-2 sensitizes endothelial cells to TNF-alpha and has a crucial role in the induction of inflammation. Nat Med 12: 235–239.
9. Lim HS, Lip GY, Blann AD (2005) Angiopoietin-1 and angiopoietin-2 in diabetes mellitus: relationship to VEGF, glycaemic control, endothelial damage/dysfunction and atherosclerosis. Atherosclerosis 180: 113–118.
10. Nadar SK, Blann A, Beevers DG, Lip GY (2005) Abnormal angiopoietins 1&2, angiopoietin receptor Tie-2 and vascular endothelial growth factor levels in hypertension: relationship to target organ damage [a sub-study of the Anglo-Scandinavian Cardiac Outcomes Trial (ASCOT)]. J Intern Med 258: 336–343.
11. Chong AY, Caine GJ, Freestone B, Blann AD, Lip GY (2004) Plasma angiopoietin-1, angiopoietin-2, and angiopoietin receptor tie-2 levels in congestive heart failure. J Am Coll Cardiol 43: 423–428.
12. David S, Kumpers P, Hellpap J, Horn R, Leitolf H, et al. (2009) Angiopoietin-2 and cardiovascular disease in dialysis and kidney transplantation. Am J Kidney Dis 53: 770–778.
13. Lee KW, Lip GY, Blann AD (2004) Plasma angiopoietin-1, angiopoietin-2, angiopoietin receptor tie-2, and vascular endothelial growth factor levels in acute coronary syndromes. Circulation 110: 2355–2360.
14. Parikh SM, Mammoto T, Schultz A, Yuan HT, Christiani D, et al. (2006) Excess circulating angiopoietin-2 may contribute to pulmonary vascular leak in sepsis in humans. PLoS Med 3: e46.
15. Kumpers P, Lukasz A, David S, Horn R, Hafer C, et al. (2008) Excess circulating angiopoietin-2 is a strong predictor of mortality in critically ill medical patients. Crit Care, 12: R147.
16. Kumpers P, Hafer C, David S, Hecker H, Lukasz A, et al. (2010) Angiopoietin-2 in patients requiring renal replacement therapy in the ICU: relation to acute kidney injury, multiple organ dysfunction syndrome and outcome. Intensive Care Med 36: 462–470.
17. David S, Kumpers P, Lukasz A, Fliser D, Martens-Lobenhoffer J, et al. (2010) Circulating angiopoietin-2 levels increase with progress of chronic kidney disease. Nephrol Dial Transplant 25: 2571–2576.
18. David S, John SG, Jefferies HJ, Sigrist MK, Kumpers P, et al. (2012) Angiopoietin-2 levels predict mortality in CKD patients. Nephrol Dial Transplant 27: 1867–1872.
19. Chang FC, Lai TS, Chiang CK, Chen YM, Wu MS, et al. (2013) Angiopoietin-2 is associated with albuminuria and microinflammation in chronic kidney disease. PloS One, 8: e54668.
20. Levey AS, Bosch JP, Lewis JB, Greene T, Rogers N, et al. (1999) A more accurate method to estimate glomerular filtration rate from serum creatinine: a new prediction equation. Modification of Diet in Renal Disease Study Group. Ann Intern Med 130: 461–470.
21. Levin A, Stevens PE (2014) Summary of KDIGO 2012 CKD Guideline: behind the scenes, need for guidance, and a framework for moving forward. Kidney Int 85: 49–61.
22. Davis B, Dei Cas A, Long DA, White KE, Hayward A, et al. (2007) Podocyte-specific expression of angiopoietin-2 causes proteinuria and apoptosis of glomerular endothelia. J Am Soc Nephrol 18: 2320–2329.
23. Woolf AS, Gnudi L, Long DA (2009) Roles of angiopoietins in kidney development and disease. J Am Soc Nephrol 20: 239–244.
24. Tryggvason K, Patrakka J, Wartiovaara J (2006) Hereditary proteinuria syndromes and mechanisms of proteinuria. N Engl J Med 354: 1387–1401.
25. Eremina V, Sood M, Haigh J, Nagy A, Lajoie G, et al. (2003) Glomerular-specific alterations of VEGF-A expression lead to distinct congenital and acquired renal diseases. J Clin Invest 111: 707–716.
26. Seron D, Alexopoulos E, Raftery MJ, Hartley B, Cameron JS (1990) Number of interstitial capillary cross-sections assessed by monoclonal antibodies: relation to interstitial damage. Nephrol dial transplant 5: 889–893.
27. Futrakul N, Butthep P, Futrakul P (2008) Altered vascular homeostasis in chronic kidney disease. Clin Hemorheol Microcirc 38: 201–207.
28. Tsai YC, Hung CC, Kuo MC, Tsai JC, Yeh SM, et al. (2012) Association of hsCRP, white blood cell count and ferritin with renal outcome in chronic kidney disease patients. PloS One, 7: e52775.
29. Rondaij MG, Bierings R, Kragt A, van Mourik JA, Voorberg J (2006) Dynamics and plasticity of Weibel-Palade bodies in endothelial cells. Arterioscler Thromb Vasc Biol 26: 1002–1007.
30. Rengo G, Cannavo A, Liccardo D, Zincarelli C, de Lucia C, et al. (2013) CVascular endothelial growth factor blockade prevents the beneficial effects of β-blocker therapy on cardiac function, angiogenesis, and remodeling in heart failure. Circ Heart Fail 6: 1259–67.
31. Chen JX, Zeng H, Reese J, Aschner JL, Meyrick B (2012) Overexpression of angiopoietin-2 impairs myocardial angiogenesis and exacerbates cardiac fibrosis in the diabetic db/db mouse model. Am J Physiol Heart Circ Physiol 302: 1003–1012.
32. Anuradha S, Mohan V, Gokulakrishnan K, Dixit M (2010) Angiopoietin-2 levels in glucose intolerance, hypertension, and metabolic syndrome in Asian Indians (Chennai Urban Rural Epidemiology Study-74). Metabolism Clinical and Experimental 59: 774–779.
33. Shurraw S, Hemmelgarn B, Lin M, Majumdar SR, Klarenbach, et al. (2011) SAssociation between glycemic control and adverse outcomes in people with diabetes mellitus and chronic kidney disease: a population-based cohort study. Arch Intern Med 171: 1920–1927.
34. Cui X, Chopp M, Zacharek A, Ye X, Roberts C, et al (2011) Angiopoietin/Tie2 pathway mediates type 2 diabetes induced vascular damage after cerebral stroke. Neurobiol Dis 43: 285–292.
35. Shroff RC, Price KL, Kolatsi-Joannou M, Todd AF, Wells D, et al. (2013) Circulating angiopoietin-2 is a marker for early cardiovascular disease in children on chronic dialysis. PLOS one 8: e56273.
36. Wever R, Boer P, Hijmering M, Stroes E, Verhaar M, et al. (1999) Nitric oxide production is reduced in patients with chronic renal failure. Arterioscler Thromb Vasc Biol 19: 1168–1172.
37. Baylis C (2012) Nitric oxide synthase derangements and hypertension in kidney disease. Curr Opin Nephrol Hypertens 21: 1–6.
38. Kielstein JT, Zoccali C (2005) Asymmetric dimethylarginine: a cardiovascular risk factor and a uremic toxin coming of age? Am J Kidney Dis 46: 186–202.

6

Vitamin D Deficiency Aggravates Chronic Kidney Disease Progression after Ischemic Acute Kidney Injury

Janaína Garcia Gonçalves, Ana Carolina de Bragança, Daniele Canale, Maria Heloisa Massola Shimizu, Talita Rojas Sanches, Rosa Maria Affonso Moysés, Lúcia Andrade, Antonio Carlos Seguro, Rildo Aparecido Volpini*

Nephrology Department, University of São Paulo School of Medicine, São Paulo, Brazil

Abstract

Background: Despite a significant improvement in the management of chronic kidney disease (CKD), its incidence and prevalence has been increasing over the years. Progressive renal fibrosis is present in CKD and involves the participation of several cytokines, including Transforming growth factor-β1 (TGF-β1). Besides cardiovascular diseases and infections, several studies show that Vitamin D status has been considered as a non-traditional risk factor for the progression of CKD. Given the importance of vitamin D in the maintenance of essential physiological functions, we studied the events involved in the chronic kidney disease progression in rats submitted to ischemia/reperfusion injury under vitamin D deficiency (VDD).

Methods: Rats were randomized into four groups: Control; VDD; ischemia/reperfusion injury (IRI); and VDD+IRI. At the 62 day after sham or IRI surgery, we measured inulin clearance, biochemical variables and hemodynamic parameters. In kidney tissue, we performed immunoblotting to quantify expression of Klotho, TGF-β, and vitamin D receptor (VDR); gene expression to evaluate renin, angiotensinogen, and angiotensin-converting enzyme; and immunohistochemical staining for ED1 (macrophages), type IV collagen, fibronectin, vimentin, and α-smooth mucle actin. Histomorphometric studies were performed to evaluate fractional interstitial area.

Results: IRI animals presented renal hypertrophy, increased levels of mean blood pressure and plasma PTH. Furthermore, expansion of the interstitial area, increased infiltration of ED1 cells, increased expression of collagen IV, fibronectin, vimentin and α-actin, and reduced expression of Klotho protein were observed. VDD deficiency contributed to increased levels of plasma PTH as well as for important chronic tubulointerstitial changes (fibrosis, inflammatory infiltration, tubular dilation and atrophy), increased expression of TGF-β1 and decreased expression of VDR and Klotho protein observed in VDD+IRI animals.

Conclusion: Through inflammatory pathways and involvement of TGF-β1 growth factor, VDD could be considered as an aggravating factor for tubulointerstitial damage and fibrosis progression following acute kidney injury induced by ischemia/ reperfusion.

Editor: Makoto Makishima, Nihon University School of Medicine, Japan

Funding: Fundação de Amparo à Pesquisa do Estado de São Paulo - FAPESP (www.fapesp.br) Grant number: 2010/52294-0. The funders had no role in study design, data collection and analysis, decision to publish, or preparation of the manuscript.

Competing Interests: The authors have declared that no competing interests exist.

* Email: rildovolpini@yahoo.com.br

Introduction

In most countries, the incidence and prevalence of chronic kidney disease (CKD) have been increasing over the years mainly due to the aging population and the presence of diabetic nephropathy [1,2]. It is well established that acute kidney injury (AKI) after ischemia/reperfusion injury (IRI) is a major cause of AKI [3]. IRI physiology involves a complex interaction among vascular, tubular and inflammatory factors followed by a repair process that can restore function and epithelial differentiation or result in CKD with progressive development of fibrosis [4,5].

It has been shown that the mortality of patients with CKD is directly related to renal function associated with cardiovascular diseases and infections [6]. However, such traditional risks explain only about half of mortality and various studies are being directed to non-traditional risk factors, such as vitamin D [6].

Vitamin D [25(OH)D] is a circulating hormone in the body indispensable for mineral homeostasis [7] and responsible for kidney protection and regulation of several physiological activities as well [8]. Thus, vitamin D deficiency (VDD) ($<$10 ng/mL) or insufficiency (10–30 ng/mL) can accelerate the progression of kidney disease [9–11]. The biologically active form of vitamin D is produced in the kidney by mitochondria of the renal proximal convoluted tubules, where 1α-hydroxylase converts 25-hydroxyvitamin D [25(OH)D] to 1,25-dihydroxyvitamin D3 [1,25 $(OH)_2D_3$] or calcitriol [12]. The classical 1,25 $(OH)_2D_3$ pathway requires the nuclear vitamin D receptor (VDR), which is a transcription factor for 1,25 $(OH)_2 D_3$ target genes [4,5,13].

The renal conversion of vitamin D into biologically active form is tightly regulated by several factors, including parathormone (PTH), phosphorus levels and fibroblast growth factor 23 (FGF-23) [12]. FGF-23 is a phosphatonin produced by osteocytes which promotes renal phosphate excretion [8,14–16] and a close relationship between FGF-23 and Klotho is described [17]. The lack of Klotho gene expression (α-klotho) is associated with premature phenotypes related to aging as well as to hyperphosphatemia and low levels of vitamin D [18]. Klotho protein forms binary complexes with fibroblast growth factor receptors (FGFR), increasing Klotho affinity and selectivity for FGF-23 [17], playing an important role in vitamin D synthesis.

Given the importance of vitamin D in essential physiological functions and the respective low levels of this hormone observed in CKD, our aim was to study the vitamin D deficiency in a murine model of CKD progression after AKI induced by ischemia/reperfusion.

Materials and Methods

Experimental Animals and Induction of I/R Injury

The study was approved by the Research Ethics Committee of the University of São Paulo – School of Medicine, protocol numbered 088/12. All procedures were developed in strict accordance with local institutional guidelines and with well-established international standards for the care and use of laboratory animals. All surgery was performed under appropriate anesthesia, and all efforts were made to minimize suffering.

Male Wistar rats (180–200 g) were provided by the University of São Paulo - School of Medicine animal facility. During the 90-day experiment, rats were maintained under standard laboratory conditions, receiving vitamin D-free or standard diets (MP Biomedicals, Irvine, CA, USA) and free access to tap water for 90 days. Rats were divided into four groups: (C) Control (n = 11), received a standard diet for 90 days and submitted to sham surgery; (VDD) Vitamin D Deficiency (n = 8), received a vitamin D-free diet for 90 days and submitted to sham surgery; (IRI) Ischemia/Reperfusion Injury (n = 10), received a standard diet for 90 days and submitted to ischemia/reperfusion injury; and (VDD+ IRI) Vitamin D Deficiency plus Ischemia/Reperfusion Injury (n = 9), received a vitamin D-free diet for 90 days and submitted to ischemia/reperfusion injury.

Sham Surgery. On day 28, rats from Control and VDD groups were anesthetized with 2,2,2-Tribromoethanol (250 mg/ Kg body weight), and a suprapubic incision was made and then sutured immediately.

Induction of Ischemia/Reperfusion Injury. As described above, on day 28, rats from IRI and VDD+IRI groups were anesthetized, a suprapubic incision was made for induction of ischemic renal injury by clamping both renal arteries for 45 min, followed by reperfusion.

Analysis of Urine Samples

On day 89, all rats were placed in individual metabolic cages, on a 12/12-h light/dark cycle, with free access to drinking water. We collected 24-h urine samples, centrifuged them and analyzed the supernatants. We measured urinary concentrations of sodium and calcium by ion-selective electrodes (ABL800 Flex Analyzer – Radiometer, Brønshøj, Denmark) and urinary phosphorus by automated enzymatic colorimetric assay (COBAS C111 Analyzer – Roche, USA). Urinary protein excretion was measured by a colorimetric system using a commercial kit (Labtest Diagnóstica, Minas Gerais, Brazil).

Inulin Clearance and Hemodynamic Studies

On day 90, the animals were anesthetized with sodium thiopental (50 mg/Kg BW) and placed on a temperature-regulated surgical table. The trachea was cannulated (PE-240 catheter) and spontaneous breathing was maintained. The jugular vein was cannulated (PE-60 catheter) for infusion of inulin and fluids. To monitor mean arterial pressure (MAP) and collect blood samples, the right carotid artery was catheterized with a PE-50 catheter. We assessed MAP with a data acquisition system (MP100; Biopac Systems, Santa Barbara, CA, USA). To collect urine samples, the urinary bladder was cannulated (PE-240 catheter) by suprapubic incision. After completion of the cannulation surgical procedure, a loading dose of inulin (100 mg/Kg body weight diluted in 1 mL of 0.9% saline) was administered through the jugular vein. Subsequently, a constant infusion of inulin (10 mg/kg body weight in 0.9% saline) was started and continued at 0.04 mL/min throughout the whole experiment. Three urine samples were collected at 30-min intervals. Blood samples were obtained at the beginning and at the end of the experiment. Inulin clearance values represent the mean of three periods. Blood and urine inulin were determined by the anthrone method, and the glomerular filtration rate (GFR) data is expressed as ml/min/100 g BW. To measure the renal blood flow (RBF), an ultrasonic flow probe was placed around the exposed renal artery (T402; Transonic Systems, Bethesda, MD, USA) and RBF was expressed as ml/min. To calculate renal vascular resistance (RVR, in mmHg/ml/min), we divided blood pressure by RBF.

Evaluation of Biochemical Parameters

To assess plasma levels of 25-hydroxyvitamin D [25(OH)D], parathormone (PTH), fibroblast growth factor 23 (FGF-23), sodium (P_{Na}), potassium (P_K), phosphate (P_P) and calcium (P_{Ca}), we collected blood samples after the clearance studies. We assessed 25(OH)D by radioimmunoassay (RIA) using a commercial kit (25-Hydroxyvitamin D[125], DiaSorin, Vercelli, Italy) and PTH by Enzyme-Linked Immunosorbet Assay (ELISA) using a commercial kit (Rat Bioactive Intact PTH, Immunotopics, CA, USA). FGF-23 levels were assessed by ELISA using a commercial kit (FGF-23 ELISA Kit, Kainos Laboratories, Tokyo, Japan). P_P and P_{Ca} were evaluated by automated enzymatic colorimetric assay (COBAS C111 Analyzer – Roche, USA) while P_{Na} and P_K were measured by ion-selective electrodes (ABL800 Flex Analyzer – Radiometer, Brønshøj, Denmark).

Tissue Sample Collection/Preparation

After blood samples collection, we perfused kidneys with phosphate-buffered solution (PBS, pH 7.4). Right kidneys were frozen in liquid nitrogen and stored at −80°C for Western blotting and real-time quantitative polymerase chain reaction (qPCR). Left kidneys were removed and weighed. Fragments of left kidney were fixed in 10% neutral-buffered formalin or methacarn's solution for 24 hours and in 70% alcohol thereafter. Kidney blocks were embedded in paraffin and cut into 4-μm sections for histological and immunohistochemical examination.

Preparation of Samples for Western Blotting

Kidney samples were homogenized in ice-cold isolation solution (200 mM manitol, 80 mM HEPES and 41 mM KOH, pH 7.5) containing a protease inhibitors cocktail (Sigma Chemical Company, St. Louis, MO, USA) using a homogenizer (Polytron - PT 10–35, Brinkmann Instruments, Westbury, NY, USA). Homogenates were centrifuged at low speed (2000×g) for 15 min at 4°C to remove nuclei and cell debris. Supernatants were isolated, and protein was determined by Bradford assay (BioAgency Laboratórios, São Paulo, Brazil).

Electrophoresis and Immunoblotting

Proteins were separated on SDS-polyacrylamide minigels by electrophoresis [19]. After transfer by electroelution to polyvinylidene difluoride (PVDF) membranes (GE Healthcare Limited, Little Chalfont, UK), blots were blocked for 60 minutes with 5% non-fat dry milk in Tris-buffered saline solution. Blots were then incubated overnight with antibodies against Actin (1:5,000), VDR (1:500), Klotho (1:500) and TGF-beta (1:200) (Santa Cruz Biotechnology, CA, USA). The labeling was visualized with horseradish peroxidase-conjugated secondary antibody (anti-rabbit IgG, diluted 1:2,000, or anti-goat, diluted 1:10,000, Sigma Chemical, St. Louis, MO, USA) and enhanced chemiluminescence (ECL) detection system (GE Healthcare Limited, Little Chalfont, UK).

Kidney protein levels. The images were obtained using an imaging system (Alliance 4.2; Uvitec, Cambridge, UK). We used densitometry to quantitatively analyze the protein levels, normalizing the bands to actin expression.

Gene Expression

We performed real-time qPCR in frozen renal tissue, assessing the following genes: renin (Rn00561847_m1), angiotensinogen (Rn00593114_m1), and angiotensin converting enzyme (Rn00561094_m1), (Applied Biosystems, Foster City, CA, USA). We extracted and prepared total RNA. For cDNA synthesis, we used total RNA and a Superscript VILO MasterMix (Invitrogen Technologies, Carlsbad, CA, USA). We performed real-time PCR using TaqMan on Step One Plus (Applied Biosystems, Foster City, CA, USA). All primers were purchased from Invitrogen. Relative gene expression values were evaluated with the $2^{-\Delta\Delta Ct}$ method [20] using GAPDH (Rn01775763_g1) as housekeeping gene.

Light Microscopy

Four-μm histological sections of kidney tissue were stained with Masson's trichome and examined under light microscope. The fractional interstitial area (FIA) of the renal cortex was determined by morphometry with a light camera connected to an image analyzer (Axiovision, Carl Zeiss, Eching, Germany). We analyzed 30 grid fields (0.087 mm^2 each) per kidney cortex. The interstitial areas were demarcated manually on a video screen, and the proportion of the field they occupied was determined by computerized morphometry [21]. The morphometric examination was blinded to minimize observer bias, i.e. the observer was unaware of the treatment group from which the tissue originated.

Immunohistochemistry

Samples were processed in 4-μm paraffin sections and then subjected to incubation overnight at 4°C according to each protocol developed for each primary antibody. We used the following antibodies: (1:500) monoclonal anti-ED1 (macrophages) (AbD Serotec, Oxford, UK); (1:200) polyclonal anti-Collagen IV (Abcam, Cambridge, UK); (1:400) polyclonal anti-FN1 (fibronec-tin) (Sigma-Aldrich, Saint Louis, MO, USA); (1:1,000) monoclonal anti-α-smooth-muscle actin (α-SMA) (Millipore, Billerica, MA, USA); and (1:50) monoclonal anti-vimentin (Dako, Glostrup, Denmark). The reaction product was detected with an avidin-biotin-peroxidase complex (Vector Laboratories, Burlingame, CA, USA). The color reaction was developed with 3,3-diaminobenzidine (Sigma Chemical, St. Louis, MO, USA) in the presence of hydrogen peroxide, and the sections were counterstained with Harris' hematoxylin.

For ED1, we analyzed 40–60 renal cortex fields. The result of the immunoreaction was quantified by couting the number of ED1 positive cells per field (0.087 mm^2 each) and averaging the number of cells per field for each section [21]. To evaluate immunoreactivity to collagen IV, fibronectin, α-SMA and vimentin, the volume ratios of positive areas of renal tissue sections, determined by the color limit, were obtained using Image-Pro Plus software (Media Cybernetics, Silver Spring, MD, USA) and the results were expressed as percentages [22].

Statistical Analysis

All quantitative data are mean±standard error of the mean (SEM). Comparisons between groups were made by unpaired t-test. Comparisons among groups were made by one-way analysis of variance followed by the Student–Newman–Keuls test. Values of $p < 0.05$ were considered statistically significant.

Results

Body weight and hemodynamics

As described in Table 1, there were no differences in body weight among the studied groups since all animals showed similar food ingestion (~25 g/day) during 90 days. The kidney weight/body weight ratio was calculated and, as expected, IRI and VDD+IRI groups presented an increase of this proportion (Table 1). We did not observe differences among the groups concerning glomerular filtration rate (GFR), renal blood flow (RBF) and renal vascular resistance (RVR). However, we found increased levels (mmHg) of mean arterial pressure (MAP) in VDD (135.2±3.4), IRI (137.3±3.6) and VDD+IRI (134.5±5.2) when compared to Control (119.4±2.3) group (p<0.05), Table 1.

Vitamin D and PTH levels

The animals were maintained on a standard or a free-vitamin D diet for 90 days. Over the experimental period, the levels of 25(OH)D from VDD and VDD+IRI groups were undetectable (< 1.5 ng/mL), while Control and IRI groups presented 15.4 and 15.0 ng/mL respectively (Table 2). Concerning PTH data, we found significant higher levels (pg/mL) of the respective hormone in VDD (1,250±155) and VDD+IRI (2,187±336), showing the negative feedback caused by vitamin D deficiency in these groups. Both VDD and VDD+IRI groups presented a significant increase of PTH levels when compared to Control (318±59) and IRI (453±96) groups. Furthermore, VDD+IRI presented significant high levels of PTH when compared to the other groups (Table 2).

Vitamin D deficiency and blood pressure control

In order to further investigate the role of vitamin D on blood pressure control, we evaluated the gene expression (qPCR) of some renin-angiotensin system (RAS) compounds and plasma aldosterone levels as well. The qPCR results showed increased gene expression of renin, angiotensinogen (AGT) and angiotensin converting enzyme (ACE) in VDD, IRI and VDD+IRI when compared to control group (Table 3). In addition, we found higher levels of aldosterone (pg/mL) in VDD (455.8±69.0), IRI

Table 1. Body weight, kidney weight, renal function and hemodynamic measurements after 90 days evaluated in Control rats (C), Vitamin D deficient rats (VDD), rats submitted to Ischemia/Reperfusion Injury (IRI), and Vitamin D deficient rats submitted to Ischemia/Reperfusion Injury (VDD+IRI).

	C	VDD	IRI	VDD+IRI
BW	519.4±11.6	551.4±19.8	515.8±13.6	510.1±14.1
KW/BW	0.36±0.01	0.35±0.01	0.42±0.02 [c,f]	0.44±0.01 [c,e]
GFR	0.62±0.02	0.56±0.04	0.57±0.04	0.57±0.02
MAP	119.4±2.3	135.2±3.4 [c]	137.3±3.6 [c]	134.5±5.2 [c]
RBF	5.61±0.02	5.82±0.06	5.62±0.08	5.83±0.07
RVR	22.02±0.52	24.82±1.09	24.72±0.67	23.4±0.91

BW, body weight (g); KW/BW. kidney weight/body weight ratio; GFR, inulin clearance (mL/min/100 g); MAP, mean arterial pressure (mmHg); RBF, renal blood flow (mL/min); RVR, renal vascular resistance (mmHg/mL/min). Values are mean ± SEM. [c] $p < 0.05$ vs. C; [e] $p < 0.01$ vs. VDD; [f] $p < 0.05$ vs. VDD.

(416.0±89.2) and VDD+IRI (502.5±134.2) when compared to Control (165.7±17.2) group (Table 2). Taken together, our results reinforce the role of vitamin D on blood pressure control.

Proteinuria, calcium, phosphorus and FGF-23 – Klotho axis

As shown in Table 2, we observed a progressive and significant ($p < 0.001$) increase of proteinuria (mg/24 h) among the studied groups: Control (5.96±0.53), VDD (17.16±1.56), IRI (23.97±1.43) and VDD+IRI (32.31±0.51). Neither calcium and phosphorus levels nor urinary volume presented differences among the groups (Table 2). Considering the fact that the levels of calcium and phosphorus are closely related to FGF-23 - Klotho axis, we investigated plasmatic levels of FGF-23 and the renal expression of Klotho. We observed decreased levels of FGF-23 (pg/mL) in VDD (41.8±14.6) and VDD+IRI (77.4±18.5) groups when compared to Control (293.1±33.8) and IRI (225.4±24.0) groups (Table 2). Also, we found a decreased expression of Klotho protein (%) in VDD (47.5±6.0), IRI (53.3±7.6) and VDD+IRI (46.7±2.5) when compared to Control (98.8±0.8) group (Figure 1). In addition, similar profile was found concerning gene expression of α-klotho (Table 3).

Histomorphological studies

Light microscopy studies revealed histological alterations such as interstitial fibrosis, tubular atrophy and dilatation, and inflammatory cell infiltrates in the renal cortex of vitamin D deficient and ischemic/reperfusion injury groups (Figure 2). The alterations were subtle, but evident in VDD animals and more prominent in IRI and VDD+IRI groups. In addition, morphometric studies were performed to evaluate the fractional interstitial area (FIA) of the renal cortex. We observed a progressive and increasing involvement of the tubulointerstitial compartment, featuring interstitial expansion and renal fibrosis as follows: Control and VDD groups showed 7.35% and 17.23% of FIA, respectively while IRI and VDD+IRI groups presented 24.41 and 34.87% of FIA, respectively. Based on our results, we could infer that vitamin D deficiency exerts an important role on interstitial expansion and fibrosis formation.

Macrophages infiltration

The number of ED1 positive cells, a marker to macrophages, was evaluated by immunohistochemical studies. We found a significant number of infiltrating ED1 positive cells/per field (0.087 mm^2) in IRI (10.92±1.89) and VDD+IRI (16.93±2.49)

Table 2. Biochemical parameters after 90 days evaluated in Control rats (C), Vitamin D deficient rats (VDD), rats submitted to Ischemia/Reperfusion Injury (IRI), and Vitamin D deficient rats submitted to Ischemia/Reperfusion Injury (VDD+IRI).

	C	VDD	IRI	VDD+IRI
25(OH)D	15.4±1.0	<1.5 (undetectable) [a]	15.0±0.6 [d]	<1.5 (undetectable) [a,g]
PTH	318±59	1,250±155 [c]	453±96 [f]	2,187±336 [a,f,g]
Aldosterone	165.7±17.2	455.8±69.0 [c]	416.0±89.2 [c]	502.5±134.2 [c]
FGF-23	293.1±33.8	41.8±14.6 [a,g]	225.4±24.0	77.4±18.5 [a,g]
P_P	4.8±0.2	5.2±0.2	5.5±0.2	5.3±0.3
P_{Ca}	9.48±0.50	8.81±0.41	9.28±0.15	8.17±0.40
P_{Na}	139.5±1.2	136±0.6	137.4±2.2	137.7±0.6
P_K	4.6±0.1	4.0±0.2	4.5±0.1	4.3±0.2
UV	14.23±0.93	13.40±1.03	14.42±1.71	11.13±1.77
$U_{Prot}V$	5.97±0.53	17.16±1.56 [a]	23.97±1.43 [a,d]	32.31±0.52 [a,d,g]

25(OH)D, 25 hydroxyvitamin D (ng/mL); PTH, parathormone (pg/mL); Aldosterone (pg/mL); FGF-23, fibroblast growth factor 23 (pg/mL); P_P, plasma phosphate concentration (mg/dL); P_{Ca}, plasma calcium concentration (mg/dL); P_{Na}, plasma sodium concentration (mEq/L); P_K, plasma potassium concentration (mEq/L); UV, urinary volume (mL/24 h); $U_{Prot}V$, urinary protein excretion (mg/24 h). Values are means ± SEM. [a] $p < 0.001$, [b] $p < 0.01$, [c] $p < 0.05$ vs. C; [d] $p < 0.001$ vs. VDD; [f] $p < 0.05$ vs. VDD; [g] $p < 0.001$ vs. IRI.

Table 3. Relative gene expression of α-klotho and renin-angiotensin system (RAS) compounds after 90 days evaluated in Control rats (C), Vitamin D deficient rats (VDD), rats submitted to Ischemia/Reperfusion Injury (IRI), and Vitamin D deficient rats submitted to Ischemia/Reperfusion Injury (VDD+IRI).

	C	VDD	IRI	VDD+IRI
renin	0.68±0.49	2.28±0.28 [b]	1.85±0.47 [c]	2.34±0.28 [c]
AGT	0.95±0.45	2.95±0.69 [c]	4.02±0.60 [b]	4.53±0.63 [b]
ACE	1.10±0.63	3.94±0.82 [c]	5.28±0.94 [c]	5.90±1.28 [c]
α-klotho	3.27±1.15	2.07±0.41	2.39±0.38	1.74±0.46

AGT, angiotensinogen; ACE, angiotensin-converting enzyme. Values are mean ± SEM. Relative gene expression values were evaluated with the $2^{-\Delta\Delta Ct}$ method using GAPDH as housekeeping gene. [b] $p<0.01$ and [c] $p<0.05$ vs. C.

when compared to VDD (2.18±0.14) and Control (1.14±0.19) groups. Vitamin D deficiency enhanced this alteration since VDD+IRI presented an increased number of ED1 positive cells than did the other groups (Figure 3).

Extracellular matrix components

As described above, our histological results showed that vitamin D deficiency is an aggravating factor for the expansion of tubulointerstitial compartment and fibrosis formation. This process is complex and involves the production and secretion of many extracellular matrix (ECM) components. So, we performed immunohistochemical studies for type IV collagen and fibronectin, two fibrous components of ECM. Our results showed increased expression of type IV collagen (Figure 4) and fibronectin (Figure 5), demonstrated as percentage of positive area, in the renal cortex of VDD, IRI and VDD+IRI groups when compared to Control group. Vitamin D deficiency enhanced the immuno-stainings for both ECM markers (Figures 4 and 5).

Phenotypic alteration of renal cells

Besides ECM markers studies, we also aimed to evaluate the presence of phenotypic alteration of renal tubular cells. We used the expression of vimentin to detect tubular injury and α-smooth muscle actin (α-SMA) as a marker for interstitial fibroblast activation. In Control group, the expression of vimentin and α-SMA was identical to that described in normal rats: vimentin was confined to smooth muscle cells and glomerular compartment (mensangial cells and podocytes), and α-SMA to arterial smooth muscle cells [23]. The percentage of positive area for vimentin was increased in IRI when compared to Control and VDD groups. Moreover, VDD+IRI group presented higher vimentin expression than did the other studied groups (Figure 6). A similar profile was found concerning α-SMA expression, even though without statistical difference between IRI and VDD+IRI groups (Figure 7). In addition, vitamin D deficiency may be involved in this cellular phenotypic alteration, since the animals from VDD+IRI groups presented a significant expression of vimentin and a slight increase of α-SMA expression when compared to IRI group (Figures 6 and 7).

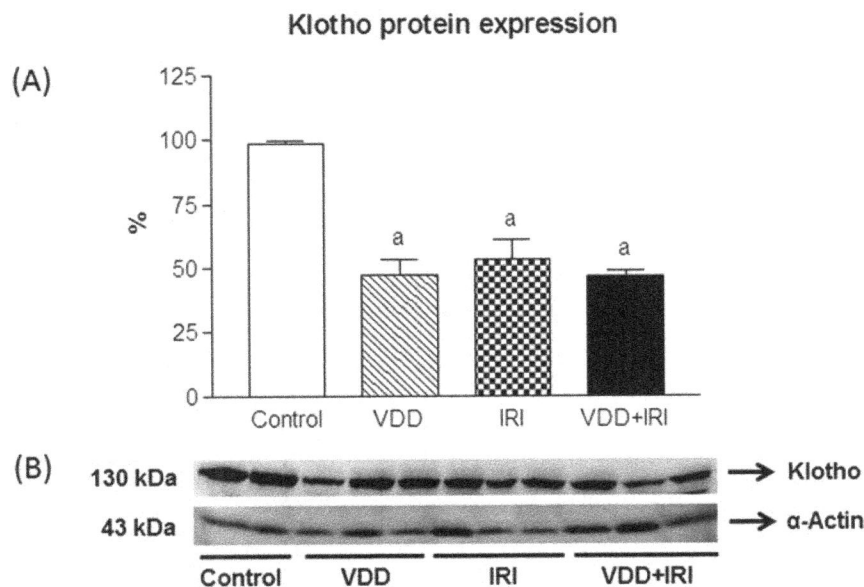

Figure 1. Semiquantitative immunoblotting of kidney fractions. (A) A densitometric analysis of samples from control (n = 4), VDD (n = 6), IRI (n = 6) and VDD+IRI (n = 6) rats is shown. (B) Immunoblots reacted with anti-Klotho revealing a 130-kDa band. Values are mean ± SEM. [a] p<0.001 vs. C.

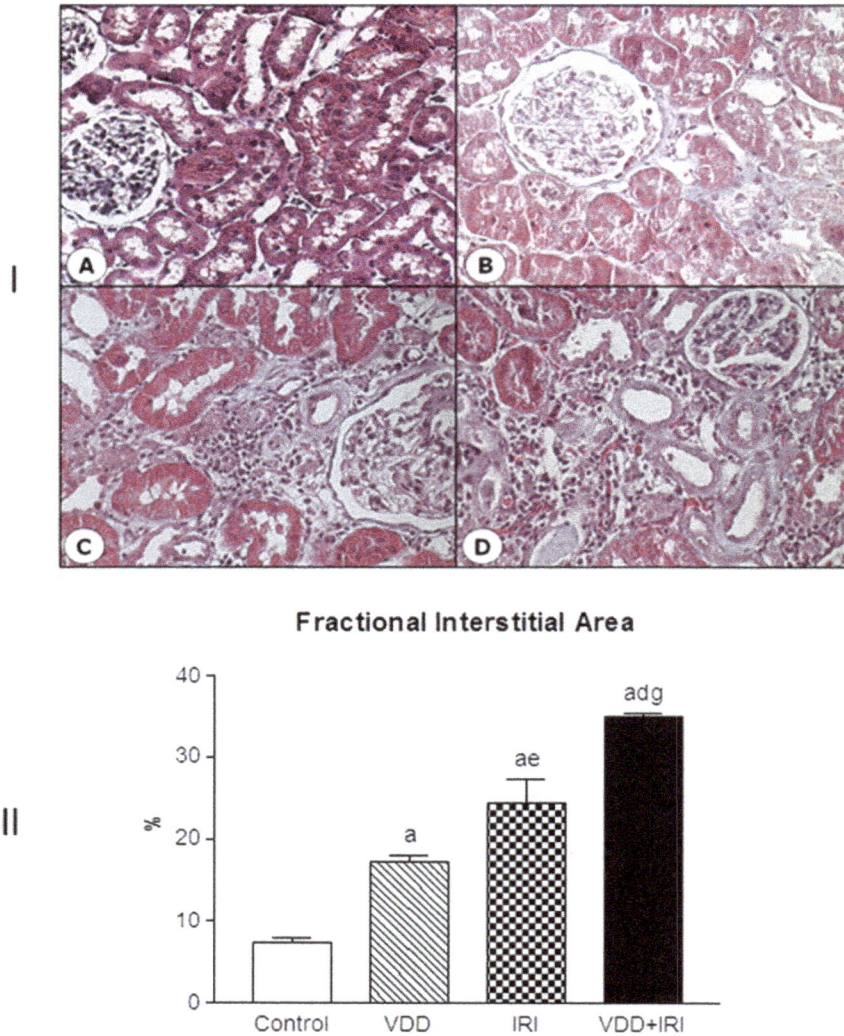

Figure 2. [I] Representative photomicrographs of renal histological changes after 90 days observed in a control rat (A), a vitamin D deficient rat (B), in a rat submitted to ischemia/reperfusion injury (C), and in a vitamin D deficient rat submitted to ischemia/ reperfusion injury (D). [II] Fractional interstitial area evaluated 90 days after in Control (C), Vitamin D Deficiency (VDD), Ischemia-Reperfusion Injury (IRI), and Vitamin D Deficiency and Ischemia/Reperfusion Injury (VDD+IRI) groups. Values are mean ± SEM. [a] $p<0.001$ vs. C; [d] $p<0.001$ vs. VDD; [e] $p<0.01$ vs. VDD; [g] $p<0.001$ vs. IRI.

Vitamin D deficiency, VDR and fibrosis formation

Our results related to histological and immunohistochemical studies revealed a potential involvement of vitamin D with renal fibrosis. To assess the possible link between vitamin D deficiency and fibrosis formation, we decided to study the role TGF-β expression, the most important pro-fibrotic cytokine, and its relationship with the vitamin D receptor (VDR). For that, we analyzed the renal expression of VDR and TGF-β in both IRI and VDD+IRI groups, since these groups presented expressive percentages of interstitial expansion and fibrosis. We observed a significant decrease in VDR expression (%) in VDD+IRI group (44.3±7.6) when compared to IRI group (100.0±22.0) (Figure 8-I). Concerning TGF-β, we found a significant increased expression (%) of this cytokine in the kidneys of VDD+IRI animals (196.3±41.9) when compared to IRI group (100.1±14.9) (Figure 8-II). So, analyzing the results, we observed that vitamin D deficiency caused a decrease in VDR expression and an increase

in TGF-β expression in VDD+IRI group, which had the highest ratio of fibrosis.

Discussion

In our experimental ischemia/reperfusion injury model, we found renal hypertrophy, increased levels of blood pressure and proteinuria in both ischemic animal groups. Furthermore, we observed enlargement of the interstitial area, including increased infiltration of ED1 positive cells and presence of fibrosis, and phenotypic modification of renal tubular cells. Vitamin D deficiency contributed to the elevation of plasma PTH and decrease of plasma FGF-23 levels as well as for important chronic tubulointerstitial changes. In addition, we found increased expression of cytokine TGF-β1 and decreased expression of VDR receptor and Klotho protein in vitamin D-deficient animals submitted to ischemia/reperfusion injury.

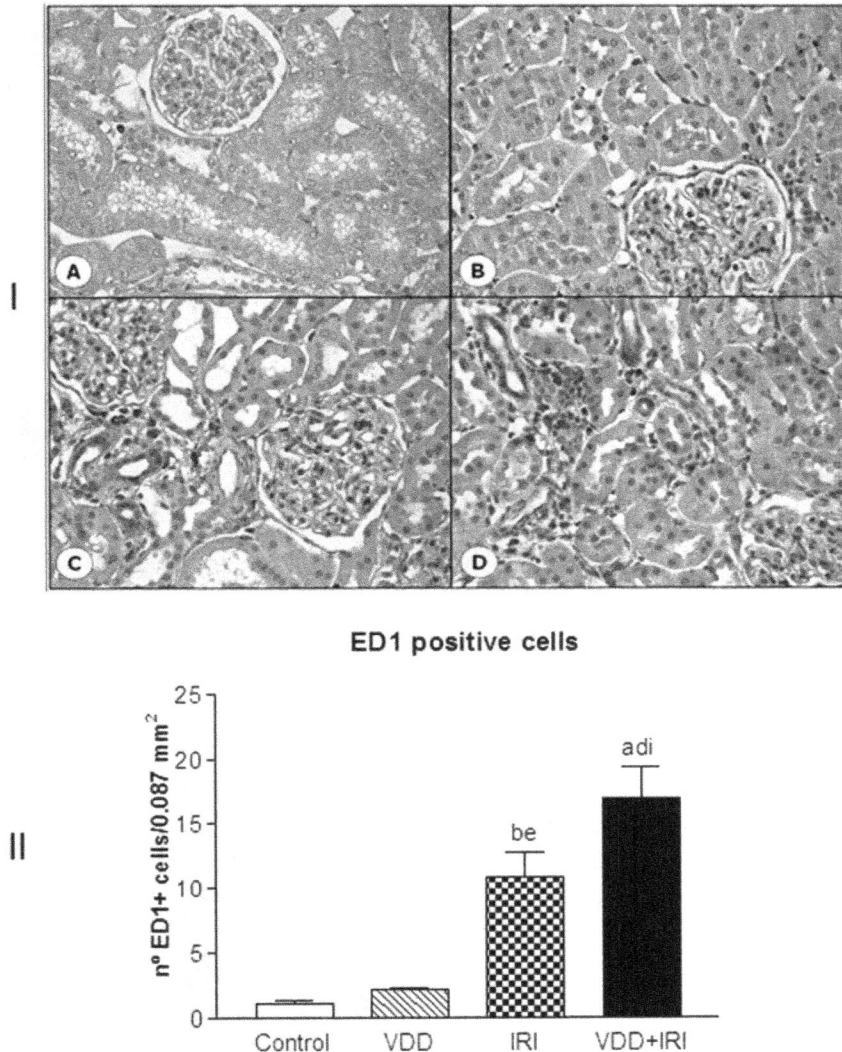

Figure 3. **[I] Expression of ED1 positive cells in the renal cortex of a control rat (A), a vitamin D deficient rat (B), in a rat submitted to ischemia/reperfusion injury (C), and in a vitamin D deficient rat submitted to ischemia/reperfusion injury (D).** [II] Number of ED1 positive cells per field (0.087 mm^2) evaluated 90 days after in Control (C), Vitamin D Deficiency (VDD), Ischemia-Reperfusion Injury (IRI), and Vitamin D Deficiency and Ischemia/Reperfusion Injury (VDD+IRI) groups. Values are mean ± SEM. [a] $p<0.001$ vs. C; [b] $p<0.01$ vs. C; [d] $p<0.001$ vs. VDD; [e] $p<0.01$ vs. VDD; [i] $p<0.05$ vs. IRI.

Our results clearly show that animals fed the vitamin D-free diet presented undetectable levels of 25(OH)D. The plasma level of 25(OH)D reflects vitamin D intake from foods and supplements, as well as cutaneous synthesis [24]. In addition to calcium and phosphorus, another important compound related to vitamin D synthesis is PTH level. Our results showed high levels of PTH in VDD, mainly in VDD+IRI group. These alterations were expected since the lack of vitamin D reduces intestinal calcium absorption, leading to a lower level of calcium and higher production of PTH by the parathyroid gland. PTH, in turn, acts on bone tissue in order to attenuate the decrease in serum calcium and the increase in phosphorus excretion [25].

We also investigated the role of vitamin D on blood pressure control. In our study, ischemic and vitamin D deficient rats showed higher levels of blood pressure. This alteration was accompanied by an increased mRNA expression of some RAS compounds, including renin, angiotensinogen and ACE. Further-more, we found increased levels of plasma aldosterone in VDD, IRI and VDD+IRI groups. So, our data reinforce an important role of vitamin D in blood pressure control. In fact, strong evidences from studies conducted in humans and animals show that vitamin D can be related to a decrease in the renin-angiotensin activity [26,27]. Also, it has been demonstrated that vitamin D deficiency can led to an upregulation of the RAS, changes in the endothelium, and vascular smooth cells as well [27–29]. Li et al [30] demonstrated that VDR knockout mice showed increased renin expression and hypertension, and these changes were suppressed by an analogue of vitamin D.

Studies have shown that vitamin D deficiency is associated with increased prevalence of proteinuria in adult population, a marker of CKD progression [31,32]. Our results showed a progressive and significant increase of proteinuria among the studied groups (C, VDD, IRI and VDD+IRI, respectively). In addition, it was noteworthy that vitamin D deficiency enhanced proteinuria in

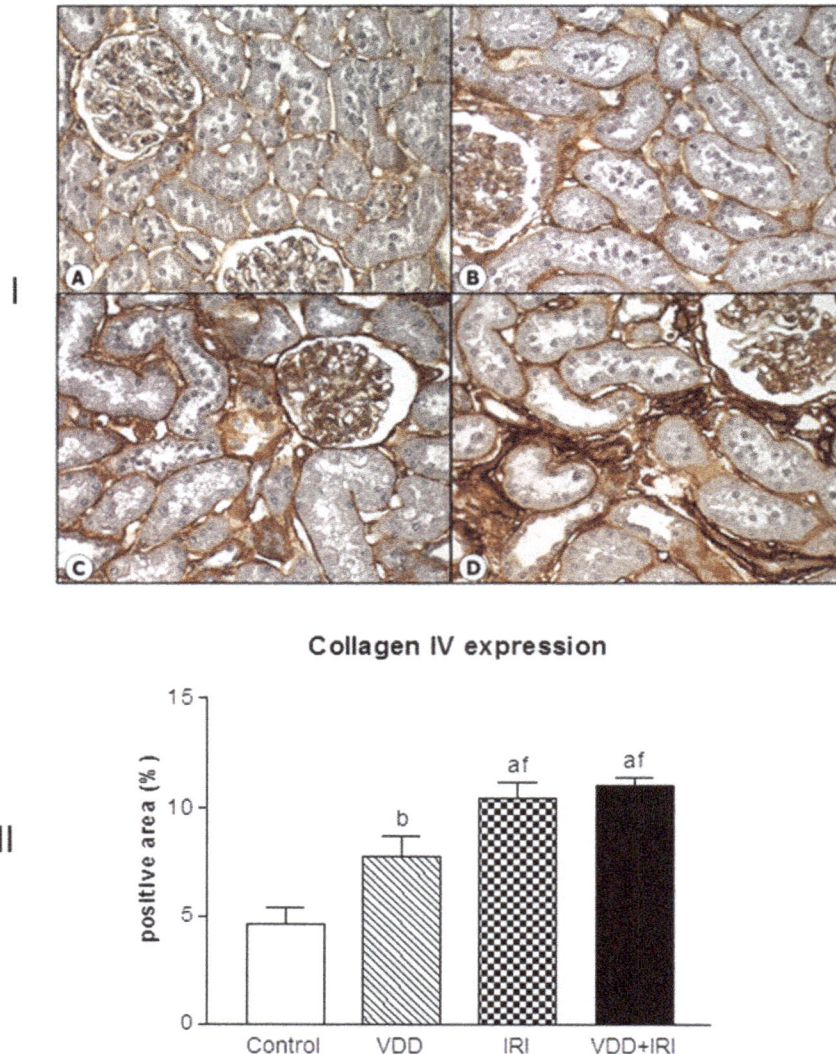

Figure 4. [I] Expression of type IV collagen in the renal cortex of a control rat (A), a vitamin D deficient rat (B), in a rat submitted to ischemia/reperfusion injury (C), and in a vitamin D deficient rat submitted to ischemia/reperfusion injury (D). [II] Evaluation of type IV collagen expression 90 days after in Control (C), Vitamin D Deficiency (VDD), Ischemia-Reperfusion Injury (IRI), and Vitamin D Deficiency and Ischemia/Reperfusion Injury (VDD+IRI) groups. Values are mean ± SEM. [a] $p<0.001$ vs. C; [b] $p<0.01$ vs. C; [f] $p<0.05$ vs. VDD.

VDD and VDD+IRI. However, the mechanisms by which proteinuria leads to reduced levels of vitamin D in the body or vice versa are not fully understood [32]. It is known that vitamin D levels can trigger proteinuria by direct and indirect factors. Through direct cellular effects, low levels of vitamin D induce loss of podocytes and development of glomerulosclerosis, damaging the integrity of the glomerular filtration membrane [33]. Indirectly, vitamin D suppresses renin transcription contributing to a reduction in proteinuria by hemodynamic effects [34].

As previously described, the conversion of vitamin D into biologically active form is tightly regulated by several factors, including FGF-23 [12]. In addition to promote renal phosphate excretion, FGF-23 suppresses the production of vitamin D by inhibition of 1-α-hydroxylase and stimulation of 24-hydroxylase [8,14–16]. Recent findings have been supporting an increasingly and important role of FGF-23 as the initial event in the development of CKD. The first step for that is featured by increased levels of FGF-23 preceding changes in calcium,

phosphorus, PTH, or even calcitriol levels [35], that is, its respective regulatory factors [36]. Curiously, in our study we found decreased levels of FGF-23 in both VDD and VDD+IRI groups. According to Rodriguez-Ortiz et al [37], this decreased FGF-23 levels could act as a compensatory response to prevent further reductions in calcitriol levels, which could exacerbate the hypocalcemia already expected by the evolution of CKD. So, a plausible explanation for our results is that we evaluated FGF-23 levels in a very early development of renal disease, without loss of renal function. Moreover, we must consider the diet used in our study for feeding the VDD and VDD+IRI animals. Besides being totally depleted of vitamin D, the diet also presented low levels of calcium and phosphorus, which may have contributed for the low levels of FGF-23 found in VDD and IRI+VDD groups.

An important partnership between FGF-23 and Klotho has been described [17]. Klotho proteins form binary complexes with FGF receptors, increasing Klotho affinity and selectivity for FGF-23 [17]. During kidney disease progression, there is reduced

Fibronectin expression

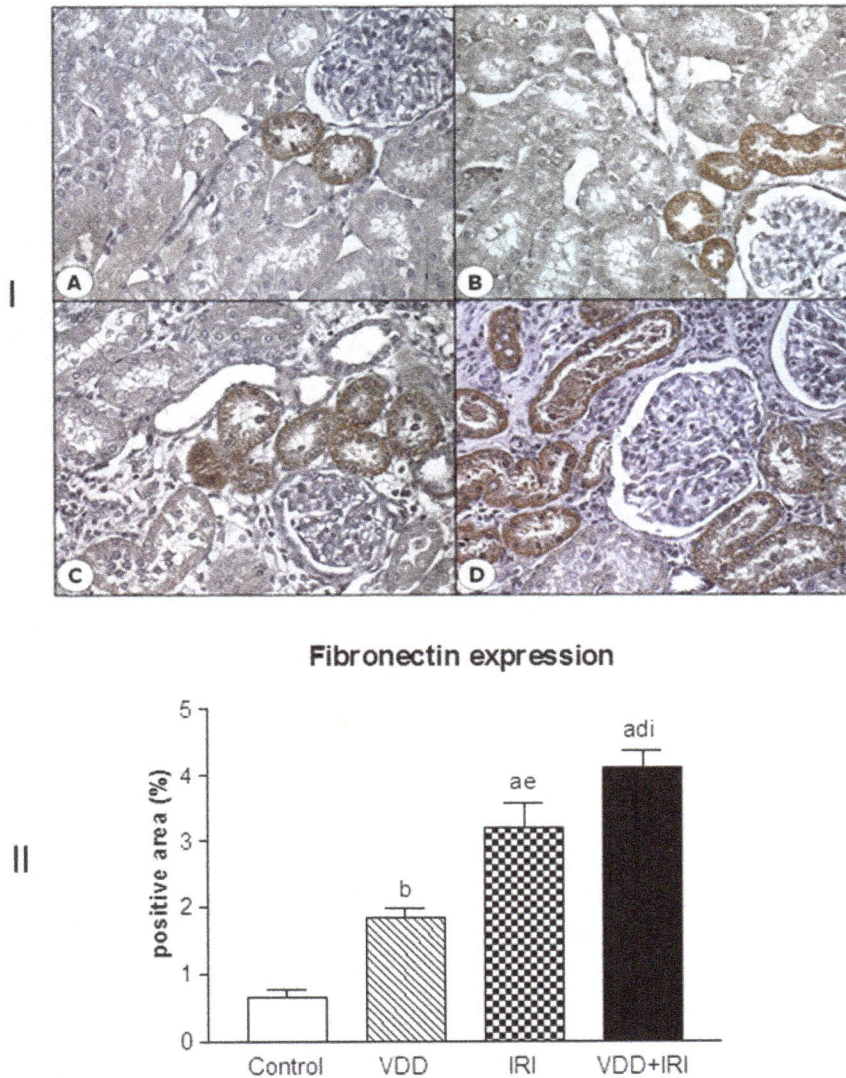

Figure 5. [I] Expression of fibronectin in the renal cortex of a control rat (A), a vitamin D deficient rat (B), in a rat submitted to ischemia/reperfusion injury (C), and in a vitamin D deficient rat submitted to ischemia/reperfusion injury (D). [II] Evaluation of fibronectin expression 90 days after in Control (C), Vitamin D Deficiency (VDD), Ischemia-Reperfusion Injury (IRI), and Vitamin D Deficiency and Ischemia/Reperfusion Injury (VDD+IRI) groups. Values are means ± SEM. [a] $p<0.001$ vs. C; [b] $p<0.01$ vs. C; [d] $p<0.001$ vs. VDD; [e] $p<0.01$ vs. VDD; [i] $p< 0.05$ vs. IRI.

expression of Klotho [38], a finding also confirmed in our study. We found a significant reduction in Klotho expression in VDD, IRI and VDD+IRI groups when compared to Control group. In addition, our data showed that vitamin D alone reduced Klotho expression in VDD animals, followed by a similar profile of gene expression for α-klotho. It is described that renal ischemia/reperfusion injury is related to Klotho deficiency. Ming-Chang Hu et al [39], using a murine model, showed that ischemic AKI was able to induce an acute and transient state of Klotho deficiency with recovery levels after seven days of injury. Most important, epidemiological studies have shown that increased levels of FGF-23, PTH and low levels of $1,25(OH)_2D_3$ are features that precede hyperphosphatemia during progression to CKD. Moreover, such alterations in FGF-23, PTH and vitamin D levels is usually followed by a progressive decrease in secreted Klotho protein in urine of CKD patients [39].

It is known that the pathological syndrome of CKD frequently does not heal but becomes self-sustaining, stimulating further kidney injury, resulting in progression of CKD [40]. In our study, a very relevant result related to morphological changes was found mainly in the kidney of vitamin D-deficient rats. Although no changes in renal function have been noticed, we observed an enlargement of the tubulointerstitial compartment associated with histological alterations (fibrosis, tubular atrophy and dilatation, and inflammatory cell infiltrates). Further, we analyzed the expression of two fibrous ECM components (fibronectin and type IV collagen) and infiltrating ED1 cells. We observed increased renal expression of both ECM markers and ED1 positive cells in VDD, IRI and VDD+IRI groups. Moreover, vitamin D deficiency enhanced the respective expressions of fibronectin, type IV collagen and ED1 cells.

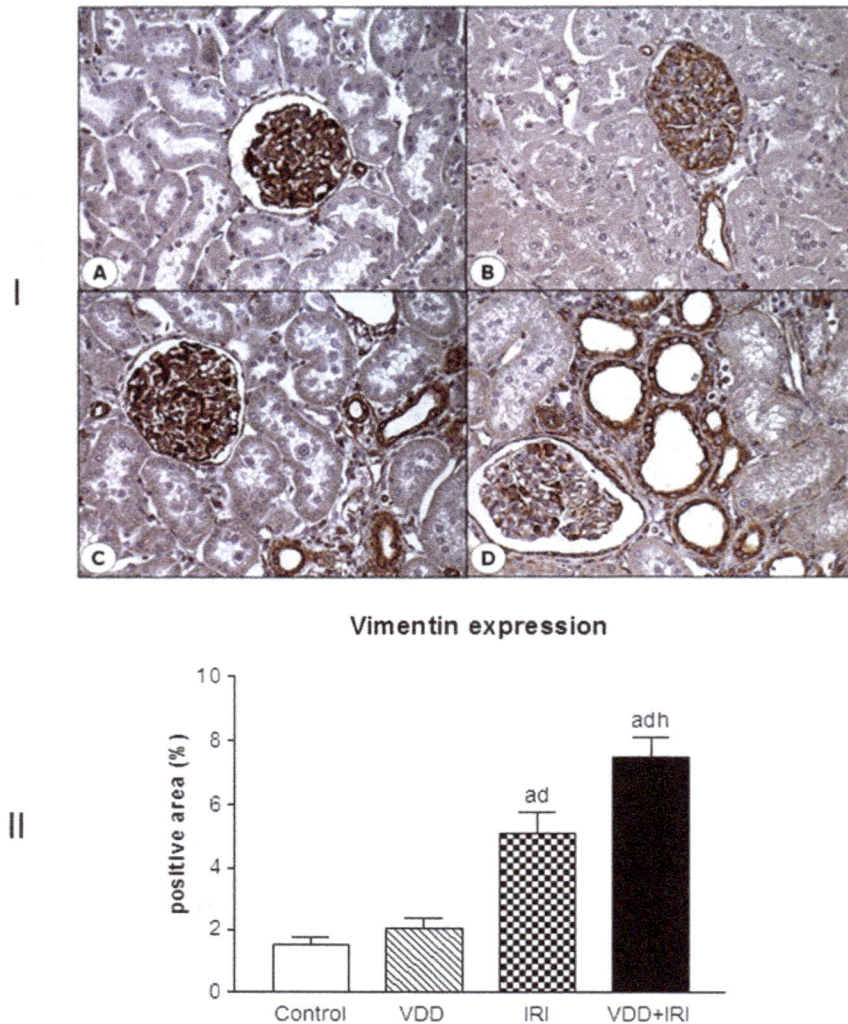

Figure 6. [I] Expression of vimentin in the renal cortex of a control rat (A), a vitamin D deficient rat (B), in a rat submitted to ischemia/reperfusion injury (C), and in a vitamin D deficient rat submitted to ischemia/reperfusion injury (D). [II] Evaluation of vimentin expression 90 days after in Control (C), Vitamin D Deficiency (VDD), Ischemia-Reperfusion Injury (IRI), and Vitamin D Deficiency and Ischemia/Reperfusion Injury (VDD+IRI) groups. Values are mean ± SEM. [a] $p<0.001$ vs. C; [d] $p<0.001$ vs. VDD; [h] $p<0.01$ vs. IRI.

Several studies have shown that the factors of initial injury to renal cell lead to: (a) vascular damage, including platelet aggregation and cytokine release; (b) activation of inflammatory responses with recruitment of neutrophils and monocytes, with subsequent pro-inflammatory cytokines releasing; and (c) fibrotic process, including pro-fibrogenic cytokine releasing such as TGF-β and CTGF (connective tissue growth factor) by macrophages and apoptotic parenchymal cells and activation of collagen-producing cells, among others [41]. These factors of initial injury can be initiated by many insults to the kidney, including toxic, ischemic, endocrine, infectious and immunological diseases [42]. In our case, we must consider two main conditions: endocrine and ischemia/reperfusion insult. As a matter of fact, our results showed morphological alterations associated with increased expression of fibrous ECM components and macrophages, including those observed in VDD group even without ischemic kidney injury. Regardless of the initial insult(s), CKD is characterized by stereotyped kidney injury responses seen pathologically as interstitial fibrosis, tubular atrophy, peritubular capillary rarefac-

tion, inflammation and glomerulosclerosis [43]. Moreover, pathologic deposition of fibrillar collagenous matrix, i.e., fibrosis, results when tissues are damaged and normal wound-healing response persist or become dysregulated, usually in response to sustained or repetitive injury. Therefore, our results allow us to infer that our VDD, IRI and VDD+IRI groups were under hemodynamic and hormonal conditions that contributed to the morphological changes found in the renal tissues.

Attempting to establish a link between fibrosis formation and vitamin D deficiency, we evaluated the expressions of TGF-β and VDR in IRI and VDD+IRI groups, both with more prominent interstitial expansion. We observed that vitamin D deficiency caused a decrease in VDR expression and an increase in TGF-β expression in VDD+IRI group, which had the highest ratio of fibrosis. Thus, our data allowed us to infer that adequate levels of vitamin D could help to slow the renal fibrosis formation. In 2006 Tan × et al [44], using the vitamin D analogue paricalcitol in a model of obstructive nephropathy, showed that paricalcitol treatment was able to suppress the expressions of TGF-β and its

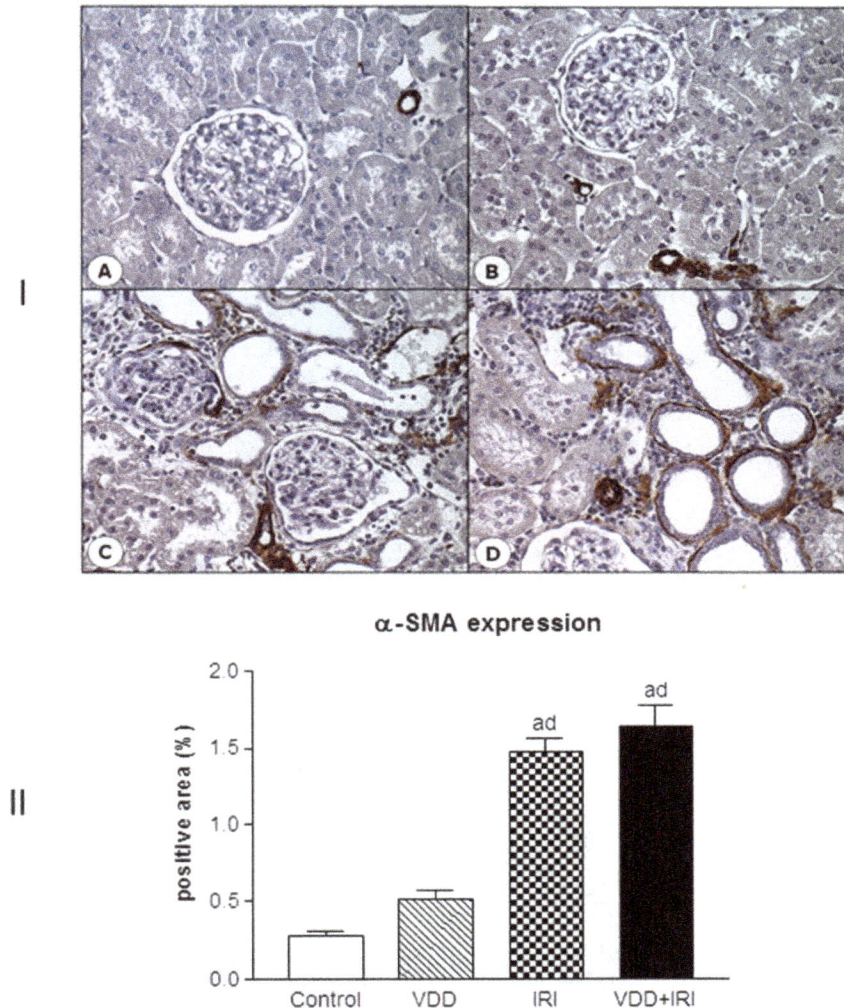

Figure 7. [I] Expression of α-SMA in the renal cortex of a control rat (A), a vitamin D deficient rat (B), in a rat submitted to ischemia/reperfusion injury (C), and in a vitamin D deficient rat submitted to ischemia/reperfusion injury (D). [II] Evaluation of α-SMA expression 90 days after in Control (C), Vitamin D Deficiency (VDD), Ischemia-Reperfusion Injury (IRI), and Vitamin D Deficiency and Ischemia/Reperfusion Injury (VDD+IRI) groups. Values are mean ± SEM. [a] $p < 0.001$ vs. C; [d] $p < 0.001$ vs. VDD.

respective receptor. In addition, paricalcitol treatment restored the expression of VDR receptor, blocked the epithelial-mesenchymal transition (EMT), and inhibited cell apoptosis and proliferation, showing that vitamin D plays a protective role on cellular integrity against cell injury process [44].

The relation of vitamin D to EMT process and our results concerning index of fibrosis in VDD+IRI group, aroused our interest to study whether renal tubule cells were under phenotypic modification. We observed a significant increase of vimentin expression in IRI and VDD+IRI groups and a similar profile of α-SMA expression, although without statistical difference. Based on that, we considered the involvement of vitamin D deficiency in cellular phenotypic alteration, since the animals from VDD+IRI groups presented more prominent expression of both markers. Xiong et al [45], showed that low expression of VDR in CKD could be a potential mechanism linking inflammation to EMT. It is known that pro-fibrotic effect of inflammation depends partly on EMT process. Such effect was possible by sustained stimulation with inflammatory cytokines (TNF-α or IL-1) on epithelial cells. According to the authors, TNF-α suppressed the expression of

VDR in various cell types, and sensitized cells to EMT process induced by TGF-β [45]. In our study, we found reduced expression of VDR and increased expression of TGF-β in VDD+IRI group, supporting the idea that vitamin D deficiency is associated with tubulointerstitial damage and interstitial fibrosis. So, a possible mechanism for that would include an association with inflammatory pathways, suggesting a combination between decreased VDR expression with increased TGF-β1 expression in our animals subjected to ischemia/reperfusion injury.

Based on our data, we can conclude that vitamin D deficiency is an aggravating factor for tubulointerstitial damage and formation of interstitial fibrosis after ischemia/reperfusion injury.

Acknowledgments

The authors thank Dr. Luciene Machado dos Reis from LIM-16 – Nephrology Department for her assistance in preparing the FGF-23 experiments.

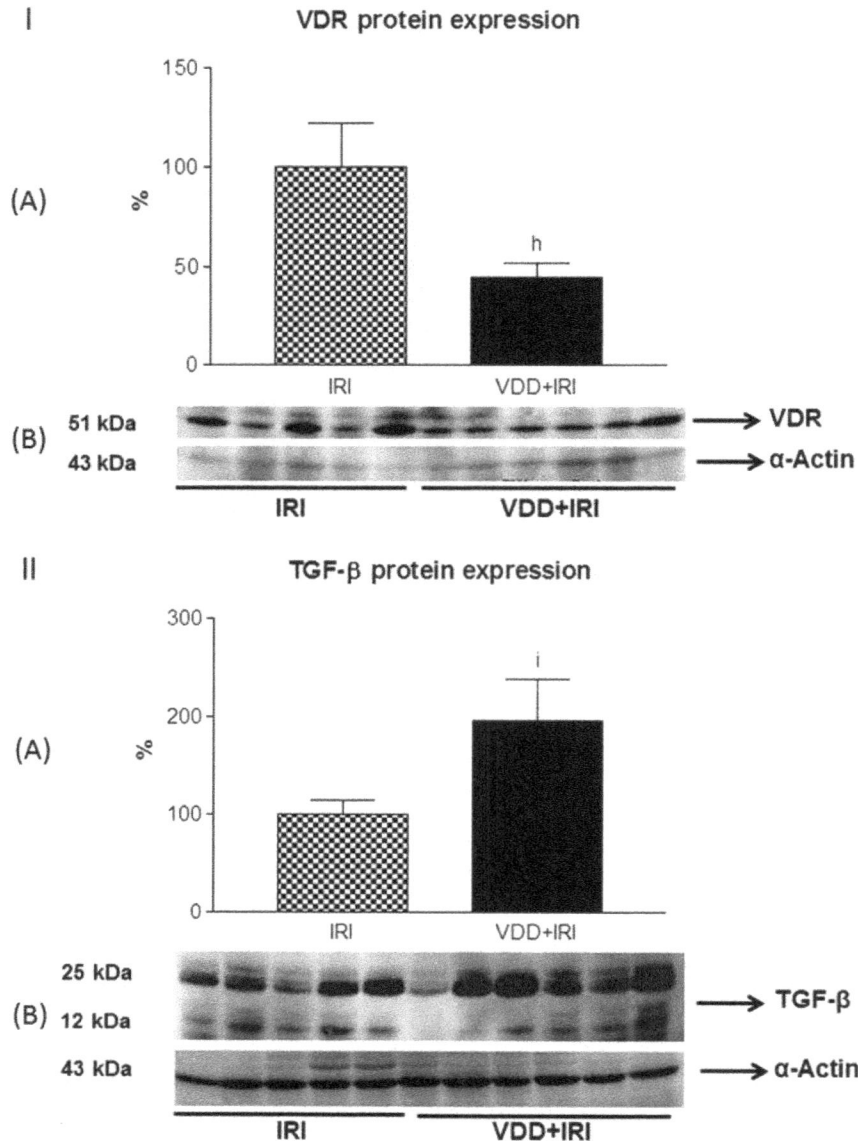

Figure 8. [I] Semiquantitative immunoblotting for VDR in kidney fractions. (A) A densitometric analysis of samples from IRI (n = 5) and VDD+IRI (n = 5) rats is shown. (B) Immunoblots reacted with anti-VDR revealing a 51-kDa band. Values are mean ± SEM. [h] p<0.01 vs. IRI. [II] Semiquantitative immunoblotting for TGF-β in kidney fractions. (A) A densitometric analysis of samples from IRI (n = 5) and VDD+IRI (n = 6) rats is shown. (B) Immunoblots reacted with anti-TGF-β revealing a 25 and 12-kDa bands. Values are mean ± SEM. [i] p<0.05 vs. IRI.

Author Contributions

Conceived and designed the experiments: RAV JGG ACS. Performed the experiments: JGG ACB DC MHMS TRS LA RAV. Analyzed the data: RAV JGG ACB LA RMAM TRS. Contributed reagents/materials/analysis tools: JGG ACB DC MHMS TRS RMAM LA ACS RAV. Contributed to the writing of the manuscript: RAV.

References

1. Francois H, Jacquet A, Beaudreuil S, Seidowsky A, Hebibi H, et al. (2011) Emerging strategies to preserve renal function. J Nephrol 24: 133–141.
2. Hagiwara S, Kantharidis P, Cooper ME (2012) What are new avenues for renal protection, in addition to RAAS inhibition? Curr Hypertens Rep 14: 100–110.
3. de Araujo M, Andrade L, Coimbra TM, Rodrigues AC, Jr., Seguro AC (2005) Magnesium supplementation combined with N-acetylcysteine protects against postischemic acute renal failure. J Am Soc Nephrol 16: 3339–3349.
4. Bonventre JV (2010) Pathophysiology of AKI: injury and normal and abnormal repair. Contrib Nephrol 165: 9–17.
5. Zhang Y, Kong J, Deb DK, Chang A, Li YC (2010) Vitamin D receptor attenuates renal fibrosis by suppressing the renin-angiotensin system. J Am Soc Nephrol 21: 966–973.
6. Patel TV, Singh AK (2009) Role of vitamin D in chronic kidney disease. Semin Nephrol 29: 113–121.
7. Baeke F, Gysemans C, Korf H, Mathieu C (2010) Vitamin D insufficiency: implications for the immune system. Pediatr Nephrol 25: 1597–1606.
8. Li YC (2011) Podocytes as target of vitamin D. Curr Diabetes Rev 7: 35–40.
9. Cuppari L, Garcia Lopes MG, Kamimura MA (2011) Vitamin D biology: from the discovery to its significance in chronic kidney disease. J Ren Nutr 21: 113–116.
10. Gonzalez EA, Sachdeva A, Oliver DA, Martin KJ (2004) Vitamin D insufficiency and deficiency in chronic kidney disease. A single center observational study. Am J Nephrol 24: 503–510.

11. Ulerich L (2010) Vitamin D in chronic kidney disease–new insights. Nephrol Nurs J 37: 429–431.
12. Holick MF (2007) Vitamin D deficiency. N Engl J Med 357: 266–281.
13. Braun AB, Christopher KB (2013) Vitamin D in acute kidney injury. Inflamm Allergy Drug Targets 12: 262–272.
14. Andress DL (2006) Vitamin D in chronic kidney disease: a systemic role for selective vitamin D receptor activation. Kidney Int 69: 33–43.
15. Perwad F, Azam N, Zhang MY, Yamashita T, Tenenhouse HS, et al. (2005) Dietary and serum phosphorus regulate fibroblast growth factor 23 expression and 1,25-dihydroxyvitamin D metabolism in mice. Endocrinology 146: 5358–5364.
16. Shimada T, Hasegawa H, Yamazaki Y, Muto T, Hino R, et al. (2004) FGF-23 is a potent regulator of vitamin D metabolism and phosphate homeostasis. J Bone Miner Res 19: 429–435.
17. Kuro-o M (2013) Klotho, phosphate and FGF-23 in ageing and disturbed mineral metabolism. Nat Rev Nephrol 9: 650–660.
18. Kuro-o M, Matsumura Y, Aizawa H, Kawaguchi H, Suga T, et al. (1997) Mutation of the mouse klotho gene leads to a syndrome resembling ageing. Nature 390: 45–51.
19. Burnette WN (1981) "Western blotting": electrophoretic transfer of proteins from sodium dodecyl sulfate–polyacrylamide gels to unmodified nitrocellulose and radiographic detection with antibody and radioiodinated protein A. Anal Biochem 112: 195–203.
20. Livak KJ, Schmittgen TD (2001) Analysis of relative gene expression data using real-time quantitative PCR and the 2(-Delta Delta C(T)) Method. Methods 25: 402–408.
21. Volpini RA, Costa RS, da Silva CG, Coimbra TM (2004) Inhibition of nuclear factor-kappaB activation attenuates tubulointerstitial nephritis induced by gentamicin. Nephron Physiol 98: p97–106.
22. Campos R, Shimizu MH, Volpini RA, de Braganca AC, Andrade L, et al. (2012) N-acetylcysteine prevents pulmonary edema and acute kidney injury in rats with sepsis submitted to mechanical ventilation. Am J Physiol Lung Cell Mol Physiol 302: L640–650.
23. Coimbra TM, Janssen U, Grone HJ, Ostendorf T, Kunter U, et al. (2000) Early events leading to renal injury in obese Zucker (fatty) rats with type II diabetes. Kidney Int 57: 167–182.
24. Powers JG, Gilchrest BA (2012) What you and your patients need to know about vitamin D. Semin Cutan Med Surg 31: 2–10.
25. Moe SM (2008) Disorders involving calcium, phosphorus, and magnesium. Prim Care 35: 215–237, v–vi.
26. Li YC (2003) Vitamin D regulation of the renin-angiotensin system. J Cell Biochem 88: 327–331.
27. Tamez H, Kalim S, Thadhani RI (2013) Does vitamin D modulate blood pressure? Curr Opin Nephrol Hypertens 22: 204–209.
28. Lucisano S, Buemi M, Passantino A, Aloisi C, Cernaro V, et al. (2013) New insights on the role of vitamin D in the progression of renal damage. Kidney Blood Press Res 37: 667–678.
29. Vaidya A, Williams JS (2012) The relationship between vitamin D and the renin-angiotensin system in the pathophysiology of hypertension, kidney disease, and diabetes. Metabolism 61: 450–458.
30. Li YC, Kong J, Wei M, Chen ZF, Liu SQ, et al. (2002) 1,25-Dihydroxyvitamin D(3) is a negative endocrine regulator of the renin-angiotensin system. J Clin Invest 110: 229–238.
31. de Boer IH, Ioannou GN, Kestenbaum B, Brunzell JD, Weiss NS (2007) 25-Hydroxyvitamin D levels and albuminuria in the Third National Health and Nutrition Examination Survey (NHANES III). Am J Kidney Dis 50: 69–77.
32. Lee DR, Kong JM, Cho KI, Chan L (2011) Impact of vitamin D on proteinuria, insulin resistance, and cardiovascular parameters in kidney transplant recipients. Transplant Proc 43: 3723–3729.
33. Kuhlmann A, Haas CS, Gross ML, Reulbach U, Holzinger M, et al. (2004) 1,25-Dihydroxyvitamin D3 decreases podocyte loss and podocyte hypertrophy in the subtotally nephrectomized rat. Am J Physiol Renal Physiol 286: F526–533.
34. Freundlich M, Quiroz Y, Zhang Z, Zhang Y, Bravo Y, et al. (2008) Suppression of renin-angiotensin gene expression in the kidney by paricalcitol. Kidney Int 74: 1394–1402.
35. Isakova T, Wolf MS (2010) FGF23 or PTH: which comes first in CKD? Kidney Int 78: 947–949.
36. Silver J, Naveh-Many T (2013) FGF-23 and secondary hyperparathyroidism in chronic kidney disease. Nat Rev Nephrol 9: 641–649.
37. Rodriguez-Ortiz ME, Lopez I, Munoz-Castaneda JR, Martinez-Moreno JM, Ramirez AP, et al. (2012) Calcium deficiency reduces circulating levels of FGF23. J Am Soc Nephrol 23: 1190–1197.
38. John GB, Cheng CY, Kuro-o M (2011) Role of Klotho in aging, phosphate metabolism, and CKD. Am J Kidney Dis 58: 127–134.
39. Hu MC, Shi M, Zhang J, Quinones H, Griffith C, et al. (2011) Klotho deficiency causes vascular calcification in chronic kidney disease. J Am Soc Nephrol 22: 124–136.
40. Campanholle G, Ligresti G, Gharib SA, Duffield JS (2013) Cellular mechanisms of tissue fibrosis. 3. Novel mechanisms of kidney fibrosis. Am J Physiol Cell Physiol 304: C591–603.
41. Kisseleva T, Brenner DA (2008) Mechanisms of fibrogenesis. Exp Biol Med (Maywood) 233: 109–122.
42. Snyder JJ, Foley RN, Collins AJ (2009) Prevalence of CKD in the United States: a sensitivity analysis using the National Health and Nutrition Examination Survey (NHANES) 1999–2004. Am J Kidney Dis 53: 218–228.
43. Grgic I, Duffield JS, Humphreys BD (2012) The origin of interstitial myofibroblasts in chronic kidney disease. Pediatr Nephrol 27: 183–193.
44. Tan X, Li Y, Liu Y (2006) Paricalcitol attenuates renal interstitial fibrosis in obstructive nephropathy. J Am Soc Nephrol 17: 3382–3393.
45. Xiong M, Gong J, Liu Y, Xiang R, Tan X (2012) Loss of vitamin D receptor in chronic kidney disease: a potential mechanism linking inflammation to epithelial-to-mesenchymal transition. Am J Physiol Renal Physiol 303: F1107–1115.

7

Indoxyl Sulfate-Induced Activation of (Pro)renin Receptor Promotes Cell Proliferation and Tissue Factor Expression in Vascular Smooth Muscle Cells

Maimaiti Yisireyili[1,3], Shinichi Saito[1], Shaniya Abudureyimu[1], Yelixiati Adelibieke[1], Hwee-Yeong Ng[4], Fuyuhiko Nishijima[2], Kyosuke Takeshita[3], Toyoaki Murohara[3], Toshimitsu Niwa[1,5]*

1 Department of Advanced Medicine for Uremia, Nagoya University Graduate School of Medicine, Nagoya, Japan, 2 Biomedical Research Laboratories, Kureha Co., Tokyo, Japan, 3 Department of Cardiology, Nagoya University Graduate School of Medicine, Nagoya, Japan, 4 Division of Nephrology, Department of Internal Medicine, Kaohsiung Chang Gung Memorial Hospital and Chang Gung University College of Medicine, Kaohsiung, Taiwan, 5 Faculty of Health and Nutrition, Shubun University, Aichi, Japan

Abstract

Chronic kidney disease (CKD) is associated with an increased risk of cardiovascular disease (CVD). (Pro)renin receptor (PRR) is activated in the kidney of CKD. The present study aimed to determine the role of indoxyl sulfate (IS), a uremic toxin, in PRR activation in rat aorta and human aortic smooth muscle cells (HASMCs). We examined the expression of PRR and renin/prorenin in rat aorta using immunohistochemistry. Both CKD rats and IS-administrated rats showed elevated expression of PRR and renin/prorenin in aorta compared with normal rats. IS upregulated the expression of PRR and prorenin in HASMCs. N-acetylcysteine, an antioxidant, and diphenyleneiodonium, an inhibitor of nicotinamide adenine dinucleotide phosphate oxidase, suppressed IS-induced expression of PRR and prorenin in HASMCs. Knock down of organic anion transporter 3 (OAT3), aryl hydrocarbon receptor (AhR) and nuclear factor-κB p65 (NF-κB p65) with small interfering RNAs inhibited IS-induced expression of PRR and prorenin in HASMCs. Knock down of PRR inhibited cell proliferation and tissue factor expression induced by not only prorenin but also IS in HASMCs.

Conclusion: IS stimulates aortic expression of PRR and renin/prorenin through OAT3-mediated uptake, production of reactive oxygen species, and activation of AhR and NF-κB p65 in vascular smooth muscle cells. IS-induced activation of PRR promotes cell proliferation and tissue factor expression in vascular smooth muscle cells.

Editor: Rudolf Kirchmair, Medical University Innsbruck, Austria

Funding: This work was supported by the research grant from Aichi Kidney Foundation, and a grant from Kureha Corporation, Japan. The funder provided support in the form of salaries for FN, but did not have additional role in the study design, data collection and analysis, decision to publish, or preparation of the manuscript. The specific role of these authors are articulated in the 'author contributions' section.

* Email: tniwa@med.nagoya.u-ac.jp

Introduction

Patients with chronic kidney disease (CKD) are at high risk for cardiovascular disease (CVD). CKD leads to accelerated atherosclerosis and consequently to a marked increase in cardiovascular morbidity and mortality [1]. Accumulation of indoxyl sulfate (IS), a protein-bound uremic toxin, is involved in the progression of not only CKD, but also CVD [2–4]. IS is a metabolite of tryptophan derived from dietary protein, and is synthesized in the liver from indole that is produced by intestinal flora including *Escherichia coli*. IS is normally excreted into urine. As renal function deteriorates, IS accumulates in serum due to its reduced renal clearance [2,5]. Because of its protein binding ability, removal by hemodialysis is not as efficient as that of non-protein bound uremic toxin. IS shows nephrotoxicity after its uptake by renal proximal tubular cells through the basolateral membrane via organic anion transporter 1 (OAT1) and OAT3 [6].

IS induces reactive oxygen species (ROS) and activates nuclear factor-κB (NF-κB) [7], p53 [8], and signal transducer and activator of transcription 3 (Stat3) [9]. Then, IS stimulates renal expression of fibrotic genes such as transforming growth factor-β1 (TGF-β1) [7,10], and α-smooth muscle actin (SMA) [7,8], and inflammatory genes such as monocyte chemotactic protein-1 (MCP-1) and intercellular adhesion molecule-1 (ICAM-1) in proximal tubular cells [11,12]. These pathophysiological changes facilitate kidney dysfunction such as interstitial fibrosis and inflammation, accelerating the progression of CKD [2,3].

Besides its negative effect on kidney, serum level of IS was associated with CVD and mortality in CKD patients [13]. IS promoted aortic calcification and senescence in hypertensive rats [14], and induced dysfunction of vascular endothelial cells [15,16], vascular smooth muscle cells [17,18], and cardiomyocytes [19,20]. Thus, IS is a nephrovascular uremic toxin [3].

Renin angiotensin system (RAS) plays an important role in CKD. (Pro)renin receptor (PRR), which binds to both renin and prorenin, is a newly discovered component of RAS, and is highly expressed not only in the kidney, but also in cardiovascular system [21–23].

Prorenin bound to PRR becomes enzymatically active, and can catalyze angiotensinogen into angiotensin (Ang) I. Further, PRR bound to prorenin or renin induces intracellular signaling and activation of mitogen-activated protein kinase (MAPK) ERK1/2, leading to activation of TGF-β1, independent of Ang II production [21,24]. PRR is expressed in the subendothelium of coronary arteries and, more precisely, in vascular smooth muscle cells [22]. Upregulation of PRR is involved in renal fibrosis [21,25], and vascular smooth muscle cell proliferation [22,26,27]. Further, recent studies revealed different roles of PRR, linked to the vacuolar H^+-ATPase (V-ATPase) activity, Wnt signaling, and autophagy [28–32]. Thus, PRR activation plays an important role in the pathophysiology of not only CKD but also CVD.

IS induces vascular smooth muscle cell proliferation through ROS and activation of p44/42 MAPK pathway [33,34]. IS induces tissue factor expression and activity in vascular smooth muscle cells [35]. Tissue factor is a crucial mediator of injury-related thrombosis and vascular smooth muscle cell proliferation, and has been implicated for stent thrombosis observed in patients with advanced CKD [35]. However, the role of IS in PRR expression in vascular smooth muscle cells has not yet been studied.

The present study aimed to clarify whether IS induces PRR expression in rat aortic tissues and human aortic smooth muscle cells (HASMCs), and whether PRR mediates IS-induced cell proliferation and tissue factor expression in HASMCs.

Methods

Reagents

Reagents and antibodies were obtained from the following companies: HASMCs were purchased from Cascade Biologics (Portland, OR, USA). Dulbecco's modified Eagle's medium (D-MEM), fetal bovine serum (FBS), penicillin–streptomycin and trypsin-EDTA solutions were purchased from Gibco (Invitrogen, Grand Island, NY, USA). IS was from Sigma Chemical (St. Louis, MO, USA). N-acetylcyteine (NAC), an antioxidant, and diphenyleneiodonium chloride (DPI), an inhibitor of nicotinamide adenine dinucleotide phosphate (NADPH) oxidase, were obtained from Calbiochem (La Jolla, CA, USA). Human prorenin was obtained from Molecular Innovations (Novi, MI, USA). Anti-PRR and anti-prorenin antibodies were from Abcam (Cambridge, UK). Anti-renin/prorenin antibody used for immunohistochemistry, which cross-reacts with renin and prorenin [36], was kindly provided by Tadashi Inagami (Department of Biochemistry, Vanderbilt University School of Medicine, Nashville, TN, USA). Anti-NF-κB p65, anti-aryl hydrocarbon receptor (AhR), and anti-tissue factor antibodies were from Santa Cruz Biotechnology (Santa Cruz, CA, USA). Anti-α-tubulin was from Calbiochem (La Jolla, CA, USA). Anti-rabbit IgG horseradish peroxidase (HRP)-linked antibody and anti-mouse IgG HRP-linked antibody were from Cell Signaling Technology (Beverly, MA, USA). CellTiter 96 Aqueous One Solution Cell Proliferation Assay was from Promega (Madison, WI, USA), and Lipofectamine RNA iMAX reagent was from Invitrogen (Life Technologies, Carsbad, CA, USA).

Animal Study 1

Experimental rats were prepared as reported previously [37]. Seven-week old male Sprague-Dawley rats (Clea, Tokyo, Japan) were used to produce CKD rats by 5/6- nephrectomy. Eleven weeks after subtotal nephrectomy, the rats were randomized into two groups, control CKD rats (n = 8), and AST-120-treated CKD rats (n = 8). AST-120 was orally administered to the rats at a dose of 4 g/kg/day with powder chow (CE-2, Clea, Tokyo, Japan) for 10 weeks, whereas powder chow alone was administered to control CKD rats. Normal rats (n = 9) were used to compare the data with CKD rats. After administration of AST-120 for 16 weeks, the rats were anesthetized, and arcuate aortas were excised for immunohistochemical study.

Animal Study 2

Experimental rats were prepared as reported previously [38]. Briefly, the animal groups consisted of: (1) Dahl normotensive rats (DN, n = 8), (2) Dahl normotensive IS-administered rats (DN+IS, n = 8), (3) Dahl hypertensive rats (DH, n = 8), and (4) Dahl hypertensive IS-administered rats (DH+IS, n = 8). IS (200 mg/kg/day in drinking water) was administered to the rats. At 48 weeks of age (32nd week of the study), their arcuate aortas were excised for immunohistochemical analysis. Serum IS levels were measured by high-performance liquid chromatography as reported previously [5]. Blood pressure was measured using the tails of the rats with a pneumatic cuff and a sphygmomanometer for small animals (UR-5000, Ueda Avancer Co., Tokyo, Japan).

The Animal Care Committee of Kureha Biomedical Research Laboratories approved these animal studies, which proceeded according to the Guiding Principles for the Care and Use of Laboratory Animals of the Japanese Pharmacological Society.

Immunohistochemistry

Immunohistochemistry was performed according to the streptavidin-biotinylated peroxidase complex (SABC) method. Aortic sections were deparaffinized with xylene, and dehydrated with ethanol. Endogenous peroxidase activity was inhibited with 0.3% H_2O_2 in methanol at room temperature for 10 min, followed by a rinse with phosphate buffered saline (PBS). All sections were incubated with 10% normal serum at room temperature for 30 min. Heat-mediated antigen retrieval method was performed twice by microwave treatment with 0.01 mol/L citrate buffer (pH 6.0) for 5 min. Then, the sections were treated at 4°C overnight with a primary antibody, anti-PRR antibody (1:100) or anti-renin/prorenin (1:50) antibody which cross reacts with renin and prorenin. Then, the sections were incubated with a secondary antibody at room temperature for 30 min followed by a rinse with PBS, and then treated with peroxidase-conjugated streptavidin (Nichirei Co) at 37°C for 30 min. Finally, localization of PRR and renin/prorenin was visualized using 3,3-diaminobenzidine tetrahydrochloride (DAB tablet; Merck KGaA, Darmstadt, Germany) at a concentration of 30 mg/mL, containing 0.03% H_2O_2. Then, the sections were counterstained with methylene green, and mounted in mounting media (Mount-quick, Daydo Sangyo Co., Saitama, Japan). All sections were photographed under light microscopy (×400) with digital camera (DN100, E-600, Nikon; Tokyo, Japan). Immunostaining-positive areas were determined using Adobe Photoshop, and quantified in 10 random fields per section using NIH Image 1.62.

Cell Culture

HASMCs were maintained in D-MEM containing 10% FBS supplemented with 100 U/mL penicillin, 100 μg/mL streptomycin at standard cell culture condition (37°C under 5% CO_2 humidified atmosphere). The medium was replaced every three days until confluence. Only cells between passages 2 to 8 were used for experiments.

Measurement of Cell Proliferation

Proliferation of HASMCs was measured using Cell Titer 96 Aqueous One Solution Cell Proliferation Assay [16]. Cells were seeded at a density of 5×10^3 cells/well on 24 well culture plate in D-MEM containing 10% FBS for 48 h. Serum-starved HASMCs (5×10^3 cells/well) in a 24-well plate were stimulated with or without IS (250 µmol/L) or prorenin (20 nmol/L) for 24 h. For gene knockdown experiment, HASMCs were transfected with siRNA for PRR (20 nmol/L) for 48 h, before IS or prorenin stimulation. Thereafter, cell proliferation reagent MTS (50 µL) was added to each well, and cells were incubated for 4 h. The absorbance was measured at 492 nm using a microplate reader (DS PharmaBiomedical Co., Ltd, Osaka, Japan).

Quantitative Real-Time Polymerase Chain Reaction (RT-PCR)

Total RNA was extracted from HASMCs lysates using TRIzol Reagent (Life Technologies, Carlsbad, CA) and subjected to reverse transcription. The cDNA was subjected to a quantitative RT-PCR analysis with the use of a Bio-Rad CFX96 RT-PCR Detection System and Power SYBR Green PCR Master Mix (Applied Biosystems, Foster City, CA). Serial dilutions of a control sample of cDNA were used as the standard curve for each reaction. All experiments were performed in triplicate. Changes in gene expression were normalized the values to the levels of glyceraldehyde 3-phosphate dehydrogenase (GAPDH). Primers (Sigma-Aldrich) used were: PRR, 5'-AAT TGG CCT ATA CCA GGA GAG C-3' (forward) and 5'-GAA ACA GGT TAC CCA CTG CGA-3' (reverse); Prorenin, 5'-CCA CCT CCG TGA TCC T-3' (forward) and 5'-GCG GAT AGT ACT GGG TGT CCA T-3' (reverse); GAPDH, 5'-ATG GGG AAG GTG AAG GTC G-3' (forward) and 5'-GGG GTC ATT GAT GGC AAC AAT A-3' (reverse).

Transfection of siRNA

Small interfering RNAs (siRNAs) specific to OAT3 (OAT3 siRNA) and AhR (AhR siRNA) were purchased from Santa Cruz Biotechnology (Santa Cruz, CA, USA). siRNAs specific to PRR (PRR siRNA) and NF-κB p65 (NF-κB p65 siRNA) were obtained from Nippon EGT (Tokyo, Japan). Lipofectamine RNA iMAX (Invitrogen, Life Technologies, Carsbad, CA, USA) was used to transfect siRNA into HASMCs cells according to a manufacturer's protocol. HASMCs were incubated with or without OAT3 siRNA (10 nmol/L), AhR siRNA (30 nmol/L), NF-κB p65 siRNA (10 nmol/L) or PRR siRNA (20 nmol/L) for 48 h. Protein expressions of OAT3, AhR, NF-κB p65, and PRR were analyzed by western blotting.

Western Blot Analysis

Serum-starved HASMCs were incubated with 250 µmol/L of IS for the indicated time periods. Cells were pretreated with 2.5 mmol/L NAC and 10 µmol/L DPI for 30 min, before IS stimulation for 24 h. For gene knock down experiment, HASMCs were transfected with siRNAs (siOAT3, siPRR, sip65 and siAhR) for 48 h, before IS stimulation. Cells were lysed in lysis buffer

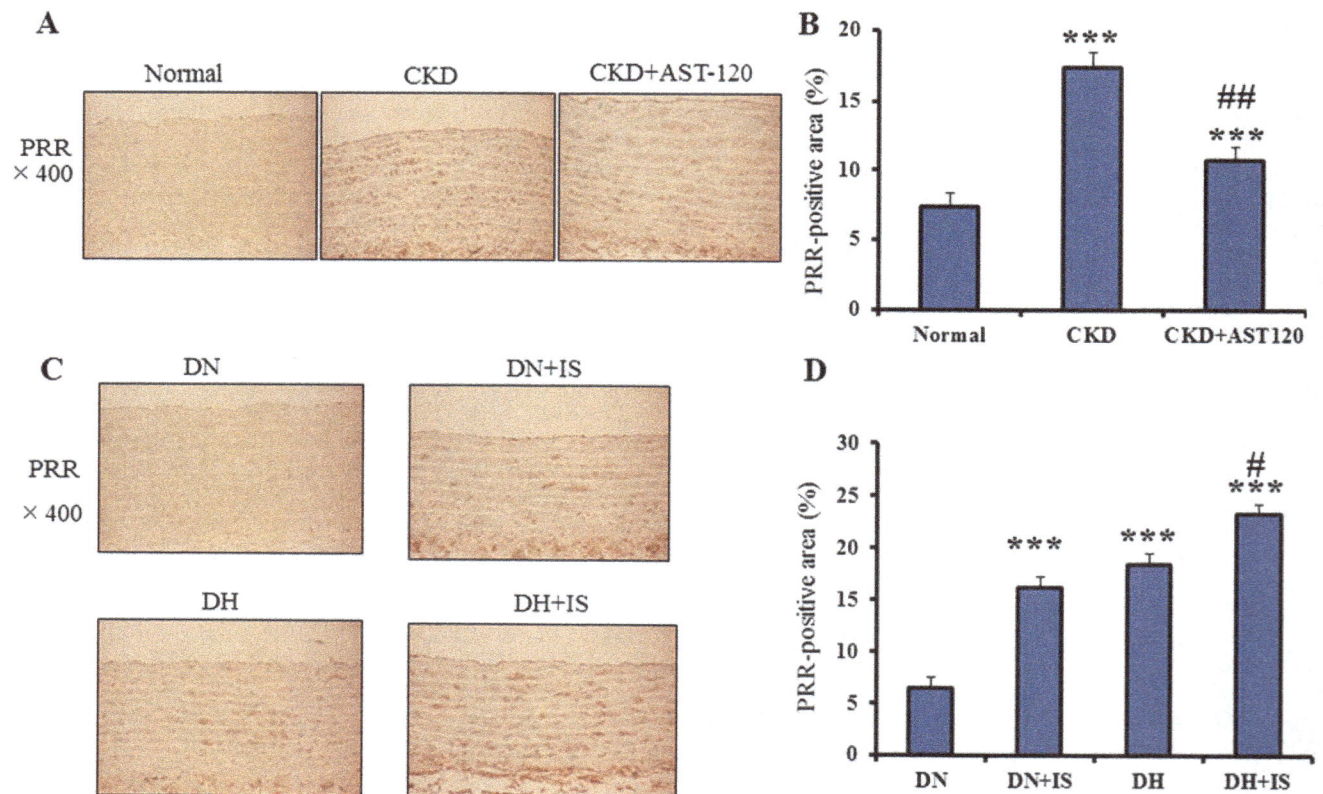

Figure 1. Immunohistochemistry of PRR in rat aorta. A. Immonohistochemical localization of PRR in the aortas of normal, CKD and AST-120-treated CKD rats. **B.** Quantitative data of PRR in the aortas of normal (n = 9), CKD (n = 8) and AST-120-treated CKD rats (n = 8) (mean±SE). ***p<0.001 vs normal, ##p<0.001 vs CKD. **C.** Immonohistochemical localization of PRR in the aortas of DN, DN+IS, DH and DH+IS rats. **D.** Quantitative data of PRR-positive area in the aorta of DN, DN+IS, DH and DH+IS rats (mean±SE, n = 8). ***p<0.001vs DN, #p<0.05 vs DH.

(65 mmol/L Tris-HCl (PH 6.8), 3.3% sodium dodecyl sulfate (SDS), 10% glycerol, 2.2% bromophenol blue) and were fractionated by SDS-polyacrylamide gel electrophoresis (PAGE) on polyacrylamide gels. Then, proteins were transferred to polyvinylidene difluoride (PVDF) membranes (Immobilon-P, Millipore Bedford, MA, USA). The membranes were blocked with 5% bovine serum albumin (BSA) in Tris-buffered saline tween-20 (TBS-T) at room temperature for 1 h. After washing with TBS-T, the membranes were treated with rabbit polyclonal anti-PRR antibody (1:1000), rabbit monoclonal anti-prorenin antibody (1:1000), rabbit polyclonal anti-OAT3 antibody (1:500), rabbit polyclonal anti-NF-κB p65 antibody (1:1000), rabbit polyclonal anti-AhR antibody (1:1000) and goat polyclonal anti-tissue factor antibody (1:1000), respectively. Then, the membranes were further incubated with HRP-linked secondary antibody (1:5000) at room temperature for 1 h. After washing with TBS-T three times, the protein expressions were visualized using the enhanced Chemi-Lumi one system (Nacalai Tesque, Kyoto, Japan). The intensity of protein bands normalized to the amount of α-tubulin (an internal control, 1:1000) is expressed as ratios (fold increase) of the control value.

Statistical Analysis

Results are expressed as mean±SE. The quantitative data among different groups were analyzed by Fisher's protected least significant difference (PLSD) test of one-way analysis of variance (ANOVA). Results were considered statistically significant when P value was <0.05.

Results

AST-120 Supresses Aortic Expression of PRR in CKD Rats

An oral absorbent (AST-120, Kremezin, Kureha Co., Tokyo, Japan) reduces serum levels of IS in CKD rats and patients [39]. To examine the effects of AST-120 on PRR expression in aorta, AST-120 was orally administered to CKD rats. Laboratory parameters of the animal study 1 were described previously [37]. Briefly, serum levels of IS were 0.008±0.007 mg/dL in normal rats, 0.52±0.16 mg/dL in CKD rats, and 0.12±0.02 mg/dL in AST-120-treated CKD rats [37].

CKD rats showed significantly increased expression of PRR in the arcuate aorta compared with normal rats (Figure 1A, B). On the other hand, AST-120-treated CKD rats revealed significantly reduced expression of PRR in the arcuate aorta compared with CKD rats (Figure 1A, B).

IS Enhances Aortic Expression of PRR in Normotensive and Hypertensive Rats

To determine the effect of IS on PRR expression in aorta, IS was orally administered to normotensive and hypertensive rats. Laboratory parameters of animal study 2 were reported previously [38]. Briefly, serum levels of IS at the 32nd weeks of the study

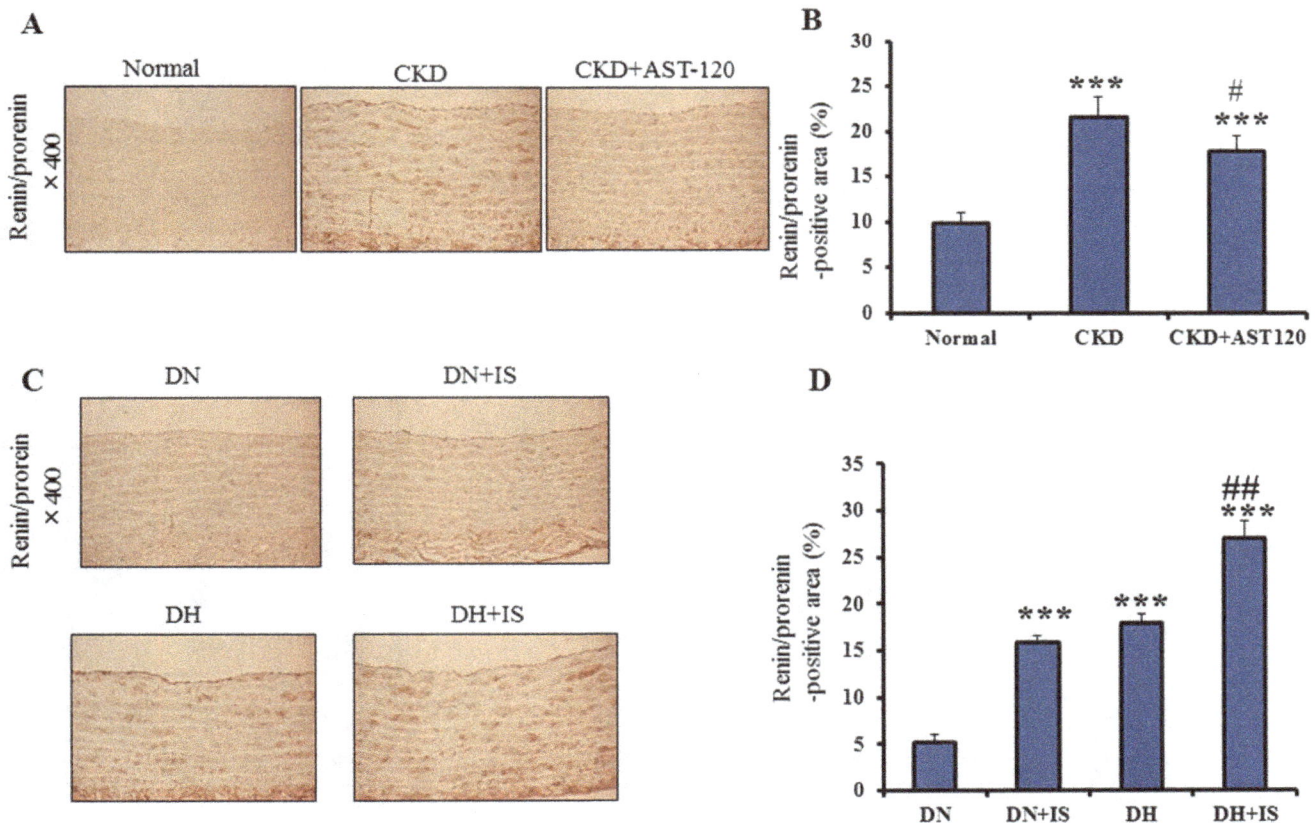

Figure 2. Immunohistochemistry of renin/prorenin in rat aorta. A. Immonohistochemical localization of renin/prorenin in the aortas of normal, CKD and AST-120-treated CKD rats. B. Quantitative data of renin/prorenin-positive area in the aortas of normal (n = 9), CKD (n = 8) and AST-120-treated CKD rats (n = 8) (Mean±SE). ***p<0.001 vs normal, #p<0.05 vs CKD. C. Immonohistochemical localization of renin/prorenin in the aortas of DN, DN+IS, DH and DH+IS rats. D. Quantitative data of renin/prorenin-positive area in the aortas of DN, DN+IS, DH and DH+IS rats (mean±SE, n = 8). ***p<0.001vs DN, ##p<0.01 vs DH.

were; 0.10±0.01 mg/dL in DN rats, 0.94±0.13 mg/dL in DN+ IS rats, 0.06±0.01 mg/dL in DH rats, and 1.89±0.26 mg/dL in DH+IS rats [38]. Systolic blood pressure levels at the 32nd weeks of the study were; 143±3 mmHg in DN rats, 141±3 mmHg in DN+IS rats, 158±5 mmHg in DH rats, and 158±9 mmHg in DH+IS rats [38].

DN+IS, DH and DH+IS rats showed significantly increased expression levels of PRR in arcuate aorta compared with DN rats (Figure 1C,D). Furthermore, DH+IS rats showed significantly elevated expression level of PRR in arcuate aorta compared with DH rats (Figure 1C,D). Taken together, IS as well as hypertension increased PRR expression in rat aorta.

Aortic Expression of Renin/prorenin is Increased in CKD Rats and IS-treated Rats

Immunohistochemical analysis was conducted to examine whether IS upregulates renin/prorenin expression in the aorta of

CKD rats and IS-treated rats. Anti-renin/prorenin antibody, which cross reacts with renin and prorenin, was used as a primary antibody [36]. Aortic expression of renin/prorenin was significantly increased in CKD rats compared with normal rats. However, AST-120-treated CKD rats reduced the expression of renin/prorenin compared with CKD rats (Figure 2A,B).

Aortic expression of renin/prorenin was significantly increased in DN+IS and DH+IS rats compared with DN and DH rat, respectively (Figure 2C,D). Taken together, CKD rats and IS-administered rats showed increased expression of renin/prorenin in the aorta.

IS Induces PRR Expression in Vascular Smooth Muscle Cells

We confirmed the effect of IS on expression of PRR by incubating HASMCs with IS at indicated time periods and concentrations. IS stimulated expression of PRR mRNA and

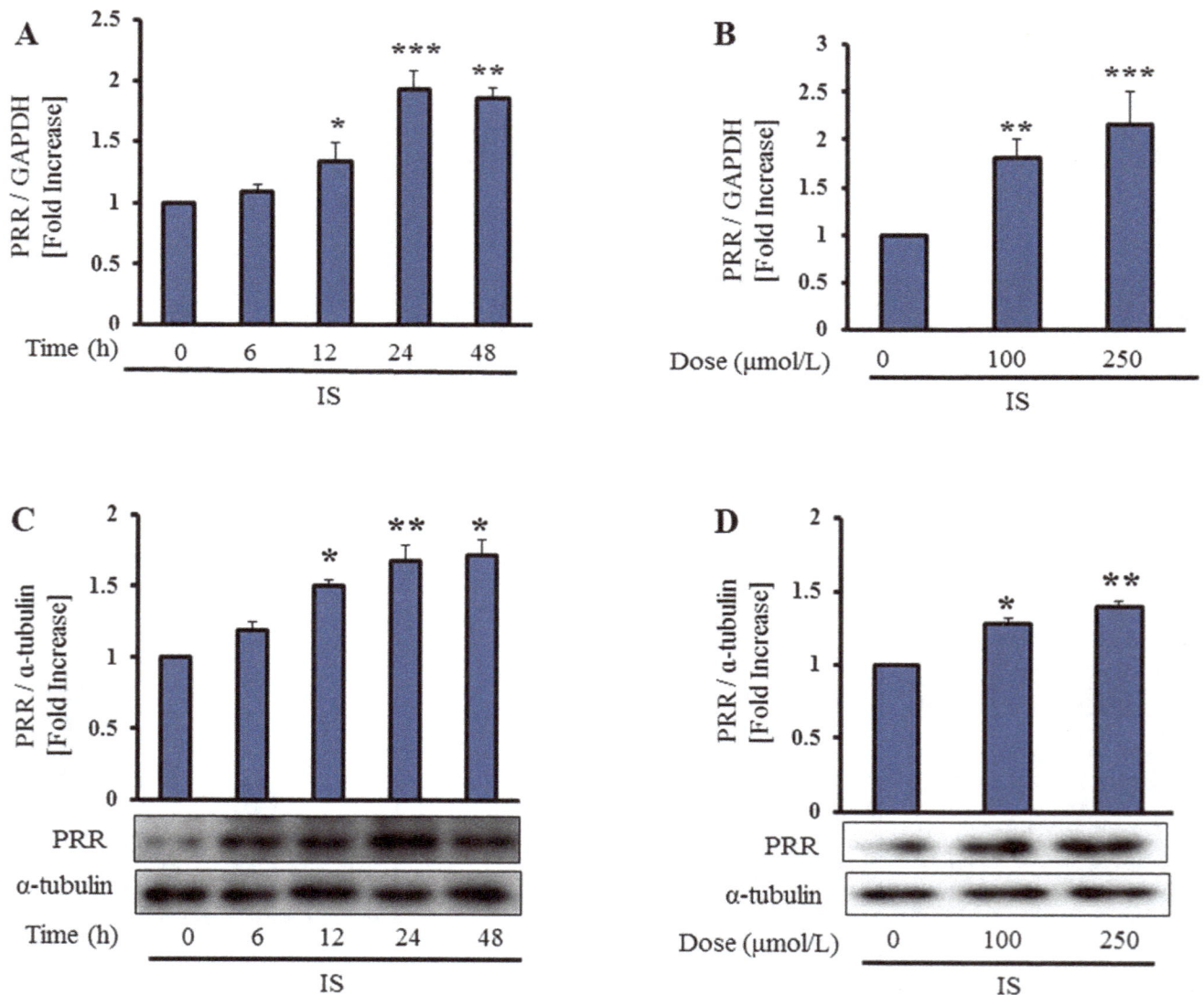

Figure 3. IS induces PRR expression in vascular smooth muscle cells. Serum-starved HASMCs were treated with IS (250 μmol/L). Incubation with IS increased PRR mRNA and protein expression in HASMCs time- (A, C) and dose- (B, D) dependently. Mean±SE (n = 3). *p<0.05, **p<0.01, ***p<0.001 vs control.

protein in a time- and dose-dependent manner in HASMCs (Figure 3A–D). The molecular weight of PRR protein was 39 kDa. PRR expression was examined at 24 h after incubating with IS at different concentrations. IS at a concentration of 250 µmol/L was used for the further *in-vitro* study, because it is comparable to the mean serum level of IS in hemodialysis patients [2].

ROS, OAT3, AhR and NF-κB p65 are Involved in IS-Induced PRR Expression in Vascular Smooth Muscle Cells

Serum-starved HASMCs were pre-incubated with 2.5 mmol/L NAC, an antioxidant, or 10 µmol/L of DPI, an inhibitor of NADPH oxidase, and then stimulated with 250 µmol/L IS for 24 h (Figure 4A,B). IS induces ROS production and expression of NADPH oxidase 4 (NOX-4) in HASMCs [16,17]. Both NAC and DPI suppressed IS-induced protein expression of PRR. Therefore, IS upregulated PRR expression in HASMCs through ROS. IS is transported into HASMCs by OAT3 [6]. OAT3 siRNA suppressed IS-induced expression of PRR in HASMCs (Figure 4D), Thus, IS is taken up by OAT3, and induces PRR expression in HASMCs.

IS was identified as an AhR agonist in human hepatocytes [40], endothelial cells [41,42], and vascular smooth muscle cells [43]. Activation of AhR mediates IS-induced expression of MCP-1 and tissue factor in endothelial cells [41]. IS activates NF-κB pathway in proximal tubular cells [7] and endothelial cells [14]. We hypothesized that IS-induced expression of PRR and prorenin is mediated by activation of AhR and NF-κB p65. Both AhR siRNA and NF-κB p65 siRNA suppressed IS-induced expression of PRR (Figure 4E,F). Thus, IS induced expression of PRR through activation of AhR and NF-κB p65 in HASMCs.

IS Induces Prorenin Expression in Vascular Smooth Muscle Cells

Prorenin which is bound to PRR, becomes enzymatically active, and then catalyzes angiotensinogen into Ang I. Further, prorenin-bound PRR induces intracellular signaling [21]. However, if prorenin does not exist, PRR could not be activated. Therefore, we examined whether IS induces prorenin expression in HASMCs. IS promoted expression of prorenin mRNA and protein in HASMCs time- and dose-dependently (Figure 5A–D). The molecular weight of prorenin was 47 kDa.

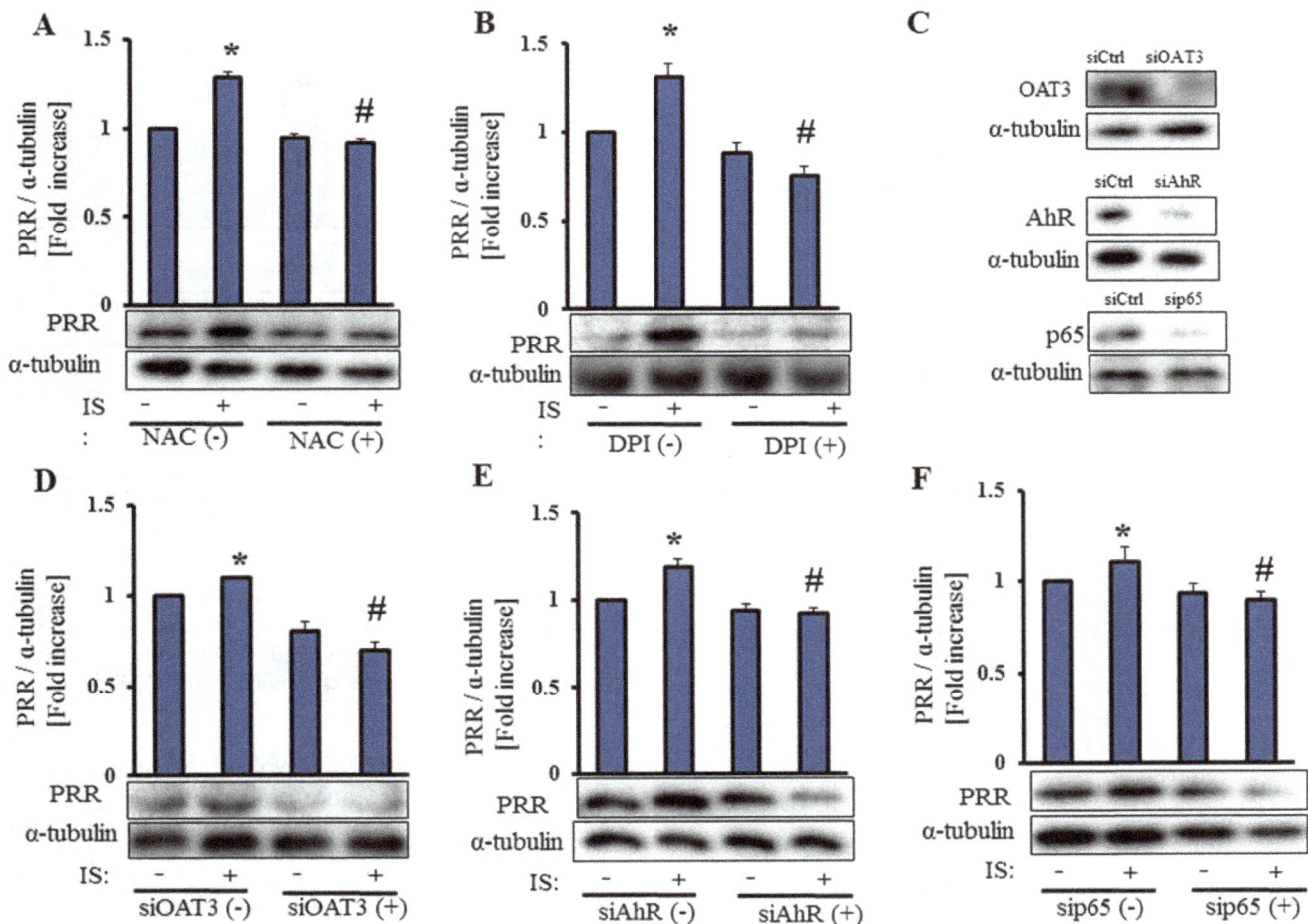

Figure 4. ROS, OAT3, AhR and NF-κB p65 are involved in IS-induced PRR expression in vascular smooth muscle cells. Serum-starved HASMCs were pretreated with NAC (2.5 mmol/L) and DPI (10 µmol/L) for 30 min before incubation with IS (250 µmol/L) for 24 h (A,B). HASMCs were transfected with or without OAT3 siRNA (10 nmol/L), AhR siRNA (30 nmol/L) or p65 siRNA (10 nmol/L), and serum starved for 24 h, followed by incubation with IS (250 µmol/L) for 24 h. Cell lysates were immunoblotted using anti-OAT3, anti-AhR, anti-p65 and anti-PRR antibodies (C–F). Mean±SE (n = 3). *p<0.05 vs control, #p<0.05 vs IS-treated group. Ctrl: control.

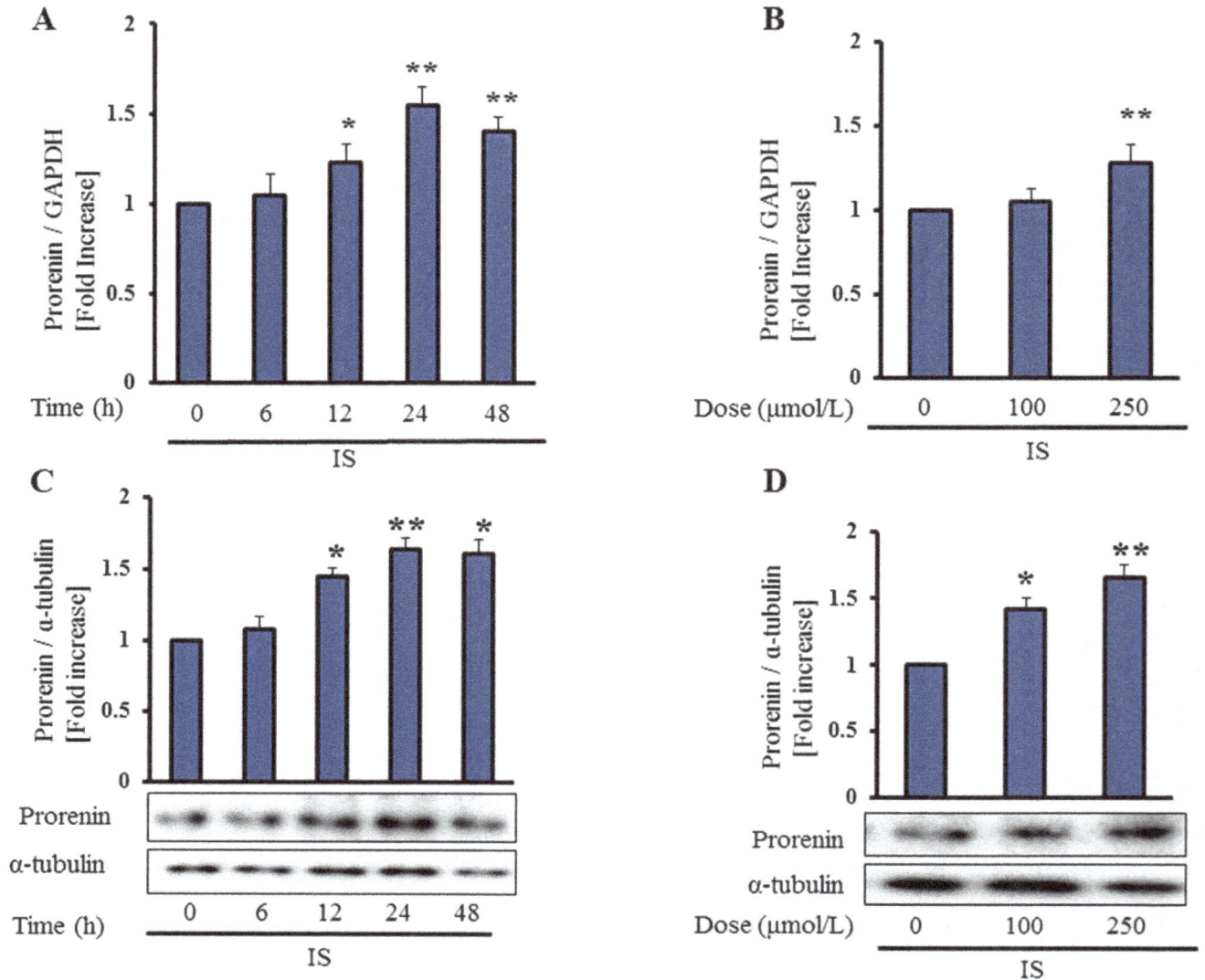

Figure 5. IS induces prorenin expression in vascular smooth muscle cells. Serum-starved HASMCs were treated with IS (250 μmol/L). Incubation with IS increased prorenin mRNA and protein expression in HASMCs time- (**A, C**) and dose- (**B, D**) dependently. Mean±SE (n = 3). *p<0.05, **p<0.01 vs control.

ROS, OAT3, AhR, and NF-κB p65 are Involved in IS-Induced Prorenin Expression in Vascular Smooth Muscle Cells

Both NAC and DPI suppressed stimulatory effects of IS on prorenin expression in HASMCs (Figure 6A, B). OAT3 siRNA, AhR siRNA and NF-κB p65 siRNA inhibited stimulatory effects of IS on prorenin expression. (Figure 6D, E, F). Therefore, IS induced prorenin expression in HASMCs through ROS, OAT3, AhR and NF-κB p65.

IS-Induced PRR Activation is Involved in Vascular Smooth Muscle Cell Proliferation

IS promotes vascular smooth muscle cell proliferation through generation of ROS and transportation by OAT3 [33,34]. Prorenin activates extracellular signal-regulated kinase (ERK) 1/2, leading to vascular smooth muscle cell proliferation, independent of Ang II generation [26,27]. We examined whether IS-induced PRR is involved in proliferation of HASMCs. PRR siRNA suppressed

IS-induced proliferation of HASMCs (Figure 7A). Prorenin (20 nmol/L) increased proliferation of HASMCs, whereas PRR siRNA suppressed prorenin-induced proliferation of HASMCs (Figure 7B). Thus, IS induces proliferation of HASMCs via prorenin/PRR pathway.

IS-Induced PRR Activation is Involved in Tissue Factor Expression in Vascular Smooth Muscle Cells

IS is positively associated with tissue factor expression in CKD [35,42]. The present study revealed that both IS and prorenin enhanced tissue factor protein expression in HASMCs. PRR siRNA suppressed IS-induced and prorenin-induced tissue factor expression in HASMCs (Figure 7D,E). Thus, IS induces tissue factor expression via prorenin/PRR pathway in HASMCs.

Discussion

The novel findings of the present study are; 1) Aortic expression of PRR and prorenin/renin was increased in CKD rats, whereas

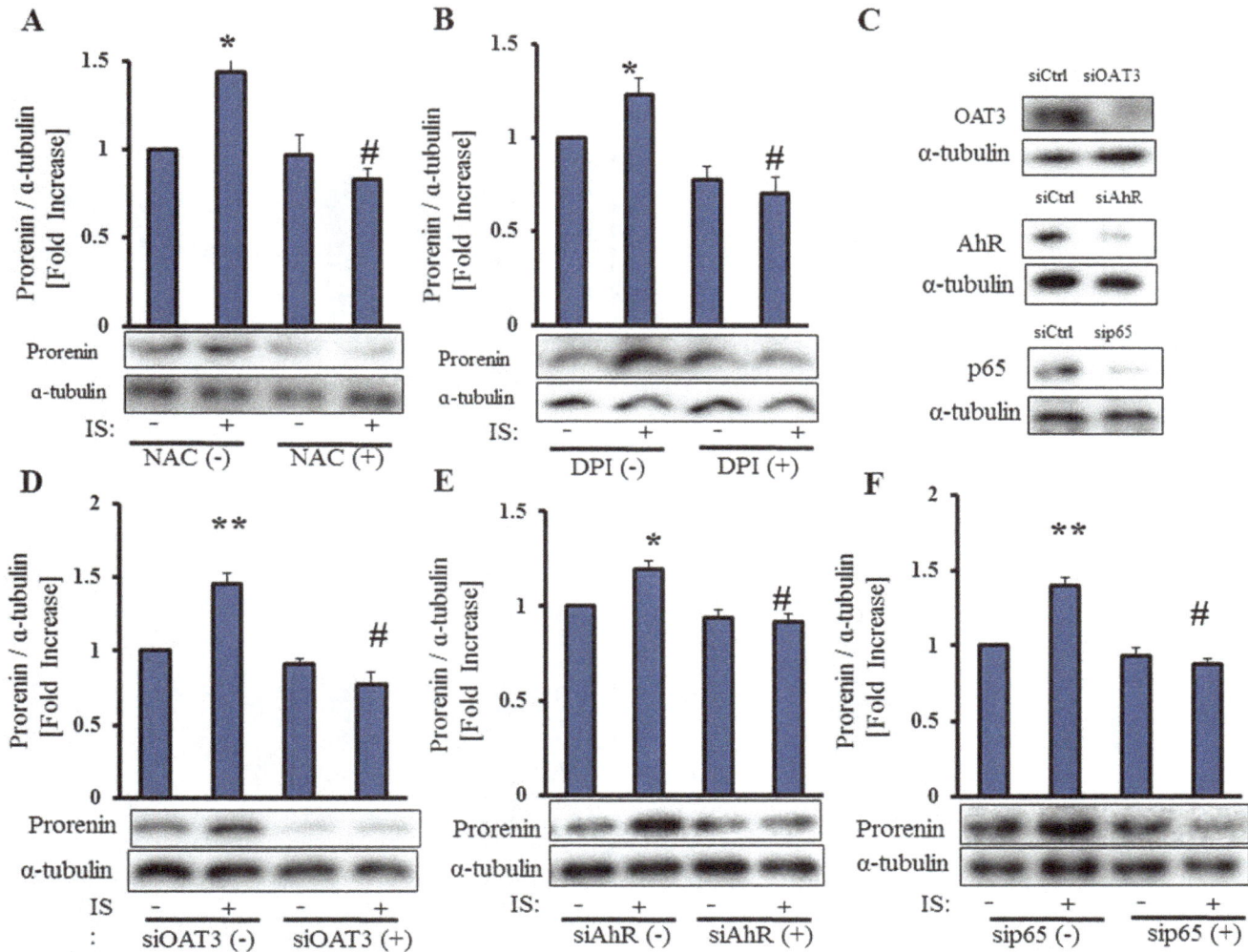

Figure 6. ROS, OAT3, AhR, and NF-κB p65 are involved in IS-induced prorenin expression in vascular smooth muscle cells. Serum starved HASMCs were pretreated with NAC (2.5 mmol/L) and DPI (10 μmol/L) for 30 min before incubation with IS (250 μmol/L) for 24 h (**A, B**). HASMCs were transfected with or without OAT3 siRNA (10 nmol/L), AhR siRNA (30 nmol/L) or p65 siRNA (10 nmol/L), and serum starved for 24 h, followed by incubation with IS (250 μmol/L) for 24 h. Cell lysates were immunoblotted using anti-OAT3, anti-AhR, anti-p65 and anti-prorenin antibodies (**C–F**). Mean±SE (n = 3). *p<0.05, **p<0.01 vs untreated group, #p<0.01 vs IS-treated group. Ctrl: control.

AST-120 reduced their expression; 2) IS increased aortic expression of PRR and prorenin/renin in rats; 3) IS increased expression of PRR and prorenin through OAT3, ROS, AhR and NF-κB in vascular smooth muscle cells; 4) IS-induced PRR activation is involved in vascular smooth muscle cell proliferation; 5) IS-induced PRR activation is involved in tissue factor expression in vascular smooth muscle cells. Taken together, IS upregulates aortic expression of prorenin/PRR in vascular smooth muscle cells through OAT3-mediated uptake, ROS production, and activation of AhR and NF-κB p65. IS-induced activation of PRR is involved in cell proliferation and tissue factor expression in vascular smooth muscle cells.

We observed aortic expression of renin/prorenin in CKD rats and IS-administered rats. Further, IS induced prorenin expression in vascular smooth muscle cells. However, previous data demonstrated that vascular renin originates largely if not completely in the kidney [44,45], and that the bulk of vascular renin is taken up from the circulation [46,47]. Taken together, our observation might suggest that aortic expression of prorenin is induced in CKD rats and IS-induced rats.

ROS induced upregulation of PRR in diabetic rat kidneys [48]. IS induces ROS generation by increasing NADPH oxidase NOX-4 and through OAT3-mediated uptake in HASMCs [16,17]. The present study revealed that NAC, DPI, and OAT3 siRNA suppressed IS-induced expression of PRR and prorenin in HASMCs. Thus, IS induced expression of PRR and prorenin through OAT3-mediated uptake and ROS production.

IS was identified as a potent endogenous ligand for AhR [40,41]. IS induces activation and translocation of AhR in endothelial cells [41]. IS-induced activation of AhR upregulates NF-κB p65 expression in vascular smooth muscle cells (unpublished data). In the present study, both AhR siRNA and NF-κB p65 siRNA suppressed IS-induced expression of PRR and prorenin. Thus, IS-induced activation of AhR/NF-κB p65 pathway simulates the expression of PRR and prorenin in vascular smooth muscle cells.

Vascular smooth muscle cell proliferation is a key event in the pathogenesis of vascular complications. Binding of PRR with prorenin induced vascular smooth muscle cell proliferation via activation of ERK1/2, independent of angiotensin II

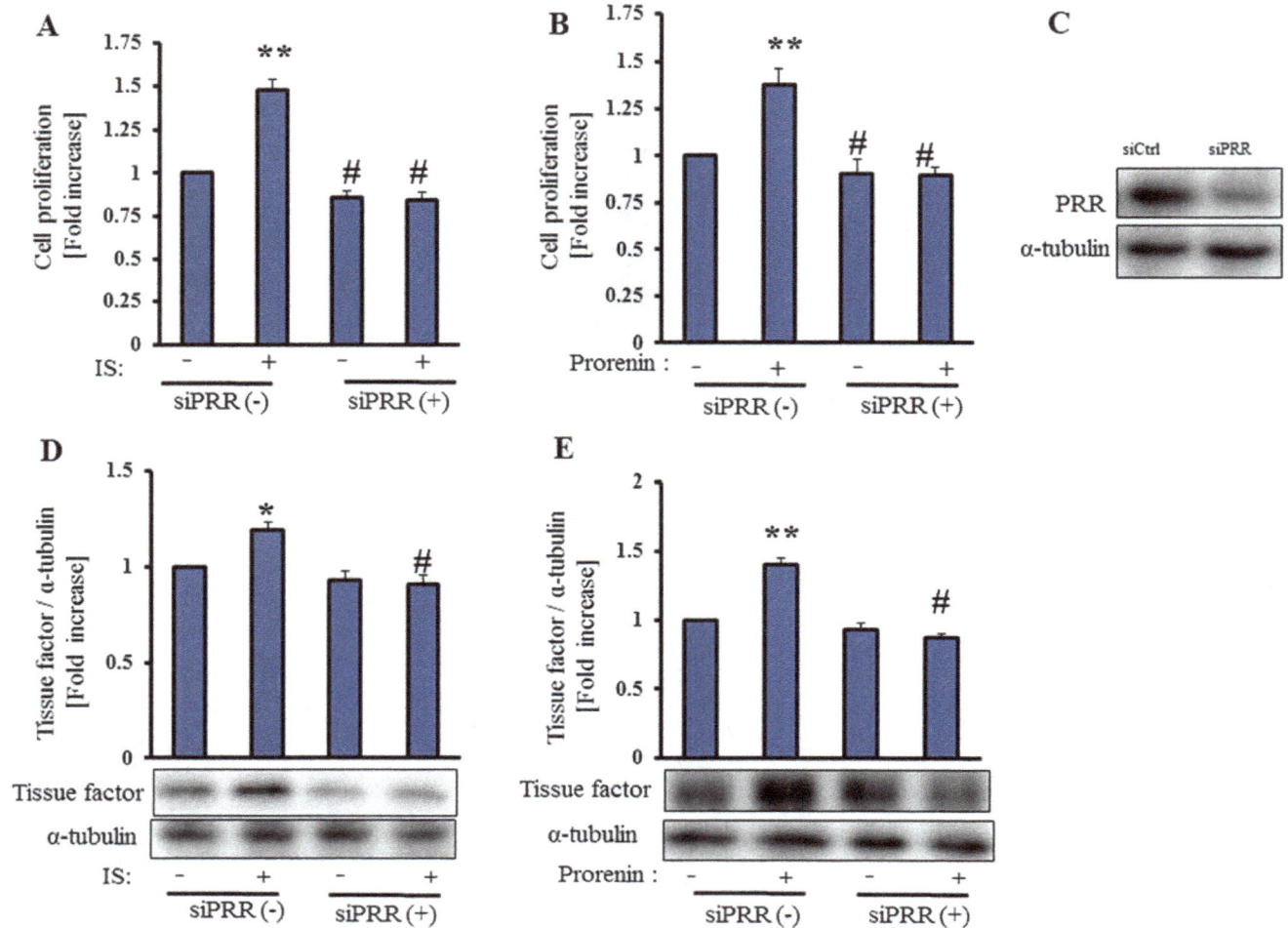

Figure 7. IS-induced PRR activation is involved in cell proliferation and tissue factor expression in vascular smooth muscle cells.
Serum-starved HASMCs (5×10^3 cells/well) in a 24-well plate were stimulated with or without IS (250 µmol/L) or prorenin (20 nmol/L) for 24 h (**A, B**). HASMCs were transfected with siPRR (20 nmol/L) for 48 h, before stimulation with IS or prorenin for 24 h. Thereafter, the cell proliferation reagent MTS (50 µL) was added to each well, and cells were incubated for 4 h. The absorbance was measured at 492 nm using a microplate reader (mean±SE, n = 3). **p<0.01 vs untreated group, #p<0.01 vs IS-treated group. HASMCs were transfected with or without PRR siRNA (20 nmol/L), and then serum starved for 24 h, followed by incubation with IS (250 µmol/L) or prorenin (20 nmol/L) for 24 h. Cell lysates were immunoblotted using anti-PRR and anti-tissue factor antibodies (**C–F**). Mean±SE (n = 3). *p<0.05, **p<0.01 vs untreated group, #p<0.05 vs IS-treated group. Ctrl: control.

[21,22,26,27]. IS promoted aortic wall thickening and aortic calcification in hypertensive rats [14]. IS stimulated vascular smooth muscle cell proliferation through ROS production [22], and directly activated ERK1/2 [21]. In the present study, PRR siRNA suppressed both IS-induced and prorenin-induced cell proliferation in HASMCs. Thus, PRR is involved in IS-induced vascular smooth muscle cell proliferation.

Tissue factor is a mediator of injury-related thrombosis, and is elevated in the serum of advanced CKD patients. IS upregulates tissue factor expression in vascular smooth muscle cells [35] and endothelial cells [42]. The present study demonstrated that PRR siRNA suppressed IS-induced upregulation of TF expression in

HASMCs. Thus, PRR is involved in IS-induced tissue factor expression in HASMCs. Taken together, IS-induced activation of prorenin-PRR pathway plays an important role in not only vascular smooth muscle cell proliferation but also tissue factor expression.

Author Contributions

Conceived and designed the experiments: TN MY. Performed the experiments: MY SS SA YA HN FN. Analyzed the data: TN MY. Contributed reagents/materials/analysis tools: TN. Wrote the paper: TN MY KT TM.

References

1. Foley RN, Parfrey PS, Sarnak MJ (1998) Clinical epidemiology of cardiovascular disease in chronic renal disease. Am J Kidney Dis 32: S112–119.
2. Niwa T, Ise M (1994) Indoxyl sulfate, a circulating uremic toxin, stimulates the progression of glomerular sclerosis. J Lab Clin Med 124: 96–104.
3. Niwa T (2010) Indoxyl sulfate is a nephro-vascular toxin. J Ren Nutr 20(Suppl 1): S2–S6.
4. Niwa T (2011) Role of indoxyl sulfate in the progression of chronic kidney disease and cardiovascular disease: experimental and clinical effects of oral sorbent AST-120. Ther Apher Dial 15: 120–124.
5. Niwa T, Takeda N, Tatematsu A, Maeda K (1988) Accumulation of indoxyl sulfate, an inhibitor of drug-binding, in uremic serum as demonstrated by

internal-surface reversed-phase liquid chromatography. Clin Chem 34: 2264–2267.

6. Enomoto A, Takeda M, Tojo A, Sekine T, Cha SH, et al. (2002) Role of organic anion transporters in the tubular transport of indoxyl sulfate and the induction of its nephrotoxicity. J Am Soc Nephrol 13: 1711–1720.

7. Shimizu H, Bolati D, Adijiang A, Muteliefu G, Enomoto A, et al. (2011) NF-κB plays an important role in indoxyl sulfate-induced cellular senescence, fibrotic gene expression, and inhibition of proliferation in proximal tubular cells. Am J Physiol Cell Physiol 301: C1201–1212.

8. Shimizu H, Bolati D, Adijiang A, Enomoto A, Nishijima F, et al. (2010) Senescence and dysfunction of proximal tubular cells are associated with activated p53 expression by indoxyl sulfate. Am J Physiol Cell Physiol 299: C1110–1117.

9. Shimizu H, Yisireyili M, Nishijima F, Niwa T (2012) Stat3 contributes to indoxyl sulfate-induced inflammatory and fibrotic gene expression and cellular senescence. Am J Nephrol 36: 184–189.

10. Miyazaki T, Ise M, Seo H, Niwa T (1997) Indoxyl sulfate increases the gene expression of TGF-β1, TIMP-1 and pro α(I) collagen in uremic rat kidneys. Kidney Int 52(Suppl 63): S15–22.

11. Shimizu H, Bolati D, Higashiyama Y, Nishijima F, Shimizu K, et al. (2012) Indoxyl sulfate upregulates renal expression of MCP-1 via production of ROS and activation of NF-κB, p53, ERK, and JNK in proximal tubular cells. Life Sci 90: 525–530.

12. Shimizu H, Yisireyili M, Higashiyama Y, Nishijima F, Niwa T (2013) Indoxyl sulfate upregulates renal expression of ICAM-1 via production of ROS and activation of NF-κB and p53 in proximal tubular cells. Life Sci 92: 143–148.

13. Barreto FC, Barreto DV, Liabeuf S, Meert N, Glorieux G, et al. (2009) Serum indoxyl sulfate is associated with vascular disease and mortality in chronic kidney disease patients. Clin J Am Soc Nephrol 4: 1551–1558.

14. Adijiang A, Goto S, Uramoto S, Nishijima F, Niwa T (2008) Indoxyl sulphate promotes aortic calcification with expression of osteoblast-specific proteins in hypertensive rats. Nephrol Dial Transplant 23: 1892–1901.

15. Tumur Z, Shimizu H, Enomoto A, Miyazaki H, Niwa T (2010) Indoxyl sulfate upregulates expression of ICAM-1 and MCP-1 by oxidative stress-induced NF-kB activation. Am J Nephrol 31: 435–441.

16. Adelibieke Y, Shimizu H, Saito S, Mironova R, Niwa T (2013) Indoxyl sulfate counteracts endothelial effects of erythropoietin through suppression of Akt phosphorylation. Circ J 77: 1326–1336.

17. Muteliefu G, Enomoto A, Jiang P, Takahashi M, Niwa T (2009) Indoxyl sulphate induces oxidative stress and the expression of osteoblast-specific proteins in vascular smooth muscle cells. Nephrol Dial Transplant 24: 2051–2058.

18. Muteliefu G, Shimizu H, Enomoto A, Nishijima F, Takahashi M, et al. (2012) Indoxyl sulfate promotes vascular smooth muscle cell senescence with upregulation of p53, p21 and prelamin A through oxidative stress. Am J Physiol Cell Physiol 303: C126–134.

19. Lekawanvijit S, Kompa AR, Wang BH, Kelly DJ, Krum H (2012) Cardio-renal syndrome: the emerging role of protein-bound uremic toxins. Circ Res 111: 1470–1483.

20. Yisireyili M, Shimizu H, Saito S, Enomoto A, Nishijima F, et al. (2013) Indoxyl sulfate promotes cardiac fibrosis with enhanced oxidative stress in hypertensive rats. Life Sci 92: 1180–1185.

21. Nguyen G, Muller DN (2010) The biology of the (pro)renin receptor. J Am Soc Nephrol 21: 18–23.

22. Greco CM, Camera M, Facchinetti L, Brambilla M, Pellegrino S, et al. (2012) Chemotactic effect of prorenin on human aortic smooth muscle cells: a novel function of the (pro)renin receptor. Cardiovasc Res 95: 366–374.

23. Batenburg WW, Lu X, Leijten F, Maschke U, Müller DN, et al. (2011) Renin- and prorenin-induced effects in rat vascular smooth muscle cells overexpressing the human (pro)renin receptor: does (pro)renin-(pro)renin receptor interaction actually occur? Hypertension 58: 1111–1119.

24. Huang Y, Wongamorntham S, Kasting J, McQuillan D, Owens RT, et al. (2006) Renin increases mesangial cell transforming growth factor-beta1 and matrix proteins through receptor-mediated, angiotensin II-independent mechanisms. Kidney Int 69: 105–113.

25. Saito S, Shimizu H, Yisireyili M, Nishijima F, Enomoto A, et al. (2014) Indoxyl sulfate-induced activation of (pro)renin receptor is involved in expression of transforming growth factor-β1 and α-smooth muscle actin in proximal tubular cells. Endocrinology en20131937.

26. Sakoda M, Ichihara A, Kaneshiro Y, Takemitsu T, Nakazato Y, et al. (2007) (Pro)renin receptor-mediated activation of mitogen-activated protein kinases in human vascular smooth muscle cells. Hypertens Res 30:1139–1146.

27. Liu G, Hitomi H, Hosomi N, Shibayama Y, Nakano D, et al. (2011) Prorenin induces vascular smooth muscle cell proliferation and hypertrophy via epidermal growth factor receptor-mediated extracellular signal-regulated kinase and Akt activation pathway. J Hypertens 29: 696–705.

28. Cruciat CM, Ohkawara B, Acebron SP, Karaulanov E, Reinhard C, et al. (2010) Requirement of prorenin receptor and vacuolar H⁺-ATPase-mediated acidification for Wnt signaling. Science 327: 459–463.

29. Oshima Y, Kinouchi K, Ichihara A, Sakoda M, Kurauchi-Mito A, et al. (2011) Prorenin receptor is essential for normal podocyte structure and function. J Am Soc Nephrol 22: 2203–2212.

30. Nguyen G, Muller DN (2010) The biology of the (pro)renin receptor. J Am Soc Nephrol 21: 18–23.

31. Kinouchi K, Ichihara A, Sano M, Sun-Wada GH, Wada Y, et al. (2010) The (pro)renin receptor/ATP6AP2 is essential for vacuolar H⁺-ATPase assembly in murine cardiomyocytes. Circ Res 107: 30–34.

32. Riediger F, Quack I, Qadri F, Hartleben B, Park JK, et al. (2011) Prorenin receptor is essential for podocyte autophagy and survival. J Am Soc Nephrol 22: 193–202.

33. Yamamoto H, Tsuruoka S, Ioka T, Ando H, Ito C, et al. (2006) Indoxyl sulfate stimulates proliferation of rat vascular smooth muscle cells. Kidney Int 69: 1780–1785.

34. Muteliefu G, Enomoto A, Niwa T (2009) Indoxyl sulfate promotes proliferation of human aortic smooth muscle cells by inducing oxidative stress. J Ren Nutr 19: 29–32.

35. Chitalia VC, Shivanna S, Martorell J, Balcells M, Bosch I, et al. (2013) Uremic serum and solutes increase post-vascular interventional thrombotic risk through altered stability of smooth muscle cell tissue factor. Circulation 127: 365–376.

36. Takii Y, Figueiredo AF, Inagami T (1985) Application of immunochemical methods to the identification and characterization of rat kidney inactive renin. Hypertension 7: 236–243.

37. Bolati D, Shimizu H, Niwa T (2012) AST-120 ameliorates epithelial-to-mesenchymal transition and interstitial fibrosis in the kidneys of chronic kidney disease rats. J Ren Nutr 22: 176–180.

38. Adijiang A, Shimizu H, Higuchi Y, Nishijima F, Niwa T (2011) Indoxyl sulfate reduces klotho expression and promotes senescence in the kidneys of hypertensive rats. J Ren Nutr 21: 105–109.

39. Niwa T, Nomura T, Sugiyama S, Miyazaki T, Tsukushi S, et al. (1997) The protein metabolite hypothesis, a model for the progression of renal failure: An oral adsorbent lowers indoxyl sulfate levels in undialyzed uremic patients. Kidney Int 52(Suppl 62): S23–28.

40. Schroeder JC, Dinatale BC, Murray IA, Flaveny CA, Liu Q, et al. (2010) The uremic toxin 3-indoxyl sulfate is a potent endogenous agonist for the human aryl hydrocarbon receptor. Biochemistry 49: 393–400.

41. Watanabe I, Tatebe J, Namba S, Koizumi M, Yamazaki J, et al. (2013) Activation of aryl hydrocarbon receptor mediates indoxyl sulfate-induced monocyte chemoattractant protein-1 expression in human umbilical vein endothelial cells. Circ J 77: 224–230.

42. Gondouin B, Cerini C, Dou L, Sallée M, Duval-Sabatier A, et al. (2013) Indolic uremic solutes increase tissue factor production in endothelial cells by the aryl hydrocarbon receptor pathway. Kidney Int 84: 733–744.

43. Sallée M, Dou L, Cerini C, Poitevin S, Brunet P, et al. (2014) The aryl hydrocarbon receptor-activating effect of uremic toxins from tryptophan metabolism: a new concept to understand cardiovascular complications of chronic kidney disease. Toxins 6: 934–949.

44. Inagami T, Murakami T, Higuchi K, Nakajo S (1991) Role of vascular wall renin: intracellular and extracellular mechanism. Blood Vessels 28: 217–223.

45. Kato H, Iwai N, Inui H, Kimoto K, Uchiyama Y, et al. (1993) Regulation of vascular angiotensin release. Hypertension 21: 446–454.

46. Hilgers KF, Hilgenfeldt U, Veelken R, Muley T, Ganten D, et al. (1993) Angiotensinogen is cleaved to angiotensin in isolated rat blood vessels. Hypertension 21: 1030–1034.

47. Müller DN, Luft FC (1998) The renin-angiotensin system in the vessel wall. Basic Res Cardiol 93 Suppl 2: 7–14.

48. Siragy HM, Huang J (2008) Renal (pro)renin receptor upregulation in diabetic rats through enhanced angiotensin AT1 receptor and NADPH oxidase activity. Exp Physiol 93: 709–714.

8

A Gene Variant in CERS2 Is Associated with Rate of Increase in Albuminuria in Patients with Diabetes from ONTARGET and TRANSCEND

Dov Shiffman[1]*, Guillaume Pare[2], Rainer Oberbauer[3], Judy Z. Louie[1], Charles M. Rowland[1], James J. Devlin[1], Johannes F. Mann[4], Matthew J. McQueen[2]

1 Celera, Alameda, CA, United States of America, 2 Population Health Research Institute, Hamilton Health Sciences and McMaster University, Hamilton, Ontario, Canada, 3 Department of Nephrology, KH Elisabethinen, Linz, Austria and Department of Nephrology, Medical University of Vienna, Vienna, Austria, 4 Department of Nephrology and Hypertension, Friedrich Alexander University, Erlangen, Germany

Abstract

Although albuminuria and subsequent advanced stage chronic kidney disease are common among patients with diabetes, the rate of increase in albuminuria varies among patients. Since genetic variants associated with estimated glomerular filtration rate (eGFR) were identified in cross sectional studies, we asked whether these variants were also associated with rate of increase in albuminuria among patients with diabetes from ONTARGET and TRANSCEND—randomized controlled trials of ramipril, telmisartan, both, or placebo. For 16 genetic variants associated with eGFR at a genome-wide level, we evaluated the association with annual rate of increase in albuminuria estimated from urine albumin:creatinine ratio (uACR). One of the variants (rs267734) was associated with rate of increase in albuminuria. The annual rate of increase in albuminuria among risk homozygotes (69% of the study population) was 11.3% (95%CI; 7.5% to 15.3%), compared with 5.0% (95%CI; 3.3% to 6.8%) for heterozygotes (27% of the population), and 1.7% (95%CI; −1.7% to 5.3%) for non-risk homozygotes (4% of the population); $P = 0.0015$ for the difference between annual rates in the three genotype groups. These estimates were adjusted for age, sex, ethnicity, and principal component of genetic heterogeneity. Among patients without albuminuria at baseline (uACR<30 mg/g), each risk allele was associated with 50% increased risk of incident albuminuria (OR = 1.50; 95%CI 1.15 to 1.95; P = 0.003) after further adjustment for traditional risk factors including baseline uACR and eGFR. The rs267734 variant is in almost perfect linkage-disequilibrium ($r^2 = 0.94$) with rs267738, a single nucleotide polymorphism encoding a glutamic acid to alanine change at position 115 of the ceramide synthase 2 (CERS2) encoded protein. However, it is unknown whether CERS2 function influences albuminuria. In conclusion, we found that rs267734 in CERS2 is associated with rate of increase in albuminuria among patients with diabetes and elevated risk of cardiovascular disease.

Editor: Hideharu Abe, University of Tokushima, Japan

Funding: The research leading to these results has received funding from the European Community's Seventh Framework Programme under the grant agreement n ° 241544. Funding for ONTARGET and TRANSCEND Studies: Boehringer Ingelheim. The funders had no role in study design, data collection and analysis, decision to publish. Co-authors DS, JZL, CMR, and JJD are employed by Celera. Celera provided support in the form of salaries for authors DS, JZL, CMR, and JJD, but did not have any additional role in the study design, data collection and analysis, decision to publish, or preparation of the manuscript. The specific roles of these authors are articulated in the 'author contributions' section.

Competing Interests: DS, JZL, CMR, and JJD are employees of Celera, a Quest Diagnostics company. DS, GP, JZL, CMR, JJD and MJM are named as inventors on the following patent application filed by Quest Diagnostics relating to the association of CERS2 variants with increased albuminuria "GENETIC POLYMORPHISMS ASSOCIATED WITH CHRONIC KIDNEY DISEASE, METHODS OF DETECTION AND USES THEREOF" Provisional applications serial no. 61/836,403 and serial no. 61/836,491). Boehringer Ingelheim has funded the ONTARGET and TRANSCEND studies.

* Email: dov.shiffman@celera.com

Introduction

Chronic kidney disease (CKD) is a common complication of type 2 diabetes and is becoming an increased burden on the medical system. Half of all patients with end stage renal disease starting dialysis suffer from type 2 diabetes mellitus [1]. In patients with diabetes, CKD frequently manifests as albuminuria prior to measurable decline in kidney function as assessed by estimated glomerular filtration rates (eGFR). It has been estimated that about 30% of patients with type 2 diabetes become either micro- or macro-albuminuric within 10 years of diagnosis [2]. However, the rate of CKD progression in patients with diabetes is modest:

on average only 2% to 5% become micro-albuminuric each year [2,3]. Identification of patients with diabetes who are at high risk for CKD progression could help focus medical resources on preventing their progression to end-stage renal disease. Several risk factors for CKD progression including systolic blood pressure, urinary albumin, plasma creatinine, and ethnicity were identified in UKPDS, an observational study of about 5,000 patients with type 2 diabetes [4].

Genetic analysis of kidney disease has largely focused on cross-sectional and case-control studies. A genome-wide meta-analysis investigated the association between genetic variants and eGFR in about 90,000 individuals from mostly population-based studies.

Table 1. Baseline characteristics.

Baseline Characteristic	Patients in Genetic Analysis		All Patients	
	ONTARGET (n = 3128)	TRANSCEND (n = 595)	ONTARGET (n = 13094)	TRANSCEND (n = 3255)
Age, years, mean (SD)	66.6 (7.2)	67.8 (7.5)	66.1 (6.9)	66.8 (7.2)
Male, n (%)	2197 (70.2)	309 (51.9)	9205 (70.3)	1772 (54.4)
Systolic blood pressure, mmHg, mean (SD)	142.5 (17.4)	141.1 (17.4)	143.2 (17.1)	142.0 (16.6)
Diastolic blood pressure, mmHg, mean (SD)	81.0 (10.3)	80.6 (9.9)	82.1 (10.3)	81.9 (10.2)
Hypertension, n (%)	1900 (60.7)	348 (58.5)	8279 (63.3)	1982 (61.0)
uACR, mg/g, median (IQR)	6.2 (2.7 to 29.4)	4.7 (2.6 to 12.7)	6.5 (2.7 to 30.5)	5.3 (2.5 to 14.5)
<30 mg/g, n (%)	2241 (71.6)	500 (84.0)	8957 (68.4)	2525 (77.6)
30 to 300 mg/g, n (%)	539 (17.2)	56 (9.4)	2196 (16.8)	387 (11.9)
>300 mg/g, n (%)	201 (6.4)	6 (1.0)	813 (6.2)	61 (1.9)
Missing baseline data, n (%)	147 (4.7)	33 (5.5)	1128 (8.6)	282 (8.7)
eGFR, ml/min/1.73 m2, mean (SD)	74.0 (21.0)	71.5 (20.5)	73.3 (20.7)	71.7 (20.1)
Ever smoked, n (%)	2071 (66.2)	327 (55.0)	8160 (62.4)	1599 (49.3)
Self-reported ethnicity				
European, n (%)	2377 (76.0)	430 (72.3)	9146 (69.9)	1879 (57.7)
Asian, n (%)	419 (13.4)	109 (18.3)	1927 (14.7)	758 (23.3)
Native Latin, n (%)	172 (5.5)	35 (5.9)	1233 (9.4)	444 (13.6)
African, n (%)	160 (5.1)	21 (3.5)	424 (3.2)	70 (2.2)
Treatment group				
Placebo, n (%)	NA	299 (50.3)	NA	1629 (50.0)
Ramipril, n (%)	1031 (33.0)	NA	4346 (33.2)	NA
Telmisartan, n (%)	1067 (34.1)	296 (49.7)	4463 (34.1)	1626 (50.0)
Ramipril and Telmisartan, n (%)	1030 (32.9)	NA	4285 (32.7)	NA
Diabetes				
Incident, n (%)	649 (20.7)	154 (25.9)	2524 (19.3)	790 (24.3)
Prevalent, n (%)	2479 (79.3)	441 (74.1)	10570 (80.7)	2465 (75.7)

SD, standard deviation. IQR, inter-quartile range. NA, not applicable.

This cross-sectional analysis identified 16 single nucleotide polymorphisms (SNPs) that were associated with eGFR at a genome-wide significance level ($P < 5 \times 10^{-8}$) [5]. The association of these 16 SNPs with incident CKD was investigated in about 26,000 individuals in eight population-based studies [6]. Only 6 of these loci were associated with incident CKD after adjustment for baseline eGFR. However, these genetic analyses were conducted in population based studies that were not enriched for patients with diabetes. More recently, these 16 SNPs were investigated in a prospective study of about 3000 patients with type 2 diabetes [7]. After correction for multiple testing, none of these SNPs was associated with incident CKD.

The association of these 16 SNPs with albuminuria was investigated in a large cross-sectional study of individuals with European ancestry [8]. In this study the minor allele of a SNP in the SHROOM3 gene was associated with low albuminuria (i.e., better kidney function), a puzzling finding since this same allele is associated with low levels of eGFR.

In this current study we investigated 16 SNPs, that were reported to be associated with eGFR, among patients with type 2 diabetes from European and non-European ancestry enrolled in two randomized controlled trials of ramipril, telmisartan, both, or placebo (ONTARGET and TRANSCEND). We asked whether these 16 SNPs are also associated with early kidney disease measured by accelerated increase in albuminuria.

Methods

Study design

This substudy of ONTARGET (ClinicalTrials.gov Identifier: NCT00153101) and TRANSCEND (ClinicalTrials.gov Identifier: NCT00153101) investigated whether 16 SNPs that were previously shown to be associated with eGFR in a cross sectional analysis are also associated with annual rate of increase in albuminuria among patients with diabetes. The ONTARGET and TRANSCEND studies were previously described [9–11]. Briefly, these studies included patients 55 years and older with atherosclerotic vascular disease or diabetes and retinopathy, left ventricular hypertrophy, micro- or macro-albuminuria, or a history of cardiac or vascular disease. Patients in ONTARGET were randomized to ramipril (10 mg/day), telmisartan (80 mg/day), or both. Patients intolerant to angiotensin converting enzyme inhibitors were included in the TRANSCEND study and were randomized to telmisartan (80 mg/day) or placebo. Patients in both studies were followed up for 56 months. This substudy included patients who had prevalent or incident diabetes and was drawn from ~10,000 patients who provided blood samples for DNA analysis. Reasonable efforts were made to collect blood samples for DNA from all ONTARGET/TRANSCEND patients. However, in some countries funding constraints and other difficulties prevented transfer of samples to the core laboratory

Table 2. SNPs associated with eGFR in cross-sectional studies.

SNP	Lead SNP	LD (r^2)	Alleles (Risk/Non-risk)	Allele Frequency (Risk)	Locus	Genes
rs267734			A/G	0.79	1q21.3	CERS2, ANXA9
rs1260326			G/A	0.59	2p23.3	GCKR
rs13538			A/G	0.78	2p13.1	NAT8
rs347685			A/C	0.73	3q23	TFDP2
rs17319721			A/G	0.42	4q21.1	SHROOM3
rs11959928			A/T	0.45	5p13.1	DAB2
rs6420094			C/T	0.33	5q35.3	SLC34A1
rs881858			A/G	0.70	6p21.1	VEGFA
rs7805747			A/G	0.28	7q36.1	PRKAG2
rs17786744	rs10109414	1	G/A	0.42	8p21.2	STC1
rs4744712			A/C	0.39	9q21.11	PIP5K1B
rs653178			G/A	0.50	12q24.12	ATXN2
rs626277			A/C	0.61	13q21.33	DACH1
rs1394125			A/G	0.35	15q24.2	UBE2Q2
rs4293393	rs12917707	1	A/G	0.82	16p12.3	UMOD
rs12460876			T/C	0.61	19q13.11	SLC7A9

LD, linkage disequilibrium.

in Hamilton, and some individual centers or investigators declined to participate. Additionally, blood samples from ~2000 patients enrolled in China were not included because authorities in Beijing would not allow export of DNA. Diabetes was defined as fasting glucose>125 mg/dl, 2 hour oral glucose tolerance test>199 mg/dl, use of antidiabetic medication, or new diabetes reported by the physician. Albuminuria was estimated from measurement of uACR from a first morning spot urine sample and eGFR was calculated from serum creatinine measurement using the Modification of Diet in Renal Disease (MDRD) formula. Genotyping was conducted using the Cardio-Metabo Chip from Illumina (San Diego CA) which interrogates about 200,000 SNPs, mostly from regions previously shown to be associated with risk of cardiovascular disease, type 2 diabetes, and related quantitative traits [12]. Quality control was performed according to Fellay et al. [13] Briefly, we excluded samples that had <99% call rate. The call rate was calculated based on a total of 189,632 SNPs (96.4% of all Metabochip SNPs) after exclusion of markers that did not achieve>99% call frequency (n = 6,281), markers that had poor signal clustering [13] (n = 783), or markers that had low signal intensity (n = 29). Genotyping reproducibility for 34 samples that were run in duplicates was>99.99%. Genotypes for SNPs in this study that were not present on the Cardio-Metabo Chip were assessed by allele-specific polymerase chain reaction (PCR) [14]. All the SNPs in this study did not deviate from Hardy-Weinberg equilibrium expectations (P>10^{-6}). This substudy of ONTARGET and TRANSCEND was approved by the Hamilton Health Sciences and McMaster University Research Ethics Board. All participants provided a written informed consent.

Statistical analysis

Participant characteristics at baseline were described by counts and percent, by medians and inter-quartile ratios, or by means and standard deviations (Table 1). Deviation from Hardy-Weinberg equilibrium expectations was assessed by an exact test for bi-allelic markers.

For regression models that included SNPs, genotypes were coded as 0, 1, or 2 pre-specified risk alleles using an additive model. Because genetic risk factors can have different magnitude in different ethnic groups, we investigated SNPs in ethnic groups separately. Specifically, SNPs were investigated in 4 ethnic groups: self-reported Europeans, Asians (including self-reported Chinese, Japanese, South Asians, other Asians, and Malaysians), Africans (self-reported Black African and Colored African) and self-reported Native Latin. Self-reported Arabs or Persians (n = 9) and others (n = 118) were excluded from the analysis. EIGENSTRAT software [15] was used to calculate the principal components of genetic variability separately in each of the 4 ethnic groups. The principal components were calculated using genotypes from about 50,000 autosomal SNPs that were selected for each ethnic group from the Cardio-Metabo Chip, such that they were not in linkage disequilibrium with one another (r^2<0.2 in each ethnic group). Patients who were identical by descent (n = 11), or those for whom the first 3 principal components of genetic variability clearly indicated that their genetic ancestry differed from their self-reported ethnicity (n = 34) were excluded. In the basic model, regression models adjusted for age, sex, and to adjust for population structure, the 10 largest ethnic-specific principal components. Results from the 4 ethnic groups were combined using random effects models [16]. The dependent variables eGFR and uACR were natural-log transformed. A fully adjusted model also included baseline hypertension (systolic blood pressure ≧140 mmHg or diastolic blood pressure ≥90 mmHg), baseline eGFR, baseline uACR, smoking status, study (ONTARGET or TRANSCEND), and treatment group. Associations between SNPs and baseline albuminuria or eGFR were assessed using linear regression models. Associations between SNPs and annual rate of change in albuminuria or change in eGFR were assessed using linear mixed models allowing for patient specific random intercepts and slopes. The fixed effects included in the linear mixed models were, visit (0, 2, or 5 years), SNP (number of risk alleles), an interaction term between visit and SNP and

Table 3. Association between SNPs and change in albuminuria.

SNP	Europeans				All Ethnic Groups			
	Annual change (%) per number of risk alleles				Annual change (%) per number of risk alleles			
	0	1	2	P value	0	1	2	P value
rs267734	1.99	4.99	8.07	0.0067	1.75	5.03	11.33	0.0015
rs1260326	8.61	7.07	5.56	0.11	8.14	9.04	11.68	0.44
rs13538	5.56	6.34	7.13	0.50	6.04	9.18	11.44	0.40
rs347685	5.23	6.31	7.41	0.31	9.00	10.28	9.97	0.45
rs17319721	6.73	6.77	6.80	0.97	11.27	7.05	6.72	0.63
rs11959928	6.20	6.85	7.51	0.50	10.25	9.93	8.01	0.57
rs6420094	5.92	7.24	8.58	0.20	9.28	11.05	10.53	0.15
rs881858	8.32	7.22	6.14	0.30	13.33	11.21	8.33	0.086
rs7805747	6.41	7.07	7.74	0.52	10.74	7.35	7.69	0.89
rs17786744	5.81	6.94	8.09	0.23	9.46	10.38	8.81	0.23
rs4744712	6.50	6.85	7.20	0.72	8.80	11.15	12.27	0.42
rs653178	7.35	6.77	6.20	0.54	10.45	7.68	6.45	0.49
rs626277	8.38	7.07	5.78	0.18	10.33	8.65	8.96	0.75
rs1394125	6.06	7.08	8.12	0.30	10.83	9.01	8.22	0.54
rs4293393	4.81	6.00	7.21	0.33	6.05	9.06	10.19	0.37
rs12460876	5.58	6.57	7.58	0.30	9.64	9.96	8.95	0.40

Results were adjusted for age, sex, 10 largest principal components of genetic variation and self-reported ethnicity (for "all ethnic groups" results).

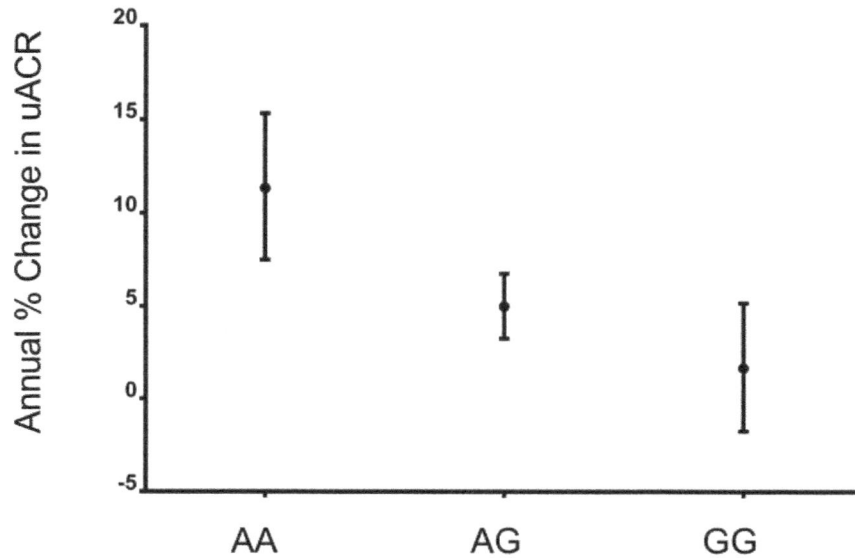

Figure 1. Whiskers denote 95% confidence intervals derived from linear mixed models adjusted for age, sex, and principal components of genetic variation.

remaining basic model variables. The general model in equation form is:

$$Y_{ij} = \beta_0 + \beta_1 \cdot SNP + \beta_2 \cdot Year + \beta_3(Year \cdot SNP) + b_{0i} + b_{1i} \cdot Year + \varepsilon_{ij}$$

where:

Y_{ij} is the observed measure of urine albumin at Year j for subject i, i = 1, …, M subjects; j = 1, …, n_i visits.

β_0 and β_1 are combined to estimate mean genotype specific population intercepts.

β_2 and β_3 are combined to estimate mean genotype specific population slopes.

b_{0i} estimates the deviation from the population intercept for subject i and are assumed independent and Gaussian with mean 0 and variance $\sigma_{b_0}^2$.

b_{1i} estimates the deviation from the population slope for subject i and are assumed independent and Gaussian with mean 0 and variance $\sigma_{b_1}^2$.

ε_{ij} represents the random deviation of the jth measurement for the ith subject and are assumed independent and Gaussian with mean 0 and variance σ_ε^2.

Additional covariates included in the models allow for additional variation in the population intercepts. The models were fit using the "lme" function found in the R package "nlme" [17–19]

A Wald test of the regression coefficient for the interaction term between visit and SNP was used to test whether the rates of change in the measurement over time differed according to the number of risk alleles. Since some mixed models did not converge when baseline uACR was included as a covariate, the fully adjusted models were evaluated using a two-stage linear regression procedure. In the first stage, a linear regression model regressing the measurement as a function of the visit (0, 2 or 5 years) was performed for each patient separately resulting in an estimated slope (rate of change in the measurement per year) for each patient. In the second stage, we used regression models to estimate the effect per risk allele on patient specific slopes. In models that

assessed the rate of change in albuminuria, patients with baseline uACR ≥100 mg/g (n = 401) were excluded because this analysis was focused on worsening albuminuria among patients that do not already have substantially elevated levels of urine albumin. Using a similar rationale, models that assessed the rate of eGFR change, patients with baseline eGFR <60 ml/min/1.73 m² were excluded (n = 960). Incident albuminuria was defined as uACR>30 mg/g in years 2 and 5, year 5 only, or year 2 when year 5 data was missing.

Results

This substudy of ONTARGET and TRANSCEND included 3128 patients from ONTARGET and 595 patients from TRANSCEND. These patients were mostly male patients (Table 1) with either prevalent (n = 2920) or incident (n = 803) diabetes. Most of the patients (75%) in this substudy were self-described Europeans. The baseline characteristics of the patients who were included in this genetic substudy of diabetic patients from ONTARGET and TRANSCEND were in general similar to the baseline characteristics of all diabetic patients in ONTARGET and TRANSCEND (Table 1). However, the fraction of patients in the European, Asian, and Native Latin self- reported ethnicities was different in study participants compared with all diabetics in ONTARGET and TRANSCEND, likely reflecting the low availability of DNA from patients recruited in Asia and Latin America.

In this substudy, we investigated 16 SNPs that were previously reported to be associated with eGFR in cross-sectional studies (Table 2). First we investigated the association of these SNPs with annual rate of increase in albuminuria among those with European ancestry and among all ethnic groups (Table 3). We found that 1 of the 16 SNPs (rs267734 in CERS2) was associated with differential annual rate of increase in albuminuria after accounting for testing 16 SNPs (P = 0.0015, Bonferroni corrected P value for α = 0.05 of 16 tests is 0.0032) and after adjustment for age, sex, ethnicity, and principal components of genetic variability. The median annual rate of increase in albuminuria in this population, regardless of genotype, was 6.8% (IQR 2.1% to

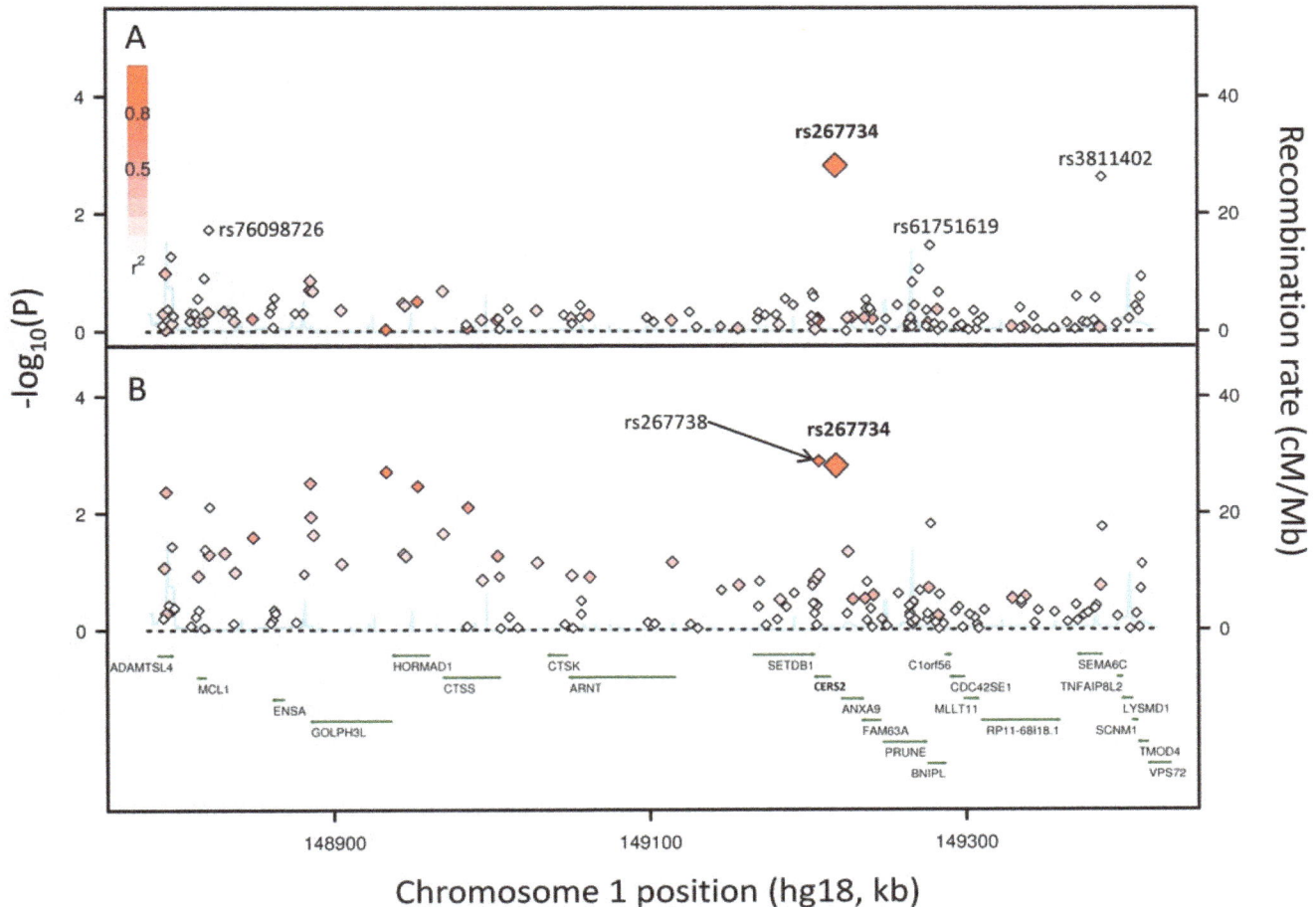

Figure 2. Regional plot for the CERS2 locus. SNPs are plotted by association P value of linear mixed models adjusted for age, sex, and principal components of genetic variation for the association between SNP and annual rate of change in albuminuria. and genomic position (NCBI Build 36). The original hit (rs267734) is labeled. The magnitude of linkage disequilibrium (r^2) between each SNP and rs267734 is indicated by the intensity of the red coloring. Estimates of recombination rates are shown by the blue line. Gene positions are indicated by green arrows. Gene names are labeled. Linkage disequilibrium and recombination rates were estimated from the Utah residents of Northern and Western European ancestry (CEU) HapMap population (release 22). Plots were prepared using SNAP [22]. Panel A: P values adjusted for rs267734. Panel B: P values not adjusted for rs267734.

12.9%). However, among carriers of 2 risk alleles of this SNP, albuminuria increased at an annual rate of 11.3% (95%CI, 7.5% to 15.3%), compared with an annual rate of 5.0% (95%CI; 3.3% to 6.8%) for carriers of one risk allele (heterozygotes), and 1.7% (95%CI, −1.7% to 5.3%) for carriers of no risk alleles (Figure 1). Further adjusting this association for baseline hypertension, eGFR, uACR, smoking, study (ONTARGET or TRANSCEND), and treatment group did not appreciably change the association of rs267734 with rate of increase in albuminuria (P = 0.0034). Among patients who were normo-albuminuric at baseline (uACR< 30 mg/g), each risk allele was associated with 50% increased risk of incident albuminuria (OR = 1.50; 95%CI 1.15 to 1.95; P = 0.003) after adjusting for age, sex, ethnicity, principal components of genetic variability, baseline hypertension, eGFR, uACR, smoking, study (ONTARGET or TRANSCEND), and treatment group.

We investigated whether other SNPs in the rs267734 locus were also associated with annual rate of increase in albuminuria (Figure 2). An investigation of 144 SNPs in this locus in the combined ethnic groups found that 19 of these SNPs were nominally associated with annual rate of increase in albuminuria (P<0.05, Table S1). However, after adjusting the associations for

the original CERS2 SNP (rs267734) only 3 SNPs remained associated with albuminuria progression (rs3811402, P = 0.0024; rs61751619, P = 0.036; and rs76098726, P = 0.019). These 3 SNPs were in low linkage disequilibrium with the original CERS2 SNP (r^2<0.02 in Europeans). Of the 19 SNPs that were associated with annual rate of increase prior to adjusting for rs267734, only one SNP in this locus (rs267738) had an association P value smaller than rs267734 (P = 0.0013). This SNP (rs267738) encodes a glutamic acid to alanine change at position 115 of the protein encoded by CERS2. These two SNPs in CERS2 (rs267734 and rs267738) are highly correlated (linkage disequilibrium r^2 = 0.94) in those with European ancestry in this substudy.

We also investigated the association of these 16 SNPs with baseline albuminuria levels (Table 4) and found that one SNP (rs13538 in NAT8) was associated with albuminuria in a combined analysis of all ethnic groups (P = 0.009), although this association did not reach statistical significance when Bonferroni correction was applied to adjust for testing 16 SNPs. Paradoxically, the rs13538 allele that was reported to be associated with low eGFR was found to be associated with low baseline albuminuria in our study.

Table 4. Association between SNPs and baseline albuminuria.

SNP	Europeans		All Ethnic Groups	
	β	P value	β	P value
rs267734	0.0043	0.94	0.015	0.78
rs1260326	−0.0439	0.34	−0.0381	0.36
rs13538	−0.1048	0.057	−0.1337	0.009
rs347685	0.0293	0.57	0.0175	0.71
rs17319721	−0.0096	0.84	−0.0684	0.51
rs11959928	0.0183	0.69	0.0111	0.79
rs6420094	0.0131	0.79	0.018	0.69
rs881858	−0.0449	0.36	−0.0598	0.18
rs7805747	−0.0651	0.19	−0.0664	0.16
rs17786744	−0.0600	0.18	−0.0258	0.74
rs4744712	−0.0462	0.32	−0.066	0.12
rs653178	0.0152	0.74	−0.0019	0.97
rs626277	−0.0069	0.88	−0.0009	0.98
rs1394125	−0.0090	0.85	0.0072	0.87
rs4293393	−0.0612	0.30	−0.0623	0.25
rs12460876	0.0021	0.96	0.0045	0.93

β is the expected change in log-transformed baseline albuminuria for each risk allele. Models are adjusted for age, sex, 10 largest principal components of genetic variation, and self-reported ethnicity.

Finally, we sought to confirm the previously reported association of these 16 SNPs with baseline eGFR in this study. Among patients with self-described European ancestry—the largest ethnic group in this substudy—we found that 3 of the 16 SNPs (rs267734 in CERS2, rs347685 in TFDP2, and rs653178 in ATXN2) were associated with baseline eGFR (P≤0.05, Table 5). As expected, patients carrying the pre-specified risk alleles of 13 of the 16 SNPs had lower eGFR than non-carriers. A combined analysis of all ethnic groups found that only one SNP (rs347685 in TFDP2) was associated with eGFR (P = 0.049) and that carriers of the risk

Table 5. Association between SNPs and baseline eGFR.

SNP	Europeans		All Ethnic Groups	
	β	P value	β	P value
rs267734	−0.0269	0.002	0.0038	0.89
rs1260326	−0.0087	0.23	−0.0195	0.33
rs13538	−0.004	0.65	0.0178	0.34
rs347685	−0.016	0.05	−0.0147	0.049
rs17319721	0.006	0.41	0.013	0.39
rs11959928	−0.0097	0.18	−0.0088	0.30
rs6420094	−0.0048	0.53	−0.0434	0.064
rs881858	−0.0147	0.062	0.0164	0.44
rs7805747	−0.013	0.10	−0.0098	0.19
rs17786744	−0.009	0.21	−0.0099	0.13
rs4744712	−0.0065	0.38	−0.0062	0.35
rs653178	−0.0144	0.046	−0.013	0.06
rs626277	0.0051	0.49	0.0044	0.52
rs1394125	−0.0056	0.45	−0.0063	0.36
rs4293393	−0.0175	0.063	−0.0172	0.047
rs12460876	0.0045	0.54	0.0028	0.67

β is the expected change in log-transformed baseline eGFR for each risk allele. Models are adjusted for age, sex, 10 largest principal components of genetic variation, and self-reported ethnicity.

Table 6. Association between SNPs and change in eGFR

| SNP | Europeans | | | | All Ethnic Groups* | | | |
| | Annual change (%) by number of risk alleles | | | | Annual change (%) by number of risk alleles | | | |
	0	1	2	P value	0	1	2	P value
rs267734	−2.53	−2.45	−2.38	0.70	−2.52	−2.45	−2.69	0.75
rs1260326	−2.37	−2.40	−2.44	0.83	−2.44	−2.73	−2.59	0.82
rs13538	−2.54	−2.46	−2.38	0.72	−2.52	−2.48	−2.70	0.80
rs347685	−2.25	−2.37	−2.49	0.54	−2.36	−2.56	−2.63	0.48
rs17319721	−2.23	−2.45	−2.66	0.22	−2.62	−2.46	−2.67	0.22
rs11959928	−2.47	−2.41	−2.35	0.71	−2.48	−3.02	−3.66	0.28
rs6420094	−2.50	−2.37	−2.25	0.50	−2.76	−2.4	−2.26	0.40
rs881858	−2.42	−2.42	−2.42	1.00	−2.44	−2.46	−2.74	0.85
rs7805747	−2.39	−2.44	−2.49	0.78	−2.61	−2.47	−2.55	0.66
rs17786744	−2.41	−2.42	−2.42	0.97	−2.49	−2.64	−2.49	0.89
rs4744712	−2.40	−2.41	−2.43	0.92	−3.05	−2.56	−2.38	0.45
rs653178	−2.50	−2.41	−2.32	0.60	−2.66	−2.89	−2.89	0.74
rs626277	−2.63	−2.45	−2.28	0.31	−2.72	−2.58	−2.32	0.40
rs1394125	−2.47	−2.40	−2.32	0.68	−2.74	−2.41	−2.33	0.60
rs4293393	−2.28	−2.36	−2.44	0.71	−2.35	−2.42	−2.66	0.73
rs12460876	−2.31	−2.40	−2.48	0.62	−2.41	−2.63	−2.55	0.51

Results were adjusted for age, sex, 10 largest principal components of genetic variation and self-reported ethnicity (for "all ethnic groups" results)

*Mixed regression models did not converge for the self-reported Native Latin group and they were excluded from the analysis.

alleles of 10 of the 16 SNPs had lower eGFR than non-carriers. None of the SNPs were associated with annual rate of eGFR change among either Europeans or in a combined analysis of all ethnic groups (Table 6).

Discussion

In a pre-specified investigation of 16 SNPs that were previously found to be associated with eGFR we found that one SNP (rs267734) in the CERS2 gene was associated with annual rate of increase in albuminuria in patients with diabetes from ONTAR-GET and TRANSCEND after adjusting for other established risk factors for CKD progression including baseline albuminuria and baseline eGFR. Each risk allele of rs267734 was associated with 50% increased risk of incident albuminuria.

This SNP was not associated with baseline albuminuria in our study. It was also not reported to be associated with baseline albuminuria in large cross sectional analysis of population-based studies [8,20]. Thus, this SNP may only be associated with rate of increase in albuminuria in this population of patients with diabetes who were predisposed to a rapid change in albuminuria. The rs267734 SNP was not associated with deterioration of eGFR—another indicator of worsening kidney function. That this SNP is associated with rate of increase in albuminuria and not with rate of deterioration of eGFR may suggest that increase in albuminuria is more rapid, or that increase in albuminuria precedes deterioration of eGFR among patients with diabetes.

CERS2 encodes ceramide synthase 2, one of 6 mammalian ceramide synthases which acylate dihydro-sphingosine to form dihydro-ceramide or sphingosine to form ceramide [21]. Ceramides are intra- and extra-cellular signaling molecules that play a role in several pathological and physiological processes including inflammation, diabetes, and angiogenesis [21]. CERS2 mRNA has been reported to be the most abundantly expressed ceramide synthase and to be highly expressed in both liver and kidney [22]. One study of CERS2 knock-out mice reported morphological changes in the kidney [23], another study reported normal kidney morphology and function [24]. The robust expression of CERS2 in mouse kidney could indicate that it might play a role in kidney physiology. However, this role might be obscured by other physiological processes in normal mice. We investigated other SNPs in the CERS2 locus and found another SNP in the CERS2 gene (rs267738) that was as strongly associated with increase in albuminuria as rs267734. These two SNPs are in strong linkage disequilibrium among Europeans; however rs267738 could conceivably be more likely to explain the association because it

encodes an amino acid change (glutamic acid to alanine) at position 115 of the CERS2 encoded protein, however, we have no functional data to indicate whether this amino acid change is associated with change in ceramide synthase activity or stability. The more common allele (glutamic acid, 80% frequency among those with European ancestry) is associated with increased rate of change in albuminuria. It would be interesting to investigate the effect of the glutamic acid to alanine substitution at this position on CERS2 activity because it could indicate whether inhibition of ceramide synthase 2 activity would inhibit or promote worsening of albuminuria.

This study has several limitations. Albuminuria was assessed from spot urine at baseline, year 2, and year 5 of follow-up. It is likely that a more accurate assessment of albuminuria and albuminuria progression would be achieved from multiple measurements on consecutive days, and from more frequent longitudinal sampling. We limited the patients in this substudy to those with prevalent or incident diabetes. However, we have no information on the duration of diabetes among those with prevalent diabetes, and thus were unable to adjust the association for potential effects of diabetes duration on albuminuria progression.

In conclusion, we found that a SNP in the CERS2 gene that was previously found to be associated with eGFR was also associated with increase in albuminuria among patients with diabetes and elevated cardiovascular risk. Although this observation has reasonable biological plausibility, it requires replication in additional studies.

Acknowledgments

The authors would like to thank ONTARGET and TRANSCEND investigators and patients. Without their contributions these studies would not have been possible.

Author Contributions

Conceived and designed the experiments: DS GP RO JJD JFM MJM. Performed the experiments: GP DS MJM. Analyzed the data: DS GP JJD JZL CMR. Contributed reagents/materials/analysis tools: GP JFM MJM. Wrote the paper: DS GP RO JJD JFM MJM.

References

1. U.S. Renal Data System (2012) USRDS 2012 annual data report: atlas of chronic kidney disease and end-stage renal disease in the United States. National Institutes of Health, National Institute of Diabetes and Digestive and Kidney Diseases 2012; Available: http://www.usrds.org/atlas12.aspx. Accessed: 2014 Jan 10.

2. Adler AI, Stevens RJ, Manley SE, Bilous RW, Cull CA, et al. (2003) Development and progression of nephropathy in type 2 diabetes: the United Kingdom Prospective Diabetes Study (UKPDS 64). Kidney Int 63: 225–232.

3. Mann JF, Gerstein HC, Yi QL, Lonn EM, Hoogwerf BJ, et al. (2003). Development of renal disease in people at high cardiovascular risk: results of the HOPE randomized study. J Am Soc Nephrol 14: 641–647.

4. Retnakaran R, Cull CA, Thorne KI, Adler AI, Holman RR (2006) Risk factors for renal dysfunction in type 2 diabetes UK Prospective Diabetes Study 74. Diabetes 55: 1832–1839.

5. Köttgen A, Pattaro C, Böger CA, Fuchsberger C, Olden M, et al. (2010) New loci associated with kidney function and chronic kidney disease. Nat Genet 42: 376–384.

6. Böger CA, Gorski M, Li M, Hoffmann MM, Huang C, et al. (2011) Association of eGFR-Related Loci Identified by GWAS with Incident CKD and ESRD. PLoS Genet 7: e1002292

7. Deshmukh HA, Palmer CN, Morris AD, Colhoun HM (2013) Investigation of known estimated glomerular filtration rate loci in patients with Type 2 diabetes. Diabet Med 30: 1230–1235.

8. Ellis JW, Chen MH, Foster MC, Liu CT, Larson MG, et al. (2012). Validated SNPs for eGFR and their associations with albuminuria. Hum Mol Genet 21: 3293–3298.

9. Teo K, Yusuf S, Sleight P, Anderson C, Mookadam F, et al. (2004) ONTARGET/TRANSCEND Investigators: Rationale, design, and baseline characteristics of 2 large, simple, randomized trials evaluating telmisartan, ramipril, and their combination in high-risk patients: the Ongoing Telmisartan Alone and in Combination with Ramipril Global Endpoint Trial/Telmisartan Randomized Assessment Study in ACE Intolerant Subjects with Cardiovascular Disease (ONTARGET/TRANSCEND) trials. Am Heart J 148: 52–61.

10. Yusuf S, Teo K, Anderson C, Pogue J, Dyal L, et al. (2008) Effects of the angiotensin-receptor blocker telmisartan on cardiovascular events in high-risk patients intolerant to angiotensin-converting enzyme inhibitors: a randomised controlled trial. Lancet 372: 1174–1183.

11. Yusuf S, Teo KK, Pogue J, Dyal L, Copland I, et al. (2008) Telmisartan, ramipril, or both in patients at high risk for vascular events. N Engl J Med 358: 1547–1559.

12. Voight BF, Kang HM, Ding J, Palmer CD, Sidore C, et al. (2012) The metabochip, a custom genotyping array for genetic studies of metabolic, cardiovascular, and anthropometric traits. PLoS Genet 8: e1002793.

13. Fellay J, Thompson AJ, Ge D, Gumbs CE, Urban TJ, et al. (2010) ITPA gene variants protect against anaemia in patients treated for chronic hepatitis C. Nature 464: 405–408.

14. Shiffman D, Ellis SG, Rowland CM, Malloy MJ, Luke MM, et al. (2005) Identification of four gene variants associated with myocardial infarction. Am J Hum Genet 77: 596–605.

15. Price AL, Patterson NJ, Plenge RM, Weinblatt ME, Shadick NA, et al. (2006) Principal components analysis corrects for stratification in genome-wide association studies Nat Genet 38: 904–909.

16. DerSimonian R, Laird N (1986) Meta-Analysis in Clinical Trials Controlled Clinical Trials 7: 177–188.

17. Pinheiro JC, Bates DM, DebRoy S, Sarkar D, R Development Core Team (2012). nlme: Linear and Nonlinear Mixed Effects Models. R package version 3.1–103.

18. Pinheiro JC, Bates DM (2000) Mixed-Effects Models in S and S-PLUS, New York: Springer-Verlag New York, Inc.

19. Laird NM, Ware JH (1982) Random-Effects Models for Longitudinal Data Biometrics, 38, 963–974.

20. Böger CA, Chen MH, Tin A, Olden M, Köttgen A, et al. (2011) CUBN is a gene locus for albuminuria. J Am Soc Nephrol 22: 555–570.

21. Hannun YA, Obeid LM (2011) Many ceramides. J Biol Chem 286: 27855–27862.

22. Laviad EL, Albee L, Pankova-Kholmyansky I, Epstein S, Park H, et al. (2008) Characterization of ceramide synthase 2: tissue distribution, substrate specificity, and inhibition by sphingosine 1-phosphate. J Biol Chem 283: 5677–5684.

23. Imgrund S, Hartmann D, Farwanah H, Eckhardt M, Sandhoff R, et al. (2009) Adult ceramide synthase 2 (CERS2)-deficient mice exhibit myelin sheath defects, cerebellar degeneration, and hepatocarcinomas. J Biol Chem 284: 33549–33560.

24. Pewzner-Jung Y, Brenner O, Braun S, Laviad EL, Ben-Dor S, et al. (2010) A critical role for ceramide synthase 2 in liver homeostasis: II. insights into molecular changes leading to hepatopathy. J Biol Chem 285: 10911–10923.

9

Circulating MiR-133a as a Biomarker Predicts Cardiac Hypertrophy in Chronic Hemodialysis Patients

Ping Wen[1], Dan Song[3], Hong Ye[1], Xiaochun Wu[1], Lei Jiang[1], Bing Tang[1], Yang Zhou[1], Li Fang[1], Hongdi Cao[1], Weichun He[1], Yafang Yang[2], Chunsun Dai[1], Junwei Yang[1]*

1 Center for Kidney Disease, Second Affiliated Hospital, Nanjing Medical University, Nanjing, China, 2 Department of Radiology, Second Affiliated Hospital, Nanjing Medical University, Nanjing, China, 3 Department of Nephrology, Affiliated Wuxi Hospital, Nanjing Medical University, Wuxi, China

Abstract

Background: MicroRNAs (miRNAs) are small ribonucleotides regulating gene expression. MicroRNAs are present in the blood in a remarkably stable form and have emerged as potential diagnostic markers in patients with cardiovascular disease. Our study aimed to assess circulating miR-133a levels in MHD patients and the relation of miR-133a to cardiac hypertrophy.

Methods: We profiled miRNAs using RNA isolated from the plasma of participants. The results were validated in 64 MHD patients and 18 healthy controls.

Results: Levels of plasma miR-133a decreased in MHD patients with LVH compared with those in healthy controls. Plasma miR-133a concentrations were negatively correlated with LVMI and IVS. After single hemodialytic treatment, plasma miR-133a levels remained unchanged. Cardiac Troponin I and T were not associated with LVMI and IVS.

Conclusions: Our observations supplied the possibility that circulating miR-133a could be a surrogate biomarker of cardiac hypertrophy in MHD patients.

Editor: Sakthivel Sadayappan, Loyola University Chicago, United States of America

Funding: This work was supported by National Science Foundation of China Grants 31171093, "973" Science Program of the Ministry of Science and Technology, China (2011CB504005) to Junwei Yang. The author Weichun He was supported by National Science Foundation of China Grants 81170659. Junwei Yang took responsibility of the design of the study and Weichun He was in charge of the preparation of the manuscript. The funders had no role in study design, data collection and analysis, decision to publish, or preparation of the manuscript.

Competing Interests: The authors have declared that no competing interests exist.

* Email: jwyang@njmu.edu.cn

Introduction

Cardiovascular disease (CVD) is the main complication in patients with chronic kidney disease (CKD) and end stage renal disease (ESRD). More importantly, CVD is the leading cause of death in ESRD patients, accounting for 50% of all deaths in renal replacement therapy patients. In ESRD patients, a major pathophysiologic process frequently occurring in uremic hearts is left ventricular hypertrophy (LVH). Even though coronary artery disease and arrhythmia are not uncommon, LVH is the most frequent cardiovascular manifestation in these patients [1,2]. In addition, LVH is a very strong independent predictor of cardiovascular mortality not only among patients with hypertension but also among ESRD patients [3,4].

To date, several imaging modalities such as echocardiography (ECHO), magnetic resonance imaging (MRI) and computerized tomography have been performed to measure LVH [5,6,7]. ECHO is widely available, noninvasive, and has been demonstrated to be of reasonable accuracy in the assessment of LVH. However, ECHO might not be able to detect LVH in all dialysis patients [8]. In addition, there are studies implied serum biomarkers like arterial vasopressin, aldosterone and cardiac Troponin T appear to predict LVH [9,10]. However, stable and accurate serum biomarkers are not found, the present study evaluates whether a new biomarker for LVH can improve detection of LVH.

Recent studies have demonstrated that microRNAs (miRNAs) are present in the human circulation in a cell-free form and can be detected in circulating blood, thus may serve as a new class of blood-based biomarkers [11]. Numerous studies reported altered plasma or serum levels of various miRNAs in patients with cardiovascular diseases, including acute myocardial infarction [12,13], myocarditis [14], acute and chronic heart failure [14,15] and stable coronary artery disease [16]. Previous studies have found that miR-133a level was decreased in hypertrophic heart [17]. In study presented here, we measured plasma miR-133a in MHD patients and healthy controls and analyzed the relationship between miR-133a level and cardiac hypertrophy.

Subjects and Methods

Ethical statement

All of the following details of the study were approval by the responsible ethics committee of Nanjing Medical University

Table 1. Clinical characteristics of the study population.

characteristics	controls	MHD without LVH	MHD with LVH
Number	18	24	40
Men, n(%)	12(66.7)	14(58.3)	26(65)
Median age(range) (yr)	42(27–59)	46(29–69)	54(44–85)
Cardiovascular history, n(%)			
Myocardial infarction	0(0)	1(4.2)	0(0)
PTCA	0(0)	1(4.2)	0(0)
CABG	0(0)	0(0)	0(0)
Pacemaker	0(0)	0(0)	1(4.2)
Hypertension	0(0)	22(91.7)	35(87.5)
Diabetes	0(0)	0(0)	6(15)
Hypercholesterolemia	3(17.6)	2(8.3)	2(5)
Anemia, n(%)	0(0)	21(87.5)	28(70)
Renal failure, n(%)	0(0)	24(100)	40(100)
Hemodialysis, n(%)	0(0)	24(100)	44(100)
Median hemodialysis duration(range) (mo)	-	81(16–165)	94(12–306)
Laboratory examinations			
Hemoglobin (g/L)	-	106.8	100.9
Product of Ca and Pi (mg^2/dl^2)	-	49.4	44.9
iPTH (ng/ml)	-	314.3	210.7
Medication, n(%)			
Aspirin	0(0)	0(0)	1(4.2)
β-blocker	0(0)	8(33.3)	11(27.5)
CCB	0(0)	5(20.8)	18(45)
ACEI	0(0)	3(12.5)	5(12.5)
ARB	0(0)	2(8.3)	4(10)
Statins	0(0)	0(0)	0(0)
Warfarin	0(0)	0(0)	0(0)

PTCA: percutaneous transluminal coronary angioplasty; CABG: coronary artery bypass grafting; β-blocker: β receptor blocker; CCB: calcium-channel blocker; ACEI: angiotensin-converting enzyme inhibitor; ARB: angiotensin II type1 receptor blocker.

(Permit Number: KY2013019). And the written informed consent was supplied by the patients before the study.

Patients

The study population consists of 64 patients with ESRD undergoing regular hemodialysis from one clinical center and 18 healthy controls from one health examination center. Two blood samples of each patient were collected: one before hemodialysis another after hemodialysis, while one blood sample was obtained from each control. All the patients were evaluated with transthoracic echocardiography and 8 of them were measured with cardiac magnetic resonance.

Left ventricular mass index estimated by echocardiography

We measured the following parameters on the M-mode echocardiogram: left ventricular diastolic dimension (LVDd, cm), interventricular septum thickness (IVS, cm), and left ventricular posterior wall thickness (LVPW, cm). LV mass was calculated according to Devereux's formula [18]: left ventricular mass (g) = $1.04 \times [(LVDd+IVS+LVPW)^3 - (LVDd)]^3 - 13.6$, where 1.04 (g/cm^3) is the specific gravity of the myocardium. It is the measurements of the peak value of R wave on the electrocardiograph. The left ventricular mass index (LVMI, g/m^2) was defined as left ventricular mass divided by body surface area (m^2).

Biochemical analyses

Plasma cardiac Troponin I (CA: DRE11443) and Troponin T (CA: DRE11403) were measured using the ELISA kit (fengxiang biotechnology company, Shanghai, China) by sandwich ELISA. The detection range were 10~300 ng/L and 5~220 ng/L respectively.

Plasma microRNA determination

Total RNA was extracted from plasma as previously described [19]. Quantitative RT-PCR was carried out using TaqMan miRNA probes (Applied Biosystems; Foster City, CA) according to the manufacturer's instructions. Real-time PCR was performed using a TaqMan PCR kit on an Applied Biosystems 7300 Sequence Detection System. The primer sequences of miR-133a was UUGGUCCCCUUCAACCAGCUGU. The mixtures of let-7d, let-7g and let-7i were used for our reference gene. To evaluate the change of miR-133a levels before and after hemodialysis, Δct was used, which can be calculated as the following equation: Δct = ct value (miR-133a)- ct value (let-7dgi).

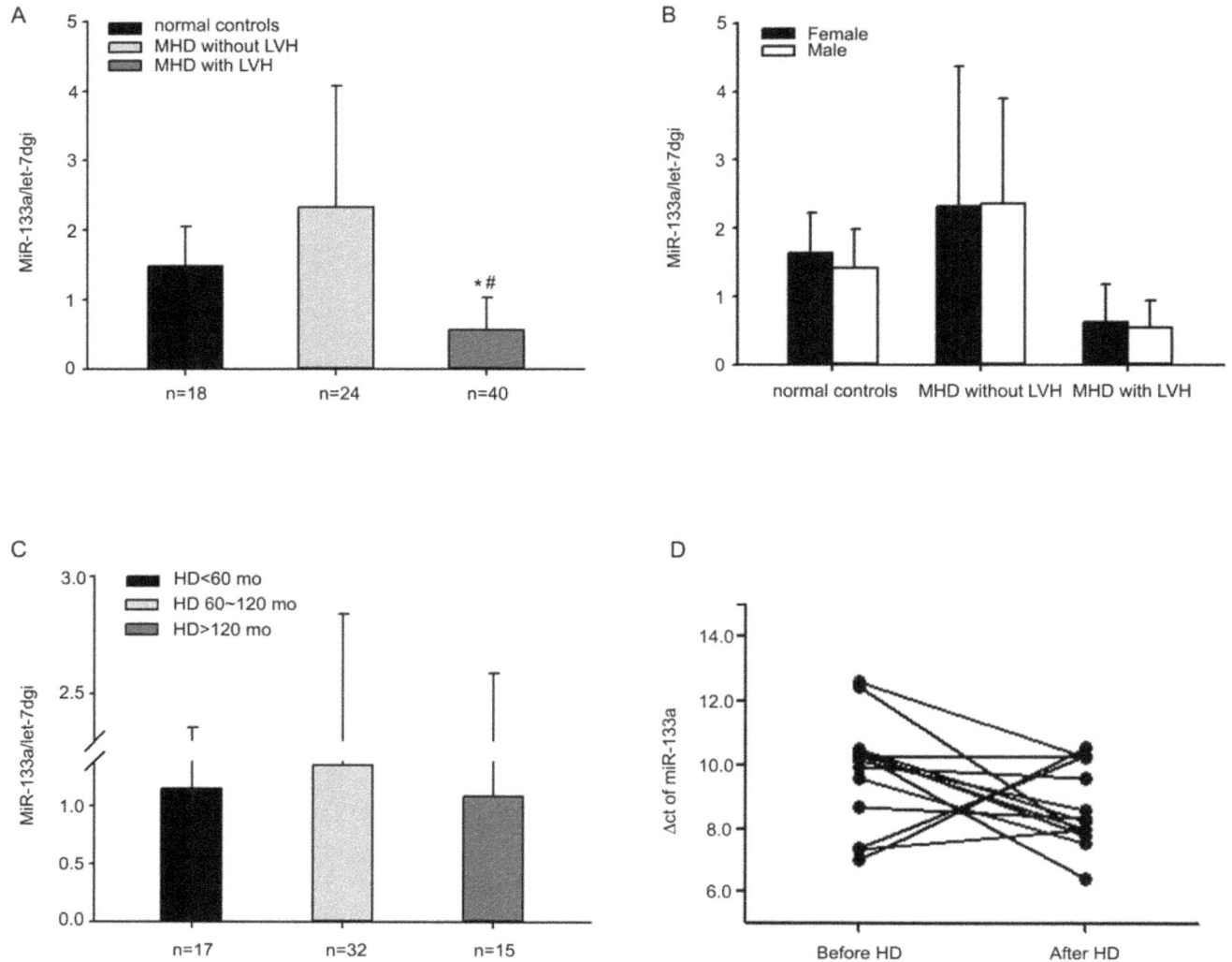

Figure 1. Plasma concentrations of miR-133a in healthy controls and MHD patients. The average miR-133a level of MHD patients with LVH was much lower than that of healthy controls and MHD patients without LVH, (0.57 ± 0.46 vs 1.48 ± 0.57, P = 0.000; 0.57 ± 0.46 vs 2.33 ± 1.75, P = $<$ 0.001) (A). There were no differences in miR-133a level between male and female in controls (1.40 ± 0.58 vs 1.63 ± 0.58, P = 0.457) and MHD patients either with LVH (0.54 ± 0.41 vs 0.63 ± 0.55, P = 0.565) or without LVH (2.34 ± 1.56 vs 2.31 ± 2.07, P = 0.961) (B). When patients were divided into three groups according to the duration of hemodialysis, there was no significant difference in miR-133a levels between groups (1.15 ± 1.21 vs 1.39 ± 1.50 vs 1.02 ± 1.48, P = 0.806) (C). Among 14 patients receiving hemodialytic treatment, miR-133a concentration remained unchanged after hemodialysis (D). Δct (ct value of 133a subtract ct value of let-7dgi) was used to evaluate the alteration. If Δct was increased, the level of miR-133a was decreased.

Statistical analyses

Data are presented as mean$\pm$SE unless otherwise described. To test the differences of miR-133a between MHD patients and healthy controls, t-test was used. Correlations were assessed using liner regression analysis and univariate logistic regression analysis method. Paired t-test was used to evaluate the change of miR-133a levels, Troponin I/T levels after hemodialysis. PASW statistics, version 18 was used to perform statistical analyses. A probability value <0.05 was considered to indicate statistical significance.

Results

Patient characteristics

A total of 82 subjects were enrolled in this study and 64 of them were ESRD patients receiving maintenance hemodialysis treatment. Clinical characteristics of all patients are shown in Table 1. 18 volunteers without documented kidney or heart diseases were used as healthy controls. Among the 64 patients, 40 had left ventricular hypertrophy which is defined as LVMI>125 g/m^2 in male and LVMI >115 g/m^2 in female. Thereby patients were divided into two groups according to the LVMI value. The traditional risk factors of LVH such as age, hypertension, and anemia were not significantly different between patients with LVH and without LVH. Among patients with LVH, there were 6 patients have diabetes. In contrast, all of the patients without LVH did not suffer the diabetes, suggesting that diabetes is a strong risk factor of LVH. There were no significant differences of laboratory indexes and medications between the two groups.

Plasma levels of miR-133a are decreased in MHD patients with LVH compared with those without LVH.

To investigate plasma miR-133a levels, blood samples were obtained from healthy controls and MHD patients before hemodialysis. The average level of plasma miR-133a was much

Table 2. Left ventricular mass index estimated by echocardiography and cardiac magnetic resonance.

patient	echocardiography			cardiac magnetic resonance		
	LVDd	IVS	LVPW(cm)	LVDd	IVS	LVPW(cm)
1	4.45	0.7	0.68	4.0	0.9	0.6
2	4.77	0.86	0.88	5.1	0.8	0.5
3	4.83	0.95	1.03	5.2	0.9	0.5
4	4.07	0.74	0.63	4.1	0.8	0.6
5	4.58	1.29	1.07	4.7	1.1	0.7
6	4.52	1.2	1.05	4.5	1.5	0.7
7	4.66	1.37	1.22	5.0	1.5	0.5
8	5.66	1.32	1.25	5.1	1.4	0.9

lower in MHD plus left ventricular hypertrophy group compared to MHD group, P = <0.001 (Figure 1A). There were no significant differences in miR-133a level between male and female both in healthy controls and MHD patients with or without LVH (Figure 1B). When patients were divided into three groups according to their duration of hemodialysis, there were no significant differences in plasma miR-133a levels between the groups (Figure 1C). The plasma miR-133a levels after hemodialysis were compared to that before hemodialysis in 14 MHD patients and it was found that miR-133a levels were not changed, P = 0.09 (Figure 1D).

Plasma miR-133a levels are negatively correlated with LVMI and IVS.

Previous study has demonstrated cardiac specific miR-133a control cardiac hypertrophy [17]. Therefore, we estimated the association between plasma miR-133a and cardiac hypertrophy. All of the patients were evaluated with ECHO while 8 of them were measured with MRI. It was confirmed that the findings from echocardiography were consistent with the results of MRI so they were credible (Table 2). To elucidate whether plasma miR-133a

concentration were associated with cardiac hypertrophy in MHD patients, the liner regression analysis was used and it indicated that plasma miR-133a level were negatively correlated with IVS and LVMI, R^2 = 0.319 and 0.383 respectively, P = <0.001 (Figure 2A, B). To further confirm the correlation between plasma miR-133a level and LVH, univariate logistic regression analysis was used to analyze the association of miR-133a level and IVS/LVMI, other clinical characteristics were also analyzed. Table 3 showed that plasma miR-133a level were only negatively correlated with IVS and LVMI, 95% confidence intervals were 0.084 to 0.677 and 0.043 to 0.396 respectively.

Plasma levels of cardiac Troponin I and Troponin T were not increased in MHD patients before hemodialysis and not correlated with cardiac hypertrophy

Cardiac Troponin I and Troponin T are common biomarkers of cardiac infarction. We assessed plasma levels of cardiac Troponin I and Troponin T in MHD patients and healthy controls. Significant differences were not found in both biomarkers between controls and patients (Figure 3A, B). There was no significant correlations between Troponin I/T levels and LVMI

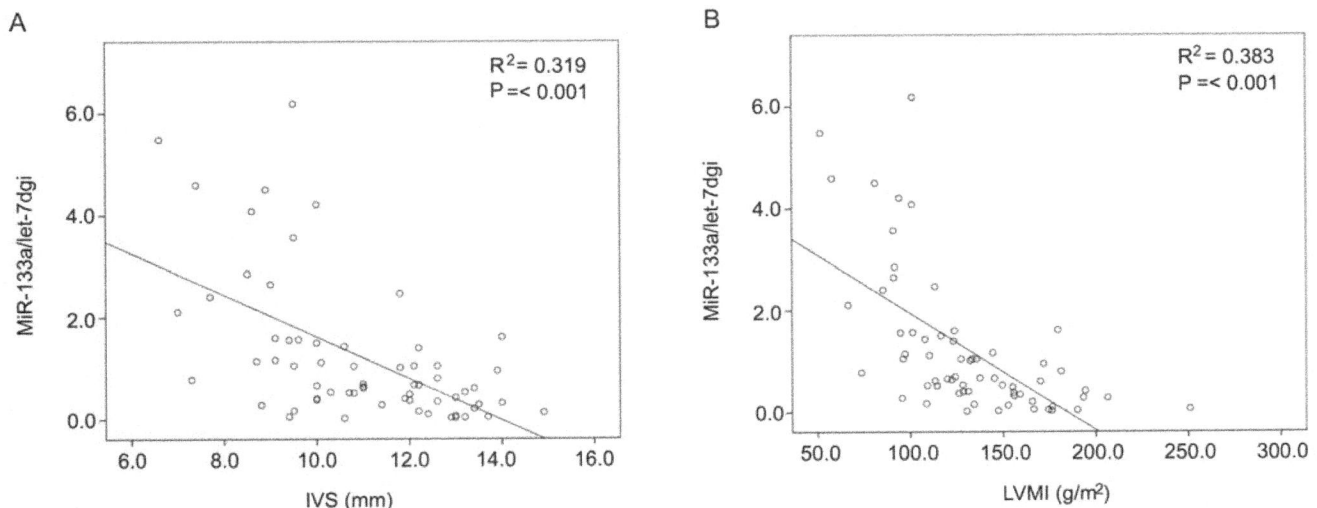

Figure 2. The correlation between plasma miR-133a level and cardiac hypertrophy in ESRD patients receiving maintenance hemodialysis treatment. Liner regression analysis showed that plasma miR-133a concentration was negatively correlated with IVS and LVMI, the correlation coefficient was 0.319 and 0.383 respectively, P = <0.001 (A, B).

Table 3. Univariate logistic regression analysis of plasma miR-133a and clinical characteristics.

Variates	95%CI
Gender	0.402–3.043
Age	0.151–1.129
Cardiovascular history	
Hypertension	0.304–7.226
Diabetes	0.074–2.567
Hypercholesterolemia	0.167–22.482
Left ventricular hypertrophy	0.044–0.461*
Anemia	0.406–7.985
Median hemodialysis duration	0.151–1.129
Medication	
β-blocker	0.269–0.306
CCB	0.215–1.686
ACEI	0.313–2.389
ARB	0.074–2.567
Laboratory index	
Troponin I	0.375–5.437
Troponin T	0.229–3.344
LVMI	0.043–0.396*
IVS	0.084–0.677*

CI: confidence interval.

(Figure 3C, D). Hemodialysis did not change Troponin I levels except that Troponin I decreased dramatically after hemodialysis in one patient (Figure 3E). Also, there was no significant difference between the Troponin T levels before and after hemodialysis, P = 0.289 (Figure 3F).

Discussion

In our study, we demonstrated that circulating miR-133a level was decreased in MHD patients compared with healthy controls. Since the expression of miR-133a in heart is decreased in cardiac hypertrophy animal model [17], we analyzed the correlation between circulating miR-133a levels and cardiac hypertrophy in MHD patients. It was found that the miR-133a level was negatively associated with LVMI, an indicator of left ventricular hypertrophy (LVH), in these patients.

The heart has capable of remodeling in response to various environmental demands and a variety of stimuli can induce it to growth or shrink. In MHD patients, primary or secondary hypertension, volume overload, hemodynamic stress and uremia toxins can alone or together induce cardiac hypertrophy.

MicroRNAs are important regulators of a wide range of cellular processes by modulating gene expression and are estimated to regulate more than 30% of the genes in a cell [20]. Recent studies both in animals and humans have demonstrated that miRNAs are present in the circulation and can be detected and quantified [11,19]. Previous studies have indicated that miR-133a is highly expressed in cardiac and skeletal muscle and is regulated in hypertrophy and failure [17,21]. Circulating miR-133a levels were measured in several studies and were consistently elevated in patients with cardiac infarction and were closely related with high-sensitivity cardiac Troponin [12,22,23,24].

In the present study, we detected circulating miR-133a levels in MHD patients and healthy controls and demonstrated that miR-

133a concentrations were decreased in MHD patients with LVH. Among 64 patients enrolled in our study, most of them (89.4%) had hypertension and about half underwent hypertension more than 5 years, but not all of them had decreased miR-133a levels. The significant association between miR-133a level and LVMI indicated that circulating miR-133a may play important role in the process of LVH and could be a biomarker of LVH. In addition, our study showed that plasma miR-133a concentrations were not changed after hemodialysis. There have been some studies investigated the influence of hemodialysis on circulating microRNA levels [25,26,27] and demonstrated different results. Daniel R. and colleagues elucidated miR-499p could be eliminated by hemodialysis [27], however, Thomas Thum [25] and Dai Y [26] indicated that circulating microRNAs could not be cleared by hemodialysis. Although the molecular weight of miRNAs is small enough to permeate the dialysis membrane, it is reported that miRNAs are likely to be transported by larger structures such as proteins and/or microvesicles [28]. Our results implied that miR-133a was not eliminated after hemodialysis. Therefore, we suggest that circulating miR-133a levels before hemodialysis treatment should be used to predict LVH.

Cardiac Troponins are considered the gold standard of biomarkers for the diagnosis of myocardial infarction at present. In our study, no patients suffered from myocardial infarction at the study time. Therefore, the plasma cardiac Troponin-I/T levels were similar to that of healthy controls. Although there was study indicated that cardiac Troponin T concentration positively correlated with left ventricular hypertrophy in hemodialysis patients and predicted lower survival rates [9], we think Troponin-T is more sensitive in cardiac infarction but not hypertrophy.

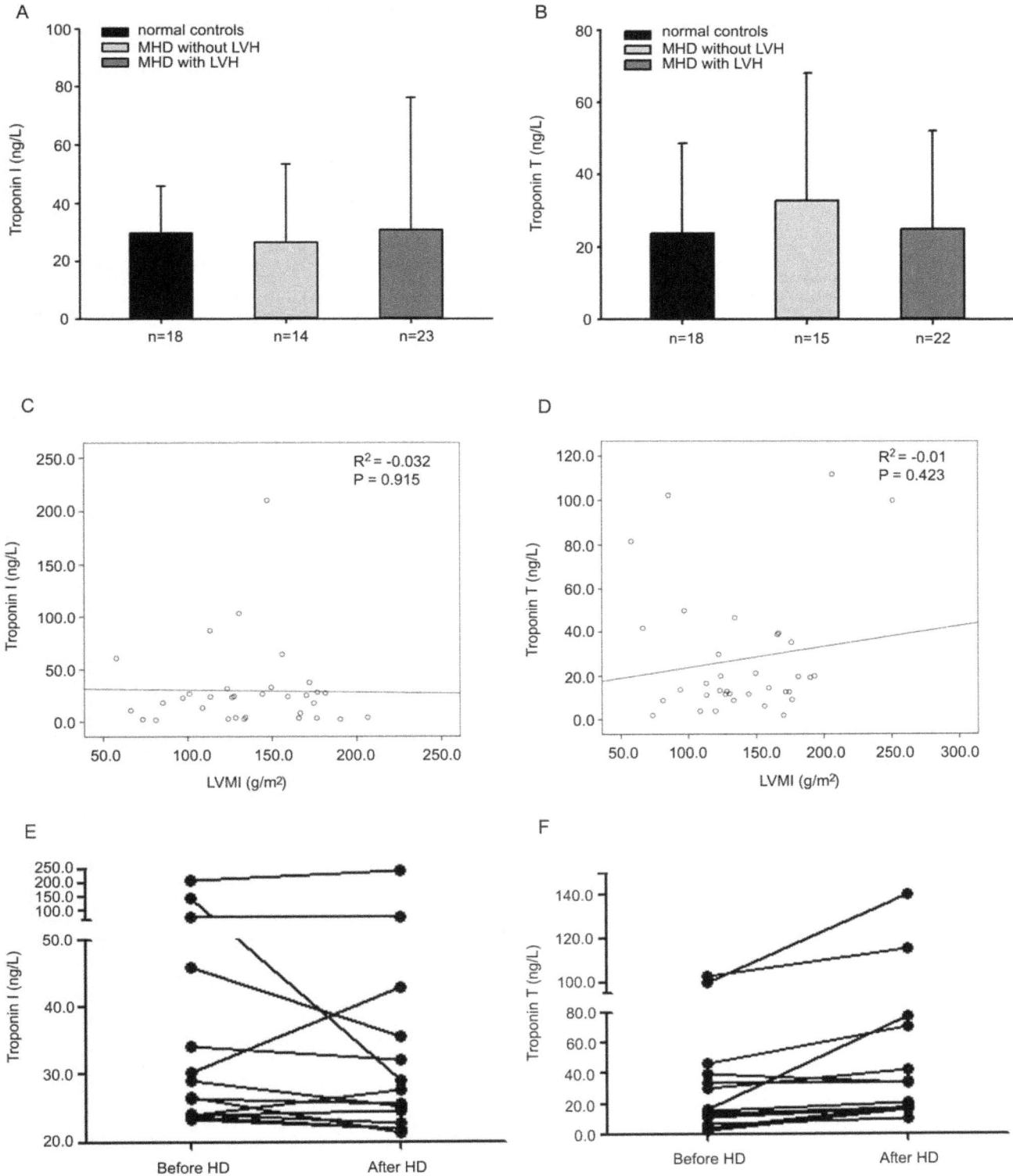

Figure 3. Plasma levels of cardiac Troponin I/T and the correlation between Troponin I/T levels and LVMI/IVS. There were no significant differences between healthy controls and MHD patients in both biomarkers before the hemodialysis treatment (cTnI: 29.72±16.16 vs 29.55±40.35, P = 0.983; cTnT: 23.85±24.67 vs 27.47±29.16, P = 0.650) (A, B). No significant differences of Troponin I/T levels were found between MHD patients plus LVH and those without LVH (cTnI: 30.85±45.46 vs 26.55±26.85, P = 0.784; cTnT: 25.22±26.92 vs 33.07±35.07, P = 0.480) (A, B). There were no correlation between LVMI and Troponin I/T before hemodialysis treatment (C, D). After hemodialysis, the cardiac Troponin I level remained unchanged in most patients except that it was evident decrease in one patient (E). There were no significant differences of the plasma Troponin T level between before and after hemodialysis (F).

This study is limited by its small size. In addition, MHD patients differed from controls in terms of age, cardiovascular history, and risk factors. More subjects need to be involved in our future study.

In conclusion, plasma miR-133a levels are decreased in MHD patients with LVH. MiR-133a levels are negatively associated with LVMI, indicating that the lower miR-133a level, the more obvious left ventricular hypertrophy. Our observations supplied the possibility that circulating miR-133a can be a blood-based biomarker for cardiac hypertrophy.

References

1. Middleton RJ, Parfrey PS, Foley RN (2001) Left ventricular hypertrophy in the renal patient. J Am Soc Nephrol 12: 1079–1084.
2. Levin A, Djurdjev O, Thompson C, Barrett B, Ethier J, et al. (2005) Canadian randomized trial of hemoglobin maintenance to prevent or delay left ventricular mass growth in patients with CKD. Am J Kidney Dis 46: 799–811.
3. Silberberg JS, Barre PE, Prichard SS, Sniderman AD (1989) Impact of left ventricular hypertrophy on survival in end-stage renal disease. Kidney Int 36: 286–290.
4. Zoccali C, Benedetto FA, Mallamaci F, Tripepi G, Giacone G, et al. (2004) Left ventricular mass monitoring in the follow-up of dialysis patients: prognostic value of left ventricular hypertrophy progression. Kidney Int 65: 1492–1498.
5. Levy D, Garrison RJ, Savage DD, Kannel WB, Castelli WP (1990) Prognostic implications of echocardiographically determined left ventricular mass in the Framingham Heart Study. N Engl J Med 322: 1561–1566.
6. Stewart GA, Foster J, Cowan M, Rooney E, McDonagh T, et al. (1999) Echocardiography overestimates left ventricular mass in hemodialysis patients relative to magnetic resonance imaging. Kidney Int 56: 2248–2253.
7. Truong QA, Ptaszek LM, Charipar EM, Taylor C, Fontes JD, et al. (2010) Performance of electrocardiographic criteria for left ventricular hypertrophy as compared with cardiac computed tomography: from the Rule Out Myocardial Infarction Using Computer Assisted Tomography trial. J Hypertens 28: 1959–1967.
8. Jakubovic BD, Wald R, Goldstein MB, Leong-Poi H, Yuen DA, et al. (2013) Comparative assessment of 2-dimensional echocardiography vs cardiac magnetic resonance imaging in measuring left ventricular mass in patients with and without end-stage renal disease. Can J Cardiol 29: 384–390.
9. Petrovic D, Obrenovic R, Stojimirovic B (2008) Cardiac troponins and left ventricular hypertrophy in hemodialysis patients. Clin Lab 54: 145–152.
10. Strand AH, Gudmundsdottir H, Fossum E, Os I, Bjornerheim R, et al. (2007) Arterial plasma vasopressin and aldosterone predict left ventricular mass in men who develop hypertension over 20 years. J Clin Hypertens (Greenwich) 9: 365–371.
11. Mitchell PS, Parkin RK, Kroh EM, Fritz BR, Wyman SK, et al. (2008) Circulating microRNAs as stable blood-based markers for cancer detection. Proc Natl Acad Sci U S A 105: 10513–10518.
12. D'Alessandra Y, Devanna P, Limana F, Straino S, Di Carlo A, et al. (2010) Circulating microRNAs are new and sensitive biomarkers of myocardial infarction. Eur Heart J 31: 2765–2773.
13. Cheng Y, Tan N, Yang J, Liu X, Cao X, et al. (2010) A translational study of circulating cell-free microRNA-1 in acute myocardial infarction. Clin Sci (Lond) 119: 87–95.
14. Corsten MF, Dennert R, Jochems S, Kuznetsova T, Devaux Y, et al. (2010) Circulating MicroRNA-208b and MicroRNA-499 reflect myocardial damage in cardiovascular disease. Circ Cardiovasc Genet 3: 499–506.
15. Tijsen AJ, Creemers EE, Moerland PD, de Windt LJ, van der Wal AC, et al. (2010) MiR423-5p as a circulating biomarker for heart failure. Circ Res 106: 1035–1039.
16. Fichtlscherer S, De Rosa S, Fox H, Schwietz T, Fischer A, et al. (2010) Circulating microRNAs in patients with coronary artery disease. Circ Res 107: 677–684.
17. Care A, Catalucci D, Felicetti F, Bonci D, Addario A, et al. (2007) MicroRNA-133 controls cardiac hypertrophy. Nat Med 13: 613–618.
18. Devereux RB, Reichek N (1977) Echocardiographic determination of left ventricular mass in man. Anatomic validation of the method. Circulation 55: 613–618.
19. Chen X, Ba Y, Ma L, Cai X, Yin Y, et al. (2008) Characterization of microRNAs in serum: a novel class of biomarkers for diagnosis of cancer and other diseases. Cell Res 18: 997–1006.
20. Lewis BP, Burge CB, Bartel DP (2005) Conserved seed pairing, often flanked by adenosines, indicates that thousands of human genes are microRNA targets. Cell 120: 15–20.
21. Chen JF, Mandel EM, Thomson JM, Wu Q, Callis TE, et al. (2006) The role of microRNA-1 and microRNA-133 in skeletal muscle proliferation and differentiation. Nat Genet 38: 228–233.
22. Wang GK, Zhu JQ, Zhang JT, Li Q, Li Y, et al. (2010) Circulating microRNA: a novel potential biomarker for early diagnosis of acute myocardial infarction in humans. Eur Heart J 31: 659–666.
23. Gidlof O, Andersson P, van der Pals J, Gotberg M, Erlinge D (2011) Cardiospecific microRNA plasma levels correlate with troponin and cardiac function in patients with ST elevation myocardial infarction, are selectively dependent on renal elimination, and can be detected in urine samples. Cardiology 118: 217–226.
24. Eitel I, Adams V, Dieterich P, Fuernau G, de Waha S, et al. (2012) Relation of circulating MicroRNA-133a concentrations with myocardial damage and clinical prognosis in ST-elevation myocardial infarction. Am Heart J 164: 706–714.
25. Martino F, Lorenzen J, Schmidt J, Schmidt M, Broll M, et al. (2012) Circulating microRNAs are not eliminated by hemodialysis. PLoS One 7: e38269.
26. Wang H, Peng W, Ouyang X, Dai Y (2012) Reduced circulating miR-15b is correlated with phosphate metabolism in patients with end-stage renal disease on maintenance hemodialysis. Ren Fail 34: 685–690.
27. Emilian C, Goretti E, Prospert F, Pouthier D, Duhoux P, et al. (2012) MicroRNAs in patients on chronic hemodialysis (MINOS study). Clin J Am Soc Nephrol 7: 619–623.
28. Lorenzen JM, Thum T (2012) Circulating and urinary microRNAs in kidney disease. Clin J Am Soc Nephrol 7: 1528–1533.

Author Contributions

Conceived and designed the experiments: JY. Performed the experiments: PW. Analyzed the data: PW DS. Wrote the paper: PW. Participated in designing the experiment: CD. In charge of the preparation of the manuscript: WH. Made some contributions in the experiments: DS. Collected the information of the patients: HY XW BT. Did part work of the experiment: LJ YZ LF HC. Analysis tools: YY.

10

Hsp72 Is a Novel Biomarker to Predict Acute Kidney Injury in Critically Ill Patients

Luis E. Morales-Buenrostro[1]*, Omar I. Salas-Nolasco[1], Jonatan Barrera-Chimal[1,2], Gustavo Casas-Aparicio[1], Sergio Irizar-Santana[1], Rosalba Pérez-Villalva[1,2], Norma A. Bobadilla[1,2]*

1 Department of Nephrology Nefrología y Metabolismo Mineral, Instituto Nacional de Ciencias Médicas y Nutrición Salvador Zubirán, México City, México, 2 Unidad de Fisiología Molecular, Instituto de Investigaciones Biomédicas, Universidad Nacional Autónoma de México, México City, México

Abstract

Background and Objectives: Acute kidney injury (AKI) complicates the course of disease in critically ill patients. Efforts to change its clinical course have failed because of the fail in the early detection. This study was designed to assess whether heat shock protein (Hsp72) is an early and sensitive biomarker of acute kidney injury (AKI) compared with kidney injury molecule (Kim-1), neutrophil gelatinase-associated lipocalin (NGAL), and interleukin-18 (IL-18) biomarkers.

Methods: A total of 56 critically ill patients fulfilled the inclusion criteria. From these patients, 17 developed AKI and 20 were selected as controls. In AKI patients, Kim-1, IL-18, NGAL, and Hsp72 were measured from 3 days before and until 2 days after the AKI diagnosis and in no-AKI patients at 1, 5 and 10 days after admission. Biomarker sensitivity and specificity were determined. To validate the results obtained with ROC curves for Hsp72, a new set of critically ill patients was included, 10 with AKI and 12 with no-AKI patients.

Results: Urinary Hsp72 levels rose since 3 days before the AKI diagnosis in critically ill patients; this early increase was not seen with any other tested biomarkers. Kim-1, IL-18, NGAL, and Hsp72 significantly increased from 2 days before AKI and remained elevated during the AKI diagnosis. The best sensitivity/specificity was observed in Kim-1 and Hsp72: 83/95% and 100/90%, respectively, whereas 1 day before the AKI diagnosis, the values were 100/100% and 100/90%, respectively. The sensibility, specificity and accuracy in the validation test for Hsp72 were 100%, 83.3% and 90.9%, respectively.

Conclusions: The biomarker Hsp72 is enough sensitive and specific to predict AKI in critically ill patients up to 3 days before the diagnosis.

Editor: Antonio C. Seguro, University of São Paulo School of Medicine, Brazil

Funding: This project was supported by grants from the Mexican Council of Science and Technology (CONACyT) (181267 to NAB), http://www.conacyt.mx/ And from the National University of Mexico (IN203412-3 to NAB), http://dgapa.unam.mx/html/papiit/papit.html. The funders had no role in study design, data collection and analysis, decision to publish, or preparation of the manuscript.

Competing Interests: Dr. Luis E. Morales Buenrostro is an speaker of Novartis, Roche, and Sanofi México. He also has participated in advisory boards of Boehringer Ingelheim México, Eli Lilly Mexico, Astra Zeneca México and Bristol-Myers Squibb, Mexico. Dr. Norma A. Bobadilla and Dr. Jonatan Barrera have presented patent applications in México Canada, China, Europe, and US (Diagnostic method for detecting acute kidney injury using Hsp72 as a sensitive biomarker, US 2013/0065239 A1).

* Email: luis_buenrostro@yahoo.com (LEMB); nab@biomedicas.unam.mx (NAB)

Introduction

Acute kidney injury (AKI) remains a common syndrome in hospitalized patients in the intensive care unit (ICU) and has consistently been associated with increased morbidity and mortality [1–3]. The major causes of AKI are ischemic and nephrotoxic injuries [4]. Nearly 15% of hospitalized patients are at risk of developing AKI; however, the incidence increases up to 40–60% in patients admitted to the intensive care unit [5–8]. During AKI, many alterations occur at the cellular and molecular level that finally leads to organ dysfunction. Moreover, there is accumulating evidence which supports that patients who survive an AKI episode have a higher risk of developing chronic kidney disease (CKD) in the following years [9–12], including the patients with a complete renal function recovery [13].

Advances in reducing this complication have long been delayed by the lack of early and sensitive biomarkers [14]. In spite of creatinine limitations, the current acute kidney injury network (AKIN) and Risk, Injury, Failure, Loss of kidney function, and End-stage kidney disease (RIFLE) classifications for diagnosing AKI are based on the elevation of serum creatinine or urine output reduction [14–16]. Over the past few years, many studies have focused on the development of accurate biomarkers for AKI because early initiation of treatment could improve the prognosis for patients with AKI [17]. Therefore, the development of sensitive renal biomarkers is crucial for the identification of new therapeutic strategies for AKI; such biomarkers will facilitate early treatment, injury stratification and monitoring the course of the disease. With the use of the innovative genomic and proteomic tools, several molecules that are up-regulated during AKI in experimental models and humans have been identified and proposed as biomarkers. Among the most commonly used are: neutrophil gelatinase-associated lipocalin (NGAL), which is almost undetectable in normal epithelial renal cells and its expression is induced during AKI [18,19]; kidney injury molecule type 1 (Kim-1), which is induced on the surface of proximal tubule cells during ischemic or nephrotoxic injury [20–22]; and interleukin 18 (IL-18), which is over-expressed in patients diagnosed with AKI [23,24]. Recently, we showed that heat shock protein 72 (Hsp72) is an early and sensitive biomarker for AKI in rats and humans. Moreover, this novel biomarker was suitable for stratifying different degrees of tubular injury and recovery, and for monitoring a renoprotective intervention in an experimental rat model of AKI [25,26]. Because in our previous study, we showed that Hsp72 could predict AKI, we designed a study for diagnostic test to evaluate the sensitivity, specificity, and predictive values of Hsp72 compared with other conventional biomarkers in the early detection of AKI in critically ill patients.

Materials and Methods

This is a diagnostic test study that was performed in accordance with national and international guidelines and regulations, and was approved by Ethics Committee, Instituto Nacional de Ciencias Médicas y Nutrición Salvador Zubiran, México (No. 166) and it was adhered to Declaration of Helsinki. All subjects or designed surrogate (when ICU patients could not sign) signed the informed consent form.

Inclusion of critically ill ICU patients

A diagnostic test study was performed with only critically ill patients who were recruited during three months in the intensive care unit from our institution and who exhibited two or more organ failures. One of the organ failures had to be respiratory with

mechanical ventilation, a glomerular filtration rate (GFR) estimated by the Modification of Diet in Renal Disease (MDRD) Study equation >60 ml/min/1.73 m^2, and with no AKI at the moment of enrollment.

An aliquot of daily fresh urine sample was collected at 7 o'clock in the morning from all critically ill patients hospitalized in the ICU and stored at $-80°C$ until the biomarkers were measured. Serum creatinine and urinary volume were monitored daily. Accordingly with our gold standard for this study (AKIN criteria), AKI was defined when urinary output was <0.5 ml/kg/h during a 6-h period or when the serum creatinine increased more than 0.3 mg/dl or 1.5- to 2-fold increase from the baseline value.

Urinary Kim-1, IL-18, NGAL, and Hsp72 levels were measured by ELISA technique from 17 patients diagnosed with AKI, from 3 days before until 2 days after the development of AKI. From the daily samples collected from all patients who did not develop AKI, we randomly selected 20 patients to be included in the study. The biomarkers were analyzed only in urine samples from days 1, 5 and 10 after ICU admission. These sampling days were chosen to ensure that the biomarkers levels were representative of all hospitalization period in no AKI patients and supported by the fact that the release of these biomarkers in the urine did not occur so fast. In addition, the mean value of the 3 different urine samples of each biomarker was used to compare the values obtained in patients diagnosed with AKI and for the Receiver Operating Characteristic (ROC) curve analysis.

NGAL, Kim-1 and IL-18 detected by ELISA

Urinary NGAL, Kim-1 and IL-18 levels were analyzed using commercially available enzyme-linked immune absorbent assay (ELISA) kits: human NGAL ELISA kit (BioPorto Diagnostics, KIT036), human kidney injury molecule 1 (Kim-1) ELISA kit (Cusabio Biotech, CSB-E08807h) and human Interleukin-18 (IL-18) ELISA Kit (Invitrogen, KHC0181). All procedures were performed according to the manufacturer's instructions.

Table 1. Summary of baseline and clinical characteristics.

Variable	Total N = 37	AKI N = 17	NO AKI N = 20	p Value
Age (y)	51.6±20.2	54.5±22.5	49.2±18.2	0.42
Male	20 (54.1)	12 (70.6)	8 (40.0)	0.12
Mortality	15 (40.5)	8 (47.1)	7 (35.0)	0.68
Cause of admission to ICU				
Severe Sepsis or Septic Shock	20 (55.6)	11 (64.7)	9 (47.4)	0.38
Cardiovascular surgery	5 (13.9)	2 (11.8)	3 (15.8)	0.84
Neurological	4 (11.1)	2 (11.8)	2 (10.5)	0.72
No cardiovascular surgery	3 (8.3)	1 (5.9)	2 (10.5)	0.88
Other	4 (11.1)	1 (5.9)	3 (15.8)	0.72
Comorbidities on admission				
Hypertension	6 (16.2)	2 (11.8)	4 (20.0)	0.66
Diabetes	9 (24.3)	4 (23.5)	5 (25.0)	1.0
Cancer	9 (24.3)	4 (23.5)	5 (25.0)	1.0
SLE-APS	4 (10.8)	2 (11.8)	2 (10.0)	1.0
Obesity	5 (13.5)	4 (23.5)	1 (5.0)	0.15

Continuous values are represented as mean ± standard deviation; dichotomous values are N (%). AKI: Acute Kidney Injury. ICU: Intensive Care Unit. SLE: Systemic Lupus Erythematosus. APS: Antiphospholipid Syndrome.

Kim-1 in critically ill patients after ICU admission

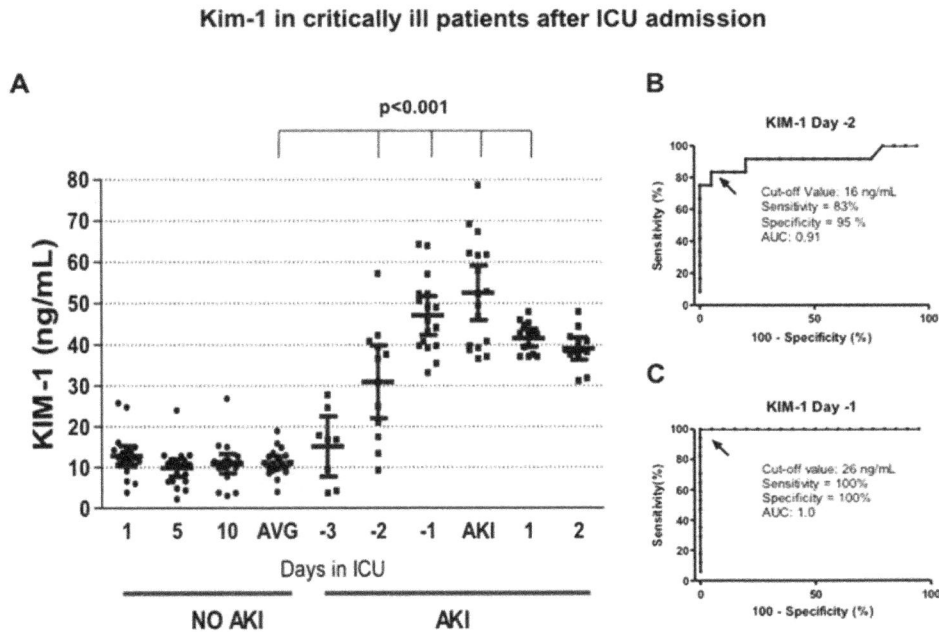

Figure 1. Kim-1 in critically ill patients after ICU admission. A) Urinary Kim-1 levels assessed by ELISA from AKI and no-AKI patients. In no-AKI patients, Kim-1 was measured at days 1, 5 and 10 of their stay in the ICU; whereas, in AKI patients Kim-1 was measured from ICU admission until two days after the diagnosis of AKI. Every point represents the biomarker value in each urine sample, and the lines depicted the mean and 95% confident interval. AVG = average of urinary Kim-1 levels in no-AKI patients determined at 1, 5, and 10 days after ICU admission. B) Specificity and sensitivity of Kim-1 to detect AKI two days before the AKIN criteria, determined by ROC analysis. C) Specificity and sensitivity of Kim-1 to detect AKI one day before the AKIN criteria, determined by ROC analysis.

NGAL in critically ill patients after ICU admission

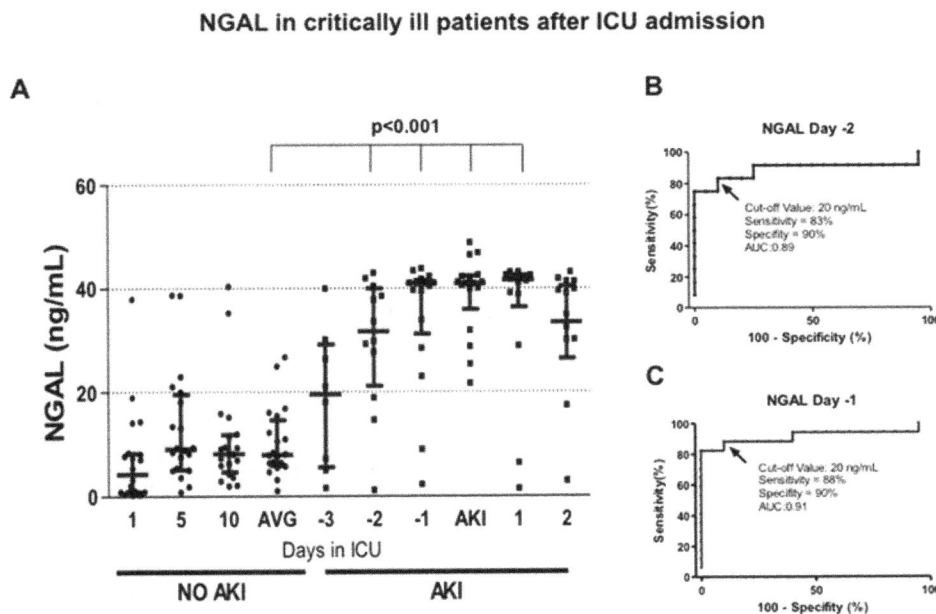

Figure 2. NGAL-1 in critically ill patients after ICU admission. A) Urinary NGAL levels assessed by ELISA from AKI and no-AKI patients. Every point represents the biomarker value in each urine sample, and the lines depicted the mean and 95% confident interval. AVG = average of urinary NGAL levels in no-AKI patients determined at 1, 5, and 10 days after ICU admission B) Specificity and sensitivity of NGAL to detect AKI two days before the AKIN criteria, as determined by ROC analysis. C) Specificity and sensitivity of NGAL to detect AKI one day before the AKIN criteria, determined by ROC analysis.

IL-18 in critically ill patients after ICU admission

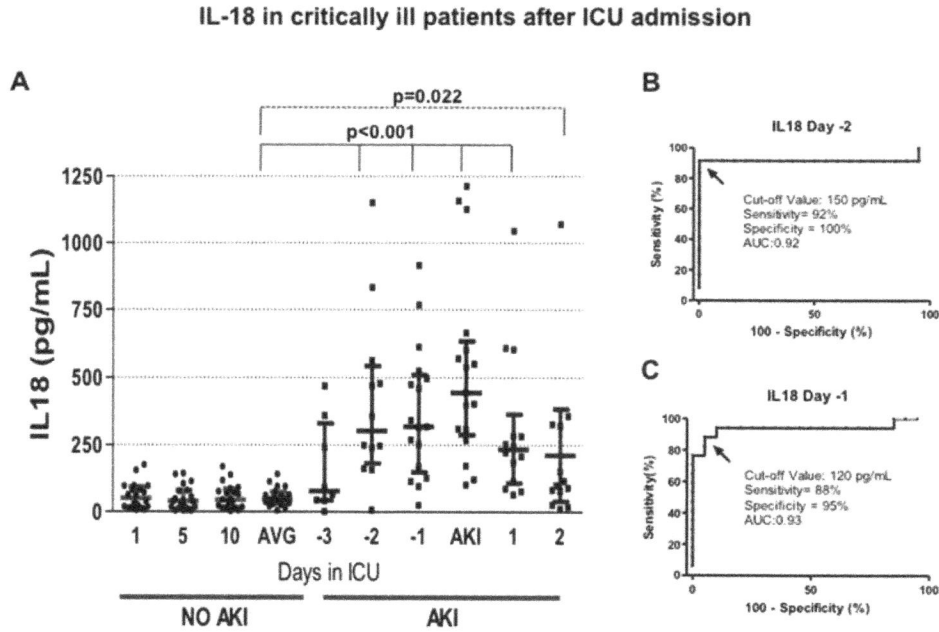

Figure 3. IL-18 in critically ill patients after ICU admission. A) Urinary IL-18 levels assessed by ELISA from AKI and no-AKI patients. Every point represents the biomarker value in each urine sample, and the lines depicted the mean and 95% confident interval. AVG = average of urinary IL-18 levels in no-AKI patients determined at 1, 5, and 10 days after ICU admission. B) Specificity and sensitivity of IL-18 to detect AKI two days before the AKIN criteria, determined by ROC analysis. C) Specificity and sensitivity of IL-18 to detect AKI one day before the AKIN criteria, determined by ROC analysis.

Urinary Hsp72 levels were assessed by ELISA

Urinary Hsp72 levels were also analyzed by ELISA, using a commercially available assay (Assay Designs ADI-EKS-715, MI, USA). Briefly, samples and standards were added to wells coated with a mouse monoclonal antibody. Hsp72 was captured by the antibody and then detected by adding a rabbit polyclonal

Hsp72 in critically ill patients after ICU admission

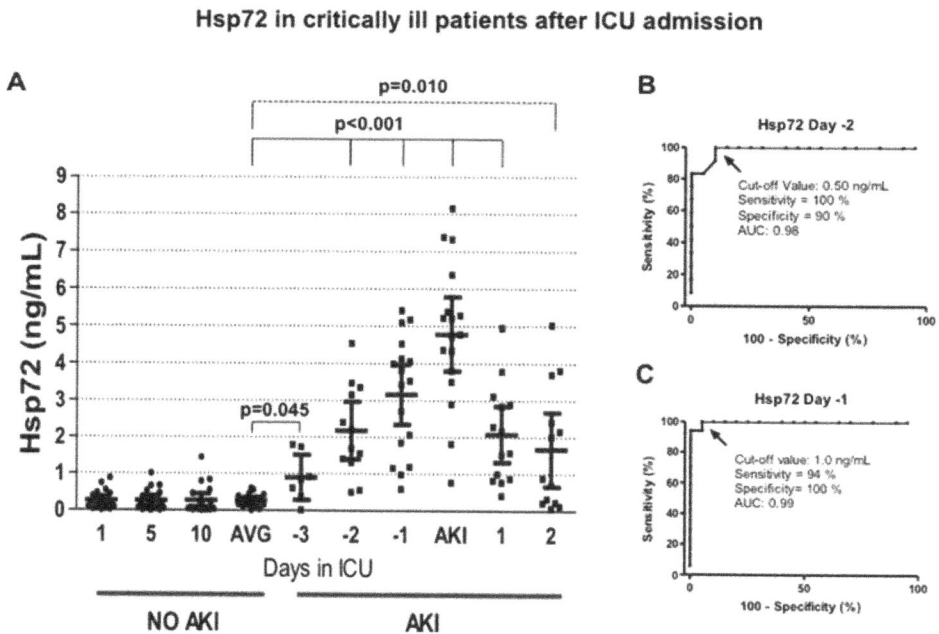

Figure 4. Hsp72 in critically ill patients after their admission at ICU. A) Urinary Hsp72 levels assessed by ELISA from AKI and no-AKI patients. Every point represents the biomarker value in each urine sample, and the lines depicted the mean and 95% confident interval. AVG = average of urinary Hsp72 levels in no-AKI patients determined at 1, 5, and 10 days after ICU admission. B) Specificity and sensitivity of Hsp72 to detect AKI two days before the AKIN criteria, determined by ROC analysis. C) Specificity and sensitivity of Hsp72 to detect AKI one day before the AKIN criteria, determined by ROC analysis.

Table 2. Validation test for Hsp72 in a similar population in ICU.

		Patients with AKI	Patients without AKI		
	Positive test	**10** (True Positive)	**2** (False Positive)	Positive Test = **12**	**PPV** = 83.3%
Hsp72 Cut-off value 1.0 ng/ml	**Negative Test**	**0** (False Negative)	**10** (True Negative)	Negative Test = **10**	**NPV** = 100%
		Total AKI = 10	**Total No AKI = 12**	**All Patients = 22**	
		Sensibility = 100%	**Specificity** = 83.3%	**Accuracy** = 90.9%	

Use of cut-off value one day before AKI diagnosis (AKIN criteria). PPV = Positive Predictive Value. NPV = Negative Predictive Value.

detection antibody. The Hsp72 antibody is specific and does not react with other members of the Hsp70 family. A horseradish peroxidase conjugate binds to the detection antibody, color development was achieved by the addition of a tetramethylbenzidine substrate, and the reaction was stopped with an acid stop solution. The optical density of samples was read at 450 nm by a plate reader and was overlapped with the standard curve generated from known concentrations of recombinant Hsp72, ranging from 0.1 to 12.5 ng/ml.

Validation test

To validate the results obtained by the ROC curves for Hsp72 in our primary phase of this study, three months after the study ended, we included a new set of patients with the same inclusion and exclusion criteria. A total of 22 patients were included, 10 with AKI and 12 with no-AKI. Because there are not previous studies evaluating Hsp72 biomarker performance for AKI in humans, we selected the cut-off value for Hsp72 according to the point in the ROC analysis at -1 day that conferred the best values for sensitivity and specificity. In addition, AUC, positive and negative predictive values were determined.

Statistical analysis

Categorical variables are shown as frequencies and proportions, whereas continuous variables were analyzed with the Kolmogorov-Smirnov test to determine the distribution. The values of the 4 biomarkers assessed showed a normal distribution; therefore, the mean and 95% confident interval for each assessed day were calculated. Comparisons of the categorical variables were performed by the x^2 test. To compare biomarker values between the AKI and no-AKI groups, we used the Student's t test. ROC curves were performed to calculate biomarkers sensitivity, specificity and area under curve (AUC) 1 and 2 days before the development of AKI. For the Hsp72 validation assay, we performed a ROC analysis with the best cut-off point (1.0 ng/ml) found in the main part of the study. Statistical significance was defined when the p value was <0.05.

Results

The development of AKI

During the study period of 3-months, a total of 56 patients fulfilled the inclusion criteria. Seventeen were diagnosed with AKI with the AKIN criteria, which represents 30.4%, whereas, 39 (69.6%) did not develop AKI. To maintain a better proportion of positive cases, no-AKI group was composed by only 20 randomly-chosen patients.

In the 17 patients who developed AKI, AKIN I was observed in 10 (58.8%), AKIN II in 7 (41.2%) and none was in the AKIN III class. For all the AKI cases, 35.3% was diagnosed on base of a reduction in urinary output, 58.8% by serum creatinine elevation, and 5.9% by the combination of both parameters.

AKI appearance was observed in 16.2% of patients after one day of ICU admission, 5.4% after two days, and 78.4% developed AKI after three days. It is important to remember that one of the inclusion criteria was a GFR>60 ml/min.

Main characteristics of critically ill patients with AKI and no-AKI

In Table 1, the baseline characteristics of the studied patients are listed. Thirty-seven patients were included: 17 with AKI and 20 with no-AKI. No differences were found in the mean age, gender or mortality between the patients who developed AKI compared with no-AKI patients in the ICU. The major cause of AKI was associated with septic shock, followed by cardiovascular surgery, neurological alterations, or miscellaneous causes. The main co-morbidities found were hypertension, diabetes, cancer, systemic lupus erythematous and obesity.

Using Kim-1, NGAL, IL-18 to establish an early diagnosis of AKI

In critically ill patients who did not developed AKI, the biomarkers were quantified on days 1, 5 and 10 of their stay in the ICU. The media from these three measurements was compared with the media from critically ill patients who developed AKI. In the AKI population, the biomarkers were measured from 3 days before the serum creatinine elevation until 2 days after the AKI diagnosis occurred. Figure 1A shows the urinary Kim-1 levels in all patients studied. Patients with no-AKI exhibited urinary Kim-1 values approximately 10 ng/ml; this value remained unaffected throughout 10 days in the ICU. In contrast, the urinary Kim-1 levels in AKI patients rose significantly from 2 days before the AKI diagnosis using the AKIN criteria (p<0.001) and remained elevated throughout the study protocol in all the AKI patients. The AUC-ROC analysis, using a cut-off value of 16 ng/ml, revealed that at -2 day, the sensitivity and specificity of Kim-1 to detect AKI was 83 and 95%, respectively, with an AUC of 0.91 (Figure 1B). At -1 day, the sensitivity and specificity improved to 100% with an AUC of 1.00 (Figure 1C), with a cut-off value of 26 ng/ml.

Regarding NGAL, greater variability was found in the urinary NGAL levels of no-AKI patient than Kim-1 in no-AKI patients. This variability was also observed in AKI patients, but there was a significant elevation in NGAL values from -2 days (p<0.001), and similar to Kim-1, these values remained elevated (Figure 2A). Similar sensitivity and specificity of Kim-1 was observed at -2 days (83 and 90%, respectively), with an AUC of 0.89 (Figure 2B). In contrast, NGAL exhibited lesser sensitivity and specificity than Kim-1 at -1 day (88 and 90%, respectively), with an AUC of 0.91 (Figure 2C). In both cases, the same cut off value was used (20 ng/ml).

In Figure 3A, the urinary IL-18 values are represented in both AKI and no-AKI patients during their staying in the ICU. Patients with no-AKI exhibited basal urinary IL-18 values of approximately 40 ng/ml that remained constant throughout 10 days in the ICU. In contrast, the urinary IL-18 levels rose by more than 5-fold from 2 days before the AKI diagnosis using the AKIN criteria (p<0.001). A progressive reduction in urinary IL-18 started after the AKI diagnosis; however, a great variability in each set of measurements was observed with this biomarker. The AUC-ROC analysis revealed that at -2 days, the Kim-1 sensitivity and specificity to detect AKI was 92 and 100%, respectively, with an AUC of 0.92, using a cut-off value of 150 pg/ml (Figure 3B). At -1 day, the sensitivity and specificity were 88 and 95%, respectively, with an AUC of 0.93, using a cut-off value of 120 pg/ml (Figure 3C).

Finally, patients with no-AKI exhibited urinary Hsp72 values of approximately 0.3 ng/ml that remained unaffected throughout 10 days in the ICU. In contrast, the urinary Hsp72 levels in AKI patients rose significantly from 3 days before AKI was diagnosed with the AKIN criteria (p = 0.045). This difference was not seen with the other 3 biomarkers. A progressive increase in urinary Hsp72 levels was observed from -3 days to the diagnosis of AKI, followed by a progressive reduction until day 2 post AKI diagnosis, the last day of assessment (Figure 4A). The ROC analysis revealed that at -2 day, the sensitivity and specificity of Hsp72 to detect AKI was 100 and 90%, respectively, with an AUC of 0.98, using a cut-off value of 0.5 ng/ml (Figure 4B). At -1 day, the sensitivity and specificity was 94 and 100%, respectively with an AUC of 99%, with a cut-off value of 1.0 ng/ml (Figure 4C).

Hsp72 validation test

For the Hsp72 validation test, a total of 22 patients were included, 10 with AKI and 12 no-AKI. The best cut-off value of Hsp72 for ROC was taken at 1 day before the AKI diagnosis. Table 2 lists the sensitivity, specificity, accuracy, and positive and negative predictive values of urinary Hsp72 in AKI and no-AKI patients. No false negatives were observed in patients with AKI and two false positives were observed in no-AKI patients. Thus, the sensibility/specificity and accuracy were 100/83.3% and 90.9%, respectively.

Discussion

This is the first diagnostic test study that showed that urinary Hsp72 detection is a sensitive and early AKI biomarker for critically ill patients. Specifically, in patients who arrived in the ICU of our institution 3 days before the AKI diagnosis, Hsp72 effectively detected AKI. This performance was not seen with other assessed biomarkers. Moreover, in the urine samples at -2 and -1 days, the best detection methods of AKI were Kim-1 and Hsp72, followed by NGAL and IL-18.

The clinical impact of AKI is very clear. AKI is associated with increased morbidity, mortality, length of hospital stay, and cost. [1,27] AKI complicates the course of disease in critically ill patients, causing several million deaths worldwide every year. Efforts to change its clinical course have failed because early detection is not possible with SCr elevation or oliguria, and novel biomarkers have not proven to be sufficiently efficacious. [28,29] As a consequence, a delay in initiating appropriate therapies contributes to disappointing prognoses. However, a major disadvantage limiting the routine use of biomarkers is low sensitivity and specificity, which generally do not exceed 70 to 75%, for detecting early kidney damage [30]. Therefore, the creation of a kit integrating several biomarkers for the accurate diagnosis of AKI in the ICU has been proposed [28,29].

We previously showed that Hsp72 is a reliable biomarker for the early detection of AKI in rats. Thus, urinary Hsp72 levels were adequately sensitive for stratifying different degrees of tubular injury and recovery, and for monitoring a renoprotective intervention in an experimental rat model of AKI induced by bilateral renal ischemia/reperfusion. [25] The clinical application of a new biomarker should be more accurate with earlier detectability than the current gold standard SCr. Here, we showed enough evidence indicating that Hsp72 is a specific and sensitive biomarker to detect AKI before SCr elevation is noted in critically ill patients.

Most of the previous studies using biomarkers have focused on and been validated in situations in which the time of renal injury can be easily known, such as during cardiac surgery, administration of intravenous contrast, or other nephrotoxic agents. [24,31,32–38] In contrast, this study was designed to focus on critically ill patients, who clinicians see in their daily practice, and there is uncertainty about the precise moment in which AKI starts. Here, we found that the increase in urinary Hsp72 levels preceded the rise in creatinine and reduction in urinary volume by up to 3 days.

Although, most of the other biomarkers assessed showed similar ability to predict AKI 24-h before the AKIN criteria were fulfilled, Hsp72 was clearly superior because it was the earliest detectable AKI biomarker and was extremely sensitive and specific.

In this study, we found that most of the cases of AKI were classified as AKIN 1, a class seen by clinicians as having little relevance or clinical impact. However, in the context of the ICU, early detection of mild cases of AKI will improve renal perfusion and can modify the natural history of AKI, with the potential to reduce the frequency of AKI and CKD development.

Although, there is uncertainty on how and when measurements of any novel biomarker should be completed because in clinical practice, this is a challenge. [39] Most critically ill patients developed AKI in the first three days after admission. Thus, to efficiently detect AKI before conventional markers, the balance between cost and benefit would favor daily urinary Hsp72 detection, from ICU admission to three to five days after ICU discharge.

To reinforce our results, we validated with a different ICU patient population and obtained similar results. The strength of our study is based in that all included patients had the same critical conditions and none healthy subject was included, thus Hsp72 elevation was not related to the clinical condition.

The ability of urinary Hsp72 levels to detect AKI could differ depending on the cause of AKI, such as contrast-induced nephropathy or post-surgical AKI. Thus, more studies are necessary to prove the applicability of Hsp72 in these entities.

The limitations of our study are the number of critically ill patients included and the exclusion of patients with pre-existing chronic kidney disease. Thus the applicability of this biomarker in this population of patients have to wait until the validation will be performed.

Our data show that Hsp72 is a sensitive biomarker for detecting early AKI in critically ill patients without pre-existing chronic kidney disease, which could be helpful to establish early interventions intended to prevent or reduce AKI severity and improve prognosis.

Acknowledgments

The results presented in this paper have not been previously published in whole or in part, except as an abstract presented at the Annual Meetings & Scientific Exposition 2012 of the American Society of Nephrology (San Diego, CA. USA).

Author Contributions

Conceived and designed the experiments: LEMB NAB. Performed the experiments: JBCH RPV OISN GCA SIS. Analyzed the data: LEMB JBCH OISN NAB. Contributed reagents/materials/analysis tools: JBCH RPV NAB. Contributed to the writing of the manuscript: LEMB NAB.

References

1. Chertow GM, Burdick E, Honour M, Bonventre JV, Bates DW (2005) Acute kidney injury, mortality, length of stay, and costs in hospitalized patients. J Am Soc Nephrol 16: 3365–3370. ASN.2004090740 [pii];10.1681/ASN.2004090740 [doi].
2. Liano F, Pascual J (1996) Epidemiology of acute renal failure: a prospective, multicenter, community-based study. Madrid Acute Renal Failure Study Group. Kidney Int 50: 811–818.
3. Waikar SS, Curhan GC, Wald R, McCarthy EP, Chertow GM (2006) Declining mortality in patients with acute renal failure, 1988 to 2002. J Am Soc Nephrol 17: 1143–1150.
4. Thadhani R, Pascual M, Bonventre JV (1996) Acute renal failure. N Engl J Med 334: 1448–1460.
5. Munshi R, Hsu C, Himmelfarb J (2011) Advances in understanding ischemic acute kidney injury. BMC Med 9: 11. 1741-7015-9-11 [pii];10.1186/1741-7015-9-11 [doi].
6. Murugan R, Kellum JA (2011) Acute kidney injury: what's the prognosis? Nat Rev Nephrol 7: 209–217. nrneph.2011.13 [pii];10.1038/nrneph.2011.13 [doi].
7. Lafrance JP, Miller DR (2010) Acute kidney injury associates with increased long-term mortality. J Am Soc Nephrol 21: 345–352. ASN.2009060636 [pii];10.1681/ASN.2009060636 [doi].
8. Kelly KJ (2006) Acute renal failure: much more than a kidney disease. Semin Nephrol 26: 105–113.
9. Jones J, Holmen J, De Graauw J, Jovanovich A, Thornton S, et al. (2012) Association of complete recovery from acute kidney injury with incident CKD stage 3 and all-cause mortality. Am J Kidney Dis 60: 402–408. S0272-6386(12)00637-3 [pii];10.1053/j.ajkd.2012.03.014 [doi].
10. Venkatachalam MA, Griffin KA, Lan R, Geng H, Saikumar P, et al. (2010) Acute kidney injury: a springboard for progression in chronic kidney disease. Am J Physiol Renal Physiol. 00017.2010 [pii];10.1152/ajprenal.00017.2010 [doi].
11. Hsu CY (2012) Yes, AKI truly leads to CKD. J Am Soc Nephrol 23: 967–969. ASN.2012030222 [pii];10.1681/ASN.2012030222 [doi].
12. Coca SG, Singanamala S, Parikh CR (2012) Chronic kidney disease after acute kidney injury: a systematic review and meta-analysis. Kidney Int 81: 442–448. ki2011379 [pii];10.1038/ki.2011.379 [doi].
13. Bucaloiu ID, Kirchner HL, Norfolk ER, Hartle JE, Perkins RM (2012) Increased risk of death and de novo chronic kidney disease following reversible acute kidney injury. Kidney Int 81: 477–485. ki2011405 [pii];10.1038/ki.2011.405 [doi].
14. Wu I, Parikh CR (2008) Screening for kidney diseases: older measures versus novel biomarkers. Clin J Am Soc Nephrol 3: 1895–1901.
15. Bagshaw SM (2010) Acute kidney injury: diagnosis and classification of AKI: AKIN or RIFLE? Nat Rev Nephrol 6: 71–73.
16. Lopes JA, Fernandes P, Jorge S, Goncalves S, Alvarez A, et al. (2008) Acute kidney injury in intensive care unit patients: a comparison between the RIFLE and the Acute Kidney Injury Network classifications. Crit Care 12: R110.
17. Lameire NH, Bagga A, Cruz D, De MJ, Endre Z, et al. (2013) Acute kidney injury: an increasing global concern. Lancet 382: 170–179. S0140-6736(13)60647-9 [pii];10.1016/S0140-6736(13)60647-9 [doi].
18. Mishra J, Ma Q, Prada A, Mitsnefes M, Zahedi K, et al. (2003) Identification of neutrophil gelatinase-associated lipocalin as a novel early urinary biomarker for ischemic renal injury. J Am Soc Nephrol 14: 2534–2543.
19. Mishra J, Dent C, Tarabishi R, Mitsnefes MM, Ma Q, et al. (2005) Neutrophil gelatinase-associated lipocalin (NGAL) as a biomarker for acute renal injury after cardiac surgery. Lancet 365: 1231–1238.
20. Vaidya VS, Ramirez V, Ichimura T, Bobadilla NA, Bonventre JV (2006) Urinary kidney injury molecule-1: a sensitive quantitative biomarker for early detection of kidney tubular injury. Am J Physiol Renal Physiol 290: F517–F529.
21. Vaidya VS, Ford GM, Waikar SS, Wang Y, Clement MB, et al. (2009) A rapid urine test for early detection of kidney injury. Kidney Int 76: 108–114.
22. Vaidya VS, Ozer JS, Dieterle F, Collings FB, Ramirez V, et al. (2010) Kidney injury molecule-1 outperforms traditional biomarkers of kidney injury in preclinical biomarker qualification studies. Nat Biotechnol 28: 478–485.
23. Melnikov VY, Ecder T, Fantuzzi G, Siegmund B, Lucia MS, et al. (2001) Impaired IL-18 processing protects caspase-1-deficient mice from ischemic acute renal failure. J Clin Invest 107: 1145–1152.
24. Parikh CR, Mishra J, Thiessen-Philbrook H, Dursun B, Ma Q, et al. (2006) Urinary IL-18 is an early predictive biomarker of acute kidney injury after cardiac surgery. Kidney Int 70: 199–203.
25. Barrera-Chimal J, Perez-Villalva R, Cortes-Gonzalez C, Ojeda-Cervantes M, Gamba G, et al. (2011) Hsp72 is an early and sensitive biomarker to detect acute kidney injury. EMBO Mol Med 3: 5–20. 10.1002/emmm.201000105 [doi].
26. Sanchez-Pozos K, Barrera-Chimal J, Garzon-Muvdi J, Perez-Villalva R, Rodriguez-Romo R, et al. (2012) Recovery from ischemic acute kidney injury by spironolactone administration. Nephrol Dial Transplant 27: 3160–3169. gfs014 [pii];10.1093/ndt/gfs014 [doi].
27. Lewington AJ, Cerda J, Mehta RL (2013) Raising awareness of acute kidney injury: a global perspective of a silent killer. Kidney Int 84: 457–467. ki2013153 [pii];10.1038/ki.2013.153 [doi].
28. Molitoris BA, Melnikov VY, Okusa MD, Himmelfarb J (2008) Technology Insight: biomarker development in acute kidney injury–what can we anticipate? Nat Clin Pract Nephrol 4: 154–165. ncpneph0723 [pii];10.1038/ncpneph0723 [doi].
29. Endre ZH, Pickering JW, Walker RJ, Devarajan P, Edelstein CL, et al. (2011) Improved performance of urinary biomarkers of acute kidney injury in the critically ill by stratification for injury duration and baseline renal function. Kidney Int 79: 1119–1130. ki2010555 [pii];10.1038/ki.2010.555 [doi].
30. Cruz DN, de Geus HR, Bagshaw SM (2011) Biomarker strategies to predict need for renal replacement therapy in acute kidney injury. Semin Dial 24: 124–131. 10.1111/j.1525-139X.2011.00830.x [doi].
31. Wagener G, Jan M, Kim M, Mori K, Barasch JM, et al. (2006) Association between increases in urinary neutrophil gelatinase-associated lipocalin and acute renal dysfunction after adult cardiac surgery. Anesthesiology 105: 485–491.
32. Parikh CR, Devarajan P, Zappitelli M, Sint K, Thiessen-Philbrook H, et al. (2011) Postoperative biomarkers predict acute kidney injury and poor outcomes after adult cardiac surgery. J Am Soc Nephrol 22: 1748–1757. ASN.2010121302 [pii];10.1681/ASN.2010121302 [doi].
33. Bennett M, Dent CL, Ma Q, Dastrala S, Grenier F, et al. (2008) Urine NGAL predicts severity of acute kidney injury after cardiac surgery: a prospective study. Clin J Am Soc Nephrol 3: 665–673. CJN.04010907 [pii];10.2215/CJN.04010907 [doi].
34. Torregrosa I, Montoliu C, Urios A, Elmlili N, Puchades MJ, et al. (2012) Early biomarkers of acute kidney failure after heart angiography or heart surgery in patients with acute coronary syndrome or acute heart failure. Nefrologia 32: 44–52. 10.3265/Nefrologia.pre2011.Sep.10988 [doi].
35. Matsui K, Kamijo-Ikemori A, Sugaya T, Yasuda T, Kimura K (2012) Usefulness of urinary biomarkers in early detection of acute kidney injury after cardiac surgery in adults. Circ J 76: 213–220. JST.JSTAGE/circj/CJ-11-0342 [pii].
36. Wagener G, Gubitosa G, Wang S, Borregaard N, Kim M, et al. (2008) Urinary neutrophil gelatinase-associated lipocalin and acute kidney injury after cardiac surgery. Am J Kidney Dis 52: 425–433. S0272-6386(08)00957-8 [pii];10.1053/j.ajkd.2008.05.018 [doi].
37. Parikh CR, Devarajan P, Zappitelli M, Sint K, Thiessen-Philbrook H, et al. (2011) Postoperative biomarkers predict acute kidney injury and poor outcomes after pediatric cardiac surgery. J Am Soc Nephrol 22: 1737–1747. ASN.2010111163 [pii];10.1681/ASN.2010111163 [doi].
38. Haase M, Bellomo R, Story D, Davenport P, Haase-Fielitz A (2008) Urinary interleukin-18 does not predict acute kidney injury after adult cardiac surgery: a prospective observational cohort study. Crit Care 12: R96. cc6972 [pii];10.1186/cc6972 [doi].
39. Gonzalez F, Vincent F (2012) Biomarkers for acute kidney injury in critically ill patients. Minerva Anestesiol 78: 1394–1403. R02127783 [pii].

11

Comparison of Estimated Glomerular Filtration Rate by the Chronic Kidney Disease Epidemiology Collaboration (CKD-EPI) Equations with and without Cystatin C for Predicting Clinical Outcomes in Elderly Women

Wai H. Lim[1,2*¶], Joshua R. Lewis[1,3¶], Germaine Wong[4,5¶], Robin M. Turner[6], Ee M. Lim[2,7], Peter L. Thompson[8], Richard L. Prince[1,3]

1 University of Western Australia School of Medicine and Pharmacology, Sir Charles Gairdner Hospital Unit, Perth, Australia, 2 Department of Renal Medicine, Sir Charles Gairdner Hospital, Perth, Australia, 3 Department of Endocrinology and Diabetes, Sir Charles Gairdner Hospital, Perth, Australia, 4 Centre for Kidney Research, Children's Hospital at Westmead, Sydney, Australia, 5 School of Public Health, Sydney Medical School, The University of Sydney, Sydney, Australia, 6 School of Public Health, The University of New South Wales, Sydney, Australia, 7 PathWest, Sir Charles Gairdner Hospital, Perth, Australia, 8 Department of Cardiovascular Medicine, Sir Charles Gairdner Hospital, Perth, Australia

Abstract

Background: Reduced estimated glomerular filtration rate (eGFR) using the cystatin-C derived equations might be a better predictor of cardiovascular disease (CVD) mortality compared with the creatinine-derived equations, but this association remains unclear in elderly individuals.

Aim: The aims of this study were to compare the predictive values of the Chronic Kidney Disease Epidemiology Collaboration (CKD-EPI)-creatinine, CKD-EPI-cystatin C and CKD-EPI-creatinine-cystatin C eGFR equations for all-cause mortality and CVD events (hospitalizations±mortality).

Methods: Prospective cohort study of 1165 elderly women aged>70 years. Associations between eGFR and outcomes were examined using Cox regression analysis. Test accuracy of eGFR equations for predicting outcomes was examined using Receiver Operating Characteristic (ROC) analysis and net reclassification improvement (NRI).

Results: Risk of all-cause mortality for every incremental reduction in eGFR determined using CKD-EPI-creatinine, CKD-EPI-cystatin C and the CKD-EPI-creatinine-cystatic C equations was similar. Areas under the ROC curves of CKD-EPI-creatinine, CKD-EPI-cystatin C and CKD-EPI-creatinine-cystatin C equations for all-cause mortality were 0.604 (95%CI 0.561–0.647), 0.606 (95%CI 0.563–0.649; p = 0.963) and 0.606 (95%CI 0.563–0.649; p = 0.894) respectively. For all-cause mortality, there was no improvement in the reclassification of eGFR categories using the CKD-EPI-cystatin C (NRI -4.1%; p = 0.401) and CKD-EPI-creatinine-cystatin C (NRI -1.2%; p = 0.748) compared with CKD-EPI-creatinine equation. Similar findings were observed for CVD events.

Conclusion: eGFR derived from CKD-EPI cystatin C and CKD-EPI creatinine-cystatin C equations did not improve the accuracy or predictive ability for clinical events compared to CKD-EPI-creatinine equation in this cohort of elderly women.

Editor: Antonio Carlos Seguro, University of São Paulo School of Medicine, Brazil

Funding: Dr. Lewis was supported by Raine Medical Research Foundation Priming Grant and Dr. Turner was supported by National Health and Medical Research Council (NHMRC) program grant #633003 to the Screening & Test Evaluation Program. The authors had full access to all of the data in the study and take responsibility for the integrity of the data and the accuracy of the data analysis. The study was supported by Kidney Health Australia, Healthway Health Promotion Foundation of Western Australia and by project grants 254627, 303169 and 572604 from the National Health and Medical Research Council of Australia. The funders had no role in study design, data collection and analysis, decision to publish, or preparation of the manuscript.

Competing Interests: The authors have declared that no competing interests exist.

* Email: wai.lim@health.wa.gov.au

¶ These authors contributed equally to this work.

¶ These authors are co-first authors on this work.

Comparison of Estimated Glomerular Filtration Rate by the Chronic Kidney Disease Epidemiology...

89

Introduction

Chronic kidney disease (CKD) is a major public health burden worldwide. Patients with CKD, especially those on dialysis, suffer from reduced life expectancy and quality of life [1]. CKD is a multi-system disease with established evidence demonstrating reduced kidney function increases the risk of cardiovascular disease (CVD) mortality [2–5], infections and cancer [6]. Previous meta-analyses reported the risk of associated disease such as CVD mortality commences with an estimated glomerular filtration rate (eGFR) of less than 60 ml/min/1.73 m^2 and increases exponentially as one approaches end-stage renal disease (ESRD) requiring dialysis. However, epidemiological studies have also shown that eGFR between 60–74.9 mL/min/1.73 m^2 is associated with a higher risk of CVD-related death compared to eGFR of $\geq$ 75 mL/min/1.73 m^2 in patients following myocardial infarction suggesting that the risk of adverse clinical events is not confined to those with eGFR of less than 60 mL/min/1.73 m^2 [7]. Although it is generally accepted that early identification of CKD may slow the progression to advanced stage kidney disease and provides a window of opportunity to prevent associated illness such as CVD and cancer [8], the threshold of reduced kidney function that prompts early intervention remains undefined suggesting that determining precise GFR in individuals may not be absolutely critical.

Chronic Kidney Disease Epidemiology Collaboration (CKD-EPI) equation [3] has been shown to be a more reliable marker of measured GFR and is superior in predicting the risk of adverse clinical outcomes such as mortality and stroke compared to Modification of Diet in Renal Disease (MDRD) [9] or the Cockcroft-Gault equations [10]. Although these equations are widely used in the community, previous studies have shown that serum creatinine-based equations may underestimate actual kidney function, especially in elderly individuals. As serum creatinine is affected by multiple factors including muscle mass and age, [11], alternative filtration markers such as cystatin C have been evaluated for GFR estimation.

Several newly-derived eGFR equations such as the CKD-EPI cystatin C and CKD-EPI creatinine-cystatin C equations have shown improvement in the precision and accuracy of determining GFR compared to CKD-EPI creatinine equation, but uncertainties remain as to the clinical significance and cost-effectiveness of using cystatin C-derived eGFR estimations over creatinine-derived eGFR estimations in the general population, particularly in elderly individuals. A recent meta-analysis of sixteen population cohorts reported both CKD-EPI cystatin C and combined CKD-EPI creatinine-cystatin C equations improved the accuracy in predicting all-cause and CVD mortality compared to CKD-EPI creatinine equation, but the majority of the included population cohorts were younger individuals of mixed gender with dissimilar proportion of muscle mass [12]. There have been no prior studies examining the clinical utility of these newly derived cystatin C equations in predicting adverse clinical outcomes exclusively in the older female population. The aims of this study were to determine the association of reduced kidney function as measured by CKD-EPI creatinine, CKD-EPI cystatin C and CKD-EPI creatinine-cystatin C equations and all-cause mortality and CVD events and also to assess the accuracy of these newly derived cystatin C-based eGFR equations in the prediction of clinical events in a cohort of elderly women mainly without prevalent CKD and with two-thirds of women with eGFR above 60 mL/min/1.73 m^2.

Subjects and Methods

Study Population

One thousand five hundred women were recruited in 1998 to a five-year prospective, randomized, controlled trial of oral calcium supplements (1.2 g of elemental calcium daily or matching placebo) to prevent osteoporotic fractures, the Calcium Intake Fracture Outcome study (CAIFOS; Australian Clinical Trials Registry Registration Number: ACTRN012607000055404) [13]. Details of recruitment are published elsewhere [13]. Our population-based study is representative of the general elderly population in Western Australia. Participants were women aged over 70 years who were selected using the electoral roll and contacted by mail. Registration on this electoral roll is a standard and compulsory requirement of citizenship in Australia. Of the 5,586 women who responded to a letter inviting participation, 1510 eligible women were randomly selected. Participants had similar disease burden and pharmaceutical consumption to the whole population of this age but they were more likely to be from higher socio-economic groups [13]. The University of Western Australia Human Ethics Committee had approved the study and written informed consents were obtained from all participants. The present study is to evaluate the utility of creatinine and/or cystatin-derived eGFR equations in a cohort of elderly women recruited in 1998 in predicting 10-year clinical outcomes up to 2008.

Baseline medical history including the presence of diabetes, hypertension, smoking history (current/former smokers or non-smokers) and medications were obtained from all participants. Blood pressure was measured on the right arm with a mercury column manometer using an adult cuff after the participants have been seated in an upright position and had rested for 5 minutes. An average of three blood pressure readings was recorded.

Fasting blood samples were collected at baseline (i.e. at time of randomisation in 1998) with sera stored in −70°C freezer until analysis. Creatinine and cystatin C measurements were performed using stored sera after 2008 and results were available in 1165 women (77%). Serum creatinine was analysed using an isotope dilution mass spectrometry (IDMS) traceable Jaffe kinetic assay for creatinine on a Hitachi 917 analyser (Roche Diagnostics GmbH, Mannheim Germany). Serum cystatin C was measured on the Siemens Dade Behring Nephelometer, traceable to the International Federation of Clinical Chemistry Working Group for Standardization of Serum cystatin C and the Institute for Reference Materials and Measurements certified reference materials. eGFR was estimated by three equations derived by *Inker et al* and these are presented in Table S1 – CKD-EPI creatinine equation, CKD-EPI cystatin C equation and CKD-EPI creatinine-cystatin C equation [14].

Assessment of clinical outcomes

Participants' general practitioners verified their medical histories and medications where possible, and were coded using the International Classification of Primary Care–Plus (ICPC-Plus) method [15]. Prevalent CVD was determined from hospital discharge data between 1980 and 1998 and were defined using diagnosis codes from the International Classification of Diseases, Injuries and Causes of Death Clinical Modification (ICD-9-CM, 309-459) [16]. Prevalent renal disease was collected between 1980 and 1998 using International Classification of Diseases, Injuries and Causes of Death Clinical Modification (ICD-9-CM) 17. These codes included glomerular diseases (ICD-9-CM codes 580–583); renal tubulo-interstitial diseases (ICD-9-CM codes 593.3–593.5, 593.7); renal failure (ICD-9-CM codes 584–586); and hypertensive renal disease (ICD-9-CM code 403). The search for renal disease hospitalizations included any diagnosis code.

The primary outcomes of the study were all-cause mortality and CVD hospitalizations and/or mortality retrieved from the Western Australian Data Linkage System (WADLS) for each of the study participants from 1998 until 10 years following their initial study visit. CVD hospitalizations and mortality were defined using primary diagnosis codes from ICD-9-CM, 390-459 [16] and the International Statistical Classification of Diseases and Related Health Problems, 10th Revision, Australian Modification (ICD-10-AM), I00-I99 [17]. All diagnosis text fields from the death certificate were used to ascertain the cause(s) of deaths where these data were not yet available from the WADLS.

Statistical Analysis

Baseline characteristics were expressed as mean and standard deviation (SD) for continuous variables or as number and proportion for categorical variables. Association between eGFR and all-cause mortality and CVD hospitalization and/or mortality was examined using Cox proportional hazard regression model and results were expressed as hazard ratio (HR) with 95% confidence interval (CI) for every incremental reduction in eGFR to allow comparison between equations. The covariates included in the Cox regression models were age, smoking history, body mass index (BMI), diabetes, antihypertensive medications, systolic blood pressure, treatment code, prevalent renal and CVD.

To assess performance of the different equations for estimating eGFR, we assessed the discrimination of the three different models using the Area Under Curve (AUC). Discrimination refers to how well the model distinguishes individuals with and without the outcomes of interests. To assess discrimination, we calculated the area under the receiver operating characteristic (ROC) curve (AUC). An area of 1 implies perfect discrimination, whereas an area of 0.5 represents random discrimination. The sidak option provides adjusted p-values comparing the ROC areas between

eGFR equations, assuming a "gold standard" being the CKD-EPI creatinine equation. For net reclassification improvement (NRI), participants were classified into three eGFR categories for all-cause and CVD hospitalization and/or mortality (≥ 75, 60–74.9 and <60 mL/min/1.73 m^2), and then reclassified into new eGFR categories with CKD-EPI cystatin C equation and CKD-EPI creatinine-cystatin C equation as compared with CKD-EPI creatinine equation. P-values of less than 0.05 in two tailed testing were considered statistically significant. The data was analysed using SPSS (version 15; SPSS Inc, Chicago, IL) and STATA (version 11 StataCorp LP, College Station, TX).

Results

Baseline characteristics

The baseline characteristics of study cohort as of 1998 are shown in table 1. The mean $\pm$ SD age of the participants was 75 ± 2.7 years. Among them, 42.7% had hypertension, 6.7% had diabetes and 36.5% were former/current smokers at the inception of the study. Using hospital discharge records, 23.4% of participants were deemed to have prevalent CVD (defined as having prior hospitalizations for CVD) and 1.5% prevalent renal disease (defined as having prior hospitalizations of any renal disease) between 1980 to study randomization. The mean $\pm$ SD eGFRs calculated by CKD-EPI creatinine equation, CKD-EPI cystatin C equation and CKD-EPI creatinine-cystatin C equation were 66.6 ± 13.3, 65.3 ± 14.8 and 65.7 ± 13.0 mL/min/1.73 m^2 respectively.

Association between eGFR, cardiovascular events and all-cause mortality

There was at least over 30% increase in CVD events between participants with eGFR of <60 mL/min/1.73 m^2 compared to those with eGFR of ≥ 75 mL/min/1.73 m^2 as measured by the CKD-EPI creatinine, CKD-EPI cystatin C and the CKD-EPI

Table 1. Baseline characteristics of the cohort.

Baseline Characteristics	All participants (n = 1,165)
Age, mean ± SD, years	75.2±2.7
Body mass index, mean ± SD, kg/m²	27.2±4.7
Systolic blood pressure, mean ± SD, mmHg	138.0±17.9
Diastolic blood pressure, mean ± SD, mmHg	73.1±11.0
Anti-hypertensive medications, No. (%)	497 (42.7)
Smoked ever, No. (%)	427 (36.5)
Diabetes, No. (%)	78 (6.7)
Cardiovascular disease at baseline (I00-I99), No. (%)	273 (23.4)
Renal disease at baseline, No. (%)	17 (1.5)
Calcium supplements, No. (%)	614 (52.7)
Biochemistry	
Creatinine, mean ± SD, mg/dL	0.9±0.2
Cystatin C, mean ± SD, mg/L	1.1±0.2
Estimated glomerular filtration rate by the CKD-EPI equations	
CKD-EPI creatinine-derived eGFR, mean ± SD, mL/min/1.73 m²	66.6±13.3
CKD-EPI Cystatin C-derived eGFR, mean ± SD, mL/min/1.73 m²	65.3±14.8
CKD-EPI Creatinine-cystatin C-derived eGFR, mean ± SD, mL/min/1.73 m²	65.7±13.0

Results are mean ± SD or number and (%). CVD cardiovascular disease, eGFR estimated glomerular filtration rate, CKD-EPI Chronic Kidney Disease EPIdemiology.

Table 2. Hazard ratios for clinical outcomes stratified by categories of eGFR in ml/min/1.73 m^2.

Characteristics (n = 1,165)	Hazard Ratio (95% CI)	P value
All-cause mortality (n = 231)		
CKD-EPI creatinine equation		0.318
≥75 ml/min/1.73 m^2	Referent	
60–74.9 ml/min/1.73 m^2	0.89 (0.63–1.26)	
<60 ml/min/1.73 m^2	1.14 (0.81–1.60)	
CKD-EPI cystatin C equation		0.208
≥75 ml/min/1.73 m^2	Referent	
60–74.9 ml/min/1.73 m^2	0.76 (0.53–1.07)	
<60 ml/min/1.73 m^2	0.96 (0.68–1.35)	
CKD-EPI creatinine-cystatin C equation		0.278
≥75 ml/min/1.73 m^2	Referent	
60–74.9 ml/min/1.73 m^2	0.80 (0.56–1.14)	
<60 ml/min/1.73 m^2	1.01 (0.71–1.45)	
Cardiovascular disease hospitalization/mortality (n = 469)		
CKD-EPI creatinine equation		0.028
≥75 ml/min/1.73 m^2	Referent	
60–74.9 ml/min/1.73 m^2	1.08 (0.84–1.39)	
<60 ml/min/1.73 m^2	1.36 (1.06–1.76)	
CKD-EPI cystatin C equation		0.031
≥75 ml/min/1.73 m^2	Referent	
60–74.9 ml/min/1.73 m^2	1.06 (0.81–1.37)	
<60 ml/min/1.73 m^2	1.35 (1.04–1.75)	
CKD-EPI creatinine-cystatin C equation		0.021
≥75 ml/min/1.73 m^2	Referent	
60–74.9 ml/min/1.73 m^2	1.21 (0.92–1.57)	
<60 ml/min/1.73 m^2	1.46 (1.11–1.91)	

Results are age and multivariable-adjusted hazard ratio (mean 95% CI) by eGFR categories by the three equations. eGFR - estimated glomerular filtration rate, CKD-EPI - Chronic Kidney Disease EPIdemiology equation. Multivariable adjustment includes age, body mass index, previous cardiovascular disease, previous renal disease, systolic blood pressure, antihypertensive medications, diabetes, smoking history and treatment.

creatinine-cystatic C equations (Table 2). However, there was no association between eGFR reduction and all-cause mortality for the three eGFR equations (Table 2). For CKD-EPI creatinine equation, the proportion of participants with prevalent renal disease in those with eGFR of <60, 60–75 and >75/mL/min/1.73 m^2 were 0.9%, 0.6% and 1.9% respectively (χ^2 3.01, p = 0.222), which was similar for CKD-EPI cystatin C and CKD-EPI creatinine-cystatin C equations.

Model discrimination

For prediction of all-cause mortality, the AUCs varied between 0.604 (95%CI 0.561, 0.647), 0.606 (95%CI 0.563, 0.649; Sidak p-value 0.963) and 0.606 (95%CI 0.563, 0.649; Sidak p-value 0.894) respectively using the CKD-EPI creatinine, CKD-EPI cystatin C and CKD-EPI creatinine-cystatin C equations adjusted for age, BMI, hypertension, diabetes, systolic blood pressure, prevalent renal disease and CVD, smoking history and treatment group (Figure 1). The correlation between the predicted probabilities of the adjusted model for all cause mortality using CKD-EPI creatinine equation compared with CKD-EPI creatinine-cystatin C equation is shown in Figure 2.

For the prediction of CVD hospitalization and/or mortality, the AUCs varied between 0.660 (95%CI 0.622, 0.712), 0.659 (95%CI 0.621, 0.710; Sidak p-value 0.974) and 0.660 (95%CI 0.622, 0.712; Sidak p-value 0.996) respectively using the CKD-EPI creatinine, CKD-EPI cystatin C and CKD-EPI creatinine-cystatin C equations adjusted for age, BMI, hypertension, diabetes, systolic blood pressure, prevalent renal disease and CVD, smoking history and treatment group (Figure 3). The correlation between the predicted probabilities of the adjusted model for CVD hospitalization and/or mortality using CKD-EPI creatinine equation compared with CKD-EPI creatinine-cystatin C equation is shown in Figure 4.

Net reclassification improvement

The reclassification of eGFR categories in predicting all-cause mortality and CVD hospitalization and/or mortality between CKD-EPI cystatin C and CKD-EPI creatinine-cystatin C equations compared with CKD-EPI creatinine equation is shown in Tables 3 and 4. For all-cause mortality, there was no significant improvement in net reclassification of eGFR categories with CKD-EPI cystatin C equation (NRI -4.1%, p = 0.401) or CKD-EPI creatinine-cystatin C equation (NRI -1.2%, p = 0.748) compared with CKD-EPI creatinine equation. For CVD hospitalization and/or mortality, there was no significant improvement in net reclassification of eGFR categories for CVD hospitalization

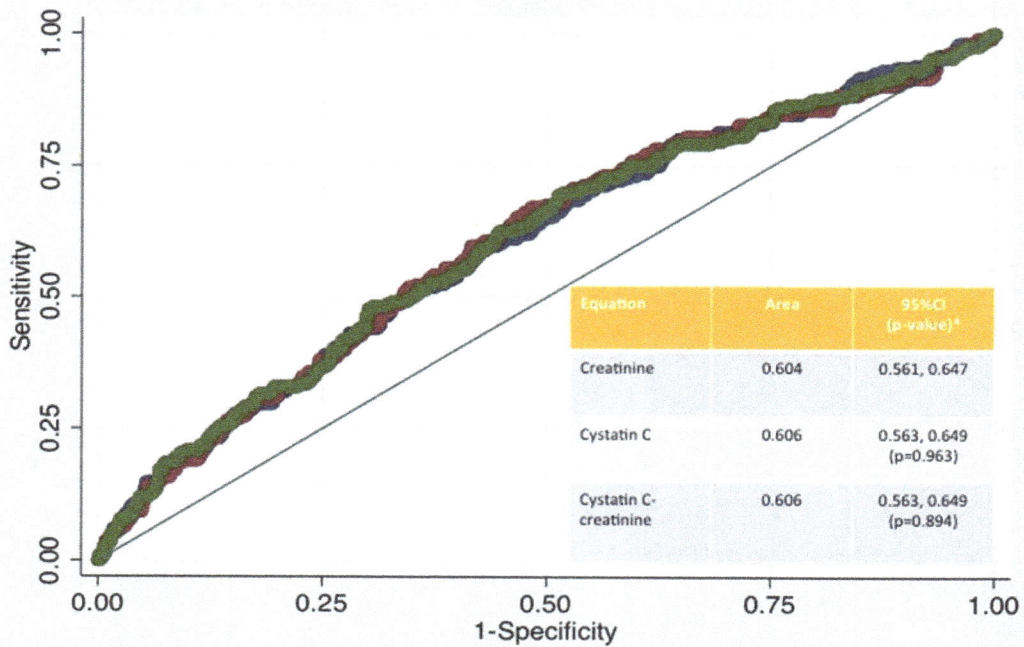

Equation	Area	95%CI (p-value)[a]
Creatinine	0.604	0.561, 0.647
Cystatin C	0.606	0.563, 0.649 (p=0.963)
Cystatin C-creatinine	0.606	0.563, 0.649 (p=0.894)

ROC adjusted for BMI, hypertension, diabetes, prevalent renal disease and CVD, smoker, treatment group
*Sidak p-value compared to creatinine eGFR

Figure 1. Receiver Operating Characteristic curves of CKD-EPI creatinine, CKD-EPI cystatin C and CKD-EPI creatinine-cystatin C eGFR equations for all-cause mortality. Fully adjusted models include body mass index, previous cardiovascular disease, previous renal disease, anti-hypertensive medications, diabetes, smoking history and treatment code.

and/or mortality with CKD-EPI cystatin C equation (NRI 2.0%, p = 0. 614) and creatinine-cystatin C equation (NRI 3.0%, p = 0.351) compared with CKD-EPI creatinine equation.

Discussion

In elderly individuals, the accurate evaluation of eGFR for CKD staging is critical to determine correct drug dosing and risk

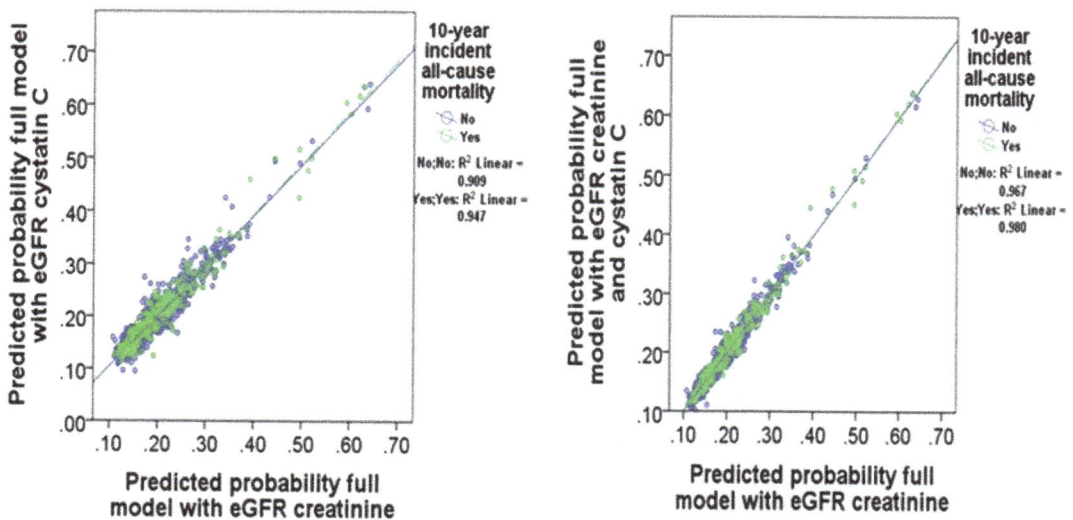

Figure 2. Receiver Operating Characteristic curves of CKD-EPI creatinine, CKD-EPI cystatin C and CKD-EPI creatinine-cystatin C eGFR equations for cardiovascular disease hospitalization and/or mortality. Fully adjusted models include body mass index, previous cardiovascular disease, previous renal disease, anti-hypertensive medications, diabetes, smoking history and treatment code.

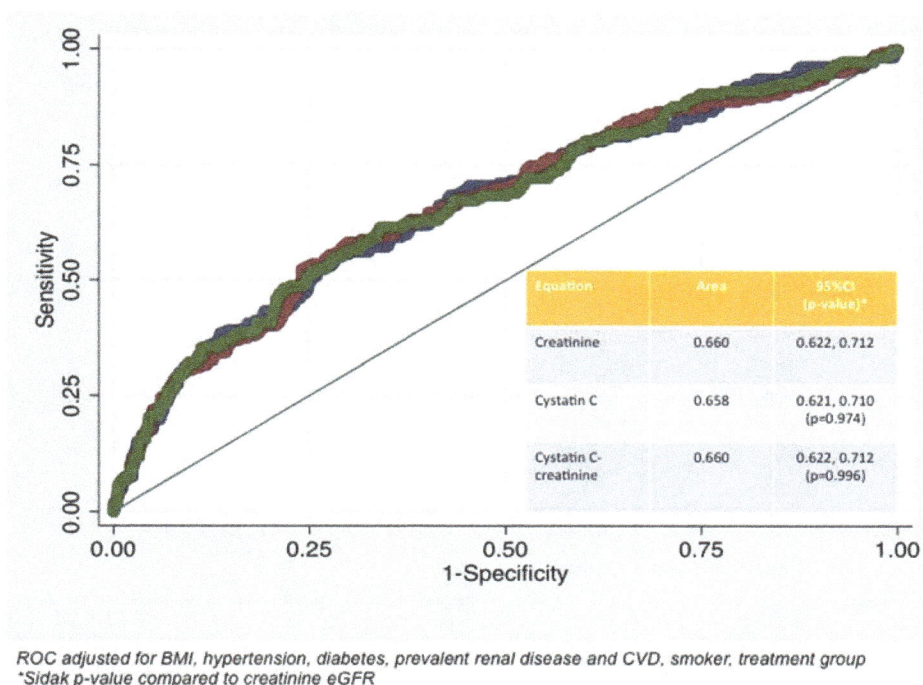

Equation	Area	95%CI (p-value)*
Creatinine	0.660	0.622, 0.712
Cystatin C	0.658	0.621, 0.710 (p=0.974)
Cystatin C-creatinine	0.660	0.622, 0.712 (p=0.996)

ROC adjusted for BMI, hypertension, diabetes, prevalent renal disease and CVD, smoker, treatment group
*Sidak p-value compared to creatinine eGFR

Figure 3. Correlation of the predicted probabilities for cardiovascular disease hospitalization and/or mortality of CKD-EPI creatinine and CKD-EPI creatinine-cystatin C equations. Fully adjusted models include body mass index, previous cardiovascular disease, previous renal disease, anti-hypertensive medications, diabetes, smoking history and treatment code.

stratification for major clinical events including CVD and all-cause mortality. Our study findings suggest that the association between reduced GFR and clinical outcomes is similar for eGFR equations with and without cystatin C. In addition, the combined CKD-EPI creatinine-cystatin C eGFR or CKD-EPI cystatin C prediction equations were not superior in predicting or reclassifying CVD hospitalization and/or mortality or all-cause mortality over the CKD-EPI creatinine eGFR equation in a cohort of elderly women.

Cystatin C appears to be a superior GFR marker compared to creatinine [18,19]. Cystatin C is a low molecular weight protein (13 kDa) that is produced at a constant rate by all cells in the body, is freely filtered by the glomeruli and is completely reabsorbed and catabolised by the proximal tubules. Unlike creatinine, cystatin C is less likely to be influenced by muscle mass or diet and therefore may be a more reliable marker of GFR, particularly in older individuals, females and those with reduced muscle mass [20]. In

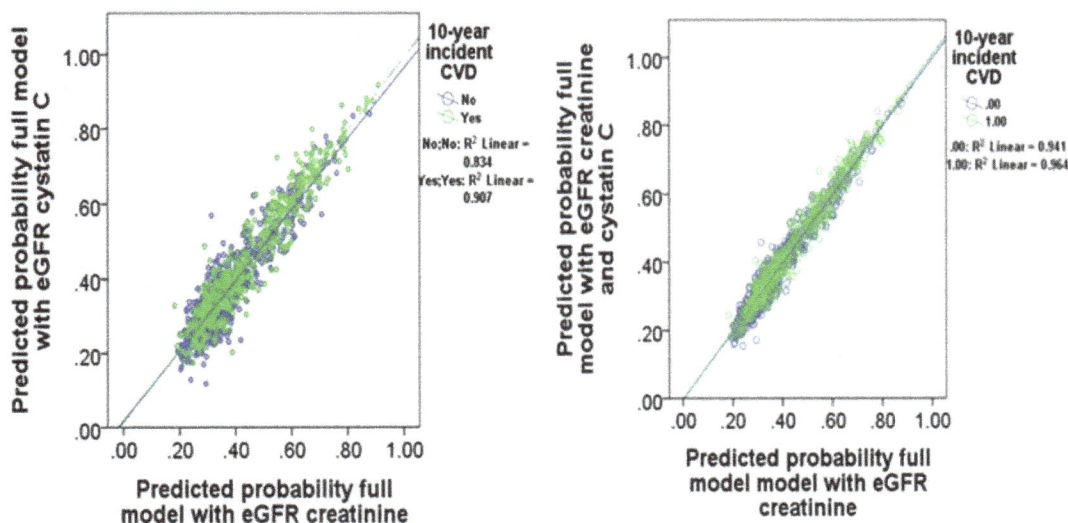

Figure 4. Correlation of the predicted probabilities for all-cause mortality of CKD-EPI creatinine and CKD-EPI creatinine-cystatin C equations. Fully adjusted models include body mass index, previous cardiovascular disease, previous renal disease, anti-hypertensive medications, diabetes, smoking history and treatment code.

Table 3. Net reclassification improvement of eGFR categories for all-cause mortality and cardiovascular disease hospitalization and/or mortality using CKD-EPI cystatin C equation compared with CKD-EPI creatinine equation.

All-cause mortality (Net reclassification improvement -4.1%, p = 0.401)

eGFR with CKD-EPI creatinine equation	eGFR with CKD-EPI cystatin C equation					
	≥75	60–74.9	<60	Reclassified higher eGFR	Reclassified lower eGFR	Correctly reclassified
Participants who died (n = 231)						
≥75	32	19	9	48 (20.8%)	50 (21.6%)	2 (0.8%)
60–74.9	22	37	22			
<60	6	20	64			
Participants who did not die (n = 934)						
≥75	124	105	38	195 (20.9%)	241 (25.8%)	46 (4.9%)
60–74.9	95	191	98			
<60	20	80	183			

Cardiovascular disease hospitalization and/or mortality (Net reclassification improvement 2.0%, p = 0.614)

eGFR with CKD-EPI creatinine equation	eGFR with CKD-EPI cystatin C equation					
	≥75	60–74.9	<60	Reclassified higher eGFR	Reclassified lower eGFR	Correctly reclassified
Participants with an event (n = 469)						
≥75	50	42	18	91 (19.4%)	116 (24.7%)	25 (5.3%)
60–74.9	37	83	56			
<60	9	45	129			
Participants without an event (n = 696)						
≥75	106	82	29	152 (21.8%)	175 (25.1%)	23 (3.3%)
60–74.9	80	145	64			
<60	17	55	118			

CVD risk factors include age, body mass index, previous cardiovascular disease, previous renal disease, systolic blood pressure, anti-hypertensive medications, diabetes, smoking history and treatment code. CVD indicates cardiovascular disease; eGFR estimated glomerular filtration rate and CKD-EPI - Chronic Kidney Disease Epidemiology equation.

several studies, compared with creatinine, cystatin C is more accurate in stratifying the risk of CVD and all-cause mortality in elderly individuals [21]. In a cohort of 3,075 participants aged over 70 years, each SD reduction (0.3 g/L) in cystatin C concentration was associated with an increased risk of all-cause mortality (HR 1.24, 95% CI 1.20, 1.28) and CVD mortality (HR 1.20, 95% CI 1.11, 1.30) [22]. In a population-based prospective observational cohort of 9988 individuals aged 45–64 years, cystatin C level was a much stronger predictor of all-cause mortality, coronary artery disease events, heart failure events and end-stage renal disease compared to estimates of GFR derived from CKD-EPI creatinine equation [23]. Other studies have corroborated these findings and have also shown that cystatin C level may identify the group of CKD patients that may not be identified by CKD-EPI equation as being at high risk of CVD events and all-cause mortality [24,25]. In contrast, a recent study by *Eriksen et al.* has shown that cystatin C was not superior in estimating measured GFR compared to creatinine in the general population [26] and other studies have suggested that the strong association between cystatin C and CVD or all-cause mortality may be related to other factors including body size and the presence of diabetes and inflammation [27]. The discrepant findings between studies may reflect dissimilar population of varying ages, differences in participants' characteristics such as BMI and presence of comorbidities.

Two recently developed CKD-EPI creatinine-cystatin C and CKD-EPI cystatin C equations were shown to perform better in predicting measured radionuclide GFR compared to CKD-EPI creatinine equation [14]. Although bias was similar in all three eGFR equations in predicting measured GFR, the combined CKD-EPI creatinine-cystatin C equation had greater precision and accuracy resulting in a more accurate classification of measured GFR as <60 ml/min/1.73 m^2. The use of the combined CKD-EPI creatinine-cystatin C equation was able to improve reclassification of individuals with creatinine-derived eGFR of 45–74 ml/min/1.73 m^2 (net reclassification index 19.4; 95% CI, 8.7 to 30.1; P<0.001), and also 17% of individuals with creatinine-based eGFR of 45–59 ml/min/1.73 m^2 to ≥60 ml/min/1.73 m^2. In a recent meta-analysis of 11 general population studies comprising of 90,750 participants, there was a more consistent linear association between reduced eGFR derived from CKD-EPI cystatin C and CKD-EPI creatinine-cystatin C equations and increased risks of all-cause and CVD mortality for all eGFR values below 85 mL/min/1.73 m^2 compared with CKD-EPI creatinine equation, well above the threshold of 60 mL/min/1.73 m^2 for the detection of CKD with CKD-EPI creatinine-based eGFR [12]. The NRI using either CKD-EPI cystatin C-derived equations for all-cause and CVD mortality was 0.23 (95%CI 0.18, 0.28) and 0.17 (95%CI 0.11, 0.23) respectively suggesting that cystatin C-derived eGFR equations strengthens the association between eGFR and clinical outcomes. However, in this

Table 4. Net reclassification improvement of eGFR categories for all-cause mortality and cardiovascular disease hospitalization and/or mortality using CKD-EPI creatinine-cystatin C equation compared with CKD-EPI creatinine equation.

All-cause mortality (Net reclassification improvement -1.2%, p = 0.748)

eGFR with CKD-EPI creatinine equation	eGFR with CKD-EPI creatinine-cystatin C equation					
	≥75	60–74.9	<60	Reclassified higher eGFR	Reclassified lower eGFR	Correctly reclassified
Participants who died (n = 231)						
≥75	41	19	0	30 (13.0%)	36 (15.6%)	6 (2.6%)
60–74.9	13	51	17			
<60	0	17	73			
Participants who did not die (n = 934)						
≥75	178	85	4	110 (11.8%)	146 (15.6%)	36 (3.8%)
60–74.9	52	275	57			
<60	0	58	225			

Cardiovascular disease hospitalization and/or mortality (Net reclassification improvement 3.0%, p = 0.351)

eGFR with CKD-EPI creatinine equation	eGFR with CKD-EPI creatinine-cystatin C equation					
	≥75	60–74.9	<60	Reclassified higher eGFR	Reclassified lower eGFR	Correctly reclassified
Participants with an event (n = 469)						
≥75	70	38	2	47 (10.0%)	72 (15.4%)	25 (5.4%)
60–74.9	16	128	32			
<60	0	31	152			
Participants without an event (n = 696)						
≥75	149	66	2	93 (13.4%)	110 (15.8%)	17 (2.4%)
60–74.9	49	198	42			
<60	0	44	146			

CVD risk factors include age, body mass index, previous cardiovascular disease, previous renal disease, systolic blood pressure, anti-hypertensive medications, diabetes, smoking history and treatment code. CVD indicates cardiovascular disease; eGFR estimated glomerular filtration rate and CKD-EPI - Chronic Kidney Disease Epidemiology equation.

meta-analysis, there were only two studies that have included exclusively elderly participants with mean age of over 70 years. The ULSAM study from Sweden included only men and the CHS study included 41% men and 17% participants were of Black race [28,29]. In both these studies, there was a large difference in mean eGFR across the three equations, with eGFR derived from CKD-EPI creatinine equation being much higher compared to both cystatin C equations. Our study has shown that the newly derived CKD-EPI cystatin C and CKD-EPI creatinine-cystatin C equations did not improve reclassification of eGFR categories that predicted the risk of CVD hospitalization and/or mortality or all-cause mortality compared to the commonly used CKD-EPI creatinine equation. The observed differences to the result of the meta-analysis may reflect dissimilar population characteristics with the studies included in the meta-analysis comprising men and women across all age categories and ethnicity compared to only elderly Caucasian women in our study. In addition, all elderly participants in this study were relatively healthy over the age of 70 with mild renal dysfunction, with the majority of participants within a relatively narrow range of eGFRs. In the two population cohorts of similar age (CHS and ULSAM studies), there were major differences in gender, race, BMI, comorbid status and baseline creatinine compared to this cohort, which may have contributed to the differences in study findings. There may also be potential errors in creatinine and cystatin C measurements and insufficient power in our study to detect significant differences

between the eGFR equations or to detect a significant associations between these equations and all-cause mortality, which all may have contributed to differences in the reported study findings.

The strengths of this study include the use of a large prospective cohort of subjects with complete and accurate data collection over a 10-year period. We were able to accurately examine the association between estimates of GFR using the newly developed cystatin C equations and clinical outcomes in a population with a low prevalence of CVD and renal diseases, which further strengthens this association. However, the strengths of the study must be balanced against the limitations, which include a lack of radionuclide GFR measurements and availability of single time-point measurements of creatinine and cystatin C to estimate baseline GFR. In addition, our study cohort only included white female participants with presumed adequate nutrition and muscle mass (BMI mean ± SD of 27 ± 5 kg/m^2) and therefore the applicability of our study findings to males, other ethnic minorities or racial groups and those with poor nutrition and low muscle mass remains unclear.

In conclusion, the newly developed CKD-EPI cystatin C and combined CKD-EPI creatinine-cystatin C-derived eGFR equations were not superior in predicting CVD events or all-cause mortality compared with the commonly used CKD-EPI creatinine-derived eGFR equation in older female subjects with no or early CKD and this data cannot be extrapolated to older individuals with more advanced CKD. With a substantial cost-difference between measurements of creatinine and cystatin C, together with the uncertainty of the value of cystatin C-derived eGFR equations in predicting clinical events over creatinine-derived eGFR equation, the utility and cost-effectiveness of cystatin C in the elderly must be investigated further prior to implementation in clinical practice.

Acknowledgments

The authors wish to thank the staff at the Data Linkage Branch, Hospital Morbidity Data Collection and Registry of Births, Deaths and Marriages

for their work on providing the data for this study.

Disclaimer: The results presented in this paper have not been published previously in whole or part, except in abstract form.

Author Contributions

Conceived and designed the experiments: WL JL GW RP. Performed the experiments: WL JL GW. Analyzed the data: WL JL GW. Contributed reagents/materials/analysis tools: WL JL GW EL. Wrote the paper: WL JL GW RT EL PT RP.

References

1. Couser WG, Remuzzi G, Mendis S, Tonelli M (2011) The contribution of chronic kidney disease to the global burden of major noncommunicable diseases. Kidney Int 80: 1258–1270.
2. Go AS, Chertow GM, Fan D, McCulloch CE, Hsu CY (2004) Chronic kidney disease and the risks of death, cardiovascular events, and hospitalization. N Engl J Med 351: 1296–1305.
3. Levey AS, Stevens LA, Schmid CH, Zhang YL, Castro AF 3rd, et al. (2009) A new equation to estimate glomerular filtration rate. Ann Intern Med 150: 604–612.
4. Ford I, Bezlyak V, Stott DJ, Sattar N, Packard CJ, et al. (2009) Reduced glomerular filtration rate and its association with clinical outcome in older patients at risk of vascular events: secondary analysis. PLoS Med 6: e16.
5. Matsushita K, Mahmoodi BK, Woodward M, Emberson JR, Jafar TH, et al. (2012) Comparison of risk prediction using the CKD-EPI equation and the MDRD study equation for estimated glomerular filtration rate. JAMA 307: 1941–1951.
6. Wong G, Hayen A, Chapman JR, Webster AC, Wang JJ, et al. (2009) Association of CKD and cancer risk in older people. J Am Soc Nephrol 20: 1341–1350.
7. Anavekar NS, McMurray JJ, Velazquez EJ, Solomon SD, Kober L, et al. (2004) Relation between renal dysfunction and cardiovascular outcomes after myocardial infarction. N Engl J Med 351: 1285–1295.
8. Drawz P, Rosenberg M (2013) Slowing progression of chronic kidney disese. Kidney Int Suppl 3: 372–376.
9. Mathew TH, Johnson DW, Jones GR (2007) Chronic kidney disease and automatic reporting of estimated glomerular filtration rate: revised recommendations. Med J Aust 187: 459–463.
10. Cockcroft DW, Gault MH (1976) Prediction of creatinine clearance from serum creatinine. Nephron 16: 31–41.
11. Swedko PJ, Clark HD, Paramsothy K, Akbari A (2003) Serum creatinine is an inadequate screening test for renal failure in elderly patients. Arch Intern Med 163: 356–360.
12. Shlipak MG, Matsushita K, Arnlov J, Inker LA, Katz R, et al. (2013) Cystatin C versus creatinine in determining risk based on kidney function. N Engl J Med 369: 932–943.
13. Prince RL, Devine A, Dhaliwal SS, Dick IM (2006) Effects of calcium supplementation on clinical fracture and bone structure: results of a 5-year, double-blind, placebo-controlled trial in elderly women. Arch Intern Med 166: 869–875.
14. Inker LA, Schmid CH, Tighiouart H, Eckfeldt JH, Feldman HI, et al. (2012) Estimating glomerular filtration rate from serum creatinine and cystatin C. N Engl J Med 367: 20–29.
15. Britt H (1997) A new coding tool for computerised clinical systems in primary care—ICPC plus. Aust Fam Physician 26 Suppl 2: S79–82.
16. World Health Organization (1977) Manual of the international statistical classification of diseases, injuries, and causes of death: based on the recommendations of the ninth revision conference, 1975, and adopted by the Twenty-ninth World Health Assembly. Geneva: World Health Organization. 2v. p.
17. World Health Organization (2004) ICD-10: international statistical classification of diseases and related health problems: tenth revision. Geneva: World Health Organization. 3v. p.
18. Dharnidharka VR, Kwon C, Stevens G (2002) Serum cystatin C is superior to serum creatinine as a marker of kidney function: a meta-analysis. Am J Kidney Dis 40: 221–226.
19. Roos JF, Doust J, Tett SE, Kirkpatrick CM (2007) Diagnostic accuracy of cystatin C compared to serum creatinine for the estimation of renal dysfunction in adults and children—a meta-analysis. Clin Biochem 40: 383–391.
20. Laterza O, Price C, Scott M (2002) Cystatin C: an improved estimator of glomerular filtration rate? Clin Chem 48: 699–707.
21. Shlipak MG, Sarnak MJ, Katz R, Fried LF, Seliger SL, et al. (2005) Cystatin C and the risk of death and cardiovascular events among elderly persons. N Engl J Med 352: 2049–2060.
22. Shlipak MG, Wassel Fyr CL, Chertow GM, Harris TB, Kritchevsky SB, et al. (2006) Cystatin C and mortality risk in the elderly: the health, aging, and body composition study. J Am Soc Nephrol 17: 254–261.
23. Astor BC, Shafi T, Hoogeveen RC, Matsushita K, Ballantyne CM, et al. (2012) Novel markers of kidney function as predictors of ESRD, cardiovascular disease, and mortality in the general population. Am J Kidney Dis 59: 653–662.
24. Peralta CA, Katz R, Sarnak MJ, Ix J, Fried LF, et al. (2011) Cystatin C identifies chronic kidney disease patients at higher risk for complications. J Am Soc Nephrol 22: 147–155.
25. Shlipak MG, Katz R, Sarnak MJ, Fried LF, Newman AB, et al. (2006) Cystatin C and prognosis for cardiovascular and kidney outcomes in elderly persons without chronic kidney disease. Ann Intern Med 145: 237–246.
26. Eriksen BO, Mathisen UD, Melsom T, Ingebretsen OC, Jenssen TG, et al. (2010) Cystatin C is not a better estimator of GFR than plasma creatinine in the general population. Kidney Int 78: 1305–1311.
27. Stevens LA, Schmid CH, Greene T, Li L, Beck GJ, et al. (2009) Factors other than glomerular filtration rate affect serum cystatin C levels. Kidney Int 75: 652–660.
28. Shlipak M, Katz R, Kestenbaum B, Fried L, Newman A, et al. (2009) Rate of kidney function decline in older adults: a comparison using creatinine and cystatin C. Am J Nephrol 30: 171–178.
29. Ingelsson E, Sundstrom J, Lind L, Riserus U, Larsson A, et al. (2007) Low-grade albuminuria and the incidence of heart failure in a community-based cohort of elderly men. Eur Heart J 28: 1739–1745.

12

Effect of Dialysis Initiation Timing on Clinical Outcomes: A Propensity-Matched Analysis of a Prospective Cohort Study in Korea

Jeonghwan Lee[1,2], Jung Nam An[3], Jin Ho Hwang[4], Yong-Lim Kim[2,5], Shin-Wook Kang[2,6], Chul Woo Yang[2,7], Nam-Ho Kim[2,8], Yun Kyu Oh[2,3], Chun Soo Lim[2,3], Yon Su Kim[2,9], Jung Pyo Lee[2,3]*

1 Department of Internal Medicine, Hallym University Hangang Sacred Heart Hospital, Seoul, Korea, 2 Clinical Research Center for End Stage Renal Disease (CRC for ESRD), Daegu, Korea, 3 Department of Internal Medicine, Seoul National University Boramae Medical Center, Seoul, Korea, 4 Department of Internal Medicine, Chung-Ang University Medical Center, Seoul, Korea, 5 Department of Internal Medicine, Kyungpook National University School of Medicine, Daegu, Korea, 6 Department of Internal Medicine, Yonsei University College of Medicine, Seoul, Korea, 7 Department of Internal Medicine, The Catholic University of Korea College of Medicine, Seoul, Korea, 8 Department of Internal Medicine, Chonnam National University Medical School, Gwangju, Korea, 9 Department of Internal Medicine, Seoul National University Hospital, Seoul National University College of Medicine, Seoul, Korea

Abstract

Background: Controversy persists regarding the appropriate initiation timing of renal replacement therapy for patients with end-stage renal disease. We evaluated the effect of dialysis initiation timing on clinical outcomes. Initiation times were classified according to glomerular filtration rate (GFR).

Methods: We enrolled a total of 1691 adult patients who started dialysis between August 2008 and March 2013 in a multi-center, prospective cohort study at the Clinical Research Center for End Stage Renal Disease in the Republic of Korea. The patients were classified into the early-start group or the late-start group according to the mean estimated GFR value, which was 7.37 ml/min/1.73 m^2. The primary outcome was patient survival, and the secondary outcomes were hospitalization, cardiovascular events, vascular access complications, change of dialysis modality, and peritonitis. The two groups were compared before and after matching with propensity scores.

Results: Before propensity score matching, the early-start group had a poor survival rate (P<0.001). Hospitalization, cardiovascular events, vascular access complications, changes in dialysis modality, and peritonitis were not different between the groups. A total of 854 patients (427 in each group) were selected by propensity score matching. After matching, neither patient survival nor any of the other outcomes differed between groups.

Conclusions: There was no clinical benefit after adjustment by propensity scores comparing early versus late initiation of dialysis.

Editor: Emmanuel A. Burdmann, University of Sao Paulo Medical School, Brazil

Funding: This study was supported by a grant from the Korea Healthcare Technology R& D Project, Ministry for Health and Welfare, Republic of Korea (A102065). The funders had no role in study design, data collection and analysis, decision to publish, or preparation of the manuscript.

Competing Interests: The authors have declared that no competing interests exist.

* Email: nephrolee@gmail.com

Introduction

Chronic kidney disease (CKD) is a major public health problem, and the number of patients requiring dialysis for end-stage renal disease (ESRD) has been increasing rapidly around the world [1]. In 2011, the prevalence of dialysis patients in the United States was 430,273 (0.2% of the general population), and the rate of ESRD cases per million population reached 1,901 [2]. Medical expenditures for patients with ESRD in the United States reached $49.3 billion in 2011, and ESRD patients accounted for 6.3% of total Medicare costs. Most cases of ESRD are complicated, with various comorbidities, and are associated with poor health outcomes. In the United States, ESRD patients were reported to

have a residual life expectancy of 6.2 years [2]. According to two large population cohort studies in Canada and Taiwan, patients aged 55 years with stage 5 CKD or who were on dialysis had life expectancies of 5.6 and 12.0 years and cardiovascular mortality rates of 58% and 71%, respectively [3–5]. Adequate dialysis therapy can relieve the burden of painful uremic symptoms and improve overall survival [6–8]. Therefore, it is important to initiate dialysis therapy at the appropriate time to prevent fatal uremic complications and improve patient survival.

However, controversy persists regarding the optimal timing for dialysis initiation. There is a conventional belief that delaying dialysis until the patient's eGFR falls below 6 ml/min/1.73 m^2

was potentially dangerous and that starting dialysis early could improve the nutritional status and survival of ESRD patients through increased uremic solute clearance, particularly in patients with diabetes or high comorbidities [9]. According to data from the United States Renal Data System (USRDS), the proportion of patients who started dialysis at an eGFR greater than 10 ml/min/ 1.73 m² had been steadily increasing up to 2009, reaching 54% of the patient population [10]. However, several observational and meta-analysis studies reported that early initiation of dialysis is associated with certain harmful clinical outcomes [11–14]. To date, there has been only one prospective, randomized, controlled study (the Initiating Dialysis Early and Late Trial; IDEAL study) on dialysis initiation time and patient survival. This study reported that planned early initiation of dialysis was not associated with improvements in either survival or clinical outcomes [15]. Recent guidelines reflecting the results of the IDEAL study emphasize that the eGFR, based on serum creatinine levels, should not be the only factor used to guide dialysis initiation time and recommend that dialysis should be preferentially deferred until the development of uremic symptoms or complications [16–18].

Clinical outcomes and mortality rates among patients initiating dialysis are known to differ according to the demographic characteristics of race or ethnicity [19]. Asian advanced CKD patients have lower mortality and cardiovascular morbidity than Caucasians despite a faster decline in GFR and a higher incidence of renal replacement therapy [20–22]. However, clinical evidence on dialysis initiation time and associated clinical outcomes is insufficient among non-Caucasian populations. Although there are a few retrospective, observational studies on dialysis initiation timing among Asian ESRD patients [23–27], single-center designs and/or insufficient adjustments in multivariate analyses attributable to limited data collection from retrospective designs make the results of these studies difficult to generalize to all populations. In the IDEAL study, most of the patients (70%) enrolled were Caucasian, and only 9.2% were Asian. Here, we aimed to compare the survival and other clinical outcomes of patients starting dialysis for ESRD according to initiation time in a Korean prospective cohort study using propensity score-matching analysis.

Methods

Study Participants

We enrolled adult patients (≥20 years old) who were started on maintenance dialysis for ESRD between August 2008 and March 2013 through an ongoing cohort study (Clinical Research Center for End Stage Renal Disease, CRC for ESRD) in South Korea. The CRC for ESRD is a nationwide, multi-center, web-based, prospective cohort of CKD patients who have started dialysis (clinicaltrial.gov NCT00931970) [28]. The CRC for ESRD cohort began to register ESRD patients on dialysis in July 2008, and 31 hospitals in South Korea are currently participating. All of the patients were informed about the study and participated voluntarily with written consent. The study was approved by the institutional review board at each center. [The Catholic University of Korea, Bucheon St. Mary's Hospital; The Catholic University of Korea, Incheon St. Mary's Hospital; The Catholic University of Korea, Seoul St. Mary's Hospital; The Catholic University of Korea, St. Mary's Hospital; The Catholic University of Korea, St. Vincent's Hospital; The Catholic University of Korea, Uijeongbu St. Mary's Hospital; Cheju Halla General Hospital; Chonbuk National University Hospital; Chonnam National University Hospital; Chung-Ang University Medical Center; Chungbuk National University Hospital; Chungnam National University Hospital; Dong-A University Medical Center; Ewha Womans

University Medical Center; Fatima Hospital; Gachon Medical School Gil Medical Center; Inje University Busan Paik Hospital; Kyungpook National University Hospital; Kwandong University College of Medicine, Myongji Hospital; National Health Insurance Corporation Ilsan Hospital; National Medical Center; Busan National University Hospital; Samsung Medical Center; Seoul National University Boramae Medical Center; Seoul National University Hospital; Seoul National University, Bundang Hospital; Yeungnam University Medical Center; Yonsei University, Severance Hospital; Yonsei University, Gangnam Severance Hospital; Ulsan University Hospital; Wonju Christian Hospital (in alphabetical order)]. All of the investigators conducted this study in accordance with the guidelines of the 2008 Declaration of Helsinki.

After the last enrollments in March 2013, participants were followed until October 2013 to observe at least 6-month mortality and clinical outcomes. Patients whose creatinine levels were missing at the time of dialysis initiation were excluded. Patients were categorized into the early-start group or the late-start group according to whether their eGFR was greater or less than the mean eGFR value at the start of dialysis. The eGFR was calculated using CKD-Epidemiology Collaboration (CKD-EPI) equations [29]. The modified Charlson co-morbidity index (mCCI) was calculated for each patient at the initiation of dialysis. The mCCI was developed to predict one-year mortality, and it has been validated in ESRD patients [30,31].

Clinical Outcomes

The primary outcome was all-cause mortality after the start of dialysis. The secondary outcomes included first hospitalization, cardiovascular events, changes in dialysis modality, vascular complications in hemodialysis patients, and peritonitis in peritoneal dialysis patients. Hospitalization was defined as admission for at least 24 hours, excluding diagnostic work-ups for transplantation. Cardiovascular events included clinical events requiring admission for ischemic heart disease, congestive heart failure, arrhythmia, or cerebrovascular disease. Changes in dialysis modality included shift from hemodialysis to peritoneal dialysis or vice versa. Vascular complications included vascular events requiring angioplasty, surgical intervention, or changes in vascular catheters for hemodialysis. Peritonitis was defined as the presence of the following conditions: 1) signs and symptoms of peritoneal inflammation; and 2) a peritoneal effluent white blood cell count greater than 100 cells/mm³ and a neutrophil percentage greater than 50%.

Statistical Analysis

The propensity scores, which were calculated from the logistic regression models, represent the probability of being assigned to either an early or a late dialysis initiation. Through the matching procedure for propensity scores, the early- and late-start groups showed similar distributions of propensity scores, indicating that the differences in covariates between the two groups were minimized. We matched propensity scores one by one using nearest neighbor methods, no replacement, and 0.2 caliper width. The characteristics of both the early- and late-start groups were compared before and after propensity score matching.

Continuous variables are expressed as the mean and standard deviation, and categorical variables are presented as frequencies with percentages. Continuous variables were compared using a t-test, and categorical variables were compared using the Chi-square test or Fisher's exact tests. Survival was compared using Kaplan-Meier curve and log-rank test. IBM SPSS software (version 21.0) was used in all descriptive and survival analysis, and R software (version 2.14.2) was used in the propensity score matching. A two-tailed P value <0.05 was considered statistically significant.

Results

Patient Characteristics

Initially, among the 4770 patients retrieved from the CRC for ESRD database, 2991 dialysis patients who had started dialysis before cohort registration were excluded (Figure 1). In addition, 88 patients without information on serum creatinine levels and/or eGFR at the time of dialysis initiation were excluded from the analysis. Ultimately, a total of 1691 adult patients who started maintenance dialysis for ESRD were enrolled. Patients were classified into the early-start group (eGFR greater than the mean value) or late-start group (eGFR less than the mean value) based

on the mean value of eGFR at the start of dialysis, which was 7.372 ml/min/1.73 m^2.

The patients' clinical and laboratory characteristics are compared and summarized in Table 1. The mean age was 56.6±14.3 years old, and 61.4% of the patients were male. Patients with diabetes as a primary cause of renal disease comprised 51.2% of the study population. Most of the patients (71.1%) received hemodialysis as the modality for renal replacement therapy. Before propensity score matching, 1051 patients were in the late-start group, and 640 patients were in the early-start group. Considering all of the participants, the mean eGFR values were 11.2±8.1 ml/min/1.73 m^2 in the early-start group and 5.0±1.4 ml/min/1.73 m^2 in the late-start group. In the early-start group, the patients were older (58.8±14.4 vs. 55.3±14.0 years old, P<0.001), and diabetic kidney disease (59.7% vs. 46.8%) was more common. A total of 69.6% of the patients in the early-start group received

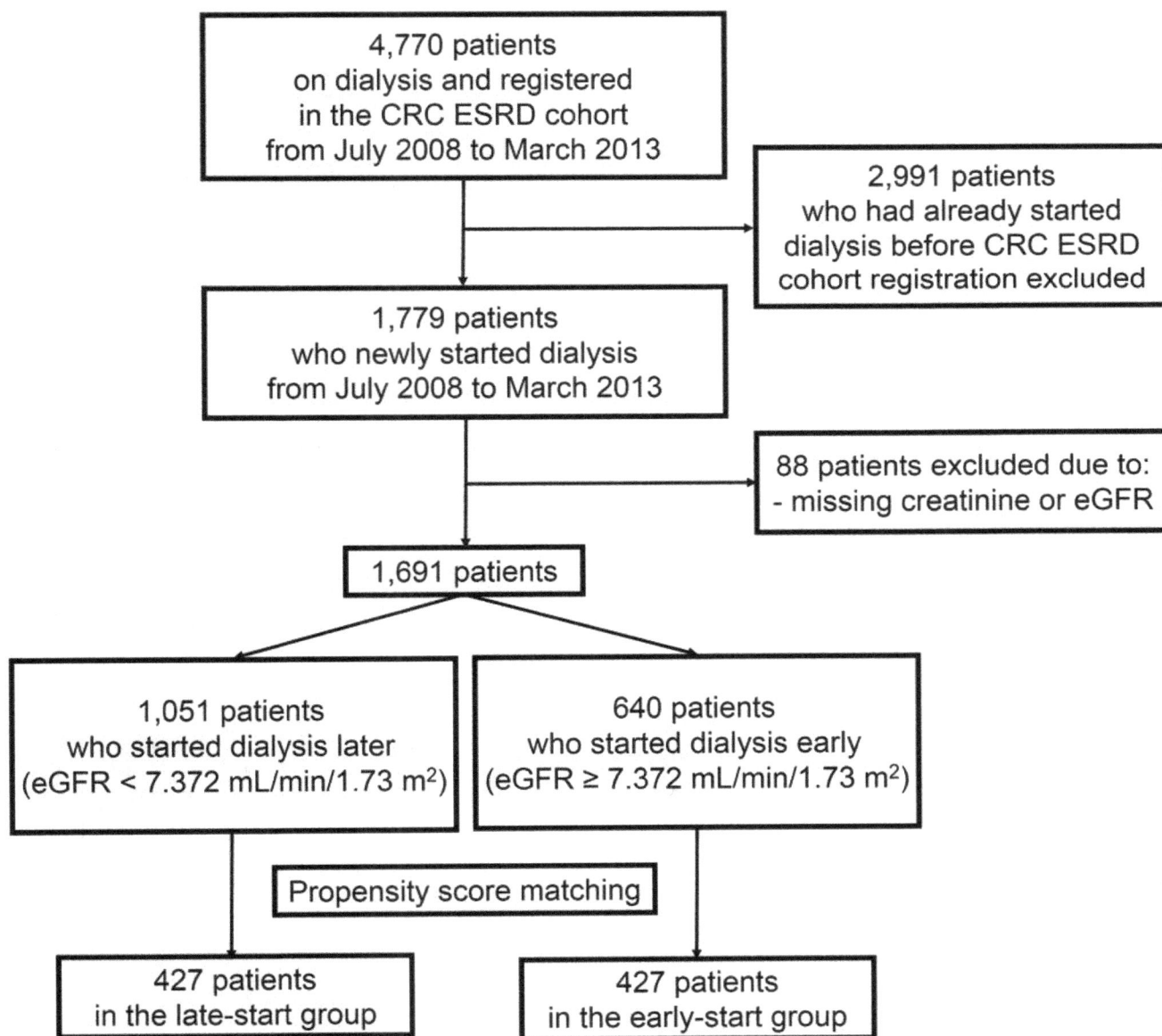

Figure 1. Flow chart of study enrollment. Between August 2008 and March 2013, 1069 dialysis patients with end-stage renal disease were initially enrolled. After propensity score matching, 854 patients remained in the final analysis.

Table 1. Patient characteristics before and after propensity score matching.

Variables	Before PSM				After PSM			
	Late Start (N=1051)	Early Start (N=640)	P	Standardized Difference	Late Start (N=427)	Early Start (N=427)	P	Standardized Difference
Age (years old)	55.3±14.0	58.8±14.4	<0.001	0.227	57.6±13.1	57.4±14.3	0.853	−0.012
Sex (male)	609 (57.9%)	430 (67.2%)	<0.001	−0.227	264 (61.8%)	272 (63.7%)	0.571	−0.040
Primary renal disease			<0.001	−0.254			0.339	−0.059
Diabetes	488 (46.8%)	377 (59.7%)			240 (56.2%)	244 (57.1%)		
Hypertension	187 (17.9%)	83 (13.2%)			57 (13.3%)	68 (15.9%)		
Glomerulonephritis	180 (17.3%)	58 (9.2%)			63 (14.8%)	44 (10.3%)		
Other	114 (10.9%)	59 (8.4%)			37 (8.7%)	38 (8.9%)		
Unknown	74 (7.1%)	54 (8.6%)			30 (7.0%)	33 (7.7%)		
Type of dialysis			0.266	0.070			0.653	−0.030
Hemodialysis	758 (72.1%)	444 (69.6%)			298 (69.8%)	304 (71.2%)		
Peritoneal dialysis	293 (27.9%)	194 (30.4%)			129 (30.2%)	123 (28.8%)		
Systolic BP (mmHg)	142.6±24.1	139.6±22.6	0.015	0.178	142.9±23.0	140.3±23.0	0.108	0.023
Diastolic BP (mmHg)	78.9±14.8	76.3±13.6	0.001	0.130	78.2±14.5	77.4±14.0	0.409	0.031
BMI (kg/m^2)	23.2±3.5	23.0±3.4	0.380	−0.055	23.2±3.3	23.1±3.5	0.742	−0.023
Charlson comorbidity index	4.69±2.25	5.80±2.66	<0.001	0.402	5.27±2.29	5.32±2.53	0.734	0.021
WBC (/mm^3)	5790±3924	5212±3956	0.004	−0.149	5319±3986	5450±3891	0.625	0.033
Hemoglobin (g/dL)	8.7±2.5	9.6±4.7	<0.001	0.178	9.1±3.3	9.2±1.5	0.510	0.023
Calcium (md/dL)	7.7±3.1	8.1±3.0	0.010	0.130	8.1±4.6	8.2±3.6	0.729	0.031
Phosphorus (md/dL)	6.2±2.8	4.6±2.6	<0.001	−0.597	4.9±1.3	4.8±1.3	0.209	−0.041
Uric acid (md/dL)	8.8±5.0	7.2±2.6	<0.001	−0.600	7.8±2.0	7.7±2.6	0.519	−0.040
Albumin (g/dL)	3.4±0.6	3.2±0.6	<0.001	−0.216	3.3±0.6	3.3±0.6	0.481	−0.046
Creatinine (md/dL)	10.45±5.91	5.35±1.35	<0.001		9.19±3.24	5.49±1.26	<0.001	
eGFR* (ml/min/1.73 m^2)	5.0±1.4	11.2±8.1	<0.001		5.5±1.2	10.4±4.9	<0.001	
Ferritin (ng/ml)	308.4±500.2	327.6±401.0	0.458		281.8±431.0	318.8±372.6	0.222	
Cholesterol (mg/dL)	159.5±48.5	155.4±51.6	0.120		158.3±48.6	156.4±48.3	0.578	
hsCRP (mg/L)	4.0±16.4	6.9±20.5	0.004		5.9±23.5	4.4±12.4	0.261	
iPTH (pg/mL)	300.4±255.6	200.0±198.0	<0.001		269.8±228.2	210.3±210.9	0.001	
Use of vitamin D	188 (17.9%)	62 (9.7%)	<0.001		67 (15.7%)	44 (10.3%)	0.025	
Use of phosphate binders	575 (54.7%)	288 (45.0%)	<0.001		233 (54.6%)	211 (49.4%)	0.212	
Single-pool Kt/V†	1.33±0.47	1.24±0.55	0.047		1.33±0.40	1.23±0.59	0.121	
Weekly Kt/V‡	2.47±1.02	2.59±1.38	0.735		2.79±1.02	2.83±1.32	0.994	

BMI, body mass index; iPTH, intact PTH; PSM, propensity score-matching; WBC, white blood cell count.
*Levels of eGFR were calculated using the CKD-EPI equation.
†Single-pool Kt/V was measured in patients with hemodialysis.
‡Weekly Kt/V was measured in patients with peritoneal dialysis.

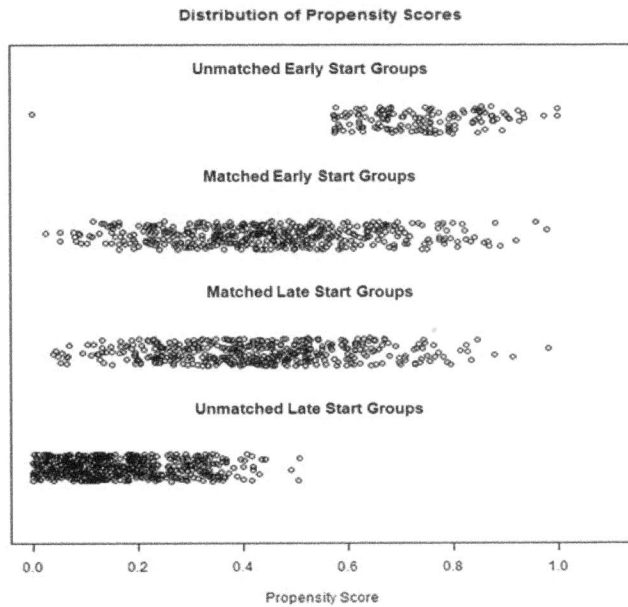

Figure 2. Distribution of propensity scores before and after propensity score matching. The propensity scores of unmatched patients were significantly different between the early- and late-start groups. The propensity scores of matched patients were almost the same between groups.

hemodialysis as the first modality of dialysis, whereas 30.4% of the patients started with peritoneal dialysis. The mCCI was higher in the early-start group. Systolic and diastolic blood pressure, serum phosphorus, uric acid, albumin, intact parathyroid hormone (iPTH), and high-sensitive C-reactive protein (hsCRP) levels, use of vitamin D or phosphate binders were lower, and hemoglobin and calcium levels were higher in the early-start group. The adequacy of hemodialysis (single-pool Kt/V) was slightly lower in the early-start group of hemodialysis patients, but the weekly Kt/V of peritoneal dialysis was not different between the two groups.

Propensity Matching of Cohort

We performed a logistic regression analysis to obtain propensity scores for dialysis initiation timing using the following covariates: age, sex, primary renal disease, type of dialysis, body mass index, mCCI, hemoglobin level, calcium level, phosphorus level, uric acid level, albumin level, and comorbidities. After propensity score matching, 854 patients (427 in each group) remained. The distributions of propensity scores before and after matching are illustrated in Figure 2. In the propensity score-matched participants, almost all of the baseline parameters, including age, sex, primary renal disease, type of dialysis, systolic and diastolic blood pressure, body mass index, mCCI, hemoglobin levels, serum calcium, phosphorus, uric acid, glucose, albumin, hsCRP levels, and adequacy of dialysis (single-pool Kt/V in hemodialysis patients and weekly Kt/V in peritoneal dialysis patients) were similar between the groups. The propensity scores of the matched patients were almost the same between the early- and late-start groups.

Survival and Clinical Outcomes

The patients' survival rates are shown in Figure 3. Before propensity score matching, the early-start group had a worse survival rate ($P < 0.001$). Hospitalization ($P = 0.195$), cardiovascular events ($P = 0.352$), vascular access complications ($P = 0.158$), changes in dialysis modality ($P = 0.660$), and peritonitis ($P = 0.833$) were not different between the groups (Figure S1). After matching, patient survival, hospitalization, cardiovascular events, vascular access complications, change of dialysis modality, and peritonitis were not different between the groups.

Subgroup analyses of all-cause mortality were performed in the propensity score-matched cohort, and the hazard ratio of starting dialysis early is illustrated in Figure 4 using a Cox proportional analysis. The hazard associated with starting dialysis early was not elevated in any subgroups except patients with diabetes. In patients with diabetes, the hazard associated with an early-start to dialysis was significantly greater (HR 2.024, 95% CI 1.025–3.996).

The causes of mortality are listed in Table 2. The distributions of the mortality causes were not different before ($P = 0.817$) and after ($P = 0.521$) propensity score matching. In propensity score-matched participants, mortality rates from cardiovascular events ($P = 0.630$), cerebrovascular accidents ($P = 0.659$), infections

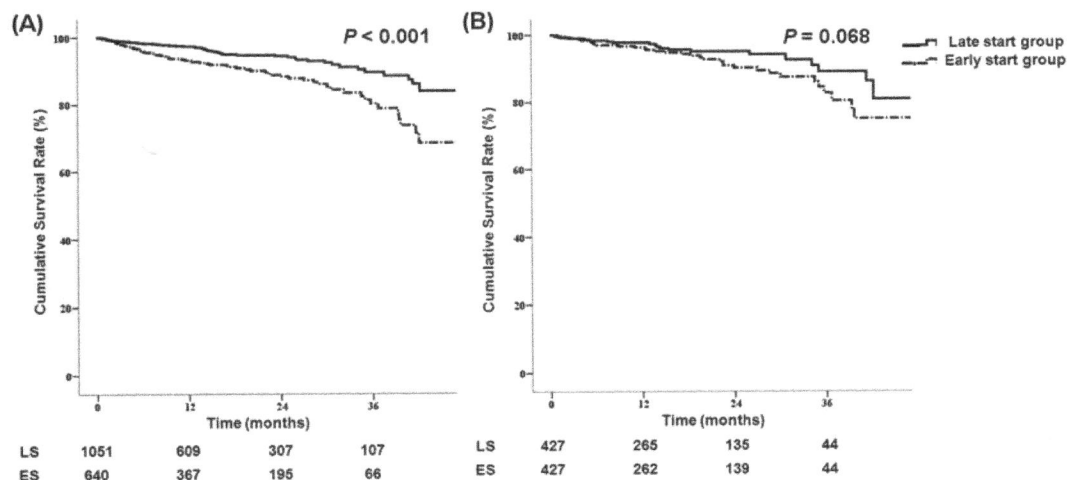

Figure 3. Kaplan-Meier patient survival curve for the timing of dialysis initiation. (A) Before matching, the patients in the early start group had poor survival. (B) After propensity score matching, patients in the early- and late-start groups showed no differences in survival.

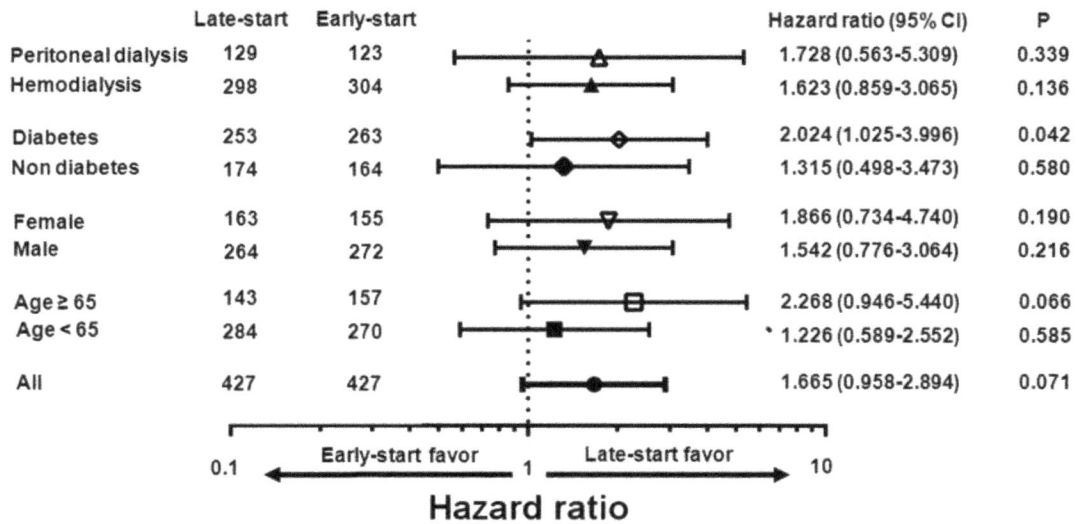

	Late-start	Early-start		Hazard ratio (95% CI)	P
Peritoneal dialysis	129	123		1.728 (0.563-5.309)	0.339
Hemodialysis	298	304		1.623 (0.859-3.065)	0.136
Diabetes	253	263		2.024 (1.025-3.996)	0.042
Non diabetes	174	164		1.315 (0.498-3.473)	0.580
Female	163	155		1.866 (0.734-4.740)	0.190
Male	264	272		1.542 (0.776-3.064)	0.216
Age ≥ 65	143	157		2.268 (0.946-5.440)	0.066
Age < 65	284	270		1.226 (0.589-2.552)	0.585
All	427	427		1.665 (0.958-2.894)	0.071

Figure 4. Hazard ratio (HR) for mortality of early dialysis initiation using a Cox proportional analysis in the propensity score-matched cohort. The hazard of early dialysis initiation was not elevated in any subgroup except patients with diabetes. In patients with diabetes, the hazard of early dialysis initiation was significantly greater (HR 2.024, 95% CI 1.025-3.996).

$(P = 0.783)$, and malignancies $(P = 0.984)$ were not different between the early- and late-start groups. Cardiovascular events, including acute myocardial infarction, arrhythmia, cardiac arrest, valvular heart disease, and congestive heart failure, were the leading causes of mortality.

Discussion

We evaluated the effects of early dialysis initiation on all-cause mortality and other clinical outcomes using a propensity score-matching analysis in an Asian prospective cohort study. Before matching, the early-start group seemed to have poorer survival than the late-start group. However, after matching, these differences in survival disappeared, and there were no significant differences in all-cause mortality or other clinical outcomes.

Comparing the entire cohort of participants, the early start-group was older than the late-start group. In addition, the proportions of male patients and cases of diabetic kidney disease were greater in the early-start group. The mCCI was also higher in the early-start group. Although systolic and diastolic blood pressure levels were lower and hemoglobin levels were higher in the early-start group, serum albumin levels were lower in the

early-start group. In summary, except for residual renal function, the demographic and laboratory parameters were worse in the early-start group. It is possible that the patients in the early-start group initiated dialysis earlier because they had more complications due to ESRD. The high burden of comorbidities in the early-start group might have been the principal cause of poor survival before matching. Indeed, after adjusting for these confounding factors using propensity score-matching methods, survival and clinical outcomes were comparable between groups.

Although the proportion of early dialysis initiation remained stable between 2009 and 2011 in the United States, the percentage of patients who started dialysis early had grown steadily until 2009, up to 54% [10]. A worldwide trend toward early dialysis initiation had been supported by the belief that increased solute clearance could improve patient survival and clinical outcomes. Prolonged uremia can decrease appetite and evoke anorexia, poor oral intake, and malnutrition [32]. Several studies had shown that decreased eGFR values at the time of dialysis initiation were closely associated with poor nutritional status and mortality [33–37]. In addition, there had been concern that delaying dialysis might fail to prevent fatal uremic complications, including severe

Table 2. Causes of patient mortality.

Causes of mortality	All participants (N = 1691)			PS-matched participants (N = 854)		
	All participants	Late-start (N = 1051)	Early-start (N = 640)	PS-matched participants	Late-start (N = 427)	Early-start (N = 427)
Cardiovascular events	34 (29.6%)	17 (33.3%)	17 (26.6%)	16 (29.1%)	7 (33.3%)	9 (26.5%)
Cerebrovascular events	7 (6.1%)	2 (3.9%)	5 (7.8%)	5 (9.1%)	2 (9.5%)	3 (8.8%)
Infections	30 (26.1%)	15 (29.4%)	15 (23.4%)	13 (23.6%)	6 (28.6%)	7 (20.6%)
Malignancies	7 (6.1%)	3 (5.9%)	4 (6.3%)	2 (3.6%)	1 (4.8%)	1 (2.9%)
Other	22 (19.1%)	8 (15.7%)	14 (21.9%)	10 (18.2%)	1 (4.8%)	9 (26.5%)
Unknown	15 (13.0%)	6 (11.8%)	9 (14.1%)	9 (16.4%)	4 (19.0%)	5 (14.7%)

hyperkalemia, uncontrolled hypertension, pulmonary edema, pericarditis, and encephalopathy. In fact, before the IDEAL study, clinical guidelines had permitted early dialysis initiation for an eGFR of over 10 ml/min/1.73 m^2 if there were relevant uremic symptoms or evidence of malnutrition [38–41]. In the United States, reflecting these guidelines, the mean eGFR at dialysis initiation increased from 8.1 ml/min/1.73 m^2 in 1997 to 10.8 ml/min/1.73 m^2 in 2007 [42]. However, the association between low eGFR at the time of dialysis initiation and poor survival cannot be used as direct evidence justifying early dialysis initiation. Almost studies reporting the benefit of early dialysis initiation were of a retrospective observational design, and the adjustments made for demographic factors and comorbid conditions were insufficient [33,34,43,44]. In addition, the possibility of lead-time bias in the studies favoring early dialysis initiation should be considered. A survival benefit of early dialysis initiation could result from the statistical misinterpretation of the fact that patients had merely started dialysis early, rather than that they actually lived longer. Korevaar et al. reported that the survival benefit of 2.5 months in the patients with early dialysis initiation was overwhelmed by the effect of delaying dialysis approximately 4.1 months in the patients with late dialysis initiation [45].

Notably, contrary to general expectations, recent observational studies have shown that early dialysis initiation was irrelevant to survival benefits or even associated with poor clinical outcomes [11,14,26,46–50]. Starting dialysis early can expose ESRD patients to dialysis-associated complications [51]. The decline in residual renal function can progress at a rapid pace, even after dialysis [52]. Dialysis therapy can also result in protein loss and aggravate nutritional status in ESRD patients [53]. Catheter- or access site-related peritoneal or bloodstream infections are increased in patients undergoing dialysis [54]. These factors can thus collectively contribute to the poor survival and negative clinical outcomes of patients with early dialysis initiation. Although there have been several lines of evidence supporting the harmful effects of early dialysis initiation, there is still a debate as to whether a high eGFR itself is the main cause of poor outcomes in patients with early dialysis initiation. Most eGFR equations are based on serum creatinine levels, so there is a possibility of overestimating the eGFR in cases of low serum creatinine levels due to low muscle mass or fluid overload [55]. Beddhu et al. reported that high eGFR values were closely associated with increased mortality, but high creatinine clearance was not [56]. In addition, survivor bias can overestimate the risk of early dialysis initiation due to the limitations of observational studies. Patients who had died before initiating dialysis were excluded from the analyses of observational studies, and the number of such patients is likely to be higher in the late-start group. Therefore, those who start dialysis later may collectively comprise a healthier group. Crew et al. minimized the lead-time and survivor bias through the enrollment of patients before the initiation of dialysis and analyzed clinical outcomes after the eGFR reached approximately 20 ml/min/1.73 m^2. This work demonstrated that patients who initiated dialysis early or late did not exhibit differences in survival [57]. Lastly, patients who had a high burden of uremic symptoms and/or comorbidities are likely to start dialysis earlier. It is known that patients who are older, male, or who had diabetes, low body mass index, high comorbidities with cardiovascular complications, or poor functional status are likely to start dialysis earlier [48,58–60]. These high risk comorbidities and demographic factors can aggravate survival and other clinical outcomes in patients with early dialysis initiation. Several investigations reported that the risk of early dialysis initiation decreased after multivariate adjustments for demographic factors, laboratory data, and comorbidities

[46,48]. Bao et al. investigated that high mortality was closely associated with frailty, including slowness or weakness, exhaustion, and low physical activity and found that the risks associated with early dialysis initiation disappeared after adjustment for frailty [61]. A recent meta-analysis showed that an early start to dialysis was associated with increased mortality and that patients with older age, diabetes, and high comorbidities seemed to start dialysis earlier [12]. The results of our study before matching are similar to the results of these studies. Patients in the early-start group of the present study were older and had more comorbidities, including diabetes. The poor survival of these patients disappeared after matching the covariates.

To date, only one randomized, controlled study has evaluated the association between dialysis initiation time and survival [15]. In the IDEAL study, Cooper et al. allocated ESRD patients to planned dialysis initiation at an eGFR greater than 10 ml/min/1.73 m^2 or conventional dialysis initiation at an eGFR less than 7 ml/min/1.73 m^2. There were no differences in survival, complications, or quality of life between the two groups. Although the actual difference in eGFR between the two groups was only approximately 2 ml/min/1.73 m^2, the patients in the late-start group could begin dialysis approximately 6 months later than those in the early-start group. When the participants in the IDEAL study were analyzed separately by dialysis modality, more adverse events associated with fluids and electrolytes were observed in the late hemodialysis group, and more patients who had been randomized to peritoneal dialysis switched to hemodialysis; however, early dialysis initiation did not provide survival or other clinical benefits [62,63]. It is difficult to generalize the results of the IDEAL study to all patients preparing for dialysis because the patients enrolled in the IDEAL study were almost all Caucasians and relatively well prepared for ESRD, with low rates of temporary vascular access and a high proportion of peritoneal dialysis. In addition, there was a high incidence of cross-over from the late dialysis group to the early dialysis group. However, the results of the IDEAL study clearly indicate that early dialysis initiation is not unconditionally beneficial for patients with ESRD and that the late initiation strategy can delay dialysis initiation for a proportion of well-prepared patients. The results of our study are consistent with those of the IDEAL study in that neither early nor late initiation of dialysis based on eGFR values was associated with mortality or clinical outcomes. Reflecting the results of recent investigations, newer guidelines recommend delaying dialysis and addressing relevant clinical signs or symptoms rather than instituting dialysis therapy solely based on eGFR values [16–18].

This study has several limitations. First, because this study is an observational cohort study beginning at the time of dialysis initiation, the possibility of survivor bias still exists. This factor can favor late dialysis initiation. In addition, because all patients enrolled were Asian, the results of this study cannot easily be generalized to all ESRD patients, as the prognosis and clinical outcomes of ESRD patients are well known to be closely associated with demographic factors and comorbid conditions. However, this study still has an advantage in that it is the only prospective and well-matched cohort study in Asian ESRD patients using propensity score-matching analysis. After matching, almost all variables, including age and comorbidities, became similar between the early- and late-start groups, except for variables associated with residual renal function. Because demographic factors, comorbid conditions, and laboratory parameters converged after matching, the possibility of bias, including lead-time bias, is minimized. In addition, because there was a substantial difference in eGFR between the groups (approximately

5 ml/min/1.73 m^2), the effects of early dialysis initiation could be explored with confidence.

We evaluated the effects of dialysis initiation timing based on eGFR on clinical outcomes using propensity score-matching analysis. Early dialysis initiation did not improve patient survival or other clinical outcomes, including hospitalization, cardiovascular events, vascular access complications, changes in dialysis modality, or peritonitis. It is appears that, rather than the eGFR at the initiation timing of dialysis, a patient's health status, including age, sex, physical activity, and comorbidities, has a greater impact on clinical outcomes in patients initiating dialysis. Although the optimal time for dialysis initiation remains controversial, dialysis initiation should not be determined based on eGFR values alone. Residual renal function, comorbidities, and uremic symptoms should be considered before starting dialysis.

Acknowledgments

A portion of this work was selected for a poster presentation, which was presented at Kidney Week 2013 at the American Society of Nephrology Annual Meeting on November 9 at the Georgia World Congress Center in Atlanta, GA. We express our gratitude to all of the participants and investigators of the cohort study (Clinical Research Center for End Stage Renal Disease, CRC for ESRD) in South Korea.

Author Contributions

Conceived and designed the experiments: JPL. Performed the experiments: JL YLK SWK CWY NHK YKO CSL YSK JPL. Analyzed the data: JL JNA JHH JPL. Contributed reagents/materials/analysis tools: YLK YKO CSL YSK JPL. Contributed to the writing of the manuscript: JL JPL.

References

1. Zhang QL, Rothenbacher D (2008) Prevalence of chronic kidney disease in population-based studies: systematic review. BMC Public Health 8: 117.
2. Collins AJ, Foley RN, Chavers B, Gilbertson D, Herzog C, et al. (2014) US Renal Data System 2013 Annual Data Report. Am J Kidney Dis 63: A7.
3. Gansevoort RT, Correa-Rotter R, Hemmelgarn BR, Jafar TH, Heerspink HJ, et al. (2013) Chronic kidney disease and cardiovascular risk: epidemiology, mechanisms, and prevention. Lancet 382: 339–352.
4. Wen CP, Cheng TY, Tsai MK, Chang YC, Chan HT, et al. (2008) All-cause mortality attributable to chronic kidney disease: a prospective cohort study based on 462293 adults in Taiwan. Lancet 371: 2173–2182.
5. Turin TC, Tonelli M, Manns BJ, Ravani P, Ahmed SB, et al. (2012) Chronic kidney disease and life expectancy. Nephrol Dial Transplant 27: 3182–3186.
6. Chandna SM, Da Silva-Gane M, Marshall C, Warwicker P, Greenwood RN, et al. (2011) Survival of elderly patients with stage 5 CKD: comparison of conservative management and renal replacement therapy. Nephrol Dial Transplant 26: 1608–1614.
7. Joly D, Anglicheau D, Alberti C, Nguyen AT, Touam M, et al. (2003) Octogenarians reaching end-stage renal disease: cohort study of decision-making and clinical outcomes. J Am Soc Nephrol 14: 1012–1021.
8. Carson RC, Juszczak M, Davenport A, Burns A (2009) Is maximum conservative management an equivalent treatment option to dialysis for elderly patients with significant comorbid disease? Clin J Am Soc Nephrol 4: 1611–1619.
9. Rosansky S, Glassock RJ, Clark WF (2011) Early start of dialysis: a critical review. Clin J Am Soc Nephrol 6: 1222–1228.
10. Rosansky SJ, Clark WF (2013) Has the yearly increase in the renal replacement therapy population ended? J Am Soc Nephrol 24: 1367–1370.
11. Crews DC, Scialla JJ, Liu J, Guo H, Bandeen-Roche K, et al. (2014) Predialysis health, dialysis timing, and outcomes among older United States adults. J Am Soc Nephrol 25: 370–379.
12. Pan Y, Xu XD, Guo LL, Cai LL, Jin HM (2012) Association of early versus late initiation of dialysis with mortality: systematic review and meta-analysis. Nephron Clin Pract 120: c121–131.
13. Susantitaphong P, Altamimi S, Ashkar M, Balk EM, Stel VS, et al. (2012) GFR at initiation of dialysis and mortality in CKD: a meta-analysis. Am J Kidney Dis 59: 829–840.
14. Stel VS, Dekker FW, Ansell D, Augustijn H, Casino FG, et al. (2009) Residual renal function at the start of dialysis and clinical outcomes. Nephrol Dial Transplant 24: 3175–3182.
15. Cooper BA, Branley P, Bulfone L, Collins JF, Craig JC, et al. (2010) A randomized, controlled trial of early versus late initiation of dialysis. N Engl J Med 363: 609–619.
16. Nesrallah GE, Mustafa RA, Clark WF, Bass A, Barnieh L, et al. (2014) Canadian Society of Nephrology 2014 clinical practice guideline for timing the initiation of chronic dialysis. CMAJ 186: 112–117.
17. KDIGO (2013) KDIGO clinical practice guideline for the evaluation and management of chronic kidney disease. Kidney Int Suppl 3: 1–150.
18. Tattersall J, Dekker F, Heimburger O, Jager KJ, Lameire N, et al. (2011) When to start dialysis: updated guidance following publication of the Initiating Dialysis Early and Late (IDEAL) study. Nephrol Dial Transplant 26: 2082–2086.
19. Arce CM, Goldstein BA, Mitani AA, Winkelmayer WC (2013) Trends in relative mortality between Hispanic and non-Hispanic whites initiating dialysis: a

retrospective study of the US Renal Data System. Am J Kidney Dis 62: 312–321.
20. Derose SF, Rutkowski MP, Crooks PW, Shi JM, Wang JQ, et al. (2013) Racial differences in estimated GFR decline, ESRD, and mortality in an integrated health system. Am J Kidney Dis 62: 236–244.
21. Conley J, Tonelli M, Quan H, Manns BJ, Palacios-Derflingher L, et al. (2012) Association between GFR, proteinuria, and adverse outcomes among White, Chinese, and South Asian individuals in Canada. Am J Kidney Dis 59: 390–399.
22. Barbour SJ, Er L, Djurdjev O, Karim M, Levin A (2010) Differences in progression of CKD and mortality amongst Caucasian, Oriental Asian and South Asian CKD patients. Nephrol Dial Transplant 25: 3663–3672.
23. Chang JH, Rim MY, Sung J, Ko KP, Kim DK, et al. (2012) Early start of dialysis has no survival benefit in end-stage renal disease patients. J Korean Med Sci 27: 1177–1181.
24. Oh KH, Hwang YH, Cho JH, Kim M, Ju KD, et al. (2012) Outcome of early initiation of peritoneal dialysis in patients with end-stage renal failure. J Korean Med Sci 27: 170–176.
25. Yamagata K, Nakai S, Iseki K, Tsubakihara Y, Committee of Renal Data Registry of the Japanese Society for Dialysis Therapy (2012) Late dialysis start did not affect long-term outcome in Japanese dialysis patients: long-term prognosis from Japanese Society for Dialysis Therapy Registry. Ther Apher Dial 16: 111–120.
26. Hwang SJ, Yang WC, Lin MY, Mau LW, Chen HC (2010) Impact of the clinical conditions at dialysis initiation on mortality in incident haemodialysis patients: a national cohort study in Taiwan. Nephrol Dial Transplant 25: 2616–2624.
27. Shiao CC, Huang JW, Chien KL, Chuang HF, Chen YM, et al. (2008) Early initiation of dialysis and late implantation of catheters adversely affect outcomes of patients on chronic peritoneal dialysis. Perit Dial Int 28: 73–81.
28. Kim do H, Kim M, Kim H, Kim YL, Kang SW, et al. (2013) Early referral to a nephrologist improved patient survival: prospective cohort study for end-stage renal disease in Korea. PLoS One 8: e55323.
29. Levey AS, Stevens LA, Schmid CH, Zhang YL, Castro AF 3rd, et al. (2009) A new equation to estimate glomerular filtration rate. Ann Intern Med 150: 604–612.
30. Charlson ME, Pompei P, Ales KL, MacKenzie CR (1987) A new method of classifying prognostic comorbidity in longitudinal studies: development and validation. J Chronic Dis 40: 373–383.
31. Hemmelgarn BR, Manns BJ, Quan H, Ghali WA (2003) Adapting the Charlson Comorbidity Index for use in patients with ESRD. Am J Kidney Dis 42: 125–132.
32. Fouque D, Kalantar-Zadeh K, Kopple J, Cano N, Chauveau P, et al. (2008) A proposed nomenclature and diagnostic criteria for protein-energy wasting in acute and chronic kidney disease. Kidney Int 73: 391–398.
33. Liu H, Peng Y, Liu F, Xiao H, Chen X, et al. (2008) Renal function and serum albumin at the start of dialysis in 514 Chinese ESRD in-patients. Ren Fail 30: 685–690.
34. Cooper BA, Aslani A, Ryan M, Ibels LS, Pollock CA (2003) Nutritional state correlates with renal function at the start of dialysis. Perit Dial Int 23: 291–295.
35. Pupim LB, Kent P, Caglar K, Shyr Y, Hakim RM, et al. (2002) Improvement in nutritional parameters after initiation of chronic hemodialysis. Am J Kidney Dis 40: 143–151.

36. Churchill DN (1997) An evidence-based approach to earlier initiation of dialysis. Am J Kidney Dis 30: 899–906.

37. Hakim RM, Lazarus JM (1995) Initiation of dialysis. J Am Soc Nephrol 6: 1319–1328.

38. Hemodialysis Adequacy 2006 Work Group (2006) Clinical practice guidelines for hemodialysis adequacy, update 2006. Am J Kidney Dis 48 Suppl 1: S2–90.

39. Peritoneal Dialysis Adequacy Work Group (2006) Clinical practice guidelines for peritoneal dialysis adequacy. Am J Kidney Dis 48 Suppl 1: S98–129.

40. Kelly J, Stanley M, Harris D, Caring for Australians with Renal Impairment (2005) The CARI guidelines. Acceptance into dialysis guidelines. Nephrology (Carlton) 10 Suppl 4: S46–60.

41. European Best Practice Guidelines Expert Group on Hemodialysis (2002) Section I. Measurement of renal function, when to refer and when to start dialysis. Nephrol Dial Transplant 17 Suppl 7: 7–15.

42. O'Hare AM, Choi AI, Boscardin WJ, Clinton WL, Zawadzki I, et al. (2011) Trends in timing of initiation of chronic dialysis in the United States. Arch Intern Med 171: 1663–1669.

43. Traynor JP, Simpson K, Geddes CC, Deighan CJ, Fox JG (2002) Early initiation of dialysis fails to prolong survival in patients with end-stage renal failure. J Am Soc Nephrol 13: 2125–2132.

44. Tang SC, Ho YW, Tang AW, Cheng YY, Chiu FH, et al. (2007) Delaying initiation of dialysis till symptomatic uraemia–is it too late? Nephrol Dial Transplant 22: 1926–1932.

45. Korevaar JC, Jansen MA, Dekker FW, Jager KJ, Boeschoten EW, et al. (2001) When to initiate dialysis: effect of proposed US guidelines on survival. Lancet 358: 1046–1050.

46. Clark WF, Na Y, Rosansky SJ, Sontrop JM, Macnab JJ, et al. (2011) Association between estimated glomerular filtration rate at initiation of dialysis and mortality. CMAJ 183: 47–53.

47. Rosansky SJ, Eggers P, Jackson K, Glassock R, Clark WF (2011) Early start of hemodialysis may be harmful. Arch Intern Med 171: 396–403.

48. Lassalle M, Labeeuw M, Frimat L, Villar E, Joyeux V, et al. (2010) Age and comorbidity may explain the paradoxical association of an early dialysis start with poor survival. Kidney Int 77: 700–707.

49. Sawhney S, Djurdjev O, Simpson K, Macleod A, Levin A (2009) Survival and dialysis initiation: comparing British Columbia and Scotland registries. Nephrol Dial Transplant 24: 3186–3192.

50. Kazmi WH, Gilbertson DT, Obrador GT, Guo H, Pereira BJ, et al. (2005) Effect of comorbidity on the increased mortality associated with early initiation of dialysis. Am J Kidney Dis 46: 887–896.

51. Wright S, Klausner D, Baird B, Williams ME, Steinman T, et al. (2010) Timing of dialysis initiation and survival in ESRD. Clin J Am Soc Nephrol 5: 1828–1835.

52. Jansen MA, Hart AA, Korevaar JC, Dekker FW, Boeschoten EW, et al. (2002) Predictors of the rate of decline of residual renal function in incident dialysis patients. Kidney Int 62: 1046–1053.

53. Mehrotra R, Duong U, Jiwakanon S, Kovesdy CP, Moran J, et al. (2011) Serum albumin as a predictor of mortality in peritoneal dialysis: comparisons with hemodialysis. Am J Kidney Dis 58: 418–428.

54. Nguyen DB, Lessa FC, Belflower R, Mu Y, Wise M, et al. (2013) Invasive methicillin-resistant Staphylococcus aureus infections among patients on chronic dialysis in the United States, 2005–2011. Clin Infect Dis 57: 1393–1400.

55. Grootendorst DC, Michels WM, Richardson JD, Jager KJ, Boeschoten EW, et al. (2011) The MDRD formula does not reflect GFR in ESRD patients. Nephrol Dial Transplant 26: 1932–1937.

56. Beddhu S, Samore MH, Roberts MS, Stoddard GJ, Ramkumar N, et al. (2003) Impact of timing of initiation of dialysis on mortality. J Am Soc Nephrol 14: 2305–2312.

57. Crews DC, Scialla JJ, Boulware LE, Navaneethan SD, Nally JV Jr, et al. (2014) Comparative effectiveness of early versus conventional timing of dialysis initiation in advanced CKD. Am J Kidney Dis 63: 806–815.

58. van de Luijtgaarden MW, Noordzij M, Tomson C, Couchoud C, Cancarini G, et al. (2012) Factors influencing the decision to start renal replacement therapy: results of a survey among European nephrologists. Am J Kidney Dis 60: 940–948.

59. Streja E, Nicholas SB, Norris KC (2013) Controversies in timing of dialysis initiation and the role of race and demographics. Semin Dial 26: 658–666.

60. Slinin Y, Guo H, Li S, Liu J, Morgan B, et al. (2014) Provider and care characteristics associated with timing of dialysis initiation. Clin J Am Soc Nephrol 9: 310–317.

61. Bao Y, Dalrymple L, Chertow GM, Kaysen GA, Johansen KL (2012) Frailty, dialysis initiation, and mortality in end-stage renal disease. Arch Intern Med 172: 1071–1077.

62. Collins J, Cooper B, Branley P, Bulfone L, Craig J, et al. (2011) Outcomes of patients with planned initiation of hemodialysis in the IDEAL trial. Contrib Nephrol 171: 1–9.

63. Johnson DW, Wong MG, Cooper BA, Branley P, Bulfone L, et al. (2012) Effect of timing of dialysis commencement on clinical outcomes of patients with planned initiation of peritoneal dialysis in the IDEAL trial. Perit Dial Int 32: 595–604.

13

Association between Combined Lifestyle Factors and Non-Restorative Sleep in Japan: A Cross-Sectional Study Based on a Japanese Health Database

Minako Wakasugi[1]*, Junichiro James Kazama[2], Ichiei Narita[3], Kunitoshi Iseki[3], Toshiki Moriyama[3], Kunihiro Yamagata[3], Shouichi Fujimoto[3], Kazuhiko Tsuruya[3], Koichi Asahi[3], Tsuneo Konta[3], Kenjiro Kimura[4], Masahide Kondo[3], Issei Kurahashi[4], Yasuo Ohashi[5], Tsuyoshi Watanabe[3]

1 Center for Inter-organ Communication Research, Niigata University Graduate School of Medical and Dental Sciences, Niigata, Japan, 2 Department of Clinical Nephrology and Rheumatology, Niigata University Graduate School of Medical and Dental Sciences, Niigata, Japan, 3 Steering Committee for "Design of the comprehensive health care system for chronic kidney disease (CKD) based on the individual risk assessment by Specific Health Checkups," Fukushima, Japan, 4 iAnalysis LLC, Tokyo, Japan, 5 Department of Integrated Science and Engineering for Sustainable Society, Chuo University, Tokyo, Japan

Abstract

Background: Although lifestyle factors such as cigarette smoking, excessive drinking, obesity, low or no exercise, and unhealthy dietary habits have each been associated with inadequate sleep, little is known about their combined effect. The aim of this study was to quantify the overall impact of lifestyle-related factors on non-restorative sleep in the general Japanese population.

Methods and Findings: A cross-sectional study of 243,767 participants (men, 39.8%) was performed using the Specific Health Check and Guidance System in Japan. A healthy lifestyle score was calculated by adding up the number of low-risk lifestyle factors for each participant. Low risk was defined as (1) not smoking, (2) body mass index<25 kg/m^2, (3) moderate or less alcohol consumption, (4) regular exercise, and (5) better eating patterns. Logistic regression analysis was used to examine the relationship between the score and the prevalence of non-restorative sleep, which was determined from questionnaire responses. Among 97,062 men (mean age, 63.9 years) and 146,705 women (mean age, 63.7 years), 18,678 (19.2%) and 38,539 (26.3%) reported non-restorative sleep, respectively. The prevalence of non-restorative sleep decreased with age for both sexes. Compared to participants with a healthy lifestyle score of 5 (most healthy), those with a score of 0 (least healthy) had a higher prevalence of non-restorative sleep (odds ratio, 1.59 [95% confidence interval, 1.29–1.97] for men and 2.88 [1.74–4.76] for women), independently of hypertension, hypercholesterolemia, diabetes, and chronic kidney disease. The main limitation of the study was the cross-sectional design, which limited causal inferences for the identified associations.

Conclusions: A combination of several unhealthy lifestyle factors was associated with non-restorative sleep among the general Japanese population. Further studies are needed to establish whether general lifestyle modification improves restorative sleep.

Editor: Mathias Basner, University of Pennsylvania Perelman School of Medicine, United States of America

Funding: This study was supported by a Health and Labor Sciences Research Grant for "Design of a comprehensive health care system for chronic kidney disease (CKD) based on individual risk assessment by Specific Health Checkups" (H24-intractible(renal)-ippan-006) from the Ministry of Health, Labor, and Welfare of Japan. The funders had no role in study design, data collection and analysis, decision to publish, or preparation of the manuscript.

Competing Interests: The authors have declared that no competing interests exist.

* Email: minakowa@med.niigata-u.ac.jp

Introduction

A combination of healthy lifestyle factors, such as abstaining from smoking, maintaining a body mass index (BMI) of less than 25 kg/m^2, consuming alcohol moderately, exercising regularly, and having a healthy diet, is reportedly associated with a significantly reduced risk of developing several diseases, such as coronary heart disease [1–2], type 2 diabetes mellitus [3], stroke [4], sudden cardiac death [5], chronic kidney disease [6], cancer [7–9], and total mortality [10]. A clear linear relationship was observed in these studies between risk reduction and the number

of healthy lifestyle factors, suggesting that an analysis of combined lifestyle factors may demonstrate their influence better than analyses based on single factors due to the complexity and multiple dimensions of habitual health behaviors. In addition, maintaining an overall healthy lifestyle throughout young adulthood was strongly associated with a low cardiovascular disease risk profile in middle age regardless of sex, race, or a parental history of myocardial infarction, suggesting that genetic factors may not be very important in determining a low risk profile [11]. Most of these studies were conducted in non-Japanese populations except for a few studies [6,9]; however, a combination of healthy lifestyle factors may play a prominent role regardless of sex, race, or genetics.

Little is known about the impact of combined lifestyle factors on inadequate sleep. There is growing evidence that inadequate sleep, which includes short sleep duration and poor sleep quality, is associated with lifestyle factors that include obesity, insufficient physical exercise, and consumption of substances such as caffeine, alcohol, and nicotine [12]. Inadequate sleep may also modify eating patterns, thereby mediating or contributing to the observed relationship between sleep disturbance and obesity [13].

Inadequate sleep is associated with several chronic diseases. Epidemiological studies have shown that short sleep duration is associated with a higher risk of lifestyle-related diseases such as obesity [14–17], type 2 diabetes mellitus [18–19], hypertension [20], dyslipidemia [21], coronary heart disease [22], and chronic kidney disease [23]. Sleep quality is important in modifying the association between sleep duration and these diseases [24–26].

We hypothesized that a combination of unhealthy lifestyle factors is associated with inadequate sleep. Evidence of a relationship could have important clinical and public health implications. If a combination of unhealthy behaviors is associated with inadequate sleep, lifestyle interventions have the potential to reduce its occurrence. We present the results of a large cross-sectional study on the prevalence of non-restorative sleep (NRS), typically defined as subjectively feeling unrefreshed upon waking

[27], and its association with a combination of lifestyle factors in the general Japanese population.

Methods

Study population and design

This cross-sectional study used baseline data from a prospective cohort study of 667,218 participants, aged 40 to 74 years, obtained from the Japanese Specific Health Check and Guidance System (SHC) created in 2008. Twenty-four of the prefectures participating in this nationwide project (Hokkaido, Miyagi, Yamagata, Fukushima, Ibaraki, Tochigi, Tokyo, Saitama, Kanagawa, Niigata, Nagano, Ishikawa, Gifu, Osaka, Okayama, Tokushima, Kochi, Fukuoka, Saga, Nagasaki, Oita, Kumamoto, Miyazaki, and Okinawa) agreed to participate in our study and were included in the present analysis. Data were sent to and verified by an independent data center, the NPO Japan Clinical Research Support Unit (Tokyo, Japan). All participants remained anonymous, and the study was conducted according to Japanese privacy protection laws and ethical guidelines for epidemiological studies published by the Ministry of Education, Science, and Culture and the Ministry of Health, Labor, and Welfare. The study protocol was approved by the ethics committee in Fukushima Medical University (No. 1485).

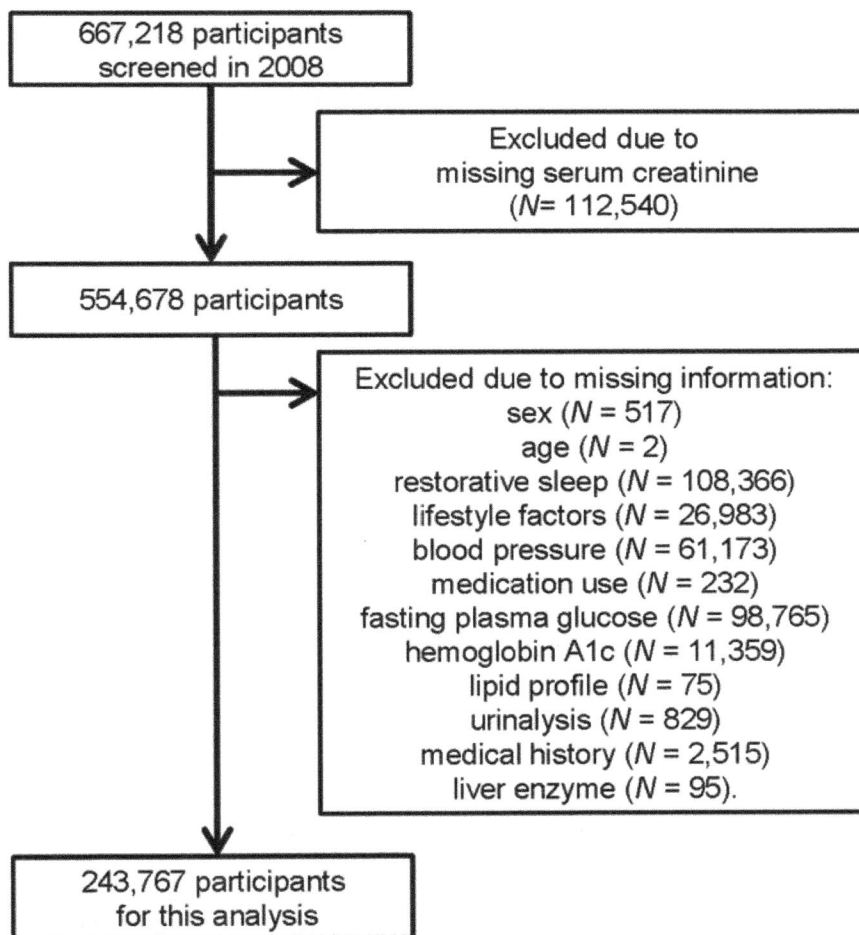

Figure 1. Flow chart of participant selection. Of the 667,218 SHC participants screened in 2008, we excluded anyone with missing information, resulting in a final sample size of 243,767.

Table 1. Clinical characteristics of male participants by restorative sleep achievement.

Characteristics	Total (N= 97,062)	Restorative sleep (N= 78,384 [80.8%])	Non-restorative sleep (N= 18,678 [19.2%])	P value
Age, years	63.9 (8.5)	64.4 (8.2)	61.7 (9.5)	<0.0001
Healthy lifestyle score, n (%)				<0.0001
0	484 (0.5)	360 (0.5)	124 (0.7)	
1	5,049 (5.2)	3,715 (4.7)	1,334 (7.1)	
2	16,986 (17.5)	13,140 (16.8)	3,846 (20.6)	
3	30,331 (31.3)	24,326 (31.0)	6,005 (32.2)	
4	31,355 (32.3)	25,735 (32.8)	5,620 (30.1)	
5	12,857 (13.3)	11,108 (14.2)	1,749 (9.4)	
Components of the healthy lifestyle score				
Current smoker, n (%)	25,359 (26.1)	20,214 (25.8)	5,145 (27.5)	<0.0001
Body mass index, kg/m²	23.6 (3.0)	23.6 (2.9)	23.7 (3.2)	0.05
Alcohol<20 g/day, n (%)	67,556 (69.6)	53,924 (68.8)	13,632 (73.0)	<0.0001
Regular exercise				
Exercise to sweat lightly, n (%)	46,069 (47.5)	39,055 (49.8)	7,014 (37.6)	<0.0001
Walking>1 hour/day, n (%)	53,950 (55.6)	45,253 (57.7)	8,697 (46.6)	<0.0001
Eating pattern				
Snacks after supper, n (%)	12,000 (12.4)	8,775 (11.2)	3,225 (17.3)	<0.0001
Skipping breakfast, n (%)	11,060 (11.4)	7,818 (10.0)	3,242 (17.4)	<0.0001
Past history, n (%)				
Stroke	4.938 (5.1)	4,003 (5.1)	935 (5.0)	0.59
Heart disease	7,964 (8.2)	6,285 (8.0)	1,679 (9.0)	<0.0001
Renal disease	552 (0.6)	417 (0.5)	135 (0.7)	0.002
Comorbidities, n (%)				
Hypertension	49,135 (50.6)	40,406 (51.5)	8,729 (46.7)	<0.0001
Diabetes	14,596 (15.0)	11,965 (15.3)	2,631 (14.1)	<0.0001
Hypercholesterolemia	33, 258 (34.3)	26,878 (34.3)	6,380 (34.2)	0.74
Chronic kidney disease	22,570 (23.3)	18,481 (23.6)	4,089 (21.9)	<0.0001
Medication, n (%)				
Antihypertensive drugs	30,756 (31.7)	25,382 (32.4)	5,374 (28.8)	<0.0001
Antidiabetic medication	6,649 (6.9)	5,457 (7.0)	1,192 (6.4)	0.005
Cholesterol-lowering drugs	10,779 (11.1)	8,856 (11.3)	1,923 (10.3)	<0.0001
Systolic pressure, mmHg	131 (17)	132 (17)	130 (17)	<0.0001
Diastolic pressure, mmHg	78 (11)	78 (11)	78 (11)	0.001
Fasting plasma glucose, mg per 100 mL	102 (25)	102 (24)	102 (26)	0.66
Hemoglobin A_{1c}, %	5.79 (0.79)	5.79 (0.77)	5.78 (0.85)	0.02
LDL cholesterol, mg per 100 mL	120.9 (30.0)	120.8 (29.9)	121.1 (30.4)	0.21
Triglycerides, mg per 100 mL	107 (77, 154)	107 (77, 153)	107 (76, 155)	0.58
HDL cholesterol, mg per 100 mL	57 (15)	57 (15)	57 (15)	0.96
Creatinine, mg per 100 mL	0.85 (0.23)	0.85 (0.23)	0.84 (0.23)	0.03
eGFR, mL min^{-1} per 1.73 m²	74.4 (16.4)	74.2 (16.3)	75.6 (16.9)	<0.0001
Proteinuria, n (%)	7,670 (7.9)	6,157 (7.9)	1,513 (8.1)	0.26

Numbers in the table are means (standard deviation) for continuous variables except triglycerides (median and interquartile range) or numbers (percentages) for categorical variables.
LDL, low-density lipoprotein; HDL, high-density lipoprotein; eGFR, estimated glomerular filtration rate.

The SHC has been previously described [6,28]. Briefly, it is a new healthcare strategy initiated by the Japanese Government in 2008 for the early diagnosis and intervention of metabolic syndrome. The proportion of men to women in the SHC does not necessarily reflect the national population. This is because the SHC is designed for people who have National Health Insurance, or dependents (e.g., spouse) of salaried workers who have health insurance. In this system, participants answer a self-administered questionnaire that covers medical history, smoking habits, alcohol intake, exercise habits, and eating patterns. Trained staff then

Table 2. Clinical characteristics of female participants by restorative sleep achievement.

Characteristics	Total (N = 146,705)	Restorative sleep (N = 108,166 [73.7%])	Non-restorative Sleep (N = 38,539 [26.3%])	P value
Age, years	63.7 (7.9)	64.2 (7.7)	62.6 (8.5)	<0.0001
Healthy lifestyle score, n (%)				<0.0001
0	63 (0.0)	35 (0.0)	28 (0.1)	
1	1,283 (0.9)	765 (0.7)	518 (1.3)	
2	9,909 (6.8)	6,502 (6.0)	3,407 (8.8)	
3	35,999 (24.5)	25,208 (23.3)	10,791 (28.0)	
4	71,637 (48.8)	53,100 (49.1)	18,537 (48.1)	
5	27,814 (19.0)	22,556 (20.9)	5,258 (13.6)	
Components of the healthy lifestyle score				
Current smoker, n (%)	9,763 (6.7)	6,655 (6.2)	3,108 (8.1)	<0.0001
Body mass index, kg/m^2	22.7 (3.4)	22.7 (3.3)	22.6 (3.5)	<0.0001
Alcohol<20 g/day, n (%)	142,216 (96.9)	105,038 (97.1)	37,178 (96.5)	<0.0001
Regular exercise				
Exercise to sweat lightly, n (%)	58,932 (40.2)	46,404 (42.9)	12,528 (32.5)	<0.0001
Walking>1 hour/day, n (%)	76,043 (51.8)	58,492 (54.1)	17,551 (45.5)	<0.0001
Eating pattern				
Snacks after supper, n (%)	20,361 (13.9)	13,630 (12.6)	6,731 (17.5)	<0.0001
Skipping breakfast, n (%)	11,791 (8.0)	7,429 (6.9)	4,362 (11.3)	<0.0001
Past history, n (%)				
Stroke	3.902 (2.7)	2,813 (2.6)	1,089 (2.8)	0.02
Heart disease	7,606 (5.2)	5,271 (4.9)	2,335 (6.1)	<0.0001
Renal disease	632 (0.4)	436 (0.4)	196 (0.5)	0.007
Comorbidities, n (%)				
Hypertension	62,034 (42.3)	46,822 (43.3)	15,212 (39.5)	<0.0001
Diabetes	11,623 (7.9)	8,625 (8.0)	2,998 (7.8)	<0.0001
Hypercholesterolemia	74,371 (50.7)	55,682 (51.5)	18,689 (48.5)	<0.0001
Chronic kidney disease	21,762 (14.8)	16,146 (14.9)	5,616 (14.6)	<0.0001
Medication, n (%)				
Antihypertensive drugs	39,592 (27.0)	29,884 (27.6)	9,708 (25.2)	<0.0001
Antidiabetic medication	5,373 (3.7)	3,960 (3.7)	1,413 (3.7)	0.96
Cholesterol-lowering drugs	28,802 (19.6)	21,771 (20.1)	7,031 (18.2)	<0.0001
Systolic pressure, mmHg	128 (18)	129 (18)	130 (18)	<0.0001
Diastolic pressure, mmHg	75 (11)	75 (11)	75 (11)	<0.0001
Fasting plasma glucose, mg per 100 mL	95 (18)	95 (17)	95 (19)	0.03
Hemoglobin A$_{1c}$, %	5.71 (0.59)	5.72 (0.58)	5.70 (0.60)	<0.0001
LDL cholesterol, mg per 100 mL	130.0 (30.3)	130.2 (30.2)	129.2 (30.8)	<0.0001
Triglycerides, mg per 100 mL	92 (68, 127)	92 (69, 127)	91 (67, 126)	<0.0001
HDL cholesterol, mg per 100 mL	65.7 (16.0)	65.5 (16.0)	66.3 (16.2)	<0.0001
Creatinine, mg per 100 mL	0.63 (0.15)	0.63 (0.15)	0.63 (0.16)	0.005
eGFR, mL min^{-1} per 1.73 m^2	75.6 (15.9)	75.4 (15.9)	76.3 (16.1)	<0.0001
Proteinuria, n (%)	5,777 (3.9)	4,169 (3.9)	1,608 (4.2)	0.006

Numbers in the table are means (standard deviation) for continuous variables except triglycerides (median and interquartile range) or numbers (percentages) for categorical variables.
LDL, low-density lipoprotein; HDL, high-density lipoprotein; eGFR, estimated glomerular filtration rate.

measure the height, weight, blood pressure, and waist circumference of each participant, after which serum and spot urine samples are collected. BMI is calculated by dividing body weight in kilograms by the square of height in meters. Blood samples are analyzed using an automated clinical chemical analyzer within 24 h of sampling. All blood analyses are conducted at a local, rather than a central, laboratory. Although the methods used for blood analyses are not calibrated between laboratories, analyses

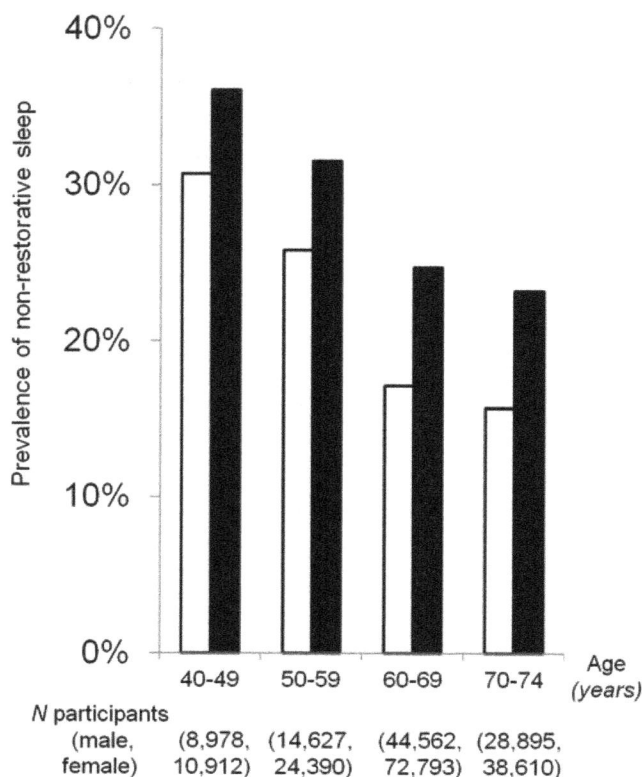

Figure 2. Prevalence of non-restorative sleep by sex and age. Trends were significant for both males (□; P<0.0001) and females (■; P<0.0001).

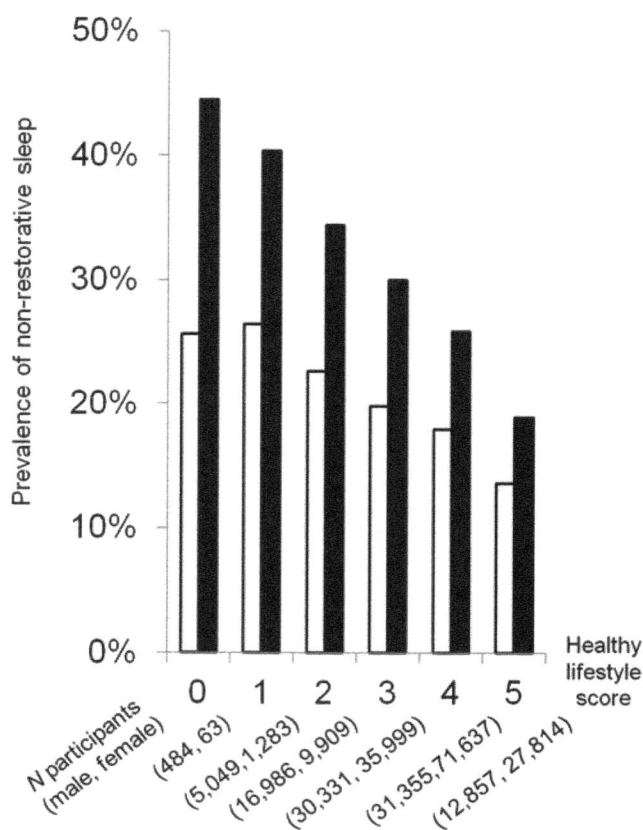

Figure 3. Prevalence of non-restorative sleep by healthy lifestyle score. Trends were significant for both males (□; P< 0.0001) and females (■; P<0.0001).

are performed according to the Japan Society of Clinical Chemistry-recommended methods for laboratory tests, which have been widely adopted by laboratories across Japan [29]. Participants diagnosed with metabolic syndrome are obligated to receive repeated lifestyle guidance over a six-month period after an annual health examination.

Participants from 40 to 74 years of age without missing information were included in this study. The complete selection process is presented in Figure 1.

Primary outcome

The primary outcome was NRS, which was assessed using this question from the self-administered questionnaire: 'Do you feel refreshed after a night's sleep?' Participants answered either yes or no. NRS was considered present when the answer was 'no'.

Lifestyle factors and covariates

For each lifestyle factor (smoking, BMI, alcohol intake, exercise habits, and eating patterns), we created a binary low-risk variable in which participants were given a score of 1 if they met the criteria for low risk or a score of 0 if otherwise, based on previous research [6]. The a priori definition of low risk was based on current literature, recommended guidelines, and realistically obtainable levels within the general population. We calculated a healthy lifestyle score by adding the total number of lifestyle factors for which each participant was at low risk. The score ranged from 0 (least healthy) to 5 (most healthy).

For smoking, we defined low risk as currently not smoking. Optimal body weight was defined as a BMI of <25 kg/m², the standard World Health Organization cutoff for healthy weight.

For alcohol, average daily consumption over 20 g was considered high risk. Alcohol consumption was assessed by the following questions: "How often do you drink alcohol (sake, shochu [distilled spirits], beer, liquor, etc.)?" to which participants responded by selecting (1) every day, (2) sometimes, or (3) rarely (can't drink); and "How much do you drink a day, in terms of glasses of refined sake? (A glass [180 mL] of refined sake is equivalent to a medium bottle [500 mL] of beer, 80 mL of shochu (alcohol content 35 percent), a glass [double, 60 mL] of whiskey, and 2 glasses [240 mL] of wine)," to which participants responded by selecting (1) <1 drink per day, (2) 1–2 drinks per day, (3) 2–3 drinks per day, or (4) ≥3 drinks per day'. The ethanol content per drink was calculated to be equivalent to 20 g. For exercise habits, two questions were asked: 'Are you in the habit of exercising to sweat lightly for over 30 minutes each time, two times weekly, for over a year?' and 'In your daily life, do you walk or do any equivalent amount of physical activity for more than one hour a day?' Low risk patients were defined as those who answered 'yes' to both questions on the basis of a current Japanese guideline [30]. For eating patterns, two questions were asked: 'Do you skip breakfast more than three times a week?' and 'Do you eat snacks after supper more than three times a week?' Low risk patients were defined as those who answered 'no' to both questions.

Hemoglobin A1c (HbA1c) was estimated as a National Glycohemoglobin Standardization Program equivalent value using the following equation [31]: HbA1c (%) = HbA1c (Japan Diabetes Society) (%)+0.4%. Diabetes was defined in accordance with American Diabetes Association guidelines [32] as a fasting plasma glucose concentration of 126 mg/dL or higher, HbA1c of

Table 3. Multivariate analysis of the relationship between categories from the healthy lifestyle score and prevalence of non-restorative sleep (N = 243,767).

Variable	Male (N= 97,062)		Female (N= 146,705)	
	Age-adjusted odds ratio (95%CI)	Multivariate odds ratio[a] (95%CI)	Age-adjusted odds ratio (95%CI)	Multivariate odds ratio[a] (95%CI)
Categories				
Current smoker				
No (ref)	1.00	1.00	1.00	1.00
Yes	0.90 (0.87–0.93)****	0.90 (0.87–0.93)****	1.09 (1.04–1.14)****	1.09 (1.04–1.14)****
Body mass index				
<25 m/kg^2 (ref)	1.00	1.00	1.00	1.00
≥25 m/kg^2	0.97 (0.93–1.00)	0.97 (0.94–1.01)	0.98 (0.95–1.00)	0.99 (0.96–1.02)
Alcohol consumption				
<20 g/day (ref)	1.00	1.00	1.00	1.00
≥20 g/day	0.83 (0.80–0.86)****	0.83 (0.80–0.86)****	1.03 (0.96–1.10)	1.03 (0.96–1.10)
Regular exercise				
Yes (ref)	1.00	1.00	1.00	1.00
No	1.57 (1.51–1.62)****	1.57 (1.51–1.63)****	1.52 (1.47–1.58)****	1.52 (1.48–1.56)****
Eating pattern				
Healthy (ref)	1.00	1.00	1.00	1.00
Less healthy	1.54 (1.48–1.60)****	1.54 (1.48–1.60)****	1.44 (1.40–1.48)****	1.44 (1.40–1.48)****
Age				
40–49 years	1.96 (1.85–2.08)****	1.95 (1.84–2.07)****	1.56 (1.48–1.63)****	1.50 (1.43–1.57)****
50–59 years	1.63 (1.55–1.71)****	1.62 (1.54–1.71)****	1.35 (1.30–1.40)****	1.32 (1.27–1.37)****
60–69 years	1.09 (1.04–1.13)****	1.09 (1.04–1.13)****	1.06 (1.03–1.09)****	1.05 (1.02–1.09)**
70–74 years (ref)	1.00	1.00	1.00	1.00
Hypertension		0.96 (0.93–1.00)*		0.94 (0.91–0.96)****
Diabetes mellitus		0.99 (0.95–1.04)		1.06 (1.02–1.11)**
Hypercholesterolemia		0.97 (0.93–1.00)		0.95 (0.92–0.97)****
Chronic kidney disease		1.04 (1.00–1.08)		1.04 (1.00–1.08)*

[a] Adjusted for age (years), sex, hypertension, diabetes, hypercholesterolemia, and chronic kidney disease.
Definitions of these factors are described in the text.
*P<0.05,
**P<0.01,
***P<0.001,
****P<0.0001.

6.5% or higher, or self-reported use of anti-hyperglycemic drugs. Hypertension was defined as using antihypertensive medications, a systolic blood pressure ≥140 mmHg, a diastolic blood pressure ≥ 90 mmHg, or both. Hypercholesterolemia was defined as using cholesterol-lowering medications, a low-density lipoprotein (LDL) cholesterol level ≥140 mg/dL, or both. Chronic kidney disease was defined as proteinuria in urinalysis, a glomerular filtration rate (GFR) less than 60 mL/min/1.73 m^2, or both [33]. Proteinuria was defined as a dipstick urinalysis score of 1+ or greater (equivalent to ≥30 mg/dL) because of poor discrimination between negative and trace positive dipstick readings [34]. Estimated GFR was calculated using the Japanese equation [35].

Statistical analysis

Data were analyzed separately by sex. First, we calculated the prevalence of NRS stratified by age categories. Age was categorized as 40–49, 50–59, 60–69, and 70–74 years. Second, we analyzed clinical and laboratory parameters stratified by the presence or absence of NRS. The chi-square test, Student's t-test, and Mann-Whitney U test were used to assess differences among participant characteristics in relation to NRS. Spearman and Pearson correlation coefficients were calculated to evaluate the relationship among each independent variable. To evaluate the association between prevalent NRS and each variable of the healthy lifestyle score, multivariable-adjusted odds ratios (ORs) and their corresponding 95% confidence intervals (CIs) were calculated using the category conventionally believed to be most healthy as the reference group. Data were initially adjusted for age. Next, we added age, hypertension, diabetes, hypercholesterolemia, and chronic kidney disease to multivariate models (Model 1). Finally, we added history of stroke, heart disease, and renal failure to Model 1 (Model 2).

To assess the robustness of the main results, we conducted several subsidiary analyses. First, subgroup analyses were stratified by age categories because age is associated with NRS. Healthy lifestyle scores from 0 (least healthy) to 1 (second-least healthy) were combined into one category because there were few cases. Age was also added as a continuous variable. Second, subgroup analyses were conducted among nonusers of medications to avoid variations in results due to medications. Nonusers of medications were defined as individuals who took no medications for diabetes, hypertension, and hypercholesterolemia. Finally, the analyses were repeated after excluding participants with obesity (BMI≥25 kg/m²) to enhance the association between healthy lifestyle and NRS, as obese participants could modify their lifestyle to lose weight. Because increased BMI may be a consequence rather than a component of an unhealthy lifestyle, another healthy lifestyle score was created to incorporate all variables except BMI. This score ranged from 0 to 4 points.

P<0.05 was considered statistically significant, and all tests were two-tailed. All analyses were performed with the SPSS for Windows statistical package (Version 18.0; SPSS, Chicago, IL, USA) and Stata/MP software (Version 12.1; Stata Corp, College Station, TX, USA).

Results

Participant flow

Of the 667,218 SHC participants screened in 2008, we excluded those who did not have serum creatinine levels measured ($n = 112,540$) because it is not mandatory for the SHC but is included independently in some areas. We also excluded anyone with missing information ($n = 310,911$), resulting in a final sample size of 243,767 (Figure 1). There were no substantial differences between included and excluded participants for characteristics such as prevalence of NRS, sex, age, and healthy lifestyle score (Table S1).

Demographic characteristics of participants

Among 97,062 men and 146,705 women, 18,678 (19.2%) and 38,539 (26.3%) were identified as having NRS, respectively. Tables 1 and 2 present the associations between various clinical characteristics and NRS. Both male and female participants with NRS were younger, had higher prevalence of current smokers, higher BMI, lower prevalence of exercise habits, and higher prevalence of less healthy eating patterns. They were also more likely to have a history of heart or renal disease and less likely to have hypertension, diabetes, and chronic kidney disease. Some differences were observed between sexes. Women with NRS were less likely to have an adequate intake of daily alcohol, while this

was more likely in men with NRS compared to those without NRS. In addition, the proportion of those with a history of stroke was significantly higher in women with NRS, but not in men with NRS.

Associations between the healthy lifestyle score and NRS

The prevalence of NRS decreased with increasing age for both men and women (P for trend <0.0001, Figure 2), and was lower among men than women for all age groups. An inverse, dose-response relationship was observed between healthy lifestyle scores and prevalence of NRS for both male and female participants (P for trend <0.0001, Figure 3).

When each variable of the healthy lifestyle score was considered individually, less healthy eating patterns and no regular exercise were associated with a higher prevalence of NRS (Table 3), but there were no apparent associations between BMI and the prevalence of NRS. Some differences were observed between men and women. Current smokers were associated with a higher prevalence of NRS in women and a lower prevalence in men. In addition, alcohol consumption was not associated with NRS in women but was associated with a lower prevalence in men.

Tables 4 and 5 show that participants with a score of 0 (least healthy) had an age-adjusted OR of 1.56 (95% CI, 1.26–1.93) for men and 2.76 (95% CI, 1.68–4.56) for women, compared to those with a score of 5 (most healthy). Additional adjustments for potential consequences of an unhealthy lifestyle (i.e., hypertension, diabetes mellitus, hypercholesterolemia, and chronic kidney disease) only partially changed risk (OR for men: 1.59, 95% CI, 1.29–1.97; OR for women: 2.88, 95% CI, 1.74–4.76). This association was not changed by additional adjustments for history of stroke, heart disease, and renal failure (Model 2).

When stratified by age categories, the association between a healthy lifestyle score and prevalence of NRS was similar when compared with the entire study population for both men and women (Figure 4). Among participants who currently took no medications for diabetes, hypertension, or hypercholesterolemia, a similar association was also observed for both sexes. Furthermore, the associations were consistent among obese and non-obese participants.

Discussion

Our findings support the hypothesis that a combination of unhealthy lifestyle factors is associated with inadequate sleep. A

Table 4. Odds ratios for the association between the healthy lifestyle score and prevalent non-restorative sleep in men ($N = 97,062$).

Healthy lifestyle score	Unadjusted	Age-adjusted	Model 1	Model 2
0	2.19 (1.77–2.70)****	1.56 (1.26–1.93)****	1.59 (1.29–1.97)****	1.60 (1.29–1.98)****
1	2.28 (2.10–2.47)****	1.73 (1.59–1.88)****	1.76 (1.62–1.91)****	1.77 (1.63–1.92)****
2	1.86 (1.75–1.98)****	1.54 (1.44–1.64)****	1.56 (1.46–1.66)****	1.56 (1.46–1.66)****
3	1.57 (1.48–1.66)****	1.40 (1.32–1.48)****	1.41 (1.33–1.49)****	1.41 (1.33–1.50)****
4	1.39 (1.31–1.47)****	1.31 (1.24–1.39)****	1.32 (1.24–1.40)****	1.32 (1.24–1.40)****
5 (ref)	1.00	1.00	1.00	1.00

Model 1: adjusted for age (years), hypertension, diabetes, hypercholesterolemia, and chronic kidney disease.
Model 2: adjusted Model 1 plus history of stroke, heart disease, and renal failure.
*$P<0.05$,
**$P<0.01$,
***$P<0.001$,
****$P<0.0001$.

Table 5. Odds ratios for the association between the healthy lifestyle score and prevalent non-restorative sleep in women ($N = 146,705$).

Healthy lifestyle score	Unadjusted	Age-adjusted	Model 1	Model 2
0	3.43 (2.09–5.65)****	2.76 (1.68–4.56)****	2.88 (1.74–4.76)****	2.88 (1.74–4.75)****
1	2.91 (2.59–2.26)****	2.43 (2.16–2.73)****	2.48 (2.21–2.79)****	2.47 (2.20–2.78)****
2	2.25 (2.14–2.37)****	2.00 (1.90–2.11)****	2.04 (1.94–2.15)****	2.03 (1.93–2.14)****
3	1.84 (1.77–1.91)****	1.71 (1.65–1.78)****	1.74 (1.67–1.81)****	1.73 (1.67–1.80)****
4	1.50 (1.45–1.55)****	1.44 (1.39–1.49)****	1.45 (1.40–1.50)****	1.44 (1.39–1.49)****
5 (ref)	1.00	1.00	1.00	1.00

Model 1: adjusted for age (years), hypertension, diabetes, hypercholesterolemia, and chronic kidney disease.
Model 2: adjusted Model 1 plus history of stroke, heart disease, and renal failure.
*$P<0.05$,
**$P<0.01$,
***$P<0.001$,
****$P<0.0001$.

combination of healthy lifestyle factors was associated with a decreased prevalence of NRS in both men and women of any age, even after adjusting for comorbidities such as hypertension, diabetes mellitus, hypercholesterolemia, chronic kidney disease, and history of stroke, heart disease, and renal failure. Although further study is needed to strengthen the association between the combined lifestyle factors and inadequate sleep, these findings raise the possibility that a healthy lifestyle could not only reduce the risk of developing several diseases but also improve sleep quality. If healthy lifestyle factors can provide restorative sleep, gaining satisfying rest would be a strong motivator for lifestyle modification.

Insomnia is an important public health issue [36] characterized by nighttime sleep problems. These may be manifest as difficulties in initiating or maintaining sleep, NRS, a combination of these complaints, or daytime symptoms [37]. Although there is a lack of consistency in the definition of NRS, and reports on NRS have been less extensive compared with other symptoms of primary insomnia (i.e., sleep latency and total sleep time), mounting evidence suggests that NRS is a frequent symptom observed in the general population. NRS prevalence was reported to be 10.8% in the non-institutionalized general population in seven European countries (France, the United Kingdom, Germany, Italy, Portugal, Spain, and Finland) [38], 35% in the participants in the Atherosclerosis Risk in Community Study in the United States [39], and 14.8% in the general South Korean population [40]. Although our methodology and questionnaire were not the same as those used in these studies, our findings were consistent in that NRS is frequently observed in the general Japanese population. The prevalence of NRS was higher in women than in men and decreased with age in our study. These results are in line with previous studies from Europe [38], the United States [36,39], South Korea [40], as well as an international survey conducted in Finland, Greece, Jordan and Lebanon, Morocco, Mexico, the Philippines, Portugal, Sweden, and Switzerland [41]. Although the prevalence of insomnia differs from one country to another [40], a decrease in NRS prevalence with age is commonly observed. This suggests that some common risk factors may be shared among young people with different racial, ethnic, cultural, and environmental background.

With regard to individual lifestyle factors, we found associations between NRS and physical inactivity or unhealthy eating patterns. Both physical activity and a healthy diet are known to be associated with sleep quality. A high level of exercise is related to better sleep patterns such as higher sleep quality, shortened sleep latency, and fewer awakenings during the night [42], while lack of habitual exercise is associated with more reported sleep complaints [43–44]. Meanwhile, skipping breakfast and a regular habit of snacking are more common in individuals with short sleep duration than in those with normal sleep duration [45]. A randomized crossover study showed that skipping breakfast in a nocturnal lifestyle, i.e., sleeping at 1:30 a.m. and waking at 8:30 a.m., was associated with decreased secretion of melatonin and leptin [46], suggesting that those lifestyle factors might be both a cause and a consequence of inadequate sleep. Although information is limited about NRS and physical inactivity or eating patterns, our findings are in line with these studies.

We found no association between NRS and BMI. Although obesity is associated with sleep apnea, little is known about its connection to NRS. Previous literature has shown that BMI is not associated with the prevalence of NRS, except in underweight individuals ($BMI<20 \text{ kg/m}^2$) who had a higher prevalence of NRS than those with normal BMI ($20–24 \text{ kg/m}^2$) [40]. A possible reason for this discrepancy is that use of a binary variable in our analysis did not detect an association between being underweight and having NRS that might only be observed when analyzed quantitatively.

Notably, sex differences were observed for smoking and alcohol consumption. Although smoking was associated with increases in NRS in women, the opposite relationship was observed in men, and adequate alcohol consumption was associated with increases in NRS among only male participants. It has generally been found that both alcohol consumption and smoking are associated with increases in sleep disorders [47–49], but associations between NRS and alcohol consumption or smoking are still controversial. Smoking has been associated with NRS in some studies [40,48] but not in another [39]. While alcohol consumption is not associated with NRS [39], some studies have found that alcohol abuse [50] and alcohol dependence [40] are connected to NRS. These inconsistencies may be primarily due to the different definitions of NRS, which only represents a single dimension or item of sleep symptoms [36]. It is also possible that using the binary variable in our study influenced results. Although associations between NRS and alcohol or smoking differed between men and women, the combined effect of healthy lifestyle factors on NRS were similar for both, suggesting that lifestyle factors cooperate with one another and are important for restorative sleep. Furthermore, a comprehensive analysis of

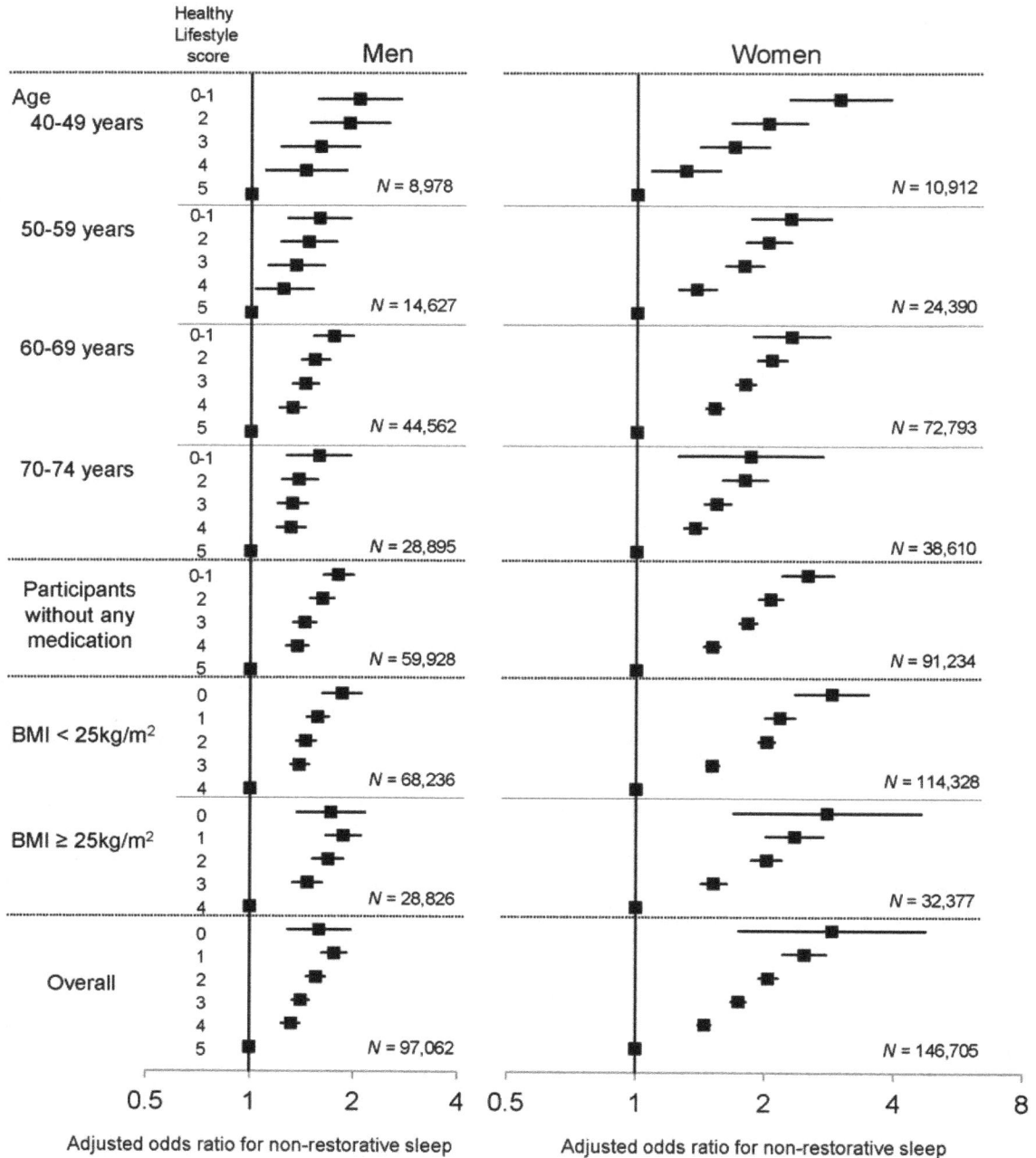

Figure 4. Subgroup analysis. Forest plot shows odds ratio with 95% confidence interval for the association between a healthy lifestyle score and prevalent non-restorative sleep in subgroups and in the entire study population. All analyses were adjusted for the following covariates: age (in years), hypertension, diabetes, hypercholesterolemia, and chronic kidney disease.

healthy lifestyle may capture influence of individual factors better than analyses based on a single factor, given the complexity and multiple dimensions of habitual health behaviors. Further investigation is needed to determine whether critical thresholds exist for each lifestyle factor and to establish combined effects and interaction effects as well as individual effects.

Patients with NRS were recently reported to have higher C-reactive protein (CRP) levels, a marker for systemic inflammation, than those without NRS [51]. Elevated CRP has also been associated with lifestyle risk factors such as obesity [52], physical inactivity [53], cigarette smoking [54], and alcohol consumption

[55,56]. These findings together suggest that participants with NRS have higher CRP levels due to unhealthy lifestyle behaviors, although no information about CRP was available in our study. It is possible that sleep deprivation [57,58] or stress [59] leads to increased CRP levels. Further investigation is warranted to clarify these aspects of the relationship between NRS and lifestyle factors.

Our study has several limitations. First, a selection bias of subjects might exist. Because participants in this cohort received annual physical checkups, they might be more health-conscious than the average Japanese population. Second, NRS was determined solely based on self-reported information and may not be accurate. A single retrospective item has limitations that need to be addressed, such as recall bias and demand characteristics. In addition, frequency (i.e., more than three times per week) and sleep duration were not included in the questionnaire used to assess NRS. However, there is no reliable and well-validated patient-reported outcome instrument currently available for evaluating NRS [27]. Third, we cannot exclude the possibility that residual confounding factors exist, which were not measured in the present study, such as marital status [38], educational level [36,50], employment status [38], work schedule [50], level of stress [50], psychiatric disorders [38], and use of sleep medications. Whether these factors affect the relationship between lifestyle factors and NRS should be assessed in the future. Fourth, we gave equal weight to each lifestyle factor to achieve the main purpose of the study. That may have resulted in conservative estimates for multiple lifestyle factors. Fifth, the nutritive content in diet could not be evaluated due to lack of information. Evidence regarding the associations between diet and NRS is scarce, although a cross-sectional study using data from the National Health and Nutrition Examination Survey (NHANES) from the United States has shown that NRS is positively associated with butanoic acid, moisture, cholesterol, and negatively associated with calcium, vitamin C, and water [60]. Sixth, odds ratios do not approximate well to the relative risk when the effect sizes are large and the prevalence of the outcome of interest is high [61]. In our study, the prevalence of NRS was relatively high, whereas the effect sizes were not large. In addition, qualitative judgments based on interpreting odds ratios as though they were relative risks are unlikely to be seriously in error [61]. Therefore, we consider that our results demonstrate important effects. Finally, the cross-sectional study design limited our ability to determine the direction of the association or causality. NRS might be the cause, rather than the consequence, of one or more unhealthy lifestyle factors.

Our study also has several strengths. First, it was a large-scale cross-sectional study with participants from all over Japan. Second, this is the first report, to the best of our knowledge, to demonstrate the prevalence of NRS in the general Japanese population and assess the association between combined lifestyle factors and NRS.

In conclusion, a combination of healthy lifestyle factors was associated with an increase in restorative sleep independently of age, sex, and comorbidities in the general Japanese population. Further studies are needed to establish whether general lifestyle modification improves restorative sleep.

Supporting Information

Table S1 Clinical characteristics of participants included and excluded in the analysis. Numbers in the table are means (standard deviation) for continuous variables except triglycerides (median and interquartile range) or numbers (percentages) for categorical variables. Note that the percentages are computed based only on the total number of non-missing cases. LDL, low-density lipoprotein; HDL, high-density lipoprotein; eGFR, estimated glomerular filtration rate.

Author Contributions

Conceived and designed the experiments: MW IN. Performed the experiments: MW JJK IN. Analyzed the data: MW. Wrote the first draft of the manuscript: MW. Contributed to drafting the manuscript: MW JJK IN. ICMJE criteria for authorship read and met: MW JJK IN KI TM KY SF KT KA TK KK MK IK YO TW. Agree with manuscript results and conclusions: MW JJK IN KI TM KY SF KT KA TK KK MK IK YO TW.

References

1. Stampfer MJ, Hu FB, Manson JE, Rimm EB, Willett WC (2000) Primary prevention of coronary heart disease in women through diet and lifestyle. N Engl J Med 343: 16–22.
2. Chiuve SE, McCullough ML, Sacks FM, Rimm EB (2006) Healthy lifestyle factors in the primary prevention of coronary heart disease among men: benefits among users and nonusers of lipid-lowering and antihypertensive medications. Circulation 114: 160–167.
3. Hu FB, Manson JE, Stampfer MJ, Colditz G, Liu S, et al. (2001) Diet, lifestyle, and the risk of type 2 diabetes mellitus in women. N Engl J Med 345: 790–797.
4. Kurth T, Moore SC, Gaziano JM, Kase CS, Stampfer MJ, et al. (2006) Healthy lifestyle and the risk of stroke in women. Arch Intern Med 166: 1403–1409.
5. Chiuve SE, Fung TT, Rexrode KM, Spiegelman D, Manson JE, et al. (2011) Adherence to a low-risk, healthy lifestyle and risk of sudden cardiac death among women. JAMA 306: 62–69.
6. Wakasugi M, Kazama JJ, Yamamoto S, Kawamura K, Narita I (2013) A combination of healthy lifestyle factors is associated with a decreased incidence of chronic kidney disease: a population-based cohort study. Hypertens Res 36: 328–333.
7. Platz EA, Willett WC, Colditz GA, Rimm EB, Spiegelman D, et al. (2000) Proportion of colon cancer risk that might be preventable in a cohort of middle-aged US men. Cancer Causes Control 11: 579–588.
8. Jiao L, Mitrou PN, Reedy J, Graubard BI, Hollenbeck AR, et al. (2009) A combined healthy lifestyle score and risk of pancreatic cancer in a large cohort study. Arch Intern Med 169: 764–770.
9. Sasazuki S, Inoue M, Iwasaki M, Sawada N, Shimazu T, et al. (2012) Combined impact of five lifestyle factors and subsequent risk of cancer: the Japan Public Health Center Study. Prev Med 54: 112–116.
10. van Dam RM, Li T, Spiegelman D, Franco OH, Hu FB (2008) Combined impact of lifestyle factors on mortality: prospective cohort study in US women. BMJ 337: a1440.
11. Liu K, Daviglus ML, Loria CM, Colangelo LA, Spring B, et al. (2012) Healthy lifestyle through young adulthood and the presence of low cardiovascular disease risk profile in middle age: the Coronary Artery Risk Development in (Young) Adults (CARDIA) study. Circulation 125: 996–1004.
12. Shochat T (2012) Impact of lifestyle and technology developments on sleep. Nature Science Sleep 4: 19–31.
13. Peuhkuri K, Sihvola N, Korpela R (2012) Diet promotes sleep duration and quality. Nutrition Research 32: 309–319.
14. Hasler G, Buysse DJ, Klaghofer R, Gamma A, Ajdacic V, et al. (2004) The association between short sleep duration and obesity in young adults: a 13-year prospective study. Sleep 27: 661–666.
15. Gangwisch JE, Malaspina D, Boden-Albala B, Heymsfield SB (2005) Inadequate sleep as a risk factor for obesity: analyses of the NHANES I. Sleep 28: 1289–1296.
16. Patel SR, Malhotra A, White DP, Gottlieb DJ, Hu FB (2006) Association between reduced sleep and weight gain in women. Am J Epidemiol 164: 947–954.
17. Chaput JP, Després JP, Bouchard C, Tremblay A (2008) The association between sleep duration and weight gain in adults: a 6-year prospective study from the Quebec Family Study. Sleep 31: 517–523.
18. Ayas NT, White DP, Al-Delaimy WK, Manson JE, Stampfer MJ, et al. (2003) A prospective study of self-reported sleep duration and incident diabetes in women. Diabetes Care 26: 380–384.
19. Gangwisch JE, Heymsfield SB, Boden-Albala B, Buijs RM, Kreier F, et al. (2007) Sleep duration as a risk factor for diabetes incidence in a large U.S. sample. Sleep 30: 1667–1673.
20. Gangwisch JE, Heymsfield SB, Boden-Albala B, Buijs RM, Kreier F, et al. (2006) Short sleep duration as a risk factor for hypertension: analyses of the first National Health and Nutrition Examination Survey. Hypertension 47: 833–839.
21. Kaneita Y, Uchiyama M, Yoshiike N, Ohida T (2008) Associations of usual sleep duration with serum lipid and lipoprotein levels. Sleep 31: 645–652.
22. Ayas NT, White DP, Manson JE, Stampfer MJ, Speizer FE, et al. (2003) A prospective study of sleep duration and coronary heart disease in women. Arch Intern Med 163: 205–209.
23. Yamamoto R, Nagasawa Y, Iwatani H, Shinzawa M, Obi Y, et al. (2012) Self-reported sleep duration and prediction of proteinuria: a retrospective cohort study. Am J Kidney Dis 59: 343–355.
24. Chang ET (2009) The impact of daytime naps on the relation between sleep duration and cardiovascular events. Arch Intern Med 169: 717. doi:10.1001/archinternmed.2009.29.
25. Chandola T, Ferrie JE, Perski A, Akbaraly T, Marmot MG (2010) The effect of short sleep duration on coronary heart disease risk is greatest among those with

sleep disturbance: a prospective study from the Whitehall II cohort. Sleep 33: 739–744.

26. Hoevenaar-Blom MP, Spijkerman AM, Kromhout D, van den Berg JF, Verschuren WM (2011) Sleep duration and sleep quality in relation to 12-year cardiovascular disease incidence: the MORGEN study. Sleep 34: 1487–1492.

27. Vernon MK, Dugar A, Revicki D, Treglia M, Buysse D (2010) Measurement of non-restorative sleep in insomnia: A review of the literature. Sleep Med Rev 14: 205–212.

28. Kohro T, Furui Y, Mitsutake N, Fujii R, Morita H, et al. (2008) The Japanese national health screening and intervention program aimed at preventing worsening of the metabolic syndrome. Int Heart J 49: 193–203.

29. Tsuruya K, Yoshida H, Nagata M, Kitazono T, Hirakata H, et al. (2014) Association of the triglycerides to high-density lipoprotein cholesterol ratio with the risk of chronic kidney disease: analysis in a large Japanese population. Atherosclerosis. 233: 260–267.

30. The Office for Lifestyle-Related Diseases Control, General Affairs Division, Health Service Bureau, Ministry of Health, Labour and Welfare of Japan (2006) Exercise and Physical Activity Guide for Health Promotion 2006 - To Prevent Lifestyle-related Diseases - <Exercise Guide 2006>Prepared in August, 2006. Available: http://www.nih.go.jp/eiken/programs/pdf/exercise_guide.pdf. Accessed 13 September 2011.

31. The Committee of Japan Diabetes Society on the diagnostic criteria of diabetes mellitus (2010) Report of the Committee on the classification and diagnostic criteria of diabetes mellitus. J Jpn Diabetes Soc 53: 450–467.

32. American Diabetes Association (2011) Diagnosis and classification of diabetes mellitus. Diabetes Care (Suppl 1): S62–S69.

33. National Kidney Foundation (2002) K/DOQI clinical practice guidelines for chronic kidney disease: evaluation, classification, and stratification. Am J Kidney Dis 39 (Suppl 1): S1–S266.

34. Harrison NA, Rainford DJ, White GA, Cullen SA, Strike PW (1989) Proteinuria: What value is the dipstick? Br J Urol 63: 202–208.

35. Matsuo S, Imai E, Horio M, Yasuda Y, Tomita K, et al. (2009) Revised equations for estimated GFR from serum creatinine in Japan. Am J Kidney Dis 53: 982–992.

36. Grandner MA, Petrov ME, Rattanaumpawan P, Jackson N, Platt A, et al. (2013) Sleep symptoms, race/ethnicity, and socioeconomic position. J Clin Sleep Med. 9: 897–905; 905A–905D.

37. Roth T, Zammit G, Lankford A, Mayleben D, Stern T, et al. (2010) Nonrestorative sleep as a distinct component of insomnia. Sleep 33: 449–458.

38. Ohayon MM (2005) Prevalence and correlates of nonrestorative sleep complaints. Arch Intern Med 165: 35–41.

39. Phillips B, Mannino D (2005) Correlates of sleep complaints in adults: the ARIC study. J Clin Sleep Med 1: 277–283.

40. Kim BS, Jeon HJ, Hong JP, Bae JN, Lee JY, et al. (2012) DSM-IV psychiatric comorbidity according to symptoms of insomnia: a nationwide sample of Korean adults. Soc Psychiatry Psychiatr Epidemiol 47: 2019–2033.

41. Léger D, Partinen M, Hirshkowitz M, Chokroverty S, EQUINOX (Evaluation of daytime QUality Impairment by Nocturnal awakenings in Outpatient's eXperience) Survey Investigators, et al. (2010) Characteristics of insomnia in a primary care setting: EQUINOX survey of 5293 insomniacs from 10 countries. Sleep Med. 11: 987–998.

42. Brand S, Gerber M, Beck J, Hatzinger M, Pühse U, et al. (2010) High exercise levels are related to favorable sleep patterns and psychological functioning in adolescents: a comparison of athletes and controls. J Adolesc Health 46: 133–141.

43. Kim K, Uchiyama M, Okawa M, Liu X, Ogihara R (2000) An epidemiological study of insomnia among the Japanese general population. Sleep 23: 41–47.

44. Morgan K (2003) Daytime activity and risk factors for late-life insomnia. J Sleep Res 12: 231–238.

45. Kim S, DeRoo LA, Sandler DP (2011) Eating patterns and nutritional characteristics associated with sleep duration. Public Health Nutr 14: 889–895.

46. Qin LQ, Li J, Wang Y, Wang J, Xu JY, et al. (2003) The effects of nocturnal life on endocrine circadian patterns in healthy adults. Life Sci 73: 2467–2475.

47. Phillips BA, Danner FJ (1995) Cigarette smoking and sleep disturbance. Arch Intern Med 155: 734–737.

48. Wetter DW, Young TB (1994) The relation between cigarette smoking and sleep disturbance. Prev Med 23: 328–334.

49. Brower KJ (2003) Insomnia, alcoholism and relapse. Sleep Med Rev 7: 523–539.

50. Ohayon MM, Hong SC (2002) Prevalence of insomnia and associated factors in South Korea. J Psychosom Res 53: 593–600.

51. Zhang J, Lamers F, Hickie IB, He JP, Feig E, et al. (2013) Differentiating nonrestorative sleep from nocturnal insomnia symptoms: demographic, clinical, inflammatory, and functional correlates. Sleep 36: 671–679.

52. Choi J, Joseph L, Pilote L (2013) Obesity and C-reactive protein in various populations: a systematic review and meta-analysis. Obes Rev 14: 232–244.

53. Kasapis C, Thompson PD (2005) The effects of physical activity on serum C-reactive protein and inflammatory markers: A systematic review. J Am Coll Cardiol 45: 1563–1569.

54. Bazzano LA, He J, Muntner P, Vupputuri S, Whelton PK (2003) Relationship between cigarette smoking and novel risk factors for cardiovascular disease in the United States. Ann Intern Med 138: 891–897.

55. Albert MA, Glynn RJ, Ridker PM (2003) Alcohol consumption and plasma concentration of C-reactive protein. Circulation 107: 443e7.

56. Averina M, Nilssen O, Arkhipovsky VL, Kalinin AG, Brox J (2006) C-reactive protein and alcohol consumption: Is there a U-shaped association? Results from a population-based study in Russia. The Arkhangelsk study. Atherosclerosis 188: 309–315.

57. van Leeuwen WM, Lehto M, Karisola P, Lindholm H, Luukkonen R, et al. (2009) Sleep restriction increases the risk of developing cardiovascular diseases by augmenting proinflammatory responses through IL-17 and CRP. PLoS One. 4: e4589.

58. Meier-Ewert HK, Ridker PM, Rifai N, Regan MM, Price NJ, et al. (2004) Effect of sleep loss on C-reactive protein, an inflammatory marker of cardiovascular risk. J Am Coll Cardiol. 43: 678–683.

59. Johnson TV, Abbasi A, Master VA (2013) Systematic review of the evidence of a relationship between chronic psychosocial stress and C-reactive protein. Mol Diagn Ther. 17: 147–164.

60. Grandner MA, Jackson N, Gerstner JR, Knutson KL (2014) Sleep symptoms associated with intake of specific dietary nutrients. J Sleep Res. 23: 22–34.

61. Davies HT, Crombie IK, Tavakoli M (1998) When can odds ratios mislead? BMJ. 316: 989–991.

14

Establishment of a Model of Renal Impairment with Mild Renal Insufficiency Associated with Atrial Fibrillation in Canines

Zhuo Liang[1]◐, Li-feng Liu[2]◐, Xin-pei Chen[2]◐, Xiang-min Shi[2], Hong-yang Guo[2], Kun Lin[2], Jian-ping Guo[2], Zhao-liang Shan[2]*, Yu-tang Wang[1]*

1 Department of Geriatric Cardiology, Chinese PLA General Hospital, Beijing, China, **2** Department of Cardiology, Chinese PLA General Hospital, Beijing, China

Abstract

Background: Chronic kidney disease and occurrence of atrial fibrillation (AF) are closely related. No studies have examined whether renal impairment (RI) without severe renal dysfunction is associated with the occurrence of AF.

Methods: Unilateral RI with mild renal insufficiency was induced in beagles by embolization of small branches of the renal artery in the left kidney for 2 weeks using gelatin sponge granules in the model group (n = 5). The sham group (n = 5) underwent the same procedure, except for embolization. Parameters associated with RI and renal function were tested, cardiac electrophysiological parameters, blood pressure, left ventricular pressure, and AF vulnerability were investigated. The activity of the sympathetic nervous system, renin-angiotensin-aldosterone system, inflammation, and oxidative stress were measured. Histological studies associated with atrial interstitial fibrosis were performed.

Results: Embolization of small branches of the renal artery in the left kidney led to ischemic RI with mild renal insufficiency. The following changes occurred after embolization. Heart rate and P wave duration were increased. Blood pressure and left ventricular systolic pressure were elevated. The atrial effective refractory period and antegrade Wenckebach point were shortened. Episodes and duration of AF, as well as atrial and ventricular rate during AF were increased in the model group. Plasma levels of norepinephrine, renin, and aldosterone were increased, angiotensin II and aldosterone levels in atrial tissue were elevated, and atrial interstitial fibrosis was enhanced after 2 weeks of embolization in the model group.

Conclusions: We successfully established a model of RI with mild renal insufficiency in a large animal. We found that RI with mild renal insufficiency was associated with AF in this model.

Editor: Nick Ashton, The University of Manchester, United Kingdom

Funding: This work was supported by the National Natural Science Foundation of China (30570737; 81270308). The funders had no role in study design, data collection and analysis, decision to publish, or preparation of the manuscript.

Competing Interests: The authors have declared that no competing interests exist.

* Email: shanzl301@sina.com (ZLS); wyt301@sina.com (YTW)

◐ These authors contributed equally to this work.

Introduction

The prevalence of atrial fibrillation (AF) in the general population is 1% [1] A recent meta-analysis showed that the prevalence of AF in end-stage renal disease patients was 11.6% [2]. The Chronic Renal Insufficiency Cohort study suggested that the prevalence of AF is 2–3-fold higher in patients with mild-to-moderate chronic kidney disease (CKD) than in the general population [3]. Concomitant CKD increases the recurrence of AF after catheter ablation of AF [4]. Renal dysfunction is also associated with an increased risk of stroke and mortality in patients with AF [5]. Therefore, exploring the inherent pathogenic mechanisms responsible for the development of AF among CKD patients and identifying effective therapeutic targets are urgent. However, few studies on animals have investigated these pathogenic mechanisms because of a lack of an appropriate animal model.

The remnant kidney model has been the most well studied model of CKD [6]. Studies have used a range of remnant kidney models, from 1/2 to 15/16 nephrectomy. Removal of tissue is generally accomplished by surgery or infarction accomplished by ligation of renal arteries. The remnant kidney model is more focused on reduced renal function, irrespective of the primary renal impairment in CKD. Most nephrons are directly removed by surgery, not injured and retained in the body. Additionally, only the remnant nephrons become impaired in the long-term, which takes several months to years, resulting from glomerular hyperperfusion, hyperfiltration, hypertension, and other factors induced by renal dysfunction. The more remnant nephrons remain, the longer it takes for impairment of remnant nephrons.

Ligation of renal arteries can lead to complete infarction, with damage to afferent and efferent nerves in the adventitia of the renal artery and area of the renal hilus. The process involved in creating the remnant kidney model causes severe trauma, which leads to a high mortality of animals, and is also complicated and time-consuming. CKD is accompanied by ischemic renal impairment (RI) and renal dysfunction. Multiple acquired factors induced by severe renal dysfunction in the remnant kidney model could account for the high prevalence of AF (e.g., hypervolemia, acidosis, hypertension, and electrolyte disturbance) [7]. The above-mentioned factors may affect the reliability of research when examining the inherent pathogenic mechanisms responsible for the development of AF among CKD patients. There is no appropriate animal model for ischemic RI and without severe renal dysfunction for examining the relationship between CKD and AF.

Therefore, in this study, we established a model of unilateral RI with mild renal insufficiency in canines. We examined whether renal impairment without severe renal dysfunction was associated with the occurrence of AF.

Materials and Methods

Ethics Statement

This study was carried out in strict accordance with the recommendations in the Guide for the Care and Use of Laboratory Animals of the National Institutes of Health (Publication No. 85-23, revised 1996). The protocol was approved by the Institutional Animal Care and Use Committee of the Chinese PLA General Hospital.

Experimental Model for RI

The experimental animals included 10 healthy, 4–5-year-old beagles weighing 10–12 kg. All dogs were anesthetized with intravenous sodium pentobarbital (20 mg/kg) and were intubated using an endotracheal tube and mechanical ventilation. Heart rate and rhythm were monitored by a continuous 3-lead electrocardiogram. A 6F sheath was placed in the right femoral artery. Systolic blood pressure (SBP) and diastolic blood pressure (DBP) were monitored via the sheath using an invasive blood pressure (BP) monitor. A bolus of heparin (4000 IU) was administered through the sheath to prevent thromboembolism. A pigtail catheter was introduced into the left ventricle (LV) through the arterial sheath to detect LV systolic pressure (LVSP) and LV end-diastolic pressure (LVEDP). A 5F multifunction catheter was introduced through the arterial sheath and renal artery angiography was performed under fluoroscopy. Following renal artery angiography, RI was induced in five dogs by transcatheter embolization of small branches of the left renal artery using gelatin sponge granules (diameter ~50 μm), whereas the main renal artery or sub-segment renal artery was kept fluent.

Electrophysiological Examinations

The right femoral vein was cannulated for catheter insertion. The tip of a multielectrode catheter was placed on the lateral right atrium to record right atrial potentials and to induce rapid atrial pacing. A train of eight basic stimuli (S1, pulse duration 1 ms) at twice the diastolic pacing threshold was followed by an extra stimulus (S2). The atrial effective refractory period (AERP) was defined as the longest S1S2 interval that failed to elicit a propagated atrial response. The AERP was measured at basic pacing cycle lengths of 300 ms and 240 ms, and the S1–S2 intervals were decreased from 200 ms to refractoriness by decrements of 5 ms (LEAD-7000, multi-channel physiology recorder; Sichuan Jinjiang Electronic Science and Technology Co., Ltd, Sichuan, China). The longest cycle length of atrial pacing causing second-degree atrioventricular nodal block (antegrade Wenckebach point) was determined. After the AERP and antegrade Wenckebach point were determined, rapid atrial pacing (basic cycle length, 60 ms) for 30 minutes was delivered (DF-5A, heart stimulator; Suzhou Dongfang Electronic Instruments Plant, Jiangsu, China) and then AERP was determined again. After the above examinations, 10 times of rapid atrial pacing were performed (60 ms of basic cycle length, 10 s in duration, four-fold threshold current) to induce AF. AF was defined as irregular atrial rates (cycle length, <200 ms; duration, >5 seconds) with irregular atrioventricular conduction. AF inductibility was defined as (the relative ratio of successful induction frequency to total frequency of pacing in each group) ×100%. All AA- and RR-intervals during AF were calculated to determine the mean atrial and ventricular rates during AF.

Plasma Measurements and Urinalysis

Blood samples were collected from the femoral vein into tubes containing EDTA, and immediately centrifuged at 2310×g for 10 minutes at 4°C, and then finally stored at −80°C until further assay. Levels of norepinephrine, renin, aldosterone, high-sensitivity C-reactive protein (hs-CRP), malondialdehyde, creatinine, urea nitrogen, lactic dehydrogenase, and lactic acid in plasma and creatinine in urine were examined by ELISA (Wuhan Beinglay Biotech Co., Ltd., Hubei, China). Sodium and potassium concentrations in plasma were examined by an Electrolyte Analyzer (HC-9883, Shenzheng Histrong Medical Equipment Co., Ltd., Shenzheng, China).

Histologic Studies

Left atria were carefully removed. Part of atrial tissue was fixed in 10% phosphate-buffered formalin, and embedded in paraffin. Deparaffined sections (5 μm thickness) were stained with Masson trichrome. Connective tissue was differentiated on the basis of its color and expressed as a percentage of the reference tissue area using Image-Pro Plus 4.5. In each atrium, 3 images with a magnification of ×400 were analyzed and averaged. Part of atrial tissue was stored at −80°C until further assay. Levels of angiotensin II and aldosterone in atrial tissue were examined by ELISA (Wuhan Beinglay Biotech Co., Ltd., Hubei, China).

Experimental Design

Dogs were divided into two groups: the model group (n = 5) and the sham group (n = 5). At baseline, an electrocardiogram, BP, and LV function were monitored. Electrophysiological examinations were performed. Plasma parameters associated with RI, renal function, the activity of the sympathetic nervous system (SNS), renin-angiotensin-aldosterone system (RAAS), inflammation, and oxidative stress were measured. After these measurements, RI was induced in the model group. In the sham group, normal saline was injected into the renal artery through a multifunction catheter after renal artery angiography as a sham procedure. After 2 weeks of feeding, the same parameters measured at baseline were measured again. Creatinine clearance (CCr) was determined by 30-min endogenous creatinine clearance method [8]. Dogs were then sacrificed humanely by an intravenous overdose of thiopental (2 g). Kidneys were removed for hematoxylin and eosin (HE) staining and morphological analysis. Hearts were removed for histologic studies.

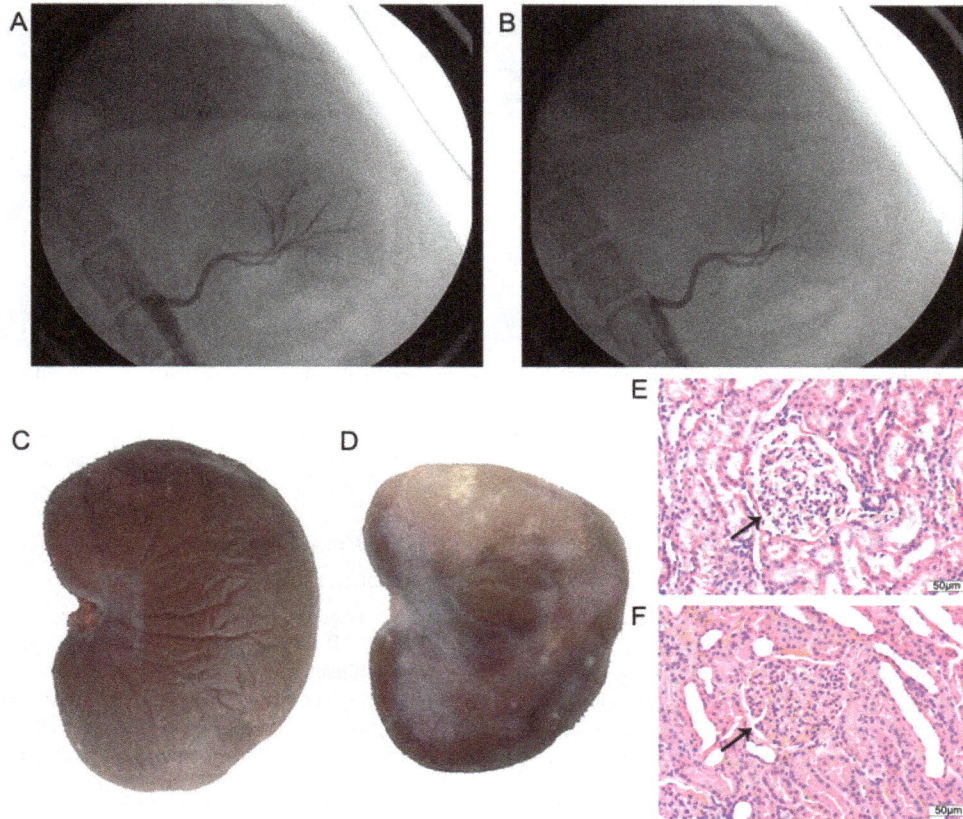

Figure 1. Images and morphological analysis of the left kidney. Images of left renal artery angiography before transcatheter embolization (A) and after transcatheter embolization (B) in the model group. Small renal artery branches were occluded, whereas the main renal artery or sub-segment renal artery remained fluent in the model group. Gross appearance of the left kidney after 2 weeks of interventional operation in the sham group (C) and the model group (D). The left kidney in the model group became pale and had atrophy and infarction. Images of HE staining of the left kidney after 2 weeks of interventional operation in the sham (E) and model (F) groups. Glomeruli were severely damaged in the model group. Arrows show a glomerulus in the sham and model groups.

Statistical Analysis

Values are shown as mean ± SD. For repeated-measures comparisons with the same baseline, repeated-measures 2-way ANOVA was used followed by the Dunnet test to compare individual mean difference if ANOVA was significant. Unpaired t tests were used to compare differences of angiotensin II, aldosterone and interstitial fibrosis in atrial tissue and CCr between sham and model groups. The chi-square test was used to compare the AF induction rate. $P \leq 0.05$ was considered statistically significant.

Table 1. Parameters associated with renal impairment and renal function.

	Sham group		Model group	
	Baseline	2 weeks	Baseline	2 weeks
Lactic dehydrogenase (U/L)	15.0±9.4	14.6±8.3	18.7±12.7	45.0±16.1[a b]
Lactic acid (mmol/L)	1.4±0.7	1.1±0.4	1.9±0.9	1.2±0.4
Creatinine (umol/L)	32.8±8.5	37.9±6.2	36.2±3.9	45.8±1.8[a b]
Creatinine clearance (ml/min/kg)		4.0±0.3		2.9±0.4[c]
Urea nitrogen (mmol/L)	2.2±0.4	2.8±0.7	3.1±1.0	4.2±1.0[a b]
Sodion (mmol/L)	148.7±2.6	151.6±1.1	148.4±3.1	149.0±3.2
Potassium (mmol/L)	5.1±0.4	4.7±0.1	4.5±0.5	4.6±0.3

[a]p<0.05 vs. baseline of model group;
[b]p<0.05 vs. 2 weeks of sham group;
[c]P<0.05 vs. 2 weeks of sham group. (mean ± standard deviation, n = 5).

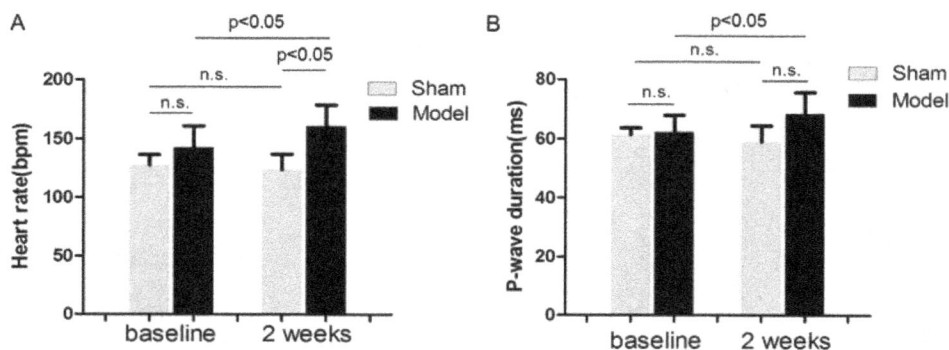

Figure 2. ECG analysis (n = 5). Effects of embolization versus sham operation on heart rate (A) and P-wave duration (B).

Results

Model of RI with Mild Renal Insufficiency

Figure 1A shows representative images of left renal artery angiography before transcatheter embolization in the model group. Small renal artery branches were occluded after transcatheter embolization, whereas the main renal artery or sub-segment renal artery remained fluent (Figure 1B). Figure 1C shows a representative gross appearance of the left kidney in the sham group. After 2 weeks of embolization in the model group, the left kidney became pale due to ischemic impairment, and had atrophy and infarction (Figure 1D). Figure 1E shows representative images of HE staining of the left kidney in the sham group. Glomeruli were severely damaged in the model group (Figure 1F), indicating that the vast majority of nephrons had lost their function. Table 1 shows some of the parameters associated with renal impairment and renal function. Lactic dehydrogenase levels were increased by 1.4-fold after 2 weeks of RI ($P<0.05$). Creatinine and urea nitrogen levels were slightly increased by 26.5% ($P<0.05$) and 26.7% ($P<0.05$) respectively after 2 weeks of RI. After 2 weeks of operation, CCr in the model group was slightly decreased by 27.5% ($P<0.05$) compared with the sham group. Lactic acid, sodium, and potassium concentrations were not changed by RI. Renal function was still in the compensatory period. These results indicate successful establishment of an animal model of RI with mild renal insufficiency.

Effects of RI with Mild Renal Insufficiency on Heart Rate and P Wave Duration

Figure 2 shows some ECG parameters in sham and model dogs during sinus rhythm. RI with mild renal insufficiency after 2 weeks of embolization resulted in a significant increase in heart rate (Figure 2A) by 12% ($P<0.05$), and prolonged the P wave duration (Figure 2B) by 12% ($P<0.05$) compared with baseline conditions in the model group. No changes were found in the sham group.

Effects of RI with Mild Renal Insufficiency on BP and LV Pressure

Figure 3 shows BP and LV pressure in sham and model dogs during sinus rhythm. After 2 weeks of embolization, SBP (Figure 3A) was increased by 17% ($P = 0.0032$), DBP (Figure 3B) was increased by 16% ($P<0.05$), and LVSP (Figure 3C) was increased by 14% ($P<0.05$) compared with baseline values in the model group. However, LVEDP (figure 3D) was unchanged in the model group. No changes in these parameters were found in the sham group. Figure 3E shows a representative pressure wave of

dogs at baseline and with RI after 2 weeks of embolization in the model group.

Effects of RI with Mild Renal Insufficiency on Atrial Refractoriness

Effects of the sham procedure, embolization and rapid pacing on the AERP are shown in Table 2. In the model group, RI with mild renal insufficiency after 2 weeks of embolization resulted in a significant decrease in AERP by 10% (basic cycle length: 300 ms, $P<0.05$) and by 8% (basic cycle length: 240 ms, $P<0.05$) at two different stimulation frequencies compared with baseline values. The AERP after 2 weeks of sham operation was unchanged in the sham group. 30 minutes of rapid pacing resulted in a decrease of AERP ($P<0.05$) at baseline and after 2 weeks of intervention in both sham and model groups. There was no difference in the decrease of AERP after 30 minutes of rapid pacing between baseline and 2 weeks in sham and model group.

Effects of RI with Mild Renal Insufficiency on Inducibility and Duration of AF

RI with mild renal insufficiency after 2 weeks of embolization resulted in a significant increase in AF inducibility (Figure 4A) by 3.2-fold ($P<0.05$) and prolonged the duration of AF (Figure 4B) by 3.8-fold ($P<0.05$) compared with baseline values in the model group. The inducibility and duration of AF were unchanged in the sham group. Figure 4C shows representative right atrial potentials and ECG recordings after 10 seconds of rapid atrial pacing at baseline and with RI after 2 weeks of embolization in the model group.

Effects of RI with Mild Renal Insufficiency on Antegrade Wenckbach Point, Atrial and Ventricular Rates during AF

RI with mild renal insufficiency after 2 weeks of embolization resulted in a significant decrease in the antegrade Wenckebach point by 10% ($P<0.05$) (Figure 5A), an increase in ventricular rate during AF (Figure 5B) by 12% ($P<0.05$) and an increase in atrial rate during AF (Figure 5C) by 13% ($P<0.05$) compared with baseline values in the model group. Antegrade Wenckebach point, ventricular and atrial rates during AF were unchanged in the sham group. Figure 5D shows representative right atrial potentials and ECG recordings after 10 seconds of rapid atrial pacing at baseline and with RI after 2 weeks of embolization in the model group.

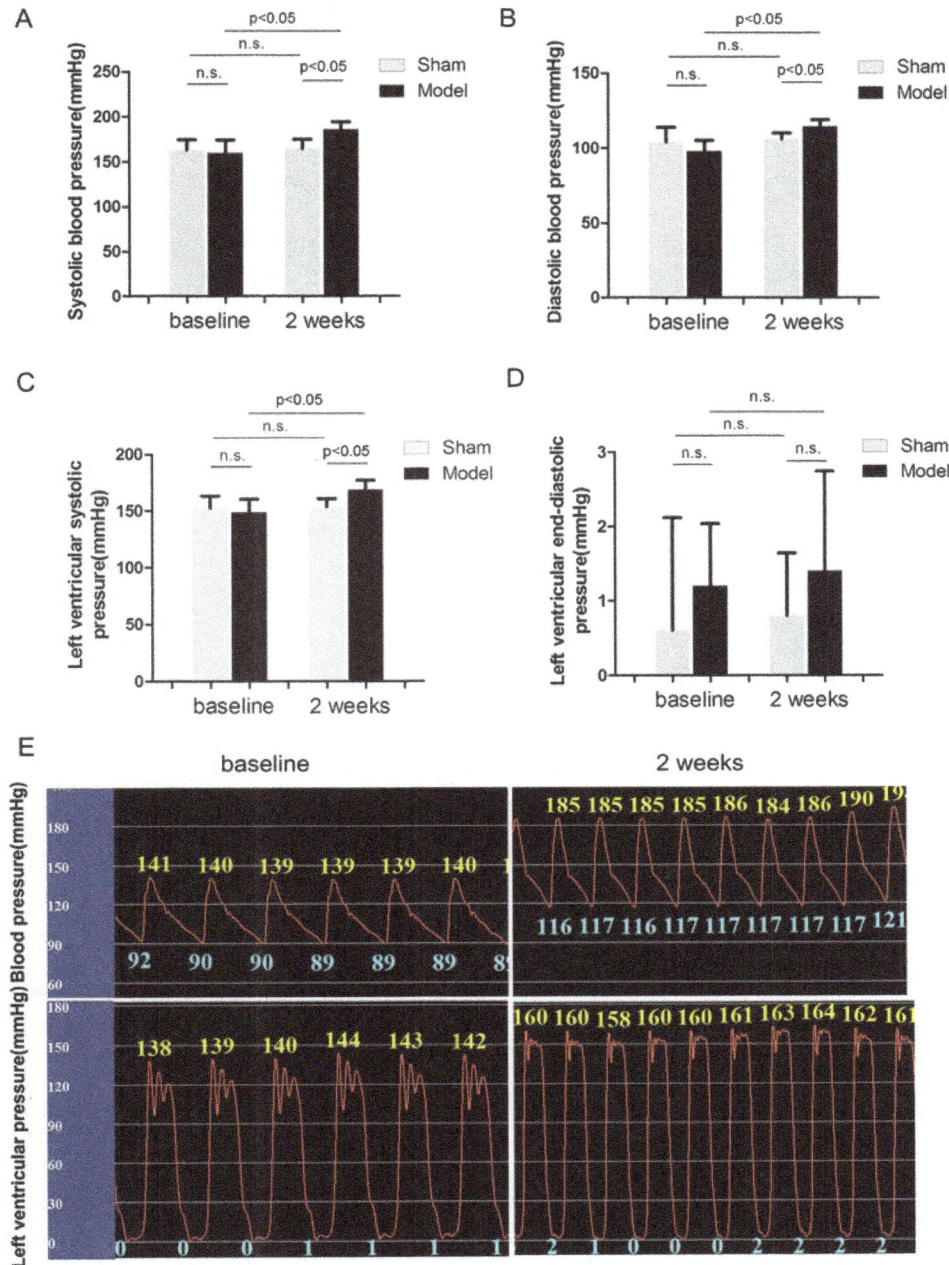

Figure 3. Analysis of BP and LV pressure (n = 5). Effects of embolization versus sham operation on SBP (A), DPB (B), LVSP (C) and LVEDP (D). Representative BP wave (upper) and LV pressure wave (lower) of dogs at baseline and with RI after 2 weeks of embolization in the model group (E).

Effects of RI with Mild Renal Insufficiency on the Systematic Activity of SNS, Inflammation and Oxidative Stress

Plasma noradrenaline levels were measured to represent systematic activity of SNS. Plasma hs-CRP levels were measured to represent activity of systematic inflammation. Plasma malondialdehyde levels were measured for activity of systematic oxidative stress. RI with mild renal insufficiency after 2 weeks of embolization resulted in a significant increase in plasma noradrenaline levels (Figure 6A) by 72% (P<0.05) compared with baseline values in the model group. Plasma noradrenaline levels were unchanged in the sham group. There was a trend for an increase in plasma hs-CRP levels after 2 weeks of embolization in the model group, but no statistical significance was found. Overall, plasma hs-CRP (Figure 6B) and malondialdehyde (Figure 6C) levels were unchanged in the model and sham groups.

Effects of RI with Mild Renal Insufficiency on RAAS

Plasma rennin and aldosterone levels were measured to represent systematic activity of the RAAS. RI with mild renal insufficiency after 2 weeks of embolization resulted in a significant increase in plasma renin levels (Figure 7A) by 61% (P<0.05), and plasma aldosterone levels (Figure 7B) by 47% (P<0.05) compared with baseline values in the model group. Plasma renin and

Table 2. Effects of embolization, sham operation and 30 minutes of rapid pacing on AERP.

	BCL	Baseline			2 weeks		
		Before pacing	After pacing	Decrease	Before pacing	After pacing	Decrease
Sham (ms)	300	144.0±17.5	136.0±14.7[a]	8.0±4.5	145.0±17.7	137.0±14.8[b]	8.0±4.5
	240	127.0±16.8	120.0±16.2[a]	7.0±2.7	127.0±14.8	120.0±15.4[b]	7.0±2.7
Model (ms)	300	149.0±12.0	142.0±10.4[a]	7.0±5.7	134.0±13.0[c]	122.0±11.5[b,d]	12.0±8.4
	240	133.0±8.4	125.0±7.9[a]	9.0±4.2	122.0±5.7[c]	111.0±5.5[b,d]	11.0±4.2

[a] p<0.05 vs. before pacing at baseline;
[b] p<0.05 vs. before pacing at 2 weeks;
[c] p<0.05 vs. before pacing at baseline;
[d] p<0.05 vs. after pacing at baseline. (mean ± standard deviation, n=5).

aldosterone levels were unchanged in the sham group. Left atrial tissue levels of angiotensin II (Figure 7C) and aldosterone (Figure 7D) were also elevated by 68% (P<0.05) and 77% (P< 0.05) respectively in the model group, compared with the sham group.

Effects of RI with Mild Renal Insufficiency on Atrial Fibrosis

Figure 8A and 8B illustrates representative images of Masson staining of the left atrial tissue after 2 weeks of interventional operation in the sham and model groups, respectively. The quantitative ratio of the area of interstitial fibrosis was summarized in Figure 8C. Compared with the Sham group (3.8%±1.6%), extensive and heterogeneous interstitial fibrosis was observed in the model group (9.3% ±3.5%, P<0.05).

Discussion

The main findings of our study were: 1) embolization of small renal artery branches of the left kidney for 2 weeks resulted in ischemic RI with mild renal insufficiency; 2) RI with mild renal insufficiency was associated with vulnerability to AF; 3) increased vulnerability of AF might be associated with increased activity of the SNS, RAAS, and atrial fibrosis in the model of RI with mild renal insufficiency.

To date, there has only been one study [9] on rats showing that CKD is associated with the development of AF. In this previous study, a classical model of CKD was created in rats with 5/6 nephrectomy. Oxidative stress may have been involved in the pathogenesis of interstitial fibrosis and enhanced vulnerability to AF in the left atrium in this CKD model. Besides the mechanism of oxidative stress, inflammation, the RAAS, and SNS activation are predicted to play important roles in the development of AF associated with CKD [10].

We established a new *in vivo* model of RI in a large animal (dogs) and found that ischemic RI with mild renal insufficiency was associated with vulnerability to AF. In Fukunaga et al's study [9], a stage 4 CKD model was created by 5/6 nephrectomy, indicating that renal function was severely damaged. In our study, unilateral diffuse ischemic RI was induced in dogs by transcatheter embolization of small renal artery branches using gelatin sponge granules. This method was simple and did not produce severe trauma in the dogs compared with 5/6 nephrectomy, and it did not cause whole organ infarction or severe renal dysfunction. Wang and Bao [11] found that renal function did not significantly change, even after 1 month of unilateral nephrectomy, indicating that the unilateral kidney could undertake compensatory function. In our study, creatinine and urea nitrogen levels were slightly increased, CCr was slightly decreased, which might be associated with the effects of persistent and unilateral RI on the normal contralateral kidney [12]. Factors induced by severe renal dysfunction were eliminated in our study because renal function in our study was still at the stage of the compensatory period.

Effects of hypertension on left atrial pressure and vulnerability to AF were not present in our study. Hypertension can be induced by severe renal dysfunction, and also by activation of the RAAS and SNS induced by RI [13]. Long-term hypertension is associated with high atrial pressure and atrial enlargement predisposing to AF [7]. LV systolic and diastolic function was not investigated in Fukunaga et al's study [9]. We found that although BP and LVSP were significantly elevated after 2 weeks of RI, LVEDP was not changed. This finding indicated that hypertension did not affect left atrial pressure and its effect on vulnerability to AF was negligible. A possible reason for this

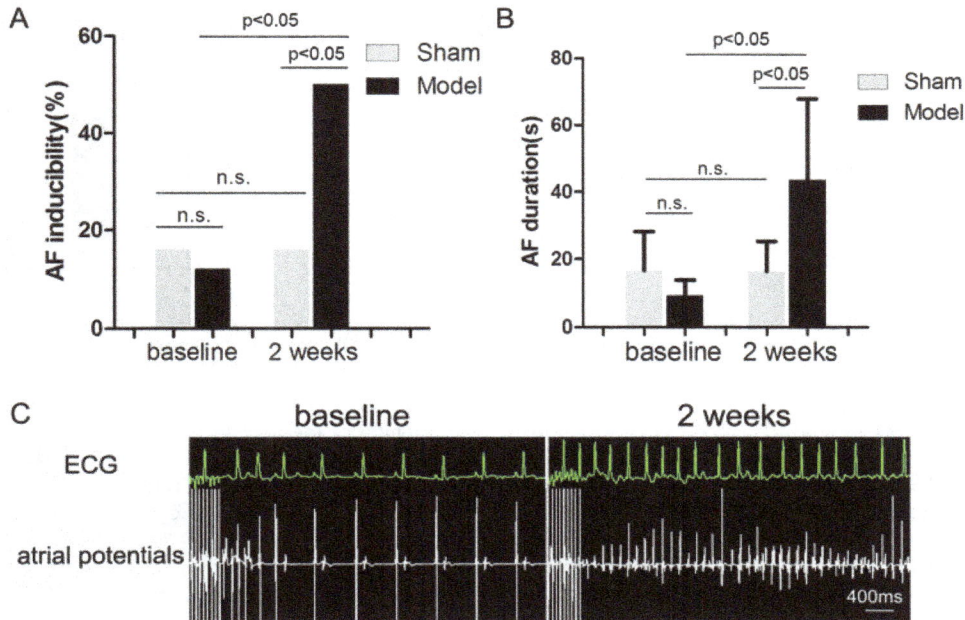

Figure 4. Effects of RI with mild renal insufficiency on the occurrence of AF (n = 5). Effects of embolization versus sham operation on inducibility of AF (A) and on the duration of induced AF episodes (B) in dogs. Representative right atrial potentials and ECG recordings after 10 seconds of rapid atrial pacing at baseline and with RI after 2 weeks of embolization in the model group (C).

finding may be because the length of time of hypertension was too short to affect left atrial pressure. Overactivity of the RAAS and SNS could contribute to elevated BP and LVSP in our model.

Heart rate was significantly increased in our study. Heart rate had a tendency to rise in a CKD model, but this was not significant in Fukunaga et al's study [9]. Ye et al [12] found that renal injury caused by phenol injection significantly increased heart rate and BP, which persisted for more than 3 weeks. Another study showed a significant increase in heart rate in a model of CKD, which was created in rats with ¾ nephrectomy. Heart rate

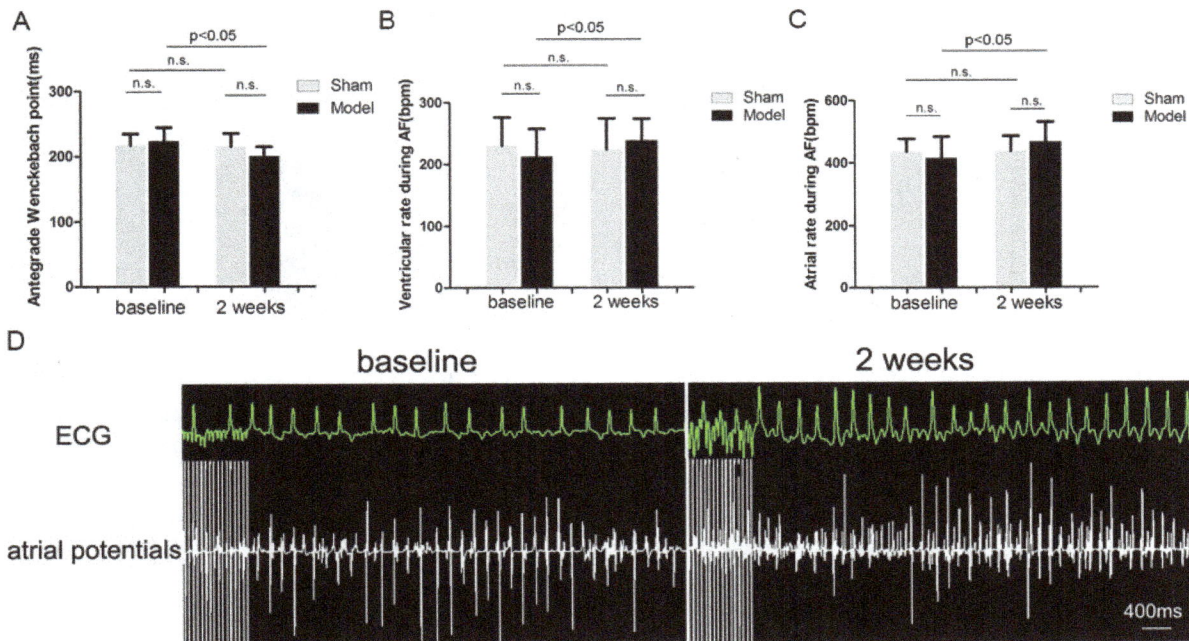

Figure 5. Electrophysiological effects of RI with mild renal insufficiency on AF and antegrade Wenckebach point (n = 5). Effects of embolization versus sham operation on antegrade Wenckebach point (A), ventricular rate during AF (B) and atrial rate during AF (C). Representative right atrial potentials and ECG recordings after 10 seconds of rapid atrial pacing at baseline and with RI after 2 weeks of embolization in the model group (D).

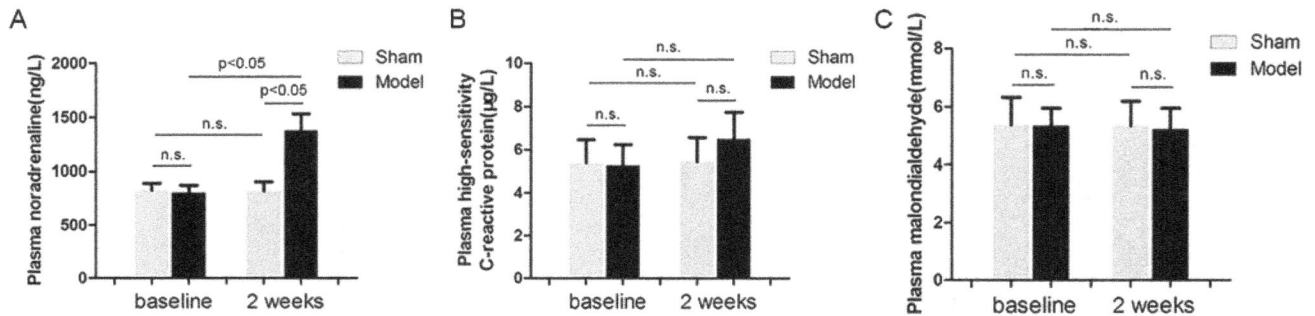

Figure 6. Effects of embolization versus sham operation on plasma noradrenaline (A), hs-CRP (B) and malondialdehyde (C) levels.

does not significantly increase in CKD patients [14], which may be associated with the baroreflex. Renal status may affect the distribution of baroreflex and nonbaroreflex activity, as well as the strength of the SBP-heart rate relationship [15]. Several studies have also found that end-stage renal disease patients have a withdrawal in parasympathetic modulation of heart rate in conjunction with an increase in sympathetic input to the sino-atrial node [16]. Activity of the SNS and sensitivity of the baroreflex might have affected heart rate in our study.

More electrophysiological parameters can be detected in large animal models than small animal models. P wave duration, and episodes and duration of AF were increased after RI compared with baseline in our study, which is consistent with Fukunaga et al's study [9]. Interstitial fibrosis might have led to prolongation of P wave duration in our study. Additionally, we found that the atrial and ventricular rates during AF were increased, and the antegrade Wenckebach point was shortened by RI with mild renal insufficiency. The increased atrial rate during AF could be the result of shortening of the effective refractory period. The increased ventricular rate during AF could be the result of

shortening of the antegrade Wenckebach point, which might be induced by overactivity of the SNS. More attention should be paid to the increased ventricular rate during AF in this model in the future, because control of this rate is important for patients with AF in clinical practice.

The design of our study is closer to the real clinical situation than other previous models. In the research field of AF, large animals, such as pigs and canines, are the most commonly used, because rats are not ideal for electrophysiological studies and catheter operations because of their fast heart rate and small size. In Fukunaga et al's study [9], hearts had to be isolated, and electrophysiological parameters and vulnerability to AF had to be detected *in vitro* because rats were used, whereas electrophysiological parameters and vulnerability to AF could be detected *in vivo* in dogs in our study.

Individual differences in electrophysiological parameters are always large. Therefore, we designed a before–after study to reduce the effect of individual differences, because large animals can be conveniently and repeatedly monitored. In Fukunaga et al's study, no significant differences were observed in the effective

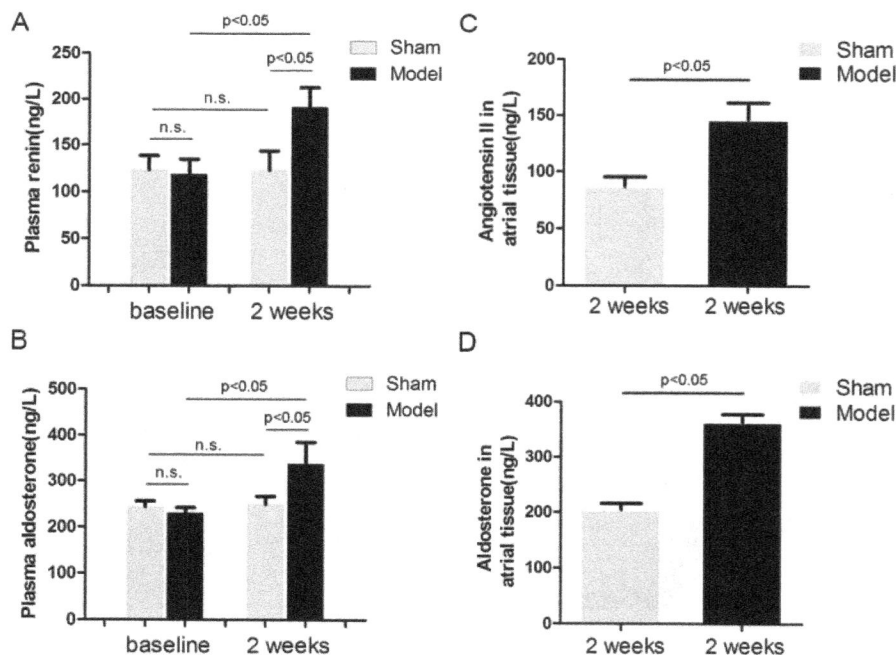

Figure 7. Effects of embolization versus sham operation on plasma renin (A) and aldosterone (B) levels, left atrial angiotensin II (C) and aldosterone (D) levels (n = 5).

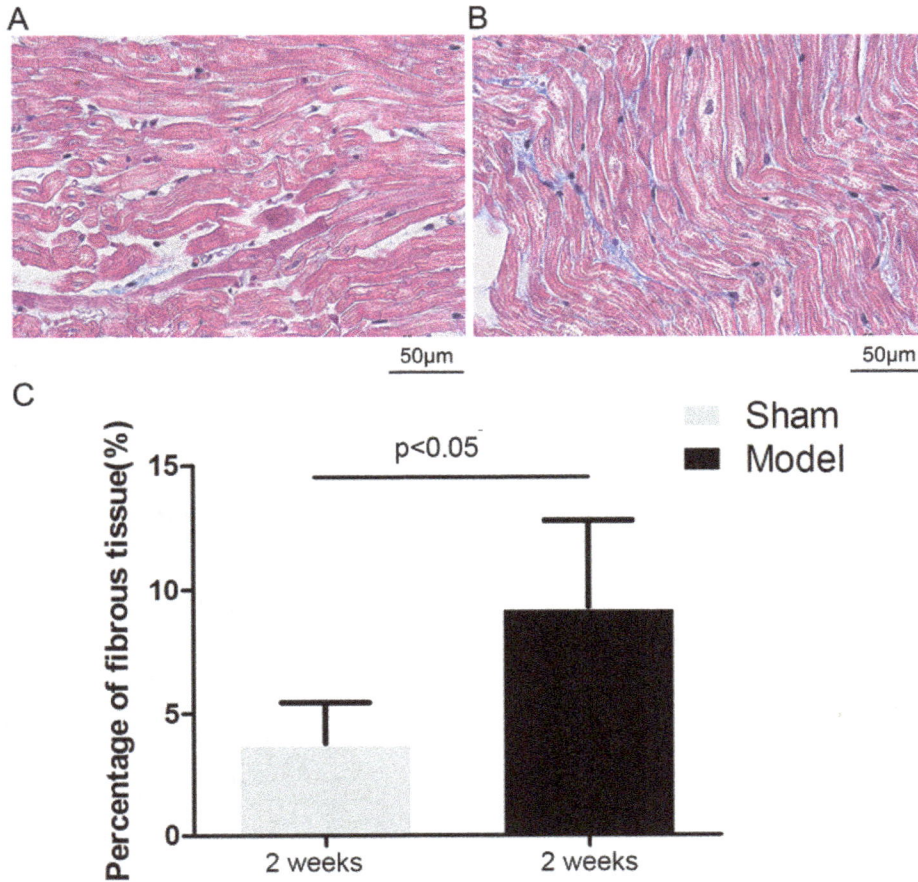

Figure 8. Analysis of atrial fibrosis. Representative images of Masson staining of the left atrial tissue after 2 weeks of interventional operation in the sham (A) and model groups (B). Mean percentage of interstitial fibrosis of the left atrium (C).

refractory period of the left atrium between the sham and model groups [9]. The effective refractory period of the right atrium also showed no significant difference between the sham and model groups in our study, whereas a significant difference was observed between baseline and 2 weeks in the model group. Overactivity of the SNS might play an important role in shortening of the effective refractory period because just adrenergic stimulation can decrease the human AERP by approximately 5% [17].

Our model was suitable for further determining the predominant factors that enhance AF vulnerability. Predicted mechanisms for the development of AF associated with CKD were observed in our study, including RAAS, SNS activation and atrial fibrosis. There was also a trend for an increase in plasma hs-CRP levels in the model group, but this was not significant. CRP, as a marker of inflammation, is elevated in chronic renal impairment [18]. Serum CRP concentrations are positively correlated with AF persistence, and predict postoperative AF occurrence [19]. The RAAS is activated by renal ischemic impairment and increased sympathetic activation in CKD [20]. The RAAS is involved in the pathogenesis of interstitial fibrosis, and they create a substrate for AF [21,22,23]. The injured kidney's afferent signals to central integrative structures in the brain lead to increased sympathetic activation [24]. Chemoreflex activation, reduced nitric oxide availability, and renalase secretion are also involved in heightened sympathetic tone and increased noradrenaline levels in patients with kidney impairment [24]. Increased sympathetic activation is found in the initial clinical stages of CKD [25], which also leads to atrial remodeling processes, possibly by neurohumoral activation and changes in atrial hemodynamics [26]. Hyper-sympathetic activity may facilitate the initiation of AF and acute atrial electrophysiological changes [27]. Understanding these mechanisms could lead to new therapeutic strategies for CKD patients combined with AF. Renal denervation, which is a new therapeutic approach to treat resistant hypertension through reducing renal norepinephrine spillover, can also prolong the antegrade Wenckebach point, and provides control of the ventricular rate during AF in normal pigs [28]. Renal denervation also inhibits pronounced shortening of the AERP and reduces susceptibility to AF in a pig model of obstructive sleep apnea or heart failure [29,30] by combined reduction of sympathetic drive and RAAS activity [31,32]. Whether this treatment has the same effects in our canine model of RI with mild renal insufficiency may be important for elucidating mechanisms and developing new therapeutic strategies for CKD-induced hypertension and atrial arrhythmogenic remodeling.

Study Limitations

The pathophysiological process and severity of renal impairment in our model is not completely in accord with the real situation of CKD. AF mainly originates from the left atrium, but AF was induced in the right atrium in our study because the left atrium is difficult to reach through a catheter operation.

Spontaneous induction of AF is too rare for systematic evaluation. Therefore, we applied fast pacing to induce AF (AF begets AF). The sensitivity of the baroreflex and the strength of sympathetic and parasympathetic modulation of the sino-atrial node in the baroreflex may influence AF vulnerability. Nonetheless, these effects could not be eliminated. Intervention measures, such as renal denervation, administration of angiotensin-converting enzyme inhibitors or β-adrenoceptor blockers need to be applied for further clarifying the related mechanisms.

Conclusions

We successfully established an *in vivo* model of RI with mild renal insufficiency in a large animal and showed that AF was associated with RI with mild renal insufficiency in this model. Increased activity of the SNS, RAAS and enhanced atrial fibrosis

may contribute to the development of AF associated with RI with mild renal insufficiency. A successful model of RI with mild renal insufficiency in canines could be used to further investigate the factors responsible for the development of AF associated with CKD in the future.

Acknowledgments

We gratefully thank Dr Jun Yi for assisting with C arm X-ray machine manipulation.

Author Contributions

Conceived and designed the experiments: ZL YTW ZLS. Performed the experiments: ZL LFL XPC. Analyzed the data: KL. Contributed reagents/materials/analysis tools: JPG. Contributed to the writing of the manuscript: XMS HYG.

References

1. Chen LY, Shen WK (2007) Epidemiology of atrial fibrillation: a current perspective. Heart Rhythm 4: S1–6.
2. Zimmerman D, Sood MM, Rigatto C, Holden RM, Hiremath S, et al. (2012) Systematic review and meta-analysis of incidence, prevalence and outcomes of atrial fibrillation in patients on dialysis. Nephrol Dial Transplant 27: 3816–3822.
3. Soliman EZ, Prineas RJ, Go AS, Xie D, Lash JP, et al. (2010) Chronic kidney disease and prevalent atrial fibrillation: the Chronic Renal Insufficiency Cohort (CRIC). Am Heart J 159: 1102–1107.
4. Naruse Y, Tada H, Sekiguchi Y, Machino T, Ozawa M, et al. (2010) Concomitant chronic kidney disease increases the recurrence of atrial fibrillation after catheter ablation of atrial fibrillation: a mid-term follow-up. Heart Rhythm 8: 335–341.
5. Guo Y, Wang H, Zhao X, Zhang Y, Zhang D, et al. (2013) Relation of renal dysfunction to the increased risk of stroke and death in female patients with atrial fibrillation. Int J Cardiol 168: 1502–1508.
6. Brown SA. (2013) Renal pathophysiology: lessons learned from the canine remnant kidney model. J Vet Emerg Crit Care (San Antonio) 23: 115–121.
7. Linz D, Neuberger HR (2012) Chronic kidney disease and atrial fibrillation. Heart Rhythm 9: 2032–2033.
8. Toshifumi W, Mika M (2007) Effects of Benazepril Hydrochloride in Cats with Experimentally Induced or Spontaneously Occurring Chronic Renal Failure. J. Vet. Med. Sci 69: 1015–1023.
9. Fukunaga N, Takahashi N, Hagiwara S, Kume O, Fukui A, et al. (2012) Establishment of a model of atrial fibrillation associated with chronic kidney disease in rats and the role of oxidative stress. Heart Rhythm 9: 2023–2031.
10. Alonso A, Lopez FL, Matsushita K, Loehr LR, Agarwal SK, et al. (2011) Chronic kidney disease is associated with the incidence of atrial fibrillation: the Atherosclerosis Risk in Communities (ARIC) study. Circulation 123: 2946–2953.
11. Wang Y, Bao X (2013) Effects of uric acid on endothelial dysfunction in early chronic kidney disease and its mechanisms. Eur J Med Res 18: 26–36.
12. Ye S, Zhong H, Yanamadala V, Campese VM (2002) Renal injury caused by intrarenal injection of phenol increases afferent and efferent renal sympathetic nerve activity. Am J Hypertens 15: 717–724.
13. Ewen S, Ukena C, Linz D, Schmieder RE, Bohm M, et al. (2013) The sympathetic nervous system in chronic kidney disease. Curr Hypertens Rep 15: 370–376.
14. Kestenbaum B, Rudser KD, Shlipak MG, Fried LF, Newman AB, et al. (2007) Kidney function, electrocardiographic findings, and cardiovascular events among older adults. Clin J Am Soc Nephrol 2: 501–508.
15. Sapoznikov D, Dranitzki Elhalel M, Rubinger D (2013) Heart rate response to blood pressure variations: sympathetic activation versus baroreflex response in patients with end-stage renal disease. PLoS One 8: e78338.
16. Chan CT (2008) Heart rate variability in patients with end-stage renal disease: an emerging predictive tool for sudden cardiac death? Nephrol Dial Transplant 23: 3061–3062.
17. Redpath CJ, Rankin AC, Kane KA, Workman AJ (2006) Anti-adrenergic effects of endothelin on human atrial action potentials are potentially anti-arrhythmic. J Mol Cell Cardiol 40: 717–724.
18. Landray MJ, Wheeler DC, Lip GY, Newman DJ, Blann AD, et al. (2004) Inflammation, endothelial dysfunction, and platelet activation in patients with chronic kidney disease: the chronic renal impairment in Birmingham (CRIB) study. Am J Kidney Dis 43: 244–253.
19. Schotten U, Verheule S, Kirchhof P, Goette A (2011) Pathophysiological mechanisms of atrial fibrillation: a translational appraisal. Physiol Rev 91: 265–325.
20. Siragy HM, Carey RM (2010) Role of the intrarenal renin-angiotensin-aldosterone system in chronic kidney disease. Am J Nephrol 31: 541–550.
21. Mayyas F, Alzoubi KH, Van Wagoner DR (2013) Impact of aldosterone antagonists on the substrate for atrial fibrillation: aldosterone promotes oxidative stress and atrial structural/electrical remodeling. Int J Cardiol 168: 5135–5142.
22. Savelieva I, Kakouros N, Kourliouros A, Camm AJ (2011) Upstream therapies for management of atrial fibrillation: review of clinical evidence and implications for European Society of Cardiology guidelines. Part II: secondary prevention. Europace 13: 610–625.
23. Thomas H, Jeffrey E (2007) Atrial Fibrosis and the Mechanisms of Atrial Fibrillation. Heart Rhythm 4: S24–S27.
24. Schlaich MP, Socratous F, Hennebry S, Eikelis N, Lambert EA, et al. (2009) Sympathetic activation in chronic renal failure. J Am Soc Nephrol 20: 933–939.
25. Grassi G, Quarti-Trevano F, Seravalle G, Arenare F, Volpe M, et al. (2011) Early sympathetic activation in the initial clinical stages of chronic renal failure. Hypertension 57: 846–851.
26. Park HW, Shen MJ, Lin SF, Fishbein MC, Chen LS, et al. (2011) Neural mechanisms of atrial fibrillation. Curr Opin Cardiol 27: 24–28.
27. Hou Y, Hu J, Po SS, Wang H, Zhang L, et al. (2013) Catheter-based renal sympathetic denervation significantly inhibits atrial fibrillation induced by electrical stimulation of the left stellate ganglion and rapid atrial pacing. PLoS One 8: e78218.
28. Linz D, Mahfoud F, Schotten U, Ukena C, Hohl M, et al. (2012) Renal sympathetic denervation provides ventricular rate control but does not prevent atrial electrical remodeling during atrial fibrillation. Hypertension 61: 225–231.
29. Linz D, Mahfoud F, Schotten U, Ukena C, Neuberger HR, et al. (2012) Renal sympathetic denervation suppresses postapneic blood pressure rises and atrial fibrillation in a model for sleep apnea. Hypertension 60: 172–178.
30. Zhao Q, Yu S, Huang H, Tang Y, Xiao J, et al. (2013) Effects of renal sympathetic denervation on the development of atrial fibrillation substrates in dogs with pacing-induced heart failure. Int J Cardiol 168: 1672–1673.
31. Linz D, Hohl M, Nickel A, Mahfoud F, Wagner M, et al. (2013) Effect of renal denervation on neurohumoral activation triggering atrial fibrillation in obstructive sleep apnea. Hypertension 62: 767–774.
32. Zhao Q, Yu S, Zou M, Dai Z, Wang X, et al. (2012) Effect of renal sympathetic denervation on the inducibility of atrial fibrillation during rapid atrial pacing. J Interv Card Electrophysiol 35: 119–125.

15

Low Ankle-Brachial Index Is Associated with Early-Stage Chronic Kidney Disease in Type 2 Diabetic Patients Independent of Albuminuria

Xuehong Dong[1]◑, Dingting Wu[1]◑, Chengfang Jia[1], Yu Ruan[1], Xiaocheng Feng[1], Guoxing Wang[1], Jun Liu[1], Yi Shen[2], Hong Li[1]*, Lianxi Li[3]*

1 Departments of Endocrinology and Metabolism, Sir Run Run Shaw Hospital, School of Medicine, Zhejiang University, Hangzhou, P. R. China, **2** Department of Epidemiology and Health Statistics School of Public Health, Zhejiang University, Hangzhou, P. R. China, **3** Department of Endocrinology and Metabolism, Shanghai Jiao Tong University Affiliated Sixth People's Hospital, Shanghai, P. R. China

Abstract

Aims: The role of low ankle-brachial index (ABI) in early-stage chronic kidney disease (CKD) is not fully known. This study was designed to investigate the prevalence of low ABI in early-stage CKD defined as an estimated glomerular filtration rate (eGFR) between 60–89 ml/min/1.73 m^2 of type 2 diabetic patients without albuminuria and to determine the association between the low ABI and mildly decreased eGFR.

Methods: The cross-sectional study enrolled 448 type 2 diabetic patients with normoalbuminuria. The patients were stratified into two groups according to the CKD-EPI eGFR level: the normal group with eGFR level ≥90 mL/min/1.73 m^2 and the lower group with eGFR of 60–89. ABI was categorized as normal (1.0–1.39), low-normal (0.9–0.99), and low (<0.9). Both stepwise forward multiple linear regression and binary logistic regression analyses were performed to examine the association between ABI categories and eGFR levels and to assess the relation of low ABI and early-stage CKD.

Results: The prevalence of low ABI in early-stage CKD of type 2 diabetic patients without albuminuria was 39.5%. Low ABI was associated with an approximate 3-fold greater risk of early-stage CKD in bivariate logistic regression analysis, and remained significantly associated with a 2.2 fold risk (95% confidence interval: 1.188–4.077; *P* = 0.012) after adjusting traditional chronic kidney disease risk factors.

Conclusions: There was a high prevalence of low ABI in early-stage CKD patients of type 2 diabetes with normoalbuminuria and a close relation between low ABI and early-stage CKD, suggesting that we should pay much more attention to the patients who have only mildly decreased eGFR and normoalbuminuria but have already had a low ABI in clinic work and consider the preventive therapy in early stage.

Editor: Karin Jandeleit-Dahm, Baker IDI Heart and Diabetes Institute, Australia

Funding: This research was supported by the National Natural Science Foundation of China for young scientists (30900703), the Doctoral Fund of Ministry of Education of China (200803351042), the Zhejiang Project of Science and Technology (2009A11), and the National Natural Science Foundation of China (81170759). The funders had no role in study design, data collection and analysis, decision to publish, or preparation of the manuscript.

Competing Interests: The authors have declared that no competing interests exist.

* Email: lihongheyi@126.com (HL); lilx@sjtu.edu.cn (LXL)

◑ These authors contributed equally to this work.

Introduction

The recently epidemic survey showed the prevalence of diabetes among a representative sample of Chinese adults at 11.6% and the population had been up to 113 million in 2010 [1]. Diabetes affecting the kidney, or diabetic nephropathy, affects approximately one third of patients with either type 1 or type 2 diabetes mellitus [2]. Our previous population-based study in Shanghai showed the prevalence of chronic kidney disease (CKD) and albuminuria were 32.7% and 44.2%, respectively [3], consistent with the data from Nanjing [4]. These data suggest diabetes may have reached an alert level in China with the potential for a major epidemic of diabetes-related complications, especially CKD.

Small amounts of albumin in the urine, or microalbuminuria is the current early biomarker. However, its association with progression to renal failure is unclear; as microalbuminuria does not always lead to progressive renal failure [5]. Ankle-brachial index (ABI) is a marker of generalized atherosclerosis that is associated with an increased risk of cardiovascular disease, cardiovascular mortality, and all-cause mortality [6]. In relation to kidney function, prior research indicated that low ABI (<0.9) was common in general populations with CKD [7,8,9] as well as in diabetic patients [10,11]. However, some of these studies examined the relation between kidney dysfunction and ABI without adjusting for albuminuria, and most of these studies defined CKD as an estimated glomerular filtration rate (eGFR) less than 60 ml/min/1.73 m^2 (CKD stage 3–5). While expert consensus proposes a level of <60 ml/min/1.73 m^2 [12], two recent studies with long-term follow-up suggested that the increased cardiovascular mortality may begin even earlier, perhaps at eGFR levels below 90 ml/min/1.73 m^2 [13,14]. The underlying risk factors and mechanisms of early-stage CKD, especially in diabetic patients who have mildly decreased eGFR, are far from completely established.

Therefore, this study aimed first to investigate the prevalence of low ABI in early-stage CKD (defined as an eGFR between 60–89 ml/min/1.73 m^2) of type 2 diabetic patients without albuminuria and second to determine the association between the low ABI and mildly decreased eGFR in these patients.

Methods

1. Study Population

This cross-sectional study was performed in a population of 1117 patients diagnosed type 2 diabetes at the department of Endocrinology and Metabolism of the Sir Run Run Shaw hospital between January 2010 and December 2012. Among these participants, 441 patients with microalbuminuria defined as urinary albumin excretion rate 30–300 mg/24 h or macroalbuminuria defined as urinary albumin excretion rate ≥300 mg/24 h [15] and 5 patients aged≤20 years were excluded from the study. 130 patients taking either angiotensin converting enzyme inhibitors or angiotensin II receptor subtype AT-1 blockers were further excluded. 41 patients with acute infection including pneumonia, diarrhea, cholecystitis, 31 patients accepted kidney operation such as nephrectomy or getting chronic kidney disease as chronic glomerulonephritis, nephropyelitis, hydronephrosis, 12 patients at the end stage of all kinds of cancers and 9 patients whose eGFR was lower than 60 mL/min/1.73 m^2 were also excluded. At last, 448 patients were enrolled in the study. All participants provided written informed consent, and the study was approved by the investigational review boards of the Sir Run Run Shaw Hospital of Zhejiang University.

2. History collection

Interviews were conducted by trained examiners who used a well-established questionnaire to collect demographic information of the study participants including date of birth, sex, smoking status, and personal medical history. Weight and height were measured while patients were dressed in light clothing. Body mass index (BMI) was calculated as weight (kg) divided by the square of the height (m). Waist circumference was measured to the nearest 0.1 cm at expiration along a horizontal plane through the abdomen at the level of the midpoint between the lowest rib and the iliac crest. Blood pressure (BP) was measured twice with the subjects in the sitting position after a 5-min rest. The lower value of two measurements was used for the study.

3. Laboratory Measurement

Venous blood samples and urinary specimens were collected in the morning following an overnight fast. HbA1c was examined using an automatic analyzer (VARIANT II, BIO-RAD Laboratories, Inc., California, USA). Lipid profiles including triglyceride, total cholesterol, high-density lipoprotein cholesterol, low-density lipoprotein cholesterol and very low density lipoprotein cholesterol, fasting blood glucose, fasting insulin, fasting C peptide, serum

creatinine, serum uric acid and C reactive protein levels were measured using another automatic analyzer (AEROSET; Abbott Laboratories, Abbott Park, Illinois, USA).

4. Diagnosis of diabetic retinopathy and neuropathy

Diabetic retinopathy (DR) was assessed by the Digital non-mydriatic fundus photography (Nonmyd; Kowa Company, Ltd.; Japan) according to the protocol previously reported [16,17]. DR was classified as none and DR containing mild non-proliferative DR, moderate non-proliferative DR, severe non-proliferative DR, proliferative DR, and diabetic macular edema by a trained ophthalmic photographer and a retinal specialist. The diagnosis of diabetic neuropathy was depending on the nerve conduction study performed by a trained physiatrist. Electrophysiological tests were done in recommended standard situations [18] for all patients by Synergy electromyograph machine (Keypoint; Dantec Dynamics A/S; Denmark), which included ulnar and median nerves (sensory and motor fibers) in upper extremities and sural (sensory), deep peroneal and tibial (motor) nerves in lower extremities. Diagnosis of diabetic neuropathy was based on at least one abnormal nerve conduction result.

5. Calculation of eGFR

eGFR was estimated using the CKD Epidemiology Collaboration (CKD-EPI) Study equation [19]. eGFR = a×(serum creatinine/b)^c×(0.993)^{age}. The variable a takes on the following values on the basis of Asia race and sex: Women = 144, Men = 141. The variable b takes on the following values on the basis of sex: Women = 0.7, Men = 0.9. The variable c takes on the following values on the basis of sex and creatinine measurement: Women: Serum creatinine≤0.7 mg/dl = −0.329, Serum creatinine> 0.7 mg/dl = −1.209; Men: Serum creatinine≤0.9 mg/dl = −0.411, Serum creatinine>0.9 mg/dl = −1.209. The enrolled patients were stratified into two groups according to the CKD-EPI eGFR level: the normal group with eGFR level ≥90 mL/min/1.73 m^2 and the lower group with eGFR of 60–89 mL/min/1.73 m^2.

6. ABI Measurement

The ABI measurements were performed in a supine position and BP was measured in the bilateral brachial and dorsalis pedis arteries with an 8-MHz Doppler probe (Vista AVS; Summit Doppler Systems, Inc., USA). According to the guidelines of American Heart Asso-ciation [20], ABI was calculated as the ratio of the higher value of the systolic BP of the two ankle ar-teries of that limb (either the anterior or the posterior tibial ar-tery) and the higher value of the two brachial systolic BP. For each patient, the lower ABI from both legs was used for further evaluation. Among the 448 enrolled patients, ABI levels ranged from 0.19 to 1.39. Therefore, we categorized ABI into 3 groups: normal (1.0–1.39), low-normal (0.9–0.99), and low (<0.9).

7. Statistical Analysis

Statistical analyses were performed using the SPSS 15.0 software package (SPSS Science, v. 15.0, Chicago, IL). The continuous variables were compared using the t test; categorical variables were compared using the x^2 test; and all variables were adjusted by age and sex. Both stepwise forward multiple linear regression and binary logistic regression analyses were performed to examine the association between ABI categories and eGFR level and to assess the relation of low ABI and early-stage CKD. For all analyses, participants with eGFR of 90 mL/min/1.73 m^2 or higher were served as the referent category with which the other

Table 1. Characteristics of the participants with normal or mildly decreased eGFR levels.

	eGFR		
	≥90 mL/min/1.73 m²	60–89 mL/min/1.73 m²	Age- and sex- adjusted P
n	362	86	
Age (years)	50±11	63±11	0.000
Male (%)	66.9	50.0	0.004
Duration of diabetes (years)	5±7	7±6	0.671
Hypertension (%)	23.5	50.0	0.071
The history of smoking (%)			
Never	53.6	72.1	
Past	8.6	13.9	0.985
Current	37.8	14.0	0.041
BMI(kg/m²)	24.4±4.3	23.4±3.2	0.195
Waist(cm)	87.7±10.1	86.8±10.1	0.799
systolic BP(mm/Hg)	125±17	128±18	0.355
diastolic BP(mm/Hg)	75±12	72±12	0.896
Diabetic retinopathy (%)	25.1	39.5	0.275
Diabetic neuropathy (%)	29.0	41.9	0.802
ABI categories(%)			
Normal	53.8	38.4	
Low normal	27.4	22.1	0.738
Abnormal	18.8	39.5	0.013
24 hMA(mg/24 H)	11.1±6.9	12.3±7.4	0.140
HbA1c (%)	9.5±2.3	8.8±2.5	0.038
FBG(mg/dl)	143±47	139±55	0.386
Fasting insulin (ulU/ml)	7.6±8.8	7.9±5.4	0.967
Fasting C peptide (pmol/l)	648±393	801±513	0.008
Triglyceride (mmol/l)	1.77±1.61	1.67±1.26	0.765
TC(mmol/l)	4.52±1.06	4.71±0.93	0.092
HDL-c (mmol/l)	1.09±0.34	1.16±0.33	0.901
LDL-c (mmol/l)	2.32±0.74	2.47±0.80	0.108
C reactive protein(mg/L)	5.5±15.9	7.6±19.4	0.855
Treatment of diabetes (%)			
None	29.3	25.6	
Oral Drugs	55.3	52.3	0.537
Insulin	5.8	11.6	0.357
Both	9.6	10.5	0.722

Abbreviations: BMI: body mass index; BP: blood pressure; MA: microalbminurine; FBG: fasting blood glucose; TC: total cholesterol; HDL-c: high-density lipoprotein cholesterol; LDL-c: Low-density lipoprotein cholesterol;
None: the patients never took anti-diabetic drugs. Both: the patients were taking oral drugs and subcutaneous injection of insulin at the same time.
Unless otherwise indicated, data are reported as mean ± SD. The referent category for P value comparisons is eGFR higher than 90 mL/min/1.73 m².

groups were compared. Differences with $P<0.05$ (two-tailed) were considered statistically significant.

Results

Characteristics of the participants

The overall prevalence of early-stage CKD defined by CKD-EPI eGFR 60–89 ml/min per 1.73 m² with normoalbuminuria was 19.2%(Table 1). Compared with participants whose eGFR levels higher than 90 mL/min/1.73 m², those with eGFR 60–89 mL/min/1.73 m² were older (50±11 VS 63±11 years, $P<0.001$), more frequently female, had a slightly lower prevalence of smoking habits (37%, and 14% respectively, $P=0.041$). After adjustment for age and sex, the lower eGFR group were more likely to have a higher level of fasting C peptide (648±393 VS

Table 2. Characteristics of the participants with different ABI categories.

ABI	normal (1.0–1.39)	low-normal (0.9–0.99)	low (<0.9)
n	228	118	102
Age (years)	50±12	51±12	57±12*[†]
Male (%)	72.4	63.6**	44.1*[††]
Duration of diabetes (years)	5.0±5.0	5.9±9.8	6.1±5.6
Hypertension (%)	23.2	28.0	41.2**[††]
The history of smoking (%)			
Never	51.8	56.8	69.6
Past	10.1	8.5	9.8
Current	38.2	34.7	20.6**[††]
BMI(kg/m²)	24.6±4.2	23.7±3.3**	24.0±4.5
Waist circumference(cm)	89.3±10.4	85.6±9.8**	85.9±9.0**
Systolic BP(mm/Hg)	124±17	124±16	131±18**[††]
Diastolic BP(mm/Hg)	74±12	73±12	76±11
Diabetic retinopathy (%)	26.3	30.5	28.4
Diabetic neuropathy (%)	33.8	25.4	33.3
eGFR(mL/min/1.73 m²)	105±15	105±17	96±16*[†]
24h MA(mg/24 H)	11.0±6.9	12.0±6.8	11.2±7.5
HbA1c (%)	9.5±2.3	9.4±2.4	9.1±2.2
FBG(mg/dl)	140±46	147±52	142±51
Fasting insulin (uIU/ml)	7.6±8.7	6.3±4.4	9.3±10.6[††]
Fasting C peptide (pmol/l)	623±370	705±463	772±466**
Triglyceride (mmol/l)	1.76±1.73	1.74±1.18	1.74±1.48
TC(mmol/l)	4.45±1.01	4.65±1.00	4.69±1.13
HDL-c (mmol/l)	1.07±0.32	1.14±0.37	1.15±0.31
LDL -c(mmol/l)	2.30±0.73	2.37±0.73	2.44±0.82
C reactive protein(mg/L)	6.2±16.8	6.7±21.0	4.4±8.8
Treatment of diabetes (%)			
None	28.9	35.6	19.6
Oral Drugs	54.8	52.5	56.9[††]
Insulin	7.5	4.2	8.8[††]
Both	8.8	7.6	14.7**[††]

*P<0.05, **P<0.001 compared with group of normal ABI.
[†]P<0.05,
[††]P<0.001 compared with group of low-normal ABI.
Abbreviations: BMI: body mass index; BP: blood pressure; MA: microalbminurine; FBG: fasting blood glucose; TC: total cholesterol; HDL-c: high-density lipoprotein cholesterol; LDL-c: Low-density lipoprotein cholesterol.

801±513 pmol/l, $P = 0.008$) and a lower level of HbA1c (9.5±2.3% VS 8.8±2.5%, $P = 0.038$). The prevalence of hypertension, diabetic neuropathy and DR of the lower eGFR group were elevated and the duration of diabetes was longer, compared with the normal eGFR group. However, these differences were all attenuated and no longer significant after multivariable adjustment. There were no other significant differences between the two groups.

Among the 448 studied participants, 22.8% (n = 102) had ABI measurements <0.90, 26.3% (n = 118) had ABI between 0.90 and 0.99, and 50.9% (n = 228) had normal ABI levels between 1.0 and 1.39, respectively. HbA1c, fasting blood glucose and lipid levels showed no differences between the three groups. Compared with the normal ABI group, the low ABI group had significantly higher

systolic BP and lower waist circumference. The patients in low ABI group were older, more frequently female, had relatively higher prevalence of hypertension, lower prevalence of smoking habits and decreased eGFR level than those in normal or low-normal group (Table 2).

Percentage of ABI categories in different eGFR groups

The prevalence of low ABI in early-stage CKD (CKD stage 2) of type 2 diabetic patients without albuminuria was 39.5%. Meanwhile, the prevalence of low ABI in normal eGFR group was only 18.8%. Normal ABI was significantly more frequent in the group showing normal eGFR levels than in those with CKD stage 2 (Figure 1). On the other side, Figure 2 showed a higher

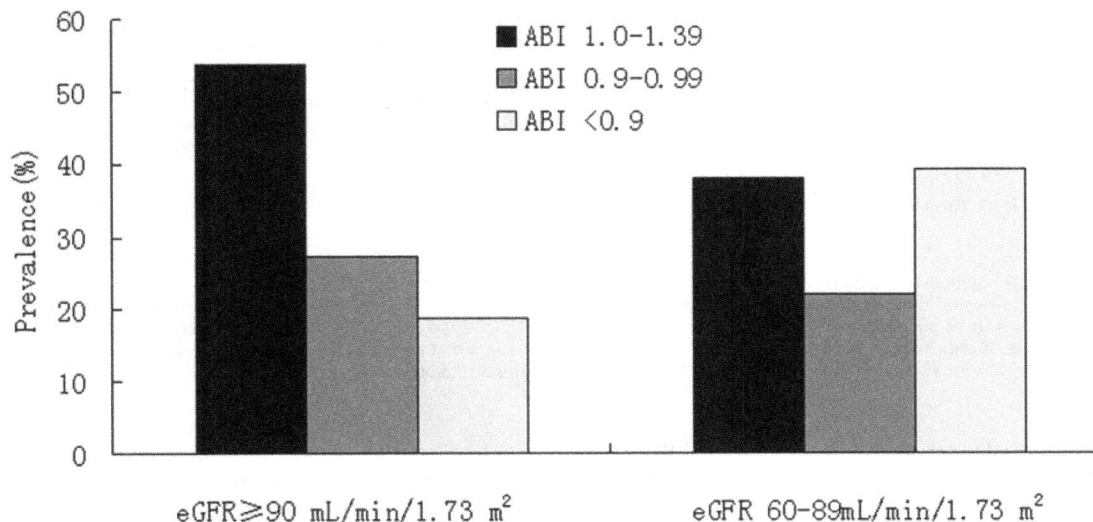

Figure 1. The distribution of ABI categories in two groups according to the eGFR level.

proportion of participants with early-stage CKD in the groups with low ABI than those with low-normal or normal ABI.

Relation between low ABI and eGFR in early-stage CKD

Low ABI was associated with an approximate 3-fold greater risk of eGFR lower than 90 in bivariate logistic regression analysis. The association of ABI <0.9 with early-stage CKD was moderately attenuated in multivariable logistic regression models, but low ABI remained significantly associated with a 2.2 fold risk (95% confidence interval [CI] 1.188–4.077; $P = 0.012$) for mildly decreased eGFR (Table 3). Furthermore, we evaluated the association of eGFR as a continuous measure with different ABI categories and found a significant relation ($\beta = -0.100$; $P = 0.043$) after adjustment for age, sex, the history of hypertension, the duration of diabetes, complications including diabetic neuropathy and retinopathy, smoking status, BMI, triglyceride and C reactive protein levels.

Discussion

A main finding of this study was the alarming high prevalence of low ABI (nearly 40%) in early-stage CKD (CKD stage 2) of type 2

diabetic patients without albuminuria. Another important finding of this study was that low ABI was significantly associated with mildly decreased eGFR after adjusting traditional chronic kidney disease risk factors. To the best of our knowledge, this is the first study to focus on the normoalbuminuric early-stage CKD and to evaluate the precise role of low ABI in eGFR declining in Chinese patients with type 2 diabetes.

The association of low ABI with cardiovascular disease has been well established in a number of populations, including diabetic patients, hypertensive patients and general subjects [21,22,23], but not until recently have several studies reported the close relation of low ABI and CKD in general population. The previous cross-sectional studies showed that low ABI was associated with ~50% higher odds of having eGFR <90 mL/min/1.73 m² compared with ABI of 1.00–1.19 [24] as well as with elevated serum creatinine level [25]. In the 3 years' ARIC study, participants with an ABI lower than 0.9 had more than 4-fold odds of experiencing a 50% rise in creatinine level compared with those with an ABI of 1 or higher, and the association persisted after adjustment for known predictors of renal functional decline [7]. The Framingham Offspring 10 year's follow-up Study showed low ABI was

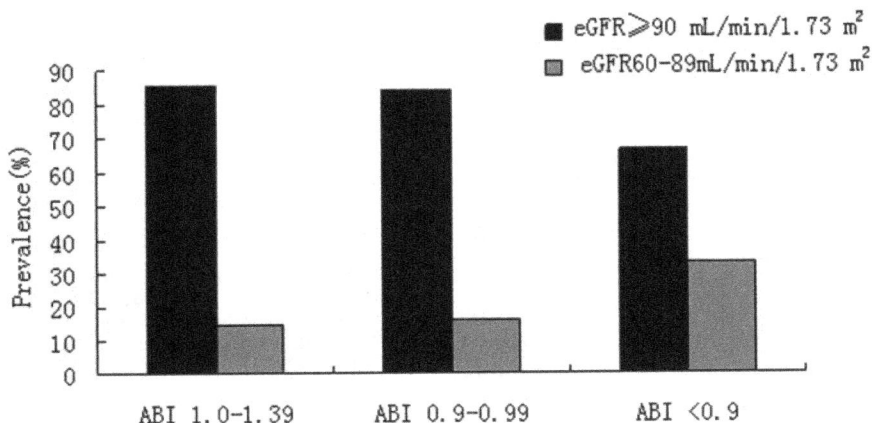

Figure 2. Proportion of the sample that developed the kidney function decline by ABI categories.

Table 3. Association of Ankle-Brachial Index(ABI) with early-stage CKD.

ABI	Bivariate OR(CI)	*P* Value	Multivariate* OR(95% CI)	*P* Value
1.0–1.39	1.0(referent)	referent	1.0(referent)	referent
0.9–0.99	1.134(0.614–2.096)	0.688	1.269(0.65–2.477)	0.485
<0.9	2.955(1.700–5.135)	0.000	2.201(1.188–4.077)	0.012
P #value for trend		0.000		0.043

Abbreviations: CI, confidence interval; OR, odds ratio.
*The following covariates ascertained at baseline were included in multivariate analysis: age, sex, the history of hypertension, the duration of diabetes, smoking status, complications including diabetic neuropathy and retinopathy, body mass index, HbA1c, HDL and LDL cholesterol values, triglyceride levels.
#The following covariates ascertained at baseline were included in regression analysis: age, sex, the history of hypertension, the duration of diabetes, smoking status, complications including diabetic neuropathy and retinopathy, BMI, triglyceride and C reactive protein levels.

associated with 5.73-fold increased odds of rapid eGFR decline and a 2.51-fold increased odds of stage 3 CKD [26]. Our findings were consistent with the current body of literature and further indicated that type 2 diabetic patients with normoalbuminuria in early-stage CKD (CKD stage 2) had a ~40% of low ABI prevalence, suggesting the importance to explore the relation of low ABI and eGFR in normoalbuminuric diabetic patients.

In the DEMAND study, 20.5% of 11,315 subjects with reported decreased kidney function were found to be normoalbuminuric [27]. In the NEFRON survey, more than half (55%) of all diabetic patients with an eGFR <60 ml/min per 1.73 m2 had normoalbuminuria and most (98%) of them were also reported as being persistently normoalbuminuric [28]. For healthy nondiabetic individuals, the rate of decline in GFR with age has been reported to range between 0.6 and 1.0 mL/min/1.73 $m^2 \cdot year^{-1}$ when estimated from serum creatinine or creatinine clearance [29,30,31]. However, Richard J. Macisaac et al showed that the rate of decline in renal function for normoalbuminuric patients (-4.6 ± 1.0 mL/min/1.73 $m^2 \cdot year^{-1}$) was clearly greater than that related to aging alone and was not different to that observed for micro- and macroalbuminuric (-2.8 ± 1.0, and -3.0 ± 0.7 mL/min/1.73 $m^2 \cdot year^{-1}$) patients [32]. Similar to our previous and other studies [3,4,33], we found that 60.5% of the overall 1117 type 2 diabetic participants were normoalbuminuric and, among them the prevalence of early-stage CKD defined by CKD-EPI eGFR 60–89 ml/min per 1.73 m^2 was 19.2%. Low ABI was associated with an approximate 3-fold greater risk of eGFR lower than 90 in bivariate logistic regression analysis, and remained significantly associated with a 2.2 fold risk for early-stage CKD after adjusting traditional chronic kidney disease risk factors. Together these findings suggest that patients with type 2 diabetes can commonly progress to a significant degree of renal impairment while remaining normoalbuminuric. Our findings further support the hypothesis that the renal manifestation of systemic arteriosclerosis can be exist in a very early stage of CKD.

In a recent study, typical glomerular changes of diabetic nephropathy were observed in 22 of 23 subjects (mean eGFR 31 mL/min/1.73 m^2) with micro- or macroalbuminuria compared with 3 of 8 subjects with normoalbuminuria [34]. By contrast, predominantly interstitial or vascular changes were seen in only 1 of 23 subjects with micro- or macroalbuminuria compared with 3 of 8 normoalbuminuric subjects. Varying degrees of arteriosclerosis were seen in seven of eight subjects with normoalbuminuria. Consistent with the previous data

[10,35], our study demonstrated that the abnormal ABI, but not other diabetic microvascular disease such as diabetic retinopathy and neuropathy, was significantly associated with mildly decreased eGFR after adjusting for other risk factors. Further studies will be needed to clarify the initial renal structural changes in early-stage CKD and explore the exact role of atherosclerosis in CKD without normoalbuminuria. An important methodological strength of the current study, as opposed to other previous population-based studies, was concerning and therefore excluding the patients with medications of the renin-angiotensin-aldosterone system inhibitors which have been demonstrated by multiple trials that can decrease proteinuria, preserve renal function, hence confuse the results [36,37,38]. Another strength of the study was that we determined the entire spectrum of patients in early-stage CKD independent of albuminuria, who were easily to be ignored in clinical work but deserved to be pay more attention to by physicians. The main limitation was the cross-sectional design that did not allow us to examine the effect of low ABI on the development of CKD. Thus, prospective studies of a larger sample should be conducted and the primary outcome of end stage renal disease incidence should be used. Other possible limitations included the incomplete records of hypoglycemia, and the hospital-based study cohort making selection bias a potential confounding factor. However, the imbalance of HbA1c levels between the two groups can also be explained by the fact that patients with different eGFR levels had diverse therapeutic regimen.

In summary, the prevalence and the important role of low ABI in early-stage CKD patients of type 2 diabetes who have normoalbuminuria have been well defined in our study. The results imply that low ABI level contributes to the risk of various degrees of renal atherosclerosis, and that we should pay much more attention to the patients who have only mildly decreased eGFR and normoalbuminuria but have already had a low ABI in clinic work and consider the preventive therapy in early stage of CKD.

Author Contributions

Conceived and designed the experiments: LXL HL XHD DTW. Performed the experiments: CFJ JL YR XCF GXW. Analyzed the data: XHD DTW YS. Contributed reagents/materials/analysis tools: XHD DTW CFJ JL YS. Contributed to the writing of the manuscript: XHD DTW HL LXL.

References

1. Bi Y, Xu Y, Ning G (2014) Prevalence of diabetes in Chinese adults–reply. JAMA 311: 200–201.

2. Reutens AT, Atkins RC (2011) Epidemiology of diabetic nephropathy. Contrib Nephrol 170: 1–7.

3. Dong X, He M, Song X, Lu B, Yang Y, et al. (2007) Performance and comparison of the Cockcroft-Gault and simplified Modification of Diet in Renal Disease formulae in estimating glomerular filtration rate in a Chinese Type 2 diabetic population. Diabet Med 24: 1482–1486.

4. Lou QL, Ouyang XJ, Gu LB, Mo YZ, Ma R, et al. (2012) Chronic kidney disease and associated cardiovascular risk factors in chinese with type 2 diabetes. Diabetes Metab J 36: 433–442.

5. Karalliedde J, Viberti G (2010) Proteinuria in diabetes: bystander or pathway to cardiorenal disease? J Am Soc Nephrol 21: 2020–2027.

6. Fowkes FG, Murray GD, Butcher I, Heald CL, Lee RJ, et al. (2008) Ankle brachial index combined with Framingham Risk Score to predict cardiovascular events and mortality: a meta-analysis. JAMA 300: 197–208.

7. O'Hare AM, Rodriguez RA, Bacchetti P (2005) Low ankle-brachial index associated with rise in creatinine level over time: results from the atherosclerosis risk in communities study. Arch Intern Med 165: 1481–1485.

8. de Vinuesa SG, Ortega M, Martinez P, Goicoechea M, Campdera FG, et al. (2005) Subclinical peripheral arterial disease in patients with chronic kidney disease: prevalence and related risk factors. Kidney Int Suppl: S44–S47.

9. Guerrero A, Montes R, Munoz-Terol J, Gil-Peralta A, Toro J, et al. (2006) Peripheral arterial disease in patients with stages IV and V chronic renal failure. Nephrol Dial Transplant 21: 3525–3531.

10. Yamashita T, Makino H, Nakatani R, Ohata Y, Miyamoto Y, et al. (2013) Renal insufficiency without albuminuria is associated with peripheral artery atherosclerosis and lipid metabolism disorders in patients with type 2 diabetes. J Atheroscler Thromb 20: 790–797.

11. Xu B, Dai M, Li M, Sun K, Zhang J, et al. (2014) Low-grade albuminuria is associated with peripheral artery disease in Chinese diabetic patients. Atherosclerosis 232: 285–288.

12. (2002) K/DOQI clinical practice guidelines for chronic kidney disease: evaluation, classification, and stratification. Am J Kidney Dis 39: S1–S266.

13. Matsushita K, van der Velde M, Astor BC, Woodward M, Levey AS, et al. (2010) Association of estimated glomerular filtration rate and albuminuria with all-cause and cardiovascular mortality in general population cohorts: a collaborative meta-analysis. Lancet 375: 2073–2081.

14. Van Biesen W, De Bacquer D, Verbeke F, Delanghe J, Lameire N, et al. (2007) The glomerular filtration rate in an apparently healthy population and its relation with cardiovascular mortality during 10 years. Eur Heart J 28: 478–483.

15. (2013) Standards of medical care in diabetes–2013. Diabetes Care 36 Suppl 1: S11–S66.

16. Murgatroyd H, Ellingford A, Cox A, Binnie M, Ellis JD, et al. (2004) Effect of mydriasis and different field strategies on digital image screening of diabetic eye disease. Br J Ophthalmol 88: 920–924.

17. Scanlon PH, Foy C, Malhotra R, Aldington SJ (2005) The influence of age, duration of diabetes, cataract, and pupil size on image quality in digital photographic retinal screening. Diabetes Care 28: 2448–2453.

18. (1992) Guidelines in electrodiagnostic medicine. American Association of Electrodiagnostic Medicine. Muscle Nerve 15: 229–253.

19. Levey AS, Stevens LA, Schmid CH, Zhang YL, Castro AR, et al. (2009) A new equation to estimate glomerular filtration rate. Ann Intern Med 150: 604–612.

20. Hirsch AT, Haskal ZJ, Hertzer NR, Bakal CW, Creager MA, et al. (2006) ACC/AHA 2005 Practice Guidelines for the management of patients with peripheral arterial disease (lower extremity, renal, mesenteric, and abdominal aortic): a collaborative report from the American Association for Vascular Surgery/Society for Vascular Surgery, Society for Cardiovascular Angiography and Interventions, Society for Vascular Medicine and Biology, Society of Interventional Radiology, and the ACC/AHA Task Force on Practice Guidelines (Writing Committee to Develop Guidelines for the Management of Patients With Peripheral Arterial Disease): endorsed by the American Association of Cardiovascular and Pulmonary Rehabilitation; National Heart, Lung, and Blood Institute; Society for Vascular Nursing; TransAtlantic Inter-Society Consensus; and Vascular Disease Foundation. Circulation 113: e463–e654.

21. Lee AJ, Price JF, Russell MJ, Smith FB, van Wijk MC, et al. (2004) Improved prediction of fatal myocardial infarction using the ankle brachial index in addition to conventional risk factors: the Edinburgh Artery Study. Circulation 110: 3075–3080.

22. Althouse AD, Abbott JD, Forker AD, Bertolet M, Barinas-Mitchell E, et al. (2014) Risk Factors for Incident Peripheral Arterial Disease in Type 2 Diabetes: Results From the Bypass Angioplasty Revascularization Investigation 2 Diabetes Trial. Diabetes Care.

23. Banerjee S, Vinas A, Mohammad A, Hadidi O, Thomas R, et al. (2014) Significance of an Abnormal Ankle-Brachial Index in Patients With Established Coronary Artery Disease With and Without Associated Diabetes Mellitus. Am J Cardiol.

24. Kshirsagar AV, Coresh J, Brancati F, Colindres RE (2004) Ankle brachial index independently predicts early kidney disease. Ren Fail 26: 433–443.

25. Turner ST, Rule AD, Schwartz GL, Kullo IJ, Mosley TH, et al. (2011) Risk factor profile for chronic kidney disease is similar to risk factor profile for small artery disease. J Hypertens 29: 1796–1801.

26. Foster MC, Ghuman N, Hwang SJ, Murabito JM, Fox CS (2013) Low ankle-brachial index and the development of rapid estimated GFR decline and CKD. Am J Kidney Dis 61: 204–210.

27. Dwyer JP, Parving HH, Hunsicker LG, Ravid M, Remuzzi G, et al. (2012) Renal Dysfunction in the Presence of Normoalbuminuria in Type 2 Diabetes: Results from the DEMAND Study. Cardiorenal Med 2: 1–10.

28. Thomas MC, Macisaac RJ, Jerums G, Weekes A, Moran J, et al. (2009) Nonalbuminuric renal impairment in type 2 diabetic patients and in the general population (national evaluation of the frequency of renal impairment co.-existing with NIDDM [NEFRON] 11). Diabetes Care 32: 1497–1502.

29. Anderson S, Brenner BM (1986) Effects of aging on the renal glomerulus. Am J Med 80: 435–442.

30. Clase CM, Garg AX, Kiberd BA (2002) Prevalence of low glomerular filtration rate in nondiabetic Americans: Third National Health and Nutrition Examination Survey (NHANES III). J Am Soc Nephrol 13: 1338–1349.

31. Kesteloot H, Joossens JV (1996) On the determinants of the creatinine clearance: a population study. J Hum Hypertens 10: 245–249.

32. MacIsaac RJ, Tsalamandris C, Panagiotopoulos S, Smith TJ, McNeil KJ, et al. (2004) Nonalbuminuric renal insufficiency in type 2 diabetes. Diabetes Care 27: 195–200.

33. Jia W, Gao X, Pang C, Hou X, Bao Y, et al. (2009) Prevalence and risk factors of albuminuria and chronic kidney disease in Chinese population with type 2 diabetes and impaired glucose regulation: Shanghai diabetic complications study (SHDCS). Nephrol Dial Transplant 24: 3724–3731.

34. Ekinci EI, Jerums G, Skene A, Crammer P, Power D, et al. (2013) Renal structure in normoalbuminuric and albuminuric patients with type 2 diabetes and impaired renal function. Diabetes Care 36: 3620–3626.

35. Retnakaran R, Cull CA, Thorne KI, Adler AI, Holman RR (2006) Risk factors for renal dysfunction in type 2 diabetes: U.K. Prospective Diabetes Study 74. Diabetes 55: 1832–1839.

36. Lewis EJ, Hunsicker LG, Bain RP, Rohde RD (1993) The effect of angiotensin-converting-enzyme inhibition on diabetic nephropathy. The Collaborative Study Group. N Engl J Med 329: 1456–1462.

37. Lewis EJ, Hunsicker LG, Clarke WR, Berl T, Pohl MA, et al. (2001) Renoprotective effect of the angiotensin-receptor antagonist irbesartan in patients with nephropathy due to type 2 diabetes. N Engl J Med 345: 851–860.

38. Parving HH, Lehnert H, Brochner-Mortensen J, Gomis R, Andersen S, et al. (2001) The effect of irbesartan on the development of diabetic nephropathy in patients with type 2 diabetes. N Engl J Med 345: 870–878.

16

Multidisciplinary Predialysis Education Reduced the Inpatient and Total Medical Costs of the First 6 Months of Dialysis in Incident Hemodialysis Patients

Yu-Jen Yu[1,2,◊], I-Wen Wu[1,2,◊], Chun-Yu Huang[3], Kuang-Hung Hsu[3], Chin-Chan Lee[1,2], Chio-Yin Sun[1,2], Heng-Jung Hsu[1,2], Mai-Szu Wu[1,4,5]*

1 Department of Nephrology, Chang Gung Memorial Hospital, Keelung, Taiwan, **2** College of Medicine, Chang Gung University, Tao-Yuan, Taiwan, **3** Laboratory for Epidemiology, Department of Health Care Management, Chang Gung University, Tao-Yuan, Taiwan, **4** Division of Nephrology, Taipei Medical University Hospital, Taipei, Taiwan, **5** School of Medicine, Taipei Medical University, Taipei, Taiwan

Abstract

Background: The multidisciplinary pre-dialysis education (MPE) retards renal progression, reduce incidence of dialysis and mortality of CKD patients. However, the financial benefit of this intervention on patients starting hemodialysis has not yet been evaluated in prospective and randomized trial.

Methods: We studied the medical expenditure and utilization incurred in the first 6 months of dialysis initiation in 425 incident hemodialysis patients who were randomized into MPE and non-MPE groups before reaching end-stage renal disease. The content of the MPE was standardized in accordance with the National Kidney Foundation Dialysis Outcomes Quality Initiative guidelines.

Results: The mean age of study patients was 63.8 ± 13.2 years, and 221 (49.7%) of them were men. The mean serum creatinine level and estimated glomerular filtration rate was 6.1 ± 4.0 mg/dL and 7.6 ± 2.9 mL·min^{-1}·1.73 m^{-2}, respectively, at dialysis initiation. MPE patients tended to have lower total medical cost in the first 6 months after hemodialysis initiation (9147.6 ± 0.1 USD/patient vs. 11190.6 ± 0.1 USD/patient, $p = 0.003$), fewer in numbers [0 (1) vs. 1 (2), $p < 0.001$] and length of hospitalization [0 (15) vs. 8 (27) days, $p < 0.001$], and also lower inpatient cost [0 (2617.4) vs. 1559,4 (5019.6) USD/patient, $p < 0.001$] than non-MPE patients, principally owing to reduced cardiovascular hospitalization and vascular access–related surgeries. The decreased inpatient and total medical cost associated with MPE were independent of patients' demographic characteristics, concomitant disease, baseline biochemistry and use of double-lumen catheter at initiation of hemodialysis.

Conclusions: Participation of multidisciplinary education in pre-dialysis period was independently associated with reduction in the inpatient and total medical expenditures of the first 6 months post-dialysis owing to decreased inpatient service utilization secondary to cardiovascular causes and vascular access–related surgeries.

Editor: Emmanuel A. Burdmann, University of Sao Paulo Medical School, Brazil

Funding: Chang Gung Memorial Hospital at Keelung provided grant support for this research (CMRPG260323/CMRPG2A0422). The funder had no role in study design, data collection and analysis, decision to publish, or preparation of the manuscript.

Competing Interests: The authors have declared that no competing interests exist.

* Email: maiszuwu@gmail.com

◊ These authors contributed equally to this work.

Introduction

The number of patients worldwide with chronic kidney disease (CKD) and end-stage renal disease (ESRD) being treated with renal replacement therapy has been continuously increasing in recent years, with a 7% rate of increase per year [1]. Aging and type 2 diabetes mellitus are the two most important factors [2]. Taiwan is the leading country in terms of ESRD prevalence, with a rate of 2447 per million population [3]. The implementation of National Health Insurance (NHI) has helped drive the growth of the ESRD populations in Taiwan [4]. However, the official prohibition of the use of aristolochic acid–containing herbs and the introduction of the nationwide CKD Preventive Project with a multidisciplinary care program have proved their effectiveness in decreasing the incidence of dialysis, and mortality and medical costs of CKD patients [5]. However, the financial benefit of this intervention has not yet been evaluated in prospective and randomized manner on patients starting hemodialysis.

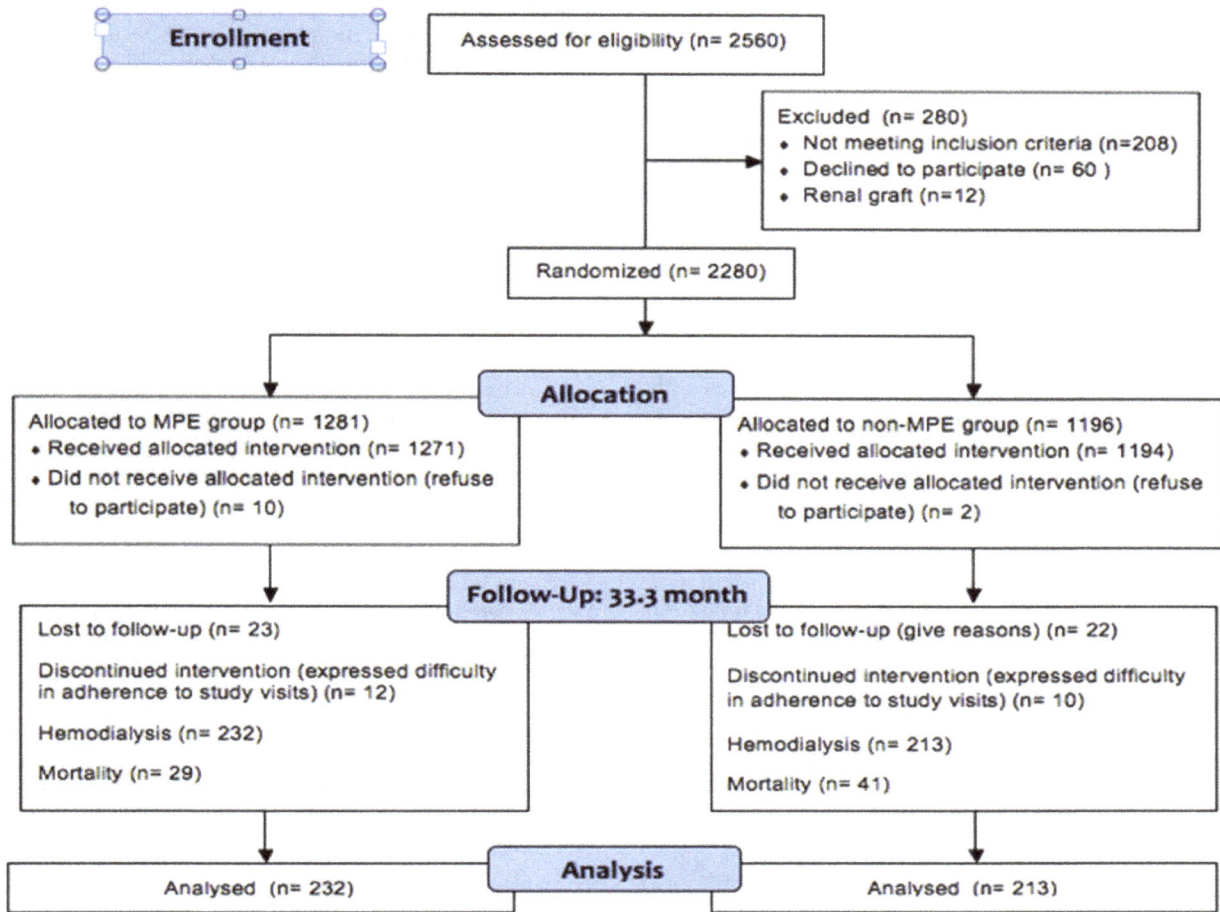

Figure 1. Enrolment scheme and patient status. MPE: multidisciplinary predialysis education.

High ESRD prevalence constitutes a large economic burden for the patient, society, and the country. Renal insufficiency represents a status of increased cardiovascular disease risk, comorbidities, and mortality [6], demanding high medical expenditures and healthcare utilization [1]. The cost for ESRD has increased to $34.3 billion, accounting for 6.3% of the total Medicare budget according to the 2013 US Renal Data System Annual Data Report [7]. Similarly, in Taiwan, the annual dialysis costs have accounted for 5.0–7.52% of the total budget of the NHI in recent years [8]. Optimal and efficient treatment strategies to combat the high prevalence of ESRD and its high cost of care are thus urgently needed.

Predialysis education can decrease the ESRD incidence and mortality in the first year of dialysis [9,10]. Nephrology-based care has also significantly improved the clinical outcomes of CKD patients in both the predialysis and postdialysis periods [11,12], especially in type 2 diabetes patients [13,14]. It has been associated with better biochemical variables, shorter hospitalization length, a higher percentage of elective construction of the arteriovenous fistula, and the availability of alternative dialysis modality [15]. Our previous controlled cohort study has confirmed that multidisciplinary predialysis education (MPE) based on the National Kidney Foundation Dialysis Outcomes Quality Initiative (NKF/DOQI) guidelines provides a better outcome with a significantly reduced incidence of ESRD and all-cause mortality [16]. The MPE program has effectively improved the quality of

pre-ESRD care, increased patients' self-care ability, and has retarded renal progression and reduced morbidities in late-stage CKD patients [17]. Multidisciplinary predialysis team care was found to decreased service utilization and saved medical costs in the 6 months before dialysis initiation and at dialysis initiation, being secondary to the early preparation of vascular access and the lack of hospitalization at dialysis initiation [18]. Predialysis nephrology–based care has been associated with reduced costs in elderly patients after the initiation of dialysis [19]. Most of these controlled or randomized trials have used the renal or patient outcome as their endpoints. However, randomized studies to evaluate the cost-saving effect of MPE in the post-dialysis period have been seldom reported to date.

Most of the medical costs associated with caring for CKD patients are incurred for the treatment of comorbidities, hospitalization, and transition into ESRD [20]. After dialysis initiation, most of the adverse outcomes occurred within the first year of hemodialysis. The all-cause mortality and mortality due to cardiovascular disease or other causes is found to peaked in the second month after initiation, and then decreased [20]. It is unclear whether the MPE program could extend the financial benefit to after the initiation of dialysis and reduces the medical costs during the first 6 months of hemodialysis initiation. We hypothesize that knowledge acquisition from MPE in the predialysis period may have a "legacy effect" during the postdialysis period. This beneficial effect of MPE may result in differences in disease patterns, reduced medical expenditure and utilization, and reduced medical costs in the immediate post-dialysis period. To further clarify this issue, we studied the medical expenditure and utilization incurred during the first 6 months of dialysis initiation in 425 incident hemodialysis patients who were randomized into MPE and non-MPE groups before reaching ESRD.

Materials and Methods

Patient cohort and settings The protocol for this trial and supporting CONSORT checklist are available as supporting information; see Checklist S1 and Protocol S1. This is an analysis of a subset population from our previously reported randomized cohort (Clinical Trials.gov NCT00644046) [16]. Briefly, the cohort includes predialysis CKD patients with an estimated glomerular filtration rate (eGFR) of <60 mL·min^{-1}·1.73 m^{-2} (determined by using the Modification of Diet in Renal Disease equation) who visited the nephrology outpatient clinics of the Department of Nephrology, Chang Gung Memorial Hospital, Keelung, from July 2007 and followed up to June 30, 2011. Patients aged 18–80 years and without renal graft failure were included in the study after obtaining informed consent from them. A total of 2280 patients were enrolled in the study and were randomly divided into the MPE group and the non-MPE group by using a random table at study entry. Four hundred and five patients reached ESRD needing hemodialysis after a mean follow-up of 33 ± 2.6 months (232 patients in the MPE group and 213 patients in the non-MPE group, as shown in Figure 1). The medical expenditure and utilization in the first 6 months of initiation of hemodialysis in these 425 patients were accurately recorded and compared between MPE and non-MPE patients. Medical service utilization was calculated as the frequency of outpatient visits and the frequency and length of hospitalization. Outpatient visits were categorized as outpatient services, preventive care (e.g., influenza vaccination and dietary counseling), and emergency services. Medical service expenditures included outpatient expenditures (all costs including physicians' and nursing fees, examinations, surgery, and medication) and inpatient expenditures (all costs including laboratory testing, imaging testing, medications, surgery and consulting, ward and administrative, nasogastric tube feeding, and hemodialysis fees). The expenditures for each participant were totaled to compute the sum of ambulatory and inpatient medical service utilization costs and expenditures. The analysis of costs in this study only included those medical costs for which our hospitals made reimbursement claims to the NHI. The salaries, overheads, and administrative costs of the care team were not included. This study was approved by the ethics committee of

Table 1. baseline characteristics of study patients.

Parameter	MPE group (n = 232)	Non-MPE group (n = 213)	p
Age, years	67.5±11.4	61.8±15.0	<0.001
Male, n (%)	116 (50.0%)	105 (49.3%)	0.882
Diabetes, n (%)	153 (65.9%)	127 (59.6%)	0.168
Hypertension, n (%)	202 (87.1%)	171 (80.3%)	0.052
Coronary artery disease, n (%)	30 (12.9%)	41 (19.2%)	0.069
Cerebrovascular disease, n (%)	30 (12.9%)	29 (13.6%)	0.832
Gout, n (%)	61 (26.3%)	44 (20.7%)	0.162
eGFR, ml/min	7.49±3.1	7.87±3.6	0.228
Serum albumin, mg/dL	3.1±0.7	3.2±0.8	0.062
Hemoglobin, g/dL	9.4±1.6	9.0±2.7	0.100
Urea reduction rate, %	0.74±0.7	0.76±0.8	0.464
Kt/V, Daugirdas	1.66±0.36	1.71±0.38	0.509
nPCR, g/Kg/day	1.13±0.37	1.20±0.32	0.371
Systolic blood pressure, mmHg	144.3±22.7	147.2±25.9	0.221
Primary renal disease			0.135
Diabetes, n (%)	139 (59.9%)	118 (55.4%)	
Hypertension, n (%)	6 (2.6%)	5 (2.3%)	
Chronic glomerulonephritis, n %	16 (6.9%)	13 (6.1%)	
Others, n %	71 (30.6%)	77 (36.2%)	
Education levels			0.650
Below elementary	42 (18.1%)	3 (1.4%)	
Elementary	151 (65.1%)	207 (97.2%)	
High school	31 (13.4%)	3 (1.4%)	
University	8 (3.4%)	0 (0%)	
Vascular access at initiation of dialysis			
Patients with vascular access created, n (%)	143 (61.6%)	100 (46.9%)	0.002
Patients without insertion of double-lumen catheter, n (%)	129 (55.6%)	96 (45.1%)	0.029

Abbreviation: eGFR, estimated glomerular filtration rate; nPCR, normalized protein catabolic rate.

Multidisciplinary Predialysis Education Reduced the Inpatient and Total Medical Costs...

137

the institutional review board of Chang Gung Memorial Hospital (Number: 100-0040A3, 96-0408B) and was conducted according to the principles expressed in the Declaration of Helsinki. All patients provided written informed consent. The registration of our cohort at Clinical Trials.gov was delayed by administrative issues (set up of Core Lab, employment of research assistance). The authors confirm that all ongoing and related trials for this drug/intervention were registered.

MPE

The MPE program was implemented in May 2006 at the Keelung Center. The team comprised a nurse for case management, social workers, dietitians, hemodialysis, peritoneal dialysis patient volunteers and 10 nephrologists. The program consisted of an integrated course involving individual lectures on renal health, delivered by the case-management nurse, according to the guidelines given in a standardized instruction booklet. The lectures focused on nutrition, lifestyle, nephrotoxin avoidance, dietary principles, and pharmacological regimens. Furthermore, the case-management nurse contacted the patients to ensure timely follow-up. Standardized interactive educational sessions were periodically conducted wherein all patients were interviewed depending on their CKD stage, determined earlier by using the NKF/DOQI guideline. Stage III or IV CKD patients were followed up every 3 months, and stage V CKD patients were followed up on a monthly basis. For stage III CKD patients, the program consisted of lectures on healthy renal function, the clinical presentation of uremia, risk factors and complications associated with renal progression, and an introduction to the various renal replacement therapies (i.e., hemodialysis, peritoneal dialysis, and renal transplantation). For stage IV CKD patients, the program included discussions on the management of complications associated with CKD, indications of renal replacement therapy, and the evaluation of vascular or peritoneal access. Patients with stage V CKD were monitored for timely initiation of renal replacement therapies, the care of vascular or peritoneal access, dialysis-associated complications, and registration for inclusion in the renal transplantation waiting list. All patients received dietary counseling biannually from a dietitian. In addition, the case-management nurse often contacted the participants by telephone to encourage them to inform their nephrologists of their symptoms and to reinforce the importance of medical visits. The MPE program was discontinued once renal replacement therapies were initiated for these patients.

Customary care

The same group of nephrologists instructed all participants about renal function, the evaluation of laboratory data, and clinical indicators of chronic renal failure, as well as about the strategies for its management and treatment. Furthermore, the nephrologists explained the general principles of hemodialysis and peritoneal dialysis when the patients exhibited an eGFR of < 30 mL·min^{-1}·1.73 m^{-2} (stage IV CKD). All patients were provided with written instructions. The nephrologists evaluated the comorbidity factors influencing each patient's condition before referral to a nurse specializing in hemodialysis or peritoneal dialysis. The nursing staff provided instructions for daily living and explained the criteria used for hemodialysis and peritoneal dialysis selection, and the difference between the two modalities.

Statistical analysis

Descriptive statistics were expressed as the mean (standard deviation) or median (interquartile range). Discrete variables were presented in terms of frequencies and percentages. The normality of numerical variables was tested using the Kolmogorov-Smirnov method, and an appropriate transformation was considered before statistical testing. The Student t-test or Mann-Whitney U-test was applied to compare mean or median values among the groups. The association between categorical variables was analyzed by using the χ^2 test. Multiple linear regression analysis was applied to calculate the unstandardized coefficients associated with MPE in both inpatient and total medical cost. All statistical tests were two-tailed, and a p value < 0.05 was considered to be statistically significant. Data were analyzed by using SPSS 17.0 for Windows XP (SPSS Inc., Chicago, IL, USA).

Results

The mean age of study patients was 63.8 ± 13.2 years, and 221 (49.7%) of them were men. The mean serum creatinine level and eGFR was 6.1 ± 4.0 mg/dL and $7.6 \pm$ mL·min^{-1}·1.73 m^{-2}, respectively, at dialysis initiation. Diabetes mellitus was identified as the leading cause of renal disease in both groups, followed by chronic glomerulonephritis. Table 1 shows the demographic and clinical characteristics of the patients in the MPE and non-MPE

Table 2. Medical utilization and expenditure between groups.

Parameter	MPE group (n = 232)	Non-MPE group (n = 213)	p
No. outpatient visits, times/patient	15.1±11.6	17.9±11.1	0.009
No. of hospitalization, times/patient	0.00 (1.00)	1.00 (2.00)	<0.001*
Frequency of hospitalization, n (%)			<0.001
Never	144 (62.1%)	86 (40.4%)	
1 time	47 (20.2%)	73 (34.2%)	
2 times	31 (13.4%)	30 (14.1%)	
≥3 times	10 (4.3%)	24 (11.3%)	
Length of hospitalization, days/patient	0.00 (15.00)	8.00 (27.00)	<0.001*
Cost of outpatient service, mean, USD/patient	6885.7±5201.2	7491.8±4200.2	0.175
Log cost of inpatient service, mean, USD/patient	3.09±4.02	4.95±4.15	<0.001
Log total cost of medical service, mean, USD/patient	6.75±4.21	8.58±2.43	<0.001

*p value using Mann-Whitney U test.

Table 3. Costs of outpatient service between groups.

Variables	MPE group (n = 232)	Non-MPE group (n = 213)	p
Hemodialysis, laboratory and imagen	6258.8±4647.2	6841.5±3883.1	0.154
Physician fee	94.4±80.1	116.9±93.4	0.007
Medication fee	512.6±120.1	510.8±75.4	0.985
Pharmacist, nursing and administrative fee	19.9±16.4	22.5±17.4	0.107

Costs were expressed in mean ± SD, USD/patient.

groups at the initiation of hemodialysis. These patients received 4 hours of hemodialysis 3 times weekly. Hemodialysis for these patients used single-use hollow-fiber dialyzers equipped with modified cellulose-based, polyamide, or polysulfone membranes. The dialysate used in all patients was a standard ionic composition and bicarbonate-based buffer. Many indices of dialysis adequacy (Urea reduction rate, Kt/V and normalized protein catabolic rate) were similar at baseline for the two groups of patients. However, the MPE group patients were more likely to have permanent vascular access created (61.6% vs. 46.9%, p = 0.002) and less insertion of double-lumen catheter at initiation of hemodialysis (55.6% vs. 45.1%, p = 0.029, Table 1).

MPE patients tended to have lower total medical cost in the first 6 months after hemodialysis initiation (9147.6±0.1 USD/patient vs. 11190.6±0.1 USD/patient, p = 0.003, Table 2). Despite the fewer outpatient visits of MPE patients, the cost of outpatient service did not differ between the groups. Most of the costs of outpatient service were spent for treatment (including hemodialysis, laboratory, and image study; Table 3). However, MPE patients were significantly fewer in numbers [mean (SD) 0.61±0.9 vs. 1.0±1.2, p<0.001; median (IQR) 0 (1) vs. 1 (2), p<0.001] and had shorter lengths [mean (SD) 10.6±21.9 days vs. 19.3±29.3 days, p<0.001; median (IQR) 0 (15) vs. 8 (27) days, p<0.001] of hospitalization than non-MPE patients. Therefore, the medical cost of inpatient service was significantly lower in MPE patients [median 0 (2617.4) or (mean 2261.8±5635.8) USD/patient in MPE patients vs. median 1559, 4 (5019.6) or (mean 3698.8±5540.9) USD/patient in non-MPE patients, respectively, p<0.001, Table 2]. The reduced cost of inpatient service observed in MPE patients was attributed to the reduction in the costs of

physicians, wards, nasogastric feeding, radiology examination, nursing, blood transfusion, hemodialysis, medication, and pharmacist service fees. Most of the costs of inpatient service were spent on hemodialysis treatment in both groups of patients (Table 4). Eighty-eight (37.9%) patients in the MPE group had at least one hospitalization, compared with 127 patients (59.6%) in the non-MPE group (p<0.001). In all first hospitalizations, 66 (75%) patients in the MPE group were admitted to the nephrology ward. Similarly, 94 (74%) of the non-MPE patients were admitted to the nephrology ward at their first hospitalization. Table 5 lists the main causes of the first hospitalization and surgery in both groups of patients. Cardiovascular disease (including uncontrolled hypertension, coronary artery disease, stroke, heart failure, and peripheral artery occlusive disease) was the main cause of first hospitalization in all patients. Participation in the MPE program reduced cardiovascular hospitalization during the first 6 months postdialysis (18.53% vs. 29.58%, p = 0.007). Among all patients, those in the MPE group were more likely to have fewer vascular access related surgeries during the first admission [35 patients (15.09%) vs. 55 (25.82%), p = 0.005]. Most first surgeries were performed for Hickman catheter–related intervention (implantation, exchange, and removal) and arteriovenous fistula/graft–related intervention (creation, thrombectomy, repair, and excision; Table 5).

Participation in MPE was independently associated with reduced inpatient cost and total medical cost in the first 6 months of dialysis initiation by using various adjustment strategies, including demographic characteristics (age and gender) in model 2, concomitant disease (diabetes mellitus and number of comorbidities) in model 3, baseline biochemistry at entry to hemodialysis

Table 4. Log-transformed costs of inpatient service between groups.

Variables	MPE group (n = 232)	Non-MPE group (n = 213)	p*
Physician fee	2.03±2.67	3.28±2.79	<0.001
Ward fee	2.49±3.26	3.99±3.38	<0.001
Laboratory examination fee	5.22±1.32	5.52±1.15	0.126
Nasogastric tube feeding fee	0.56±1.61	1.40±2.36	<0.001
Radiology examination fee	1.17±2.05	1.84±2.29	<0.001
Nursing fee	1.78±2.69	2.83±2.91	<0.001
Surgery fee	1.89±3.82	3.31±4.58	<0.001
Blood transfusion fee	1.04±1.93	1.89±2.39	<0.001
Hemodialysis fee	2.65±3.46	4.13±3.58	<0.001
Medication fee	2.16±2.94	3.45±3.08	<0.001
Pharmacist service fee	1.48±1.98	2.32±2.04	<0.001

Costs were expressed in mean ± SD, USD/patient.

Table 5. Main cause of first hospitalization and surgery.

	MPE group	Non-MPE group
Cause of first hospitalization, n		
Renal-related disease	12 (5.17%)	26 (12.21%)
Cardiovascular disease	43 (18.53%)	63 (29.58%)
Vascular access infection	9 (3.88%)	11 (5.16%)
Acute pulmonary edema	3 (1.29%)	4 (1.88%)
Other	21 (9.05%)	23 (10.8%)
No hospitalization	144 (62.07%)	86 (40.38%)
Cause of first surgery, n		
Hickman catheter related	25 (10.78%)	36 (16.9%)
Arteriovenous fistula/graft related	24 (10.34%)	39 (18.31%)
Limb amputation	2 (0.86%)	3 (1.41%)
Hemothorax/pneumothorax	1 (0.43%)	6 (2.82%)
Other	15 (6.47%)	4 (1.88%)
No surgery	165 (71.12%)	125 (58.69%)

Cardiovascular disease includes uncontrolled hypertension, coronary artery disease, stroke, heart failure, and peripheral artery occlusive disease.

(eGFR, hemoglobin, and serum albumin levels) in model 4 and status of use of double-lumen catheter at initiation of hemodialysis (model 5, Table 6).

Discussion

In this prospective study, we examined the medical expenditure and utilization incurred in the first 6 months of dialysis initiation in 425 incident hemodialysis patients who were randomized into MPE and non-MPE groups before reaching ESRD. We found that participation in a multidisciplinary education program at the predialysis period was associated with reduced inpatient service utilization, reduced inpatient cost, and reduced total medical cost in the first 6 months of hemodialysis. The reduction of cost in inpatient service was attributed to the reduction in cardiovascular disease and vascular access–related surgery during hospitalization. The decreased inpatient cost and total medical cost of service associated with MPE were independent of patients' demographic characteristics, concomitant disease, baseline biochemistry at entry to hemodialysis and use of double-lumen catheter at initiation of

hemodialysis. The findings of the present study provide evidence supporting the implementation of MPE as part of integrative CKD care to combat the high economic burden and financial impact of hemodialysis on patients.

A previous prospective controlled study demonstrated that MPE based on the NKF/DOQI guidelines effectively reduced the incidence of ESRD and all-cause mortality with a significantly reduced overall hospitalization rate among MPE patients [16]. In our study, the delivery of MPE was stopped once the patient started hemodialysis therapy. After the initiation of hemodialysis, all patients received dietary counseling in the hemodialysis room on a monthly basis. On the basis of these assumptions, knowledge acquisition from a multidisciplinary education program in the predialysis period might be one of the factors that influence the disease pattern and health-care utilization in the postdialysis period. The positive effect of MPE in the postdialysis period could be the result of many factors, such as increased knowledge about self-care [17], better diet and fluid control, medication compliance, better preparation of vascular access, the adoption of a healthier lifestyle, and greater awareness about the use of

Table 6. Multiple linear regression analysis of effect of MPE on inpatient and total medical cost.

	Inpatient cost		Total cost	
	Unstandardized Coefficients	**p**	**Unstandardized Coefficients**	**p**
Model 1	−43109.74	0.007	−61289.80	0.003
Model 2	−46226.19	0.005	−60200.11	0.005
Model 3	−44575.46	0.005	−62959.92	0.003
Model 4	−44447.13	0.001	−54490.22	0.013
Model 5	−33826.85	0.029	−52241.43	0.011

Both of the two dependent variables in these models were the log transformation of inpatient costs and total costs.
Model 1: crude.
Model 2: adjusted for age and gender.
Model 3: adjusted for diabetes status and number of comorbidities.
Model 4: adjusted for eGFR, hemoglobin and serum albumin levels at initation of hemodialysis.
Model 5: adjusted for insertion of double-lumen catheter at initiation of hemodialysis.

nephrotoxin. The transition period into ESRD and the first year of dialysis therapy represented the most vulnerable point that demands the highest health-care expenditure and utility in CKD patients [20]. The cost-saving effect of MPE in terms of inpatient and total medical service in this immediate postdialysis period was confirmed by the regression models with the adjustment of different covariates. The total medical cost of the first 6 months of hemodialysis in MPE participants was 18% less than that of nonparticipants (9147.6 USD/patient vs. 11190.6 USD/patient). For a total of 8000 incident hemodialysis patients each year in Taiwan [3], the crude estimation of cost-saving could be up to 16.3 million USD per 6 months if each incident patient was to be provided with the MPE program before reaching ESRD.

MPE is certainly beneficial in lowering the enormous cost for the care of hemodialysis patients. Although the long-term economic impact of MPE has not been studied, the findings of the present study suggest the need for a universal and efficient delivery of multidisciplinary education to all CKD patients as early as possible.

Several studies have reported on the cost-saving effect of MPE in the hospitalization of CKD patients; however, only a few retrospective studies have addressed the financial benefits of MPE in the postdialysis period [18,19]. From this prospective study, we have found that hemodialysis and the diseases associated with this treatment (cardiovascular disease and noninfectious vascular access complication) were responsible for most of the health-care cost incurred in both inpatient and outpatient services (Tables 3 and 4). Taking into account the beneficial effect of MPE in reducing renal progression [17], the incidence of ESRD [16], and cardiovascular hospitalization and vascular access surgery in the postdialysis period in our study, the implementation of MPE could result in an overall reduction in the medical utilization and expenditure of CKD patients. Similarly, Wei et al., in their retrospective observational study, found that participants in the CKD care program had lower medical costs at dialysis initiation and lower medical cost for the total period of observation than nonparticipants because of the early preparation of vascular access and the lack of hospitalization at dialysis initiation [18]. A retrospective observational study described fewer hospital days and lower total health-care costs during the year after dialysis initiation in patients receiving predialysis nephrology care [19]. We have reported a reduction in the 1-year hospitalization rate (2.8% vs. 16.4%) in recipients of MPE in a controlled prospective cohort. However, the reason for hospitalization for these patients did not differ significantly between them [16]. In a 3-year prospective study, participation in multidisciplinary care was associated with a 40% reduction in the risk of infection-related hospitalization in the predialysis period [21]. A propensity score matched cohort study found that MPE participants had less unplanned urgent dialysis, shorter hospital days, and a lower incidence of cardiovascular events than non-MPE patients during the observation period [22]. A novel finding of our study was that patients with MPE had reduced cardiovascular-related hospitalization in their postdialysis period. This finding could possibly be attributed to better control of cardiovascular risk factors, better medical adherence, fluid control, and compliance with dietary restriction in the postdialysis period with a prior acquisition of renal knowledge.

Our study included a comprehensive analysis of medical service utilization and expenditures with detailed information about outpatient and inpatient costs in patients with comparable baseline characteristics derived from a randomized cohort. The delivery of MPE was standardized according to the NKF/DOQI guidelines. A single nurse conducted the MPE program for all patients to limit interpersonal variability. This single-center study has been conducted in a university-afflicted teaching hospital. All enrolled participants were patients who visited the nephrology outpatient clinics of Chang Gung Memorial Hospital at Keelung and underwent dialysis treatment at the hemodialysis unit of the same hospital. This hospital is a group practice institution comprised 10 nephrologists and only one hemodialysis unit. Furthermore, variation within dialysis units did not exist, because the single hemodialysis unit setting. In this group practice setting, all nephrologists followed the same institutional regulation. All nephrologists were subject to the same criteria of reimbursement under a single NHI system of government of Taiwan. These 10 nephrologists took care of all renal patients at outpatient and inpatient departments. The same group of 10 nephrologists instructed the MPE and non-MPE patients at their predialysis education and also continuous their medical care in the post-dialysis period at our hemodialysis unit. For these reasons, confounding effects by practice pattern of individual nephrologists might be neglected. Despite the several advantages of MPE presented in our investigation, several limitations should be addressed. First, the study represented a secondary cost analysis of a subset of patients who started hemodialysis and were randomized into MPE and non-MPE groups before reaching ESRD. Second, patients who had died before reaching ESRD were excluded. It was unclear how MPE could influence the postdialysis health-care expenditure and utility costs of these critically ill patients. Third, the age of patients in the two groups was not comparable at the baseline. However, despite the older age of the MPE patients, the outcome of interest was consistently better than that of the non-MPE patients. In addition, the adjustment for age in the regression model has indicated no significance of this factor in our outcome. Finally, although this study examined the economic impact of MPE for the first 6 months of dialysis, its long-term effect remains unclear. Further investigations with a large-scale population, including other treatment modalities (peritoneal dialysis or renal transplantation) and a longer duration would be needed to demonstrate the cost benefit of MPE for an extended period.

In conclusion, in this prospective study, we demonstrated the lowered inpatient and total medical costs in the first 6 months postdialysis in patients receiving the MPE program. This cost reduction was attributed to decreased inpatient service utilization, and principally concerning services used because of cardiovascular causes and vascular access–related surgeries. This reduction in cost was independent of the patients' demographic characteristics, concomitant disease, baseline biochemistry and status of use of double-lumen catheter at entry to hemodialysis. This valuable information confirmed the legacy effect of the MPE program on the economic outcome in the postdialysis period. Although the optimal dose and duration of MPE remains debated, an efficient and universal delivery of multidisciplinary education should be considered as part of the integrative care of CKD patients. This simple strategy could be an ideal resolution to the problem of the increasing financial burden of renal failure worldwide.

Author Contributions

Conceived and designed the experiments: YJU IWW MSW. Performed the experiments: YJU IWW. Analyzed the data: IWW CYH KHH. Contributed reagents/materials/analysis tools: YJU IWW CCL CYS HJH. Wrote the paper: YJU IWW.

References

1. Lysaght MJ (2002) Maintenance dialysis population dynamics: current trends and long-term implications. J Am Soc Nephrol 13 Suppl 1: S37–40.
2. Meguid El Nahas A, Bello AK (2005) Chronic kidney disease: the global challenge. Lancet 365: 331–340.
3. Wu MS, Wu IW, Shih CP, Hsu KH (2011) Establishing a platform for battling end-stage renal disease and continuing quality improvement in dialysis therapy in Taiwan - Taiwan Renal Registry Data System (TWRDS). Acta Nephrologica 25: 148–153.
4. Yang WC, Hwang SJ, Taiwan Society of Nephrology (2008) Incidence, prevalence and mortality trends of dialysis end-stage renal disease in Taiwan from 1990 to 2001: the impact of national health insurance. Nephrol Dial Transplant 23: 3977–3982.
5. Hwang SJ, Tsai JC, Chen HC (2010) Epidemiology, impact and preventive care of chronic kidney disease in Taiwan. Nephrology (Carlton) 15 Suppl 2: 3–9.
6. Muntner P, He J, Hamm L, Loria C, Whelton PK (2002) Renal insufficiency and subsequent death resulting from cardiovascular disease in the United States. J Am Soc Nephrol 13: 745–753.
7. Collins AJ, Foley RN, Chavers B, Gilbertson D, Herzog C, et al. (2014) US Renal Data System 2013 Annual Data Report. Am J Kidney Dis 63: A7.
8. Department of Health. National Health Insurance Annual Statistical Report 2012. Taiwan: Department of Health, 2014. Available: http://www.nhi.gov.tw. Accessed 2014 September 2.
9. Goldstein M, Yassa T, Dacouris N, McFarlane P (2004) Multidisciplinary predialysis care and morbidity and mortality of patients on dialysis. Am J Kidney Dis 44: 706–714.
10. Devins GM, Mendelssohn DC, Barre PE, Taub K, Binik YM (2005) Predialysis psychoeducational intervention extends survival in CKD: a 20-year follow-up. Am J Kidney Dis 46: 1088–1098.
11. Bradbury BD, Fissell RB, Albert JM, Anthony MS, Critchlow CW, et al. (2007) Predictors of early mortality among incident US hemodialysis patients in the Dialysis Outcomes and Practice Patterns Study (DOPPS). Clin J Am Soc Nephrol 2: 89–99.
12. Jungers P, Massy ZA, Nguyen-Khoa T, Choukroun G, Robino C, et al. (2001) Longer duration of predialysis nephrological care is associated with improved long-term survival of dialysis patients. Nephrol Dial Transplant 16: 2357–2364.
13. Wu MS, Lin CL, Chang CT, Wu CH, Huang JY, et al. (2003) Improvement in clinical outcome by early nephrology referral in type II diabetics on maintenance peritoneal dialysis. Perit Dial Int 23: 39–45.
14. Tseng CL, Kern EF, Miller DR, Tiwari A, Maney M, et al. (2008) Survival benefit of nephrologic care in patients with diabetes mellitus and chronic kidney disease. Arch Intern Med 168: 55–62.
15. Dogan E, Erkoc R, Sayarlioglu H, Durmus A, Topal C (2005) Effects of late referral to a nephrologist in patients with chronic renal failure. Nephrology (Carlton) 10: 516–519.
16. Wu IW, Wang SY, Hsu KH, Lee CC, Sun CY, et al. (2009) Multidisciplinary predialysis education decreases the incidence of dialysis and reduces mortality–a controlled cohort study based on the NKF/DOQI guidelines. Nephrol Dial Transplant 24: 3426–3433.
17. Chen SH, Tsai YF, Sun CY, Wu IW, Lee CC, et al. (2011) The impact of self-management support on the progression of chronic kidney disease–a prospective randomized controlled trial. Nephrol Dial Transplant 26: 3560–3566.
18. Wei SY, Chang YY, Mau LW, Lin MY, Chiu HC, et al. (2010) Chronic kidney disease care program improves quality of pre-end-stage renal disease care and reduces medical costs. Nephrology (Carlton) 15: 108–115.
19. Stroupe KT, Fischer MJ, Kaufman JS, O'Hare AM, Sohn MW, et al. (2011) Predialysis nephrology care and costs in elderly patients initiating dialysis. Med Care 49: 248–256.
20. U.S. Renal Data System, USRDS 2013. Annual Data Report: Atlas of Chronic Kidney Disease and End-Stage Renal Disease in the United States, National Institutes of Health, National Institute of Diabetes and Digestive and Kidney Diseases, Bethesda, MD, 2013.
21. Chen YR, Yang Y, Wang SC, Chiu PF, Chou WY, et al. (2013) Effectiveness of multidisciplinary care for chronic kidney disease in Taiwan: a 3-year prospective cohort study. Nephrol Dial Transplant 28: 671–682.
22. Cho EJ, Park HC, Yoon HB, Ju KD, Kim H, et al. (2012) Effect of multidisciplinary pre-dialysis education in advanced chronic kidney disease: Propensity score matched cohort analysis. Nephrology (Carlton) 17: 472–479.

17

Fluctuation between Fasting and 2-H Postload Glucose State Is Associated with Glomerular Hyperfiltration in Newly Diagnosed Diabetes Patients with HbA1c < 7%

Xinguo Hou[1], Chuan Wang[1], Shaoyuan Wang[2], Weifang Yang[2], Zeqiang Ma[3], Yulian Wang[4], Chengqiao Li[4], Mei Li[4], Xiuping Zhang[5], Xiangmin Zhao[5], Yu Sun[1], Jun Song[1], Peng Lin[1], Kai Liang[1], Lei Gong[1], Meijian Wang[1], Fuqiang Liu[1], Wenjuan Li[1], Fei Yan[1], Junpeng Yang[1], Lingshu Wang[1], Meng Tian[1], Jidong Liu[1], Ruxing Zhao[1], Shihong Chen[6], Li Chen[1]*

1 Department of Endocrinology of Qilu Hospital, Shandong University, Jinan, Shandong, China, 2 Lukang Hospital of Jining, Jining, Shandong, China, 3 China National Heavy Duty Truck Group Corporation Hospital, Jinan, Shandong, China, 4 Department of Endocrinology, Second People's Hospital of Jining, Jining, Shandong, China, 5 Shantui Community Health Center, Jining, Shandong, China, 6 Department of Endocrinology, the Second Hospital of Shandong University, Jinan, Shandong, China

Abstract

Objective: To investigate whether fluctuations between the fasting and 2-h postload glucose ([2-hPBG]-fasting blood glucose [FBG]) states are associated with glomerular hyperfiltration (GHF) in middle-aged and elderly Chinese patients with newly diagnosed diabetes.

Design and Methods: In this study, we included 679 newly diagnosed diabetes patients who were ≥40 years old. All the subjects were divided into two groups; those with HbA1c<7% and ≥7%. The Chronic Kidney Disease Epidemiology Collaboration (CKD-EPI) equation was used to estimate the glomerular filtration rate (GFR). GHF was defined as an eGFR ≥ the 90th percentile. First, a multiple linear regression analysis was used to estimate the association of 2-hPBG-FBG with eGFR. Then, a generalized additive model was used to explore the possible nonlinear relationship between 2-hPBG-FBG and eGFR. Next, the 2-hPBG-FBG values were divided into four groups as follows: 0–36, 36–72, 72–108 and ≥108 mg/dl. Finally, a multiple logistic regression analysis was used to investigate the association of 2-hPBG-FBG with the risk of GHF.

Results: For the group with HbA1c<7%, the eGFR and the percentage of GHF were significantly higher compared with the group with HbA1c≥7%. After adjusting for age, gender, body mass index (BMI), systolic blood pressure (BP), diastolic BP, fasting insulin, cholesterol, triglycerides, smoking, drinking and glycated hemoglobin (HbA1c), 2-hPBG-FBG was significantly associated with increased eGFR and an increased risk of GHF (the GHF risk increased by 64.9% for every 36.0 mg/dl [2.0 mmol/L] 2-hPBG-FBG increase) only in those patients with HbA1c<7%. Additionally, 2-hPBG-FBG and eGFR showed a nonlinear association ($P<0.001$).

Conclusions: Increased fluctuations between the fasting and 2-h postload glucose states are closely associated with increased eGFR and an increased risk of GHF in newly diagnosed diabetes patients with HbA1c<7%.

Editor: Mohammad E. Khamseh, Institute of Endocrinology and Metabolism, Islamic Republic of Iran

Funding: This study was supported by grants from the Chinese Society of Endocrinology and National Clinical Research Center for Metabolic Diseases, the National Natural Science Foundation of China (No. 81100617), the Medical and Health Science and Technology Development Projects of Shandong Province (2011HD005), the National Science and Technology Support Plan (2009BAI80B04), the Natural Science Foundation of Shandong Province (ZR2012HM014), the International Science and Technology Projects of Shandong Province (2012GGE27126), the Business Plan of Jinan Students Studying Abroad (20110407), and the Special Scientific Research Fund of Clinical Medicine of the Chinese Medical Association (12030420342). The funders had no roles in the study design, data collection or analysis, in the decision to publish, or in the preparation of the manuscript.

Competing Interests: ZM is an employee of China National Heavy Duty Truck Group Corporation Hospital. There are no patents, products in development or marketed products to declare.

* Email: wangchuansdu.edu@163.com

Introduction

Diabetic nephropathy (DN), which is characterized by an initial period of glomerular hyperfiltration (GHF) followed by progressively increasing proteinuria and a gradual decline in the glomerular filtration rate (GFR), is the leading cause of chronic kidney disease (CKD) and is associated with increased cardiovascular mortality in diabetic patients worldwide [1,2]. As a functional change occurring during the early stage of diabetes, GHF is likely to correlate with the progression of DN and may even contribute to the initiation of this disease [3,4]. The prevalence of GHF reported in type 2 diabetic patients has varied

Table 1. Characteristics of study participants grouped by HbA1c category.

Characteristics	Total n = 679	HbA1c (%) <7 n = 364	HbA1c (%) ≥7 n = 315	P-value
Female (%)	423 (62.3%)	236 (64.8%)	187 (59.4%)	0.142
Age (years)	60.58±9.38	60.75±9.72	60.39±8.99	0.611
BMI (kg/m²)	27.09±3.35	26.80±3.40	27.44±3.27	**0.014**
Systolic BP (mmHg)	146.61±20.27	146.41±20.33	146.85±20.22	0.778
Diastolic BP (mmHg)	82.52±12.38	82.83±12.44	82.16±12.32	0.480
FBG (mg/dl)	150.87±45.21	132.56±25.23	172.03±53.30	**<0.001**
2-hPBG (mg/dl)	231.54±73.19	203.17±51.87	264.33±80.29	**<0.001**
2-hPBG-FBG (mg/dl)	80.67±48.73	70.60±47.91	92.30±47.13	**<0.001**
HbA$_{1c}$ (%)	7.32±1.69	6.23±0.47	8.59±1.71	**<0.001**
Fasting insulin (mIU/L)	9.60 (6.60–13.60)	10.00 (6.83–13.70)	9.20 (6.30–13.50)	0.324
HOMA-IR index	3.43 (2.34–4.91)	3.20 (2.16–4.55)	3.81 (2.62–5.73)	**<0.001**
Cholesterol (mg/dl)	218.91±40.29	217.29±39.68	220.78±40.97	0.260
Triglycerides (mg/dl)	140.87 (99.68–198.46)	132.01 (95.68–179.86)	155.05 (111.64–217.07)	**<0.001**
Smoking (%)	97 (14.3%)	41 (11.3%)	56 (17.8%)	**0.016**
Drinking (%)	124 (18.3%)	54 (14.8%)	70 (22.2%)	**0.013**
Creatinine (mg/dl)	0.77±0.14	0.76±0.13	0.78±0.14	**0.012**
eGFR (mL/min/1.73 m²)	85.10±14.68	86.17±14.51	83.87±14.81	**0.042**
GHF (%)	68 (10.0%)	46 (12.6%)	22 (7%)	**0.014**

Data are presented as the means ± SD or as numbers (%). BMI, body mass index; BP, blood pressure; FBG, fasting blood glucose; 2-hPBG, 2-h postload blood glucose; HOMA-IR, homeostasis model assessment of insulin resistance; eGFR, estimated glomerular filtration rate; GHF, glomerular hyperfiltration.

widely from 7 to 73% [5,6,7,8]. Therefore, the screening for risk factors of GHF during the early stage of type 2 diabetes is critical for DN prevention.

Hyperglycemia is closely related to the development of the vascular complications of diabetes and can be prevented by the strict control of blood glucose [9,10]. As a relatively objective indicator of average blood glucose within the past two or three months, glycated hemoglobin (HbA1c) has been used as the standard for glucose control. However, the incidence of diabetic complications increases more rapidly in proportion to postprandial glucose or to peak glucose levels compared with average blood glucose levels, indicating the important role of blood glucose fluctuations in the development of diabetic complications [11,12,13,14]. A growing body of research has suggested that glucose fluctuations may accelerate the renal complications associated with diabetes independent of the presence of hyperglycemia; however, the results are inconsistent. One study of type 1 diabetes patients has revealed that glucose fluctuations do not predict the development of nephropathy [15]. In contrast, two other studies have indicated that glucose fluctuations may affect the severity of CKD in patients with type 2 diabetes [16,17]. Therefore, it is necessary to further clarify the influence of glucose fluctuations on the changes in renal function that occur in association with diabetes, particularly during the early stage of the disease (as indicated by GHF).

However, the definition of glucose fluctuation is currently uncertain, and the monitoring of glucose fluctuation is complicated in clinical practice and large epidemiological studies. Because the most common glucose fluctuations occur following meals, differences between the fasting and postprandial glucose levels may reflect the state of glucose fluctuation (to some extent). Therefore, it should be determined whether these differences are related to GHF. However, the total calorie intake often differs between subjects because of dietary variations. To standardize

calorie intake to evaluate glycemic control, we performed the 75-g oral glucose tolerance test (OGTT) in a representative sample of the Chinese population and used 2-h postload blood glucose (2-hPBG) to represent the postprandial glucose levels. We investigated whether the fluctuations between fasting blood glucose (FBG) and 2-hPBG-FBG were associated with GHF in middle-aged and elderly Chinese patients newly diagnosed with diabetes.

Materials and Methods

Ethics statement

This work was performed as part of the baseline survey of the REACTION study assessing the association of diabetes and cancer, which included 259,657 adults (40 years of age and older) from 25 communities across mainland China from 2011 to 2012 [18]. This study was approved by the Ruijin Hospital Ethics Committee of the Shanghai Jiao Tong University School of Medicine. Written informed consent was obtained from all participants.

Study population

For this screening study, 10,028 subjects were randomly recruited who were ≥40 years old and resided in the Shandong province from January 2012 to April 2012. A 75-g OGTT was performed for all participants. We first selected the 2044 subjects whose 75-g OGTT results were indicative of diabetes (see below). Then, 1181 previously diagnosed diabetic patients were excluded based on their medical histories. Further exclusion criteria were as follows: (1) lower 2-hPBG than FBG levels; (2) missing data for the calculation of the eGFR; (3) previously diagnosed kidney disease, including autoimmune or drug-induced kidney disease, nephritis, renal fibrosis or renal failure, or prior kidney transplant and current dialysis treatment; (4) previously diagnosed hepatic disease, including fatty liver, liver cirrhosis and autoimmune hepatitis; and

(5) any malignant disease. A total of 679 subjects (423 women) were eligible for the analysis.

Data collection

Demographic characteristics, lifestyle information and previous medical histories were obtained by trained investigators through a standard questionnaire. BMI was calculated as weight (kg) divided by height squared (m^2). Blood pressure (BP) was measured 3 times consecutively (OMRON Model HEM-752 FUZZY, Omron Company, Dalian, China), and the average reading was used for the analysis. After an overnight fast, venous blood samples were collected for measurements of FBG, fasting insulin, cholesterol, triglycerides and creatinine. 2-hPBG was measured after subjects had completed the 75-g OGTT. HbA1c was measured by high-performance liquid chromatography (VARIANT II and D-10 Systems, BIO-RAD, USA). The homeostasis model assessment of insulin resistance (HOMA-IR) index was calculated as follows: fasting insulin concentration (mIU/L)×FPG concentration (mmol/L)/22.5 [19]. The eGFR was calculated from the creatinine level using the following formulas according to the Chronic Kidney Disease Epidemiology Collaboration (CKD-EPI) [20].

Definition

There is no standard definition of hyperfiltration. Previous studies have arbitrarily used eGFR thresholds of 125 to 140 mL/min/1.73 m^2 as the defining criteria for hyperfiltration. However, GFRs decrease with age [21]. The present study contained only middle-aged and elderly subjects, who were expected to present with relatively low eGFRs. Therefore, GHF was defined as an eGFR ≥ the 90th percentile (101.81 mL/min/1.73 m^2) in this study.

Newly diagnosed diabetes has been defined by the World Health Organization (WHO) in 1999 [22] as FBG≥126 mg/dl (7.0 mmol/L) and/or 2-hPBG≥200 mg/dl (11.1 mmol/L) without a history of diabetes. For newly diagnosed diabetes patients who are not receiving antidiabetic drug therapy, HbA1c levels may be reflective of the clinical course of diabetes. Therefore, we divided all subjects into two groups according to the target value of HbA1c [23] as follows: patients with HbA1c<7% were considered to be at the very early stage, and those with HbA1c ≥7% were considered to be at a comparably later stage.

Statistical analysis

Normally distributed continuous variables are expressed as the mean±SD, and variables with non-normal distributions are presented as the median (interquartile range). Categorical variables are presented as numbers (%). The differences between the HbA1c groups were detected by Student's t test (normally distributed continuous variables), Mann-Whitney U test (skewed continuous variables), or chi-square test (categorical variables). After verifying the assumption of a linear relationship between the dependent and independent variables that were introduced into the linear regression model (assessed using a histogram of the residuals, together with a scatterplot of the standardized residuals versus the standardized predicted values in the different models), a multiple linear regression analysis was used to estimate the association of 2-hPBG-FBG with eGFR. Three models were constructed as follows: the first was not adjusted; the second was adjusted for age, gender, BMI, systolic BP and diastolic BP; and the third was adjusted for age, gender, BMI, systolic BP, diastolic BP, Log (fasting insulin), cholesterol, Log (triglyceride), smoking, drinking and HbA1c. We used a generalized additive model to explore the possible nonlinear association of 2-hPBG-FBG with

eGFR after adjusting for the aforementioned factors. The 25th, 50th, and 75th percentiles of 2-hPBG-FBG were 37.8 mg/dl (2.1 mmol/L), 75.6 mg/dl (4.2 mmol/L) and 108 mg/dl (6.0 mmol/L), respectively. To facilitate the use of the 2-hPBG-FBG values in clinical practice, they were divided into four groups according to 36 mg/dl (2.0 mmol/L) intervals as follows: 0–36, 36–72, 72–108 and ≥108 mg/dl. Then, the association of 2-hPBG-FBG (the four groups of 2-hPBG-FBG were introduced as ordinal dummy variables) with the risk of GHF was estimated using a multiple logistic regression analysis for the same three models. $P<0.05$ was considered statistically significant. The analysis of the generalized additive models was performed using Empower Stats 2.13.0. The data were analyzed using SPSS 16.0 (SPSS Inc., Chicago. IL).

Results

Characteristics of study participants

We included 679 subjects (423 women) with newly diagnosed diabetes who were divided into two groups based on HbA1c, using 7% as the cut-off value. As shown in Table 1, BMI, FBG, 2-hPBG, 2-hPBG-FBG, HbA1c, HOMA-IR, triglycerides, creatinine and the percentages of smoking and drinking subjects were significantly lower in the group with HbA1c<7%. In contrast, the eGFR and the percentage of GHF were higher compared with the subjects with HbA1c≥7%.

2-hPBG-FBG is closely associated with eGFR in newly diagnosed diabetes patients with HbA1c<7%

As shown in Table 2, we constructed three models to analyze the association of 2-hPBG-FBG with eGFR (the calculation of HOMA-IR and 2-hPBG-FBG both involved FBG, so we adjusted for fasting insulin rather than for HOMA-IR in model 3). The linearity of the relationship was assessed using a histogram of the residuals for each model together with a scatterplot of the standardized residuals versus the standardized predicted values, which indicated an approximately linear relationship. Interestingly, a significantly positive association of 2-hPBG-FBG with eGFR was observed in all three models for the newly diagnosed diabetes patients with HbA1c<7% only, which was independent of age, gender, BMI, systolic BP, diastolic BP, fasting insulin, cholesterol, triglycerides, smoking, drinking and HbA1c. Moreover, we found a nonlinear association of 2-hPBG-FBG and eGFR using a generalized additive model after multivariable adjustment ($P<0.001$; Fig. 1). In contrast, a negative relationship between HbA1c and eGFR was observed in the patients with HbA1c (%) ≥7.

2-hPBG-FBG is closely associated with increased risk of GHF in newly diagnosed diabetes patients with HbA1c<7%

As shown in Table 3, we analyzed the association of increased 2-hPBG-FBG with the risk of GHF for the three models. As expected, 2-hPBG-FBG significantly increased the risk of GHF in the newly diagnosed diabetes patients with HbA1c<7% but not in the subjects with HbA1c≥7%. In model 1, a 38.2% increase in GHF risk for every 36 mg/dl (2.0 mmol/L) 2-hPBG-FBG increase was observed. After adjusting for age, gender, BMI, systolic BP and diastolic BP, the GHF risk increased by 61.4% for every 36 mg/dl (2.0 mmol/L) 2-hPBG-FBG increase. Further adjustments for fasting insulin, cholesterol, triglycerides, smoking, drinking and HbA1c revealed a 64.9% increase in the GHF risk. In contrast, HbA1c (an indicator of average blood glucose) was not associated with an increased risk of GHF.

Table 2. Multiple linear regression analysis of association of 2-hPBG-FBG with eGFR.

| Model | Independent variable | HbA1c (%) <7 | | HbA1c (%) ≥7 | |
		β Coefficient (95% CI)	P-value	β Coefficient (95% CI)	P-value
Model 1	2-hPBG-FBG, per mg/dL	0.041 (0.010 to 0.072)	**0.009**	−0.026 (−0.061 to 0.009)	0.146
Model 2	2-hPBG-FBG, per mg/dL	0.040 (0.019 to 0.061)	**<0.001**	−0.010 (−0.035 to 0.015)	0.419
Model 3	2-hPBG-FBG, per mg/dL	0.036 (0.015 to 0.057)	**0.001**	0.010 (−0.014 to 0.037)	0.492
	HbA1c, per % unit	−1.272 (−3.424 to 0.880)	0.246	−0.779 (−1.547 to −0.011)	**0.047**

Model 1: not adjusted; Model 2: adjusted for age, gender, BMI, systolic BP and diastolic BP; Model 3: Model 2 plus Log (fasting insulin), cholesterol, Log (triglycerides), smoking and drinking.

Discussion

Because GHF is a phenomenon occurring early in the clinical course of diabetes that may lead to the development of DN due to its associated glomerular damage, it is crucial to screen for risk factors of GHF during the early stage of diabetes. Therefore, we selected newly diagnosed diabetes patients as our study population. In addition, to further subdivide these patients, they were placed into two groups based on their HbA1c values. Interestingly, we found that the fluctuations between the fasting and 2-hPBG-FBG states were closely associated with eGFR and the increased risk of GHF in the patients with very early-stage diabetes only (HbA1c< 7%), which indicated the importance of glucostasis between the fasting and 2-h postload states. This association was not observed for those patients with poorly controlled diabetes, which may have been because for newly diagnosed diabetics, HbA1c may be essentially reflective of the clinical course of diabetes. Those patients with higher HbA1c levels may have had diabetes for a longer period of time and thus may not have been at the very early

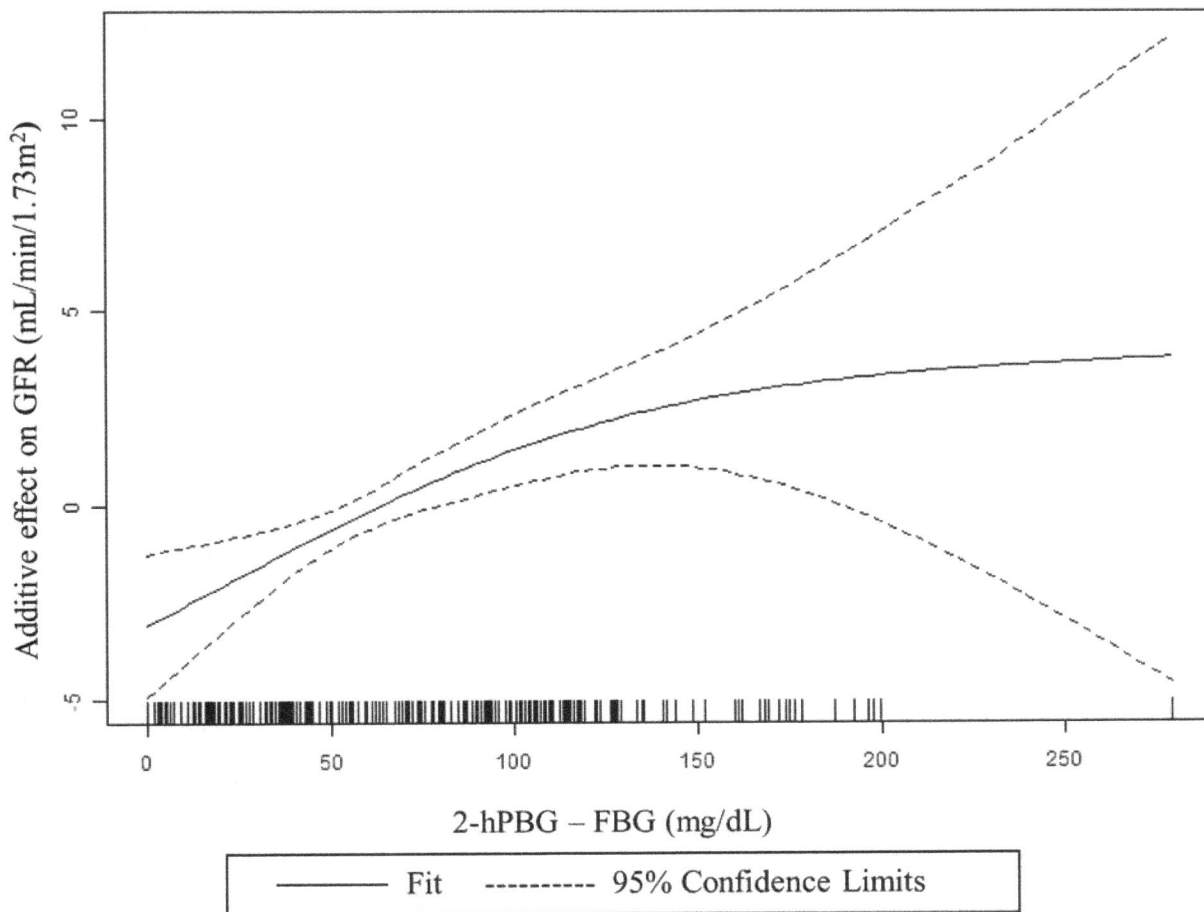

Figure 1. Nonlinear association of the difference between 2-h postload blood glucose and fasting blood glucose (2-hPBG-FBG) in association with estimated glomerular filtration rate (eGFR). The association was analyzed in a generalized additive model (df = 3, P<0.001) adjusted for age, gender, BMI, systolic BP, diastolic BP, fasting insulin, cholesterol, triglycerides, smoking, drinking and HbA1c.

Table 3. Multiple logistic regression analysis of association of 2-hPBG-FBG with GHF.

Model	Independent variable	HbA1c (%) <7		HbA1c (%) ≥7	
		Odds ratio (95% CI)	*P*-value	Odds ratio (95% CI)	*P*-value
Model 1	2-hPBG-FBG, per 36 mg/dL	1.382 (1.051 to 1.818)	**0.021**	0.520 (0.333 to 0.814)	**0.004**
Model 2	2-hPBG-FBG, per 36 mg/dL	1.614 (1.068 to 2.440)	**0.023**	0.721 (0.372 to 1.396)	0.332
Model 3	2-hPBG-FBG, per 36 mg/dL	1.649 (1.061 to 2.565)	**0.026**	0.742 (0.347 to 1.589)	0.442
	HbA1c, per % unit	0.889 (0.299 to 2.638)	0.831	0.928 (0.606 to 1.421)	0.731

Model 1: not adjusted; Model 2: adjusted for age, gender, BMI, systolic BP and diastolic BP; Model 3: Model 2 plus fasting insulin, cholesterol, triglycerides, smoking and drinking.

stage of the disease. Because GHF is always present at the very early stage of diabetes, those patients with higher HbA1c levels may not have possessed GHF any longer. In contrast, they may have presented with decreased eGFR.

The two main risk factors for DN are hyperglycemia and arterial hypertension [24]. Therefore, we adjusted for HbA1c, which is reflective of the average blood glucose level within the past two to three months, in addition to BP to analyze the association of blood glucose fluctuations with GHF. The traditional risk factors for DN also include sex, age, smoking, drinking, dyslipidemia and insulin resistance [24]. Thus, we further adjusted for the above risk factors in model 3 to verify the relationship between blood glucose fluctuations and GHF. Notably, because the calculations of HOMA-IR and 2-hPBG-FBG both involve FBG, we added fasting insulin rather than HOMA-IR to model 3. Interestingly, the GHF risk increased by 64.9% for every 36 mg/dl (2.0 mmol/L) 2-hPBG-FBG increase after adjusting for age, gender, BMI, systolic BP, diastolic BP, fasting insulin, cholesterol, triglycerides, smoking, drinking and HbA1c. In contrast, average blood glucose (HbA1c) was not associated with GHF.

Two recent studies have revealed that HbA1c fluctuation independently affects the development of CKD in type 2 diabetes patients [16,17], reflecting the effects of long-term glycemic fluctuations on renal complications. The Renal Insufficiency And Cardiovascular Events (RIACE) Italian multicenter study [16] has shown that in patients with type 2 diabetes, HbA1c fluctuations affect (albuminuric) CKD more than average HbA1c levels. In addition, a study [17] conducted in Hong Kong has found that long-term glycemic fluctuations as expressed by the SD of HbA1c predict the development of renal and cardiovascular complications. Although the effects of long-term glycemic fluctuations on renal complications have been investigated in some studies, population studies of the influences of short-term glycemic fluctuations, and particularly those of glucose fluctuations, between the fasting and 2-h postload states on renal function are scarce, and few studies have been conducted using animal models, which have shown that blood glucose fluctuations may induce renal pathological changes in diabetic rodents [25,26]. Blood glucose fluctuation may accelerate the development of kidney fibrosis in diabetic mice by increasing collagen production and inhibiting collagen degradation, and both the ERK/MAPK and TGF-β/Smad signaling pathways seem to play roles in its development, leading to changes in the GFR [25]. Moreover, a more serious degree of glomerular sclerosis has been observed in association with blood glucose fluctuations in mice compared with those with sustained high blood glucose levels [26]. The influences of glucose fluctuations on endothelial function have also been explored [27,28]. Glucose fluctuations may induce the production of reactive oxygen species (ROSs) in endothelial cells, facilitating the development of vascular endothelial dysfunction in rats with type 2 diabetes [27,28]. In the present study, we also observed that glucose fluctuations led to the increased risk of GHF during the early stage of diabetes.

Creatinine-based equations for estimating the GFR include the Cockcroft-Gault equation, the Modification of Diet in Renal Disease (MDRD) equation and the CKD-EPI equation. Currently, the Cockcroft-Gault equation has been supplanted by the latter two equations [29]. In addition, the CKD-EPI equation is more accurate and precise in estimating the GFR than the MDRD equation in middle-aged and older South Asians [30]. Therefore, we selected the CKD-EPI equation to calculate the eGFR.

Our study contains some limitations. First, a cross-sectional study cannot infer causality between 2-hPBG-FBG and GHF. Second, fluctuations between the fasting and 2-h postload glucose (2-hPBG-FBG) states do not precisely reflect glucose fluctuations. However, as a simple indicator of glucose fluctuations, 2-hPBG-FBG may be easily applicable in clinical practice. Third, our study contained only middle-aged and older Chinese people; age and ethnic differences should be taken into account when assessing these results. Fourth, we diagnosed diabetes based on one 75-g OGTT, which should be repeated and confirmed. Finally, the GFR based on creatinine levels and estimated by the CKD-EPI equation may not accurately reflect kidney function, which may have affected the accuracy of the GHF estimation. However, the gold standard method for measuring the GFR (the isotope clearance measurement) is very expensive and time-consuming, so the use of creatinine-based equations to estimate the GFR is logical for large epidemiological studies.

In conclusion, we found that fluctuations between the fasting and 2-hPBG-FBG states are associated with an increased risk of GHF in newly diagnosed diabetes patients with HbA1c<7% but not in subjects with HbA1c≥7%. For newly diagnosed diabetics, HbA1c as well as 2-hPBG-FBG should be strictly controlled to prevent diabetes complications. In addition, longitudinal studies are needed to explore the extent to which the 2-hPBG-FBG value should be controlled in clinical practice to effectively aid in the prevention of DN.

Author Contributions

Conceived and designed the experiments: XH. Performed the experiments: XH CW SW WY ZM YW CL ML X. Zhang X. Zhao YS JS PL KL LG MW FL WL FY JY LW MT JL RZ SC LC. Analyzed the data: XH. Contributed reagents/materials/analysis tools: XH. Contributed to the writing of the manuscript: XH SC LC.

References

1. Reutens AT, Atkins RC (2011) Epidemiology of diabetic nephropathy. Contrib Nephrol 170: 1–7.
2. Valmadrid CT, Klein R, Moss SE, Klein BE (2000) The risk of cardiovascular disease mortality associated with microalbuminuria and gross proteinuria in persons with older-onset diabetes mellitus. Arch Intern Med 160: 1093–1100.
3. Magee GM, Bilous RW, Cardwell CR, Hunter SJ, Kee F, et al. (2009) Is hyperfiltration associated with the future risk of developing diabetic nephropathy? A meta-analysis. Diabetologia 52: 691–697.
4. Brenner BM, Hostetter TH, Olson JL, Rennke HG, Venkatachalam MA (1981) The role of glomerular hyperfiltration in the initiation and progression of diabetic nephropathy. Acta Endocrinol Suppl (Copenh) 242: 7–10.
5. Bruce R, Rutland M, Cundy T (1994) Glomerular hyperfiltration in young Polynesians with type 2 diabetes. Diabetes Res Clin Pract 25: 155–160.
6. Keller CK, Bergis KH, Fliser D, Ritz E (1996) Renal findings in patients with short-term type 2 diabetes. J Am Soc Nephrol 7: 2627–2635.
7. Lebovitz HE, Palmisano J (1990) Cross-sectional analysis of renal function in black Americans with NIDDM. Diabetes Care 13: 1186–1190.
8. Lee KU, Park JY, Hwang IR, Hong SK, Kim GS, et al. (1995) Glomerular hyperfiltration in Koreans with non-insulin-dependent diabetes mellitus. Am J Kidney Dis 26: 722–726.
9. Stratton IM, Adler AI, Neil HA, Matthews DR, Manley SE, et al. (2000) Association of glycaemia with macrovascular and microvascular complications of type 2 diabetes (UKPDS 35): prospective observational study. BMJ 321: 405–412.
10. The Diabetes Control and Complications Trial Research Group (1993) The effect of intensive treatment of diabetes on the development and progression of long-term complications in insulin-dependent diabetes mellitus. The Diabetes Control and Complications Trial Research Group. N Engl J Med 329: 977–986.
11. Gerich JE (2003) Clinical significance, pathogenesis, and management of postprandial hyperglycemia. Arch Intern Med 163: 1306–1316.
12. Ceriello A, Hanefeld M, Leiter L, Monnier L, Moses A, et al. (2004) Postprandial glucose regulation and diabetic complications. Arch Intern Med 164: 2090–2095.
13. Heine RJ, Balkau B, Ceriello A, Del Prato S, Horton ES, et al. (2004) What does postprandial hyperglycaemia mean? Diabet Med 21: 208–213.
14. Meigs JB, Nathan DM, D'Agostino RB, Sr., Wilson PW (2002) Fasting and postchallenge glycemia and cardiovascular disease risk: the Framingham Offspring Study. Diabetes Care 25: 1845–1850.
15. Kilpatrick ES, Rigby AS, Atkin SL (2006) The effect of glucose variability on the risk of microvascular complications in type 1 diabetes. Diabetes Care 29: 1486–1490.
16. Penno G, Solini A, Bonora E, Fondelli C, Orsi E, et al. (2013) HbA1c variability as an independent correlate of nephropathy, but not retinopathy, in patients with type 2 diabetes: the Renal Insufficiency And Cardiovascular Events (RIACE) Italian multicenter study. Diabetes Care 36: 2301–2310.
17. Luk AO, Ma RC, Lau ES, Yang X, Lau WW, et al. (2013) Risk association of HbA1c variability with chronic kidney disease and cardiovascular disease in type 2 diabetes: prospective analysis of the Hong Kong Diabetes Registry. Diabetes Metab Res Rev 29: 384–390.
18. Ning G (2012) Risk Evaluation of cAncers in Chinese diabeTic Individuals: a lONgitudinal (REACTION) study. J Diabetes 4: 172–173.
19. Matthews DR, Hosker JP, Rudenski AS, Naylor BA, Treacher DF, et al. (1985) Homeostasis model assessment: insulin resistance and beta-cell function from fasting plasma glucose and insulin concentrations in man. Diabetologia 28: 412–419.
20. Levey AS, Stevens LA, Schmid CH, Zhang YL, Castro AF, 3rd, et al. (2009) A new equation to estimate glomerular filtration rate. Ann Intern Med 150: 604–612.
21. Hoy WE, Douglas-Denton RN, Hughson MD, Cass A, Johnson K, et al. (2003) A stereological study of glomerular number and volume: preliminary findings in a multiracial study of kidneys at autopsy. Kidney Int Suppl: S31–37.
22. Alberti KG, Zimmet PZ (1998) Definition, diagnosis and classification of diabetes mellitus and its complications. Part 1: diagnosis and classification of diabetes mellitus provisional report of a WHO consultation. Diabet Med 15: 539–553.
23. American Diabetes Association (2009) Standards of medical care in diabetes–2009. Diabetes Care 32 Suppl 1: S13–61.
24. Zelmanovitz T, Gerchman F, Balthazar AP, Thomazelli FC, Matos JD, et al. (2009) Diabetic nephropathy. Diabetol Metab Syndr 1: 10.
25. Cheng X, Gao W, Dang Y, Liu X, Li Y, et al. (2013) Both ERK/MAPK and TGF-Beta/Smad signaling pathways play a role in the kidney fibrosis of diabetic mice accelerated by blood glucose fluctuation. J Diabetes Res 2013: 463740.
26. Wang H, Wang A, Lei M, Liao J, Hu W (2013) [Effect of blood glucose fluctuation and the sustained high blood glucose on renal pathological change and collagen IV expression in diabetic rats]. Zhong Nan Da Xue Xue Bao Yi Xue Ban 38: 818–823.
27. Wang JS, Yin HJ, Guo CY, Huang Y, Xia CD, et al. (2013) Influence of high blood glucose fluctuation on endothelial function of type 2 diabetes mellitus rats and effects of Panax Quinquefolius Saponin of stem and leaf. Chin J Integr Med 19: 217–222.
28. Ge QM, Dong Y, Zhang HM, Su Q (2010) Effects of intermittent high glucose on oxidative stress in endothelial cells. Acta Diabetol 47 Suppl 1: 97–103.
29. Delanaye P, Mariat C (2013) The applicability of eGFR equations to different populations. Nat Rev Nephrol 9: 513–522.
30. Jessani S, Levey AS, Bux R, Inker LA, Islam M, et al. (2014) Estimation of GFR in South Asians: a study from the general population in Pakistan. Am J Kidney Dis 63: 49–58.

18

Efficacy and Safety of Dipeptidyl Peptidase-4 Inhibitors in Type 2 Diabetes Mellitus Patients with Moderate to Severe Renal Impairment

Dongsheng Cheng, Yang Fei, Yumei Liu, Junhui Li, Yuqiang Chen, Xiaoxia Wang, Niansong Wang*

Department of Nephrology and Rheumatology, Shanghai Jiaotong University Affiliated Sixth People's Hospital, Shanghai, P.R. China

Abstract

Objective: To perform a systematic review and meta-analysis regarding the efficacy and safety of dipeptidyl peptidase-4 (DDP-4) inhibitors ("gliptins") for the treatment of type 2 diabetes mellitus (T2DM) patients with moderate to severe renal impairment.

Methods: All available randomized-controlled trials (RCTs) that assessed the efficacy and safety of DDP-4 inhibitors compared with placebo, no treatment, or active drugs were identified using PubMed, EMBASE, Cochrane CENTRAL, conference abstracts, clinical trials.gov, pharmaceutical company websites, the FDA, and the EMA (up to June 2014). Two independent reviewers extracted the data, and a random-effects model was applied to estimate summary effects.

Results: Thirteen reports of ten studies with a total of 1,915 participants were included in the final analysis. Compared with placebo or no treatment, DPP-4 inhibitors reduced HbA1c significantly (−0.52%, 95%CI −0.64 to −0.39) and had no increased risk of hypoglycemia (RR 1.10, 95%CI 0.92 to 1.32) or weight gain. In contrast to glipizide monotherapy, DPP-4 inhibitors showed no difference in HbA1c lowering effect (−0.08%, 95% CI −0.40 to 0.25) but had a lower incidence of hypoglycemia (RR 0.40, 95%CI 0.23 to 0.69). Furthermore, DPP-4 inhibitors were well-tolerated, without any additional mortality and adverse events. However, the quality of evidence was mostly as low, as assessed using the GRADE system for each outcome.

Conclusions: DPP-4 inhibitors are effective at lowering HbA1c in T2DM patients with moderate to severe renal impairment. DPP-4 inhibitors also have a potential advantage in lowering the risk of adverse events. Regarding the low quality of the evidence according to GRADE, additional well-designed randomized trials that focus on the safety and efficacy of DPP-4 inhibitors in various CKD stages are needed urgently.

Editor: Jaap A. Joles, University Medical Center Utrecht, Netherlands

Funding: This research is supported by grant from the Project of National Nature Science Foundation of China (81270824), Shanghai Science and Technology Project (11DZ1921904 and 11410708500). The funders played no role in the study design, data collection and analysis, decision to publish, and preparation of the manuscript.

Competing Interests: The authors have declared that no competing interests exist.

* Email: wangniansong2012@163.com

Introduction

The prevalence of type 2 diabetes mellitus (T2DM) and chronic kidney disease (CKD) is increasing steadily. Diabetes is the leading cause of CKD, which might progress to end-stage renal disease and increase the risk of death [1]. It is known that good glycemic control might delay the deterioration in kidney function [2]. However, antihyperglycemic therapy, including the use of metformin, sulfonylureas, thiazolidinediones, and insulin, in T2DM patients with renal impairment remains controversial regarding its tolerability and safety. Metformin might no longer be the first choice for CKD patients because of the risk of lactic acidosis. The KDIGO recommended that metformin could be continued in individuals with a glomerular filtration rate (GFR)> 45 ml/min/1.73 m^2, should be reviewed in those with a GFR 30–44 ml/min/1.73 m^2, and should be discontinued in patients with a GFR<30 ml/min/1.73 m^2 [3]. Selected sulfonylureas are associated with a higher risk of hypoglycemia, which can be worse in CKD patients [4]. For thiazolidinediones, although there is no higher risk of hypoglycemia or dose adjustment in renal failure patients, they might cause fluid retention and edema, which are common manifestations of kidney disease [5]. Although insulin is used widely, its dose has to be adjusted occasionally based on blood glucose to avoid hypoglycemia because it is partially metabolized by the kidney [6].

Dipeptidyl peptidase-4 (DPP-4) inhibitors are a novel type of oral glucose-lowering agents that modulate fasting plasma glucose, postprandial glucose, and HbAlc levels by decreasing the inactivation of incretins such as glucagon-like peptide 1 and glucose-dependent insulinotropic polypeptide to stimulate the release of insulin in a glucose-dependent manner [7–8]. Since most DPP-4 inhibitors are eliminated by the kidney, a dose reduction is required for patients with moderate to severe renal impairment, except for linagliptin because of its relatively reduced renal metabolism [9–10]. Giorda et al [9] conducted a systematic review on the pharmacokinetics, safety, and efficacy of DPP-4 inhibitors in patients with both T2DM and renal impairment, and suggested that DDP-4 inhibitors could be appropriate drugs for patients with renal impairment. However, their study lacked sufficient randomized trials; therefore, a further meta-analysis is needed.

The aim of the current study was to perform a systematic review and meta-analysis of the safety and efficacy of DPP-4 inhibitors for the treatment of T2DM patients with moderate to severe renal impairment.

Methods

This review was conducted and reported according to PRISMA (Preferred Reporting Items for Systematic Reviews and Meta-Analysis; Table S1) [11].

Search Strategy

Literature searches were performed using PubMed, EMBASE, and Cochrane CENTRAL to identify studies published before June 20, 2014, with no language restrictions. The main search term was a combination of MESH terms and text words for DPP-4 inhibitors and renal impairment. The details of the search are presented in File S1. To find additional relevant studies, a full search was conducted of the references lists of the identified studies and abstracts from the 2011 to 2013 annual meetings of the American Diabetes Association and the European Association for the Study of Diabetes. Additional unpublished trials were searched from clinicaltrials.gov (www.clinicaltrials.gov) and relevant pharmaceutical company websites. Finally, the Food and Drug Administration (FDA; www.fda.gov) and European Medicines Agency (EMA; www.ema.europa.eu) websites were searched for medical reviews of DPP-4 inhibitors (alogliptin, linagliptin, saxagliptin, and sitagliptin in the FDA, and vildaligptin in the EMA).

Eligibility criteria for the inclusion in the meta-analysis

The inclusion criteria were as follows: (1) randomized controlled trials, (2) duration ≥12 weeks, (3) studies assessing T2DM patients with moderate or severe renal insufficiency, including dialysis patients, and (4) a comparison of DPP-4 inhibitors with placebo, no treatment, or other active drugs.

The degree of renal impairment was classified as non-dialysis patients including moderate renal insufficiency (estimated glomerular filtration rate [eGFR] 30–60 ml/min or ml/min/1.73 m^2), severe renal insufficiency (eGFR<30 ml/min or ml/min/1.73 m^2, not on dialysis), and persons receiving dialysis.

Study selection

The titles, abstracts, and/or full-text were assessed independently by DC and YL using the abovementioned inclusion criteria. Discrepancies were resolved by consensus, and the reasons for exclusion were recorded. Endnote X4 was used for literature management and selection.

Data extraction

Data were extracted independently by DC and YL using electronic extraction forms. The extracted data included the authors, study title, publication year, study design, number of participants, mean age of the participants, follow-up duration, completeness, inclusion criteria, baseline HbA1C, intervention type, intervention dose, sponsor information, and pre-specified outcomes. The main outcome for efficacy was the mean change in HbA1c from baseline. Other efficacy outcomes included the mean changes in glycated albumin, fasting blood glucose (FPG), 2-h postprandial glucose, and the proportion of participants that achieved the goal of an HbA1c<7%. The parameters used to assess safety included the incidence of hypoglycemia, the mean change in body weight and renal function, the incidence of cardiovascular disease events, mortality, the incidence of any adverse events (AE), serious adverse events (SAE), drug-related AE, drug-related SAE, and the discontinuation rate. In the current meta-analysis, data from the longest follow-up report were extracted. For studies that contained a 12-week placebo treatment as the initial control and an extended 40–42-week sulfonylurea treatment, only the data from the first period were extracted.

Risk of bias assessment and grading the quality of the evidence

The risk of bias was evaluated using the Cochrane Collaboration's "risk of bias" tool [12]. The overall risk of bias was classified into three grades: low risk of bias if all bias domains were low, high risk if any bias domain was high, and the remaining cases were judged as unclear. The quality of evidence for each outcome was assessed using Grading of Recommendations Assessment, Development, and Evaluation (GRADE) [13], and GRADEprofiler was used to create a GRADE evidence profile (Version 3.6.1, GRADE Working Group).

Data analysis and synthesis

The mean difference (MD) and its 95% confidence interval (CI) were applied for continuous variables, whereas the risk ratio (RR) and its 95%CI were used for dichotomous outcomes. All analyses were based on a random-effects model. Statistical heterogeneity across trials was analyzed using χ^2 tests ($p<0.10$) and I^2 tests [14]. I^2 values of 25%, 50%, and 75% corresponded to low, medium, and high levels of heterogeneity, respectively [15]. Subgroup analyses were performed to investigate potential sources of heterogeneity (such as participants, interventions, and study quality). Sensitivity analyses were performed to assess changes in HbA1c by excluding reports at high risk of bias, eliminating unpublished reports, removing open label studies, and using fixed effects models. Publication bias for the main outcome was assessed primarily using funnel plots. Egger's and Begg's tests were applied to provide statistical evidence of funnel graph symmetry. In addition, the trim and fill method was applied to evaluate the influence of missing studies. Meta analyses were performed using Review Manager Software (Version 5.1. The Cochrane Collaboration, 2011). Funnel plots, Egger's and Begg's tests, and the trim and fill method were performed using Stata software (Version 11, College Station, TX).

Results

Search results and study characteristics

Figure 1 shows the flow diagram of trial selection. From the initial 607 records in the electronic databases, a total of 28 articles were examined in full, among which nine reports on seven studies (seven primary reports and two extensions) [16–24] were finally selected. Furthermore, four additional unpublished reports (three primary reports and one extension) [25–28] obtained from conference abstracts, ClinicalTrials.gov and company website were selected, yet one trial on gemigliptin conducted in October 2013 identified in ClinicalTrials.gov was excluded [29]. Ultimately, thirteen reports on ten RCT studies were included in this systematic review.

The characteristics of the included trials are presented in Table 1. With the exception of one open label study, all trials were designed as double-blinded parallel studies and included a total of 1,915 participants; the enrollment sizes ranged from 51–369

individuals. The reports were published between 2008 and 2013, with durations of 12–54 weeks. The mean baseline HbA1c varied from 6.7% to 8.5%.

Among the enrolled articles, six studies (or eight reports) focused mainly on non-dialysis patients, two assessed dialysis patients, and two (or three reports) analyzed both types of patients. The study by Kothny et al. [21], which contained only two hemodialysis subjects, was included in the non-dialysis group. The studies also differed in the type of DPP-4 inhibitors used: five (or six reports) on sitagliptin, three (or four reports) on vildagliptin, two on linagliptin, and one (or two reports) on saxagliptin.

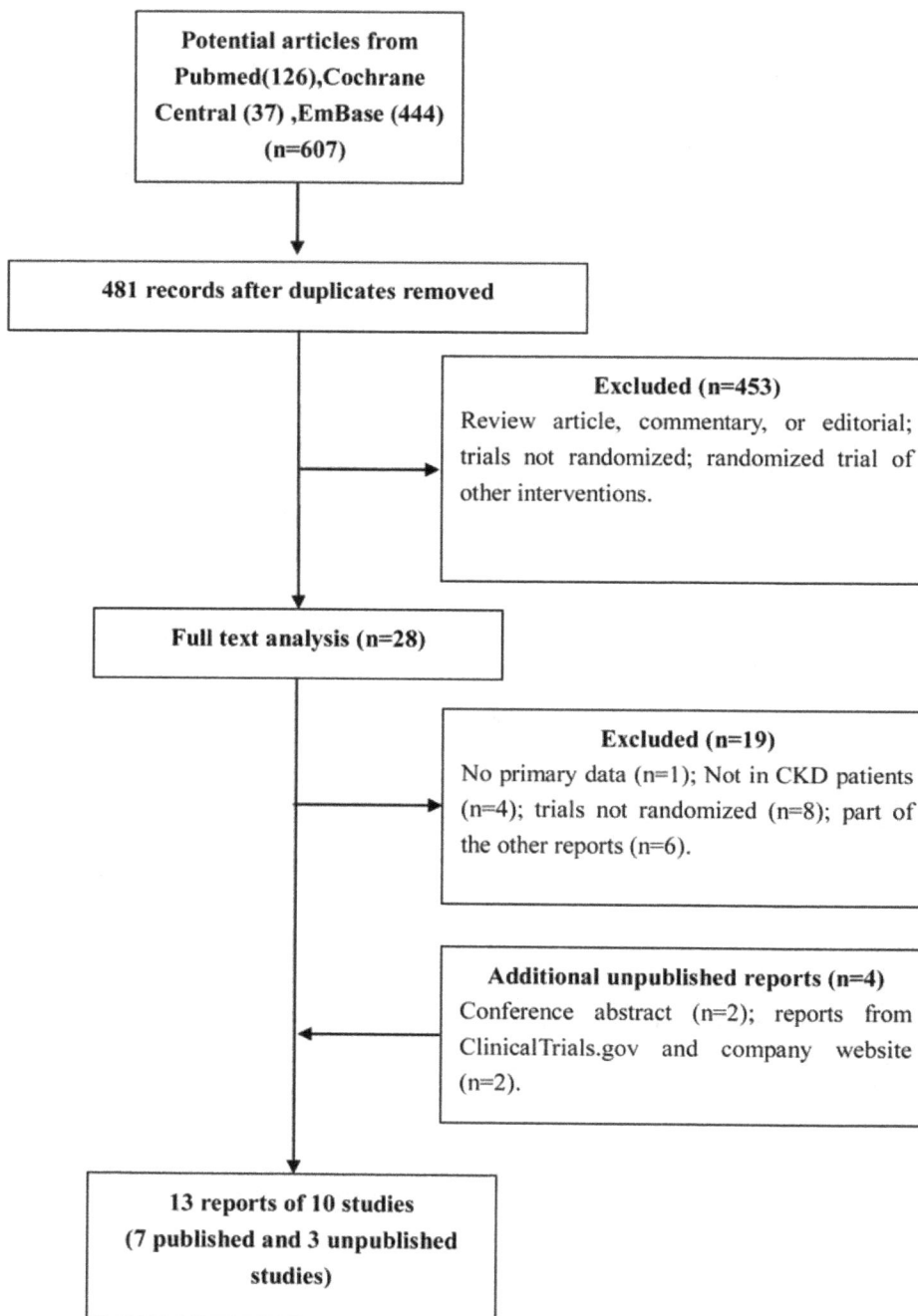

Figure 1. Study flow diagram for trial selection and exclusion.

Table 1. Characteristics of the randomized controlled clinical trials included in this analysis.

Trial	Design	Extension periods	Participant details		Renal status	Type of prevention		Follow-up details	
			Total number	Baseline HbA1C		I	C	Duration	Completeness
DPP-4 inhibitor vs. placebo or no treatment									
Chan, 2008 [16]*	Double blinded RCT	NA	91	I, 7.6% vs. C, 7.8%	eGFR<50 ml/min, including HD and PD patients	Sitagliptin (25–50 mg/day)+SBT	Placebo+SBT	12 weeks	I, 70.8% vs. C, 76.9%
Ito, 2011 [17]	Open label RCT	NA	51	I, 6.7% vs. C, 6.7%	HD patients	Vildagliptin (50–100 mg/day)+SBT	SBT	24 weeks	I, 100% vs. C, 100%
Nowicki, 2011a [18]	Double blinded RCT	Nowicki 2011b [19]	170	I, 8.5% vs. C, 8.1%	eGFR<50 ml/min, including HD patients	Saxagliptin (2.5 mg/day)+SBT	Placebo+SBT	52 weeks (12+40)	I, 49% vs. C, 58%
Lukashevich, 2011 [20]	Double blinded RCT	Kothny 2012 [21]	369	I, 7.8% vs. C, 7.8%	eGFR<50 ml/min/1.73 m², including HD patients	Vildagliptin (50 mg/day)+SBT	Placebo+SBT	52 weeks (24+28)	I, 67.8% vs. C, 60.8%
McGill, 2013 [22]	Double blinded RCT	NA	133	I, 8.2% vs. C, 8.2%	eGFR<30 ml/min/1.73 m², not requiring dialysis	Linagliptin (5 mg/day)+SBT	Placebo+SBT	52 weeks	I, 72.1% vs. C, 73.8%
Laakso, 2013 [23]*	Double blinded RCT	NA	235	I, 8.1% vs. C, 8.0%	eGFR<60 ml/min/1.73 m², not requiring dialysis	Linagliptin (5 mg/day)+SBT	Placebo+SBT	12 weeks	NR
DPP-4 inhibitor vs. glipizide									
Ferreira, 2013a [24]	Double blinded RCT	NA	422	I, 7.8% vs. C, 7.8%	eGFR<50 ml/min/1.73 m², not requiring dialysis	Sitagliptin (25–50 mg/day)+ glipizide matching placebo	Glipizide (2.5–20 mg/day)+ sitagliptin matching placebo	54 weeks	I, 77.7% vs. C, 80.2%
Ferreria, 2013b [25]	Double blinded RCT	NA	129	I, 7.9% vs. C, 7.8%	HD and PD patients	Sitagliptin (25 mg/day)+ glipizide matching placebo	Glipizide (2.5–20 mg/day)+ sitagliptin matching placebo	54 weeks	I, 73% vs. C, 69%
DPP-4 inhibitor vs. GLP-1 receptor agonist albiglutide									
Leiter, 2013 [26]#	Double blinded RCT	NA	231	I, 8.2% vs. C, 8.2%	eGFR 15–60 ml/min/1.73 m²	Sitagliptin (25–100 mg/day)+ albiglutide matching placebo+SBT	Albiglutide (30 mg/week)+ sitagliptin matching placebo +SBT	26 weeks	NR
Vildagliptin vs. sitagliptin									
Novartis, 2011a [27]	Double blinded RCT	Novartis, 2011b [28]	84	NR	eGFR<30 ml/min/1.73 m²	Vildagliptin (50 mg/day)+ sitagliptin matching placebo +SBT	Sitagliptin (25 mg/day)+ vildagliptin matching placebo+SBT	52 weeks (24+28)	NR

I, DPP-4 inhibitor group; C, control group; NA, not applicable; NR, not reported; HD, hemodialysis; PD, peritoneal dialysis; eGFR, estimated glomerular filtration rate; SBT, stable background therapy.

*For studies that used placebo as the comparison group for the first period of time (12 weeks) and sulfonylureas for an extended 40–42 weeks, only data from the first period were extracted for the meta-analyses.

#Only data for subjects with moderate to severe renal impairment in this trial were extracted for analysis.

Four studies (or six reports) compared DPP-4 inhibitors with placebo or no treatment in patients who were already treated with a stable antidiabetic therapy [17–22]. Two studies compared DPP-4 inhibitor monotherapy with glipizide monotherapy [24–25]. In addition, two studies used placebo as a control for the first period (12 weeks) followed by an extended 40–42-week sulfonylurea treatment, which was ignored because of the potential influence of the first period [16,23]. The final two studies also compared two different types of DPP-4 inhibitors [27–28] and compared the DPP-4 inhibitor with GLP-1 receptor agonist [26].

Risk of bias in the included studies and quality of the evidence

Random sequence generation was adequate in four of the ten trials (40%). The allocation concealment was stated clearly in one trial (10%). Nine trials (90%) blinded the participants, investigators, and outcome assessors. The outcome data were incomplete in five trials (50%), and selective reporting was not found. The loss to follow-up rate ranged from 0 to 51%. The risk of bias domains of the included studies are shown in Figures 2 and S1. The quality of evidence assessed using the GRADE approach ranged from moderate for any AE to low or very low for all other outcomes (Files S2 and S3).

Glycemic efficacy

HbA1c. The efficacy of the DPP-4 inhibitors was analyzed thoroughly and compared with the placebo or no treatment group. A statistically significant improvement was observed in HbA1c in individuals treated with DPP-4 inhibitors (random MD -0.52, 95%CI -0.64 to -0.39; $p < 0.00001$) without heterogeneity ($I^2 = 0\%$; $p = 0.70$) (Figure 3A). The HbA1c change was not significantly different in groups with varied dialysis statuses (test for subgroup differences $p = 0.94$). The mean change was -0.50 in the non-dialysis group, compared with -0.49 in the dialysis group (Figure S2). Sensitivity analyses were performed to assess the change in HbA1c by excluding reports at a high risk of bias, eliminating unpublished reports, removing open-label studies, and using fixed-effects models. The results revealed that all the effect sizes were similar in magnitude and direction to the overall estimates (Table S2). The funnel plot (Figure 4) for this outcome was asymmetrical, which was confirmed using Egger's and Begg's tests ($p = 0.013$ and $p = 0.039$, respectively). The trim and fill method was also used to evaluate the influence of the possible missing studies. However, no trimming was performed and the data were unchanged.

According to the two trials (398 participants) that compared monotherapy using DPP-4 inhibitor or glipizide, there was no significant difference in HbA1c reduction between groups (random MD -0.08, 95%CI -0.40 to 0.25; $p = 0.65$). The heterogeneity was moderate ($I^2 = 52\%$; $p = 0.15$) (Figure 3B). A subgroup analysis in another study that compared the efficacy of sitagliptin and albiglutide revealed a significant difference in HbA1c reduction in moderate renal insufficiency patients (-0.53, 95%CI -0.80 to -0.26), whereas no difference was found in the severe renal insufficiency group (-0.47, 95%CI -1.12 to 0.18).

Responder rates: achieving an HbA1c of <7%. Four studies (838 participants) used achieving an HbA1c target of <7% as an outcome. Compared with the placebo or no treatment groups, the DPP-4 inhibitor groups had a higher proportion of patients who achieved the HbA1c goal (461 participants, random RR 1.94, 95%CI 1.40 to 2.70; $p < 0.0001$). Heterogeneity was absent ($I^2 = 0\%$; $p = 0.94$) (Figure 5A).

There was no difference in the proportion of patients receiving glipizide monotherapy and DPP-4 inhibitor monotherapy that

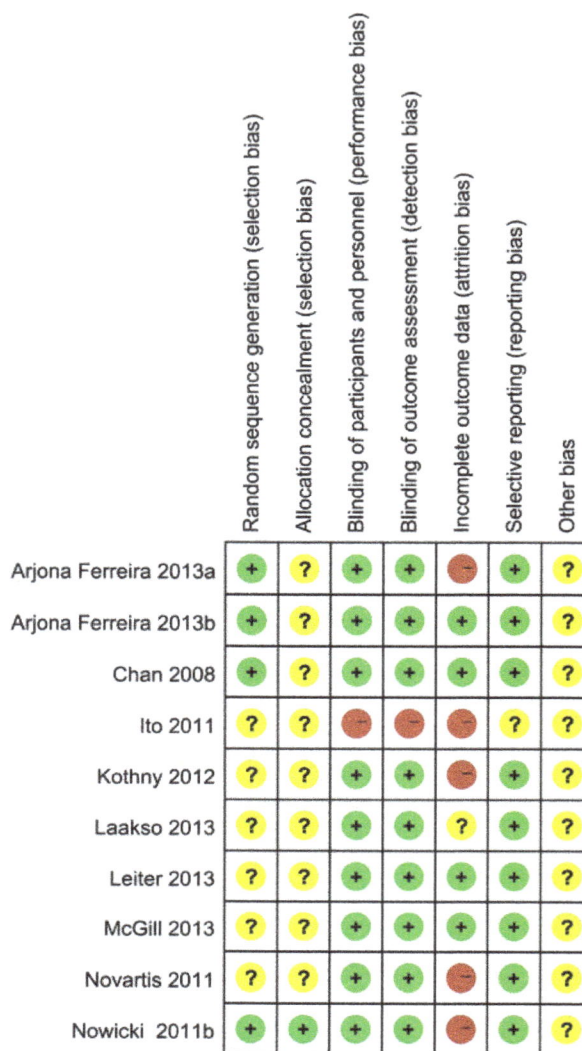

Figure 2. Risk of bias summary of the included studies.

achieved an HbA1c <7% (random RR 0.96, 95%CI 0.66 to 1.40; $p = 0.84$); the heterogeneity was moderate ($I^2 = 64\%$; $p = 0.09$) (Figure 5B).

Fasting blood glucose (FBG). Changes in FBG from baseline were described in six studies. As shown in Figure 6A, there was no significant decrease in FBG between the DPP-4 inhibitor and placebo groups, and the heterogeneity was moderate (522 participants, random MD -0.66, 95%CI -1.35 to 0.02, $p = 0.06$; $I^2 = 48\%$). The result remained consistent after excluding reports at a high risk of bias (random MD -0.61, 95%CI -1.95 to 0.73, $p = 0.37$; $I^2 = 76\%$), and dialysis patients (random MD -0.64, 95%CI -1.30 to 0.01, $p = 0.05$; $I^2 = 32\%$). There was also no significant difference between DPP-4 inhibitor monotherapy and glipizide monotherapy (random MD 0.38, 95%CI -0.11 to 0.86; $p = 0.13$); there was no heterogeneity ($I^2 = 0\%$; $p = 0.60$) (Figure 6B).

Glycated albumin and 2-h postprandial glucose. Only one study (51 dialysis participants) that compared a DPP-4 inhibitor with a no treatment group reported glycated albumin and 2-h postprandial glucose. After 24 weeks of intervention with vildagliptin, the mean glycated albumin levels were decreased

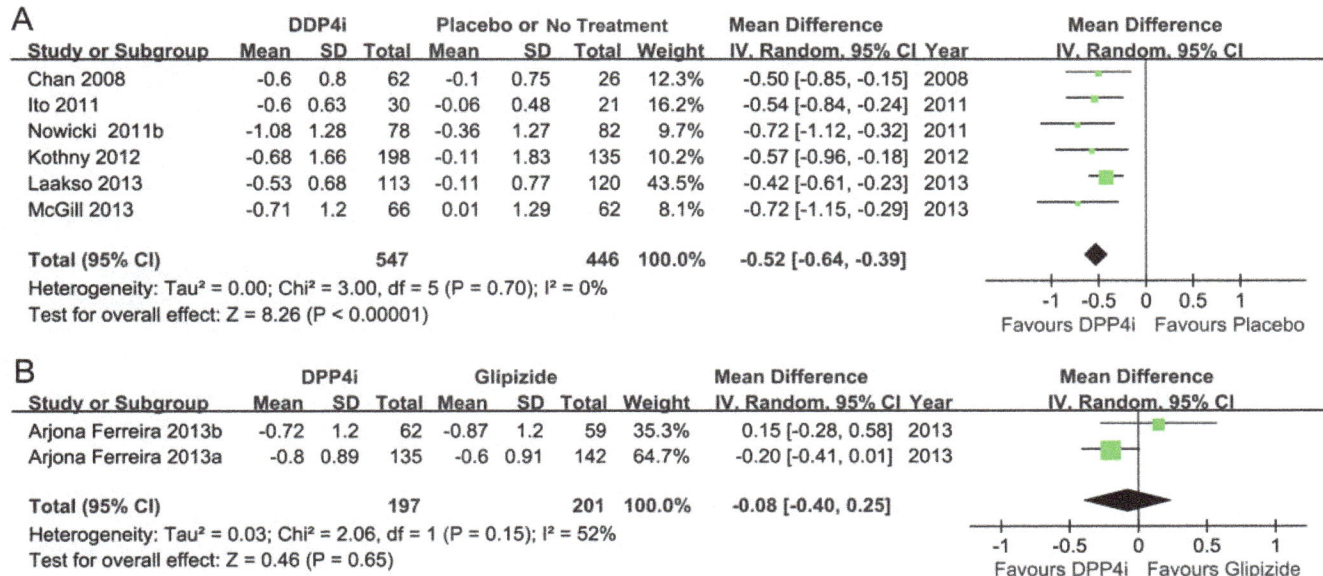

A

Study or Subgroup	DDP4i Mean	SD	Total	Placebo or No Treatment Mean	SD	Total	Weight	Mean Difference IV. Random, 95% CI	Year
Chan 2008	-0.6	0.8	62	-0.1	0.75	26	12.3%	-0.50 [-0.85, -0.15]	2008
Ito 2011	-0.6	0.63	30	-0.06	0.48	21	16.2%	-0.54 [-0.84, -0.24]	2011
Nowicki 2011b	-1.08	1.28	78	-0.36	1.27	82	9.7%	-0.72 [-1.12, -0.32]	2011
Kothny 2012	-0.68	1.66	198	-0.11	1.83	135	10.2%	-0.57 [-0.96, -0.18]	2012
Laakso 2013	-0.53	0.68	113	-0.11	0.77	120	43.5%	-0.42 [-0.61, -0.23]	2013
McGill 2013	-0.71	1.2	66	0.01	1.29	62	8.1%	-0.72 [-1.15, -0.29]	2013
Total (95% CI)			**547**			**446**	**100.0%**	**-0.52 [-0.64, -0.39]**	

Heterogeneity: Tau² = 0.00; Chi² = 3.00, df = 5 (P = 0.70); I² = 0%
Test for overall effect: Z = 8.26 (P < 0.00001)

B

Study or Subgroup	DPP4i Mean	SD	Total	Glipizide Mean	SD	Total	Weight	Mean Difference IV. Random, 95% CI	Year
Arjona Ferreira 2013b	-0.72	1.2	62	-0.87	1.2	59	35.3%	0.15 [-0.28, 0.58]	2013
Arjona Ferreira 2013a	-0.8	0.89	135	-0.6	0.91	142	64.7%	-0.20 [-0.41, 0.01]	2013
Total (95% CI)			**197**			**201**	**100.0%**	**-0.08 [-0.40, 0.25]**	

Heterogeneity: Tau² = 0.03; Chi² = 2.06, df = 1 (P = 0.15); I² = 52%
Test for overall effect: Z = 0.46 (P = 0.65)

Figure 3. Meta-analysis for changes in HbA1c levels. A, DPP-4 inhibitor vs. placebo or no treatment. B, DPP-4 inhibitor vs. glipizide.

significantly from 24.5% at baseline to 20.5%, and the mean postprandial glucose levels decreased from 186 mg/dl at baseline to 140 mg/dl (all $p<0.0001$) [17].

Safety

Body weight. Seven trials reported changes in body weight, but only five trials (809 participants) were included in the pooled analysis. Compared with the placebo group, the DPP-4 inhibitor group had a neutral weight profile (432 participants, random MD -0.20, 95%CI -1.22 to 0.83; $p=0.71$). The heterogeneity was moderate ($I^2=64\%$; $p=0.06$) (Figure 7A). There were no significant differences in the non-dialysis group (341 participants;

random MD -0.61, 95%CI -1.26 to 0.03; $p=0.06$). There was no heterogeneity ($I^2=0\%$; $p=0.46$). The dialysis group was excluded from the analysis because of its effect on dry weight.

DPP-4 inhibitor, but not glipizide monotherapy, treatment resulted in decreased body weight (377 participants, random MD -1.43, 95%CI -2.66 to -0.20; $p=0.02$). There was no heterogeneity ($I^2=0\%$; $p=0.52$) (Figure 7B).

Hypoglycemia. All studies reported the incidence of hypoglycemia, and seven of 10 studies also mentioned severe hypoglycemia; eight cases occurred in the DPP-4 inhibitor groups (464 participants), and ten occurred in the placebo groups (350 participants). Compared with placebo or no treatment, DPP-4

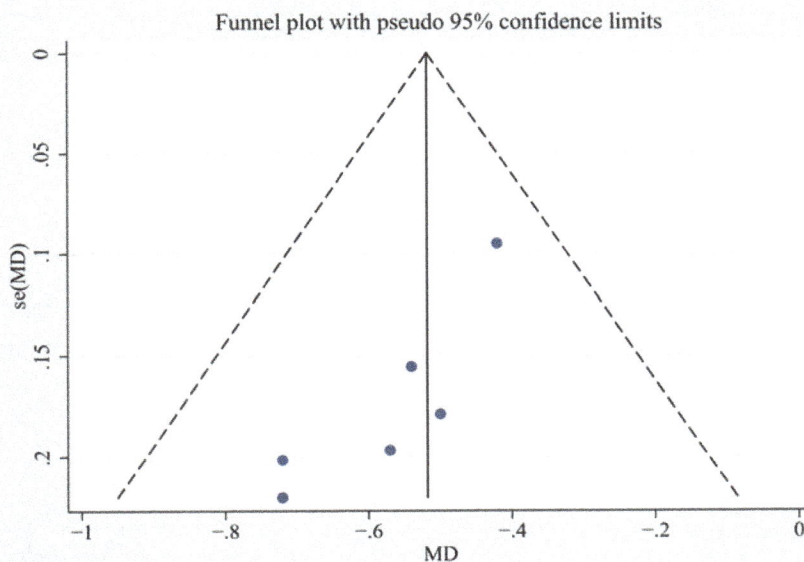

Figure 4. Funnel plot for mean difference (MD) in the change in HbA1c (DPP-4 inhibitor vs. placebo or no treatment).

A

Study or Subgroup	DPP4i Events	DPP4i Total	Placebo Events	Placebo Total	Weight	Risk Ratio M-H, Random, 95% CI	Year
Kothny 2012	86	198	30	135	87.1%	1.95 [1.37, 2.78]	2012
McGill 2013	12	66	6	62	12.9%	1.88 [0.75, 4.70]	2013
Total (95% CI)		264		197	100.0%	1.94 [1.40, 2.70]	
Total events	98		36				

Heterogeneity: Tau² = 0.00; Chi² = 0.01, df = 1 (P = 0.94); I² = 0%
Test for overall effect: Z = 3.95 (P < 0.0001)

Risk Ratio M-H, Random, 95% CI — 0.02 0.1 1 10 50 — Favours Placebo Favours DPP4i

B

Study or Subgroup	DPP4i Events	DPP4i Total	Glipizide Events	Glipizide Total	Weight	Risk Ratio M-H, Random, 95% CI	Year
Arjona Ferreira 2013a	64	135	59	142	55.5%	1.14 [0.88, 1.49]	2013
Arjona Ferreira 2013b	27	62	33	59	44.5%	0.78 [0.54, 1.12]	2013
Total (95% CI)		197		201	100.0%	0.96 [0.66, 1.40]	
Total events	91		92				

Heterogeneity: Tau² = 0.05; Chi² = 2.79, df = 1 (P = 0.09); I² = 64%
Test for overall effect: Z = 0.20 (P = 0.84)

Risk Ratio M-H, Random, 95% CI — 0.02 0.1 1 10 50 — Favours Glipizide Favours DPP4i

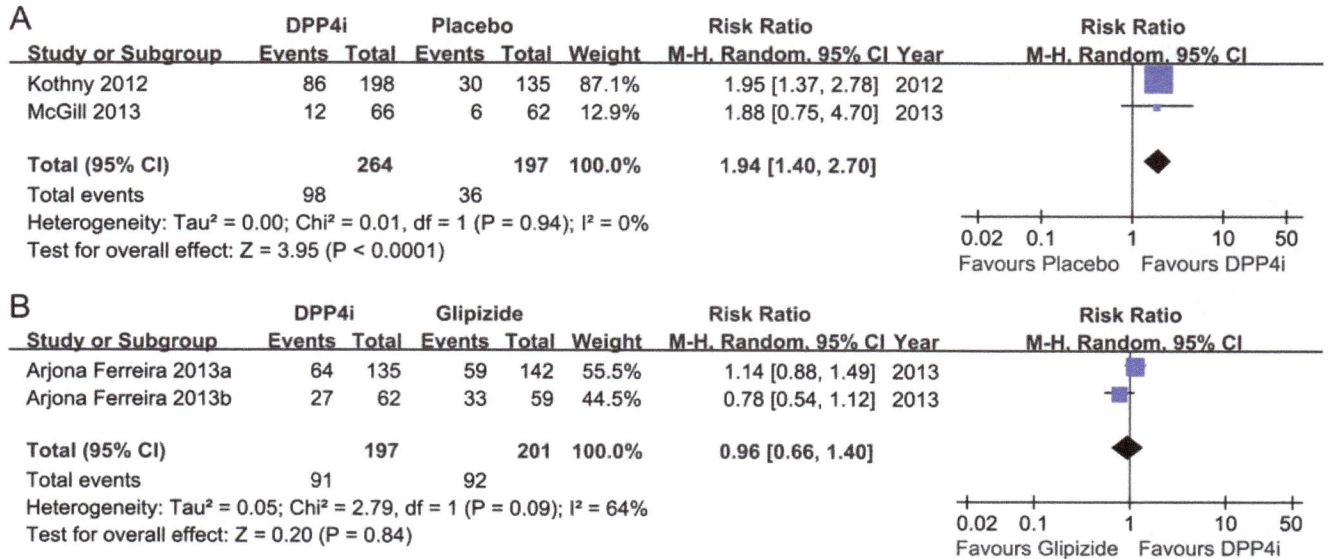

Figure 5. Risk ratio for achieving an HbA1c<7%. A, DPP-4 inhibitor vs. placebo. B, DPP-4 inhibitor vs. glipizide.

inhibitor therapy did not increase the incidence of hypoglycemia (1,049 participants, random RR 1.10, 95%CI 0.92 to 1.32; $p = 0.30$) (Figure 8A), and there was no heterogeneity ($I^2 = 0\%$; $p = 0.43$). Subgroup analyses according to dialysis status were not performed due to insufficient data.

Only two articles compared the effects of DPP-4 inhibitor and glipizide on hypoglycemia. Data revealed that the DPP-4 inhibitor group had a lower incidence of hypoglycemia than did the glipizide group (551 participants, random RR 0.40, 95%CI 0.23 to 0.69; $p = 0.0009$; there was no heterogeneity ($I^2 = 0\%$; $p = 0.42$) (Figure 8B). Compared with glipizide, the DPP-4 inhibitor

reduced the incidence of severe hypoglycemia in dialysis patients significantly (five of 64 participants vs. 0 of 64, respectively) but not in non-dialysis patients (six cases of 212 participants vs. three cases of 210 participants). In contrast, there was no significant difference between vildagliptin and sitagliptin regarding their risk of causing hypoglycemia (0 cases of 46 participants vs. two of 38 participants, respectively).

Renal function and cardiovascular disease events. Seven studies assessed the relationship between DPP-4 inhibitors and renal function in non-dialysis patients using several parameters such as changes in eGFR (four studies), serum creatinine (one

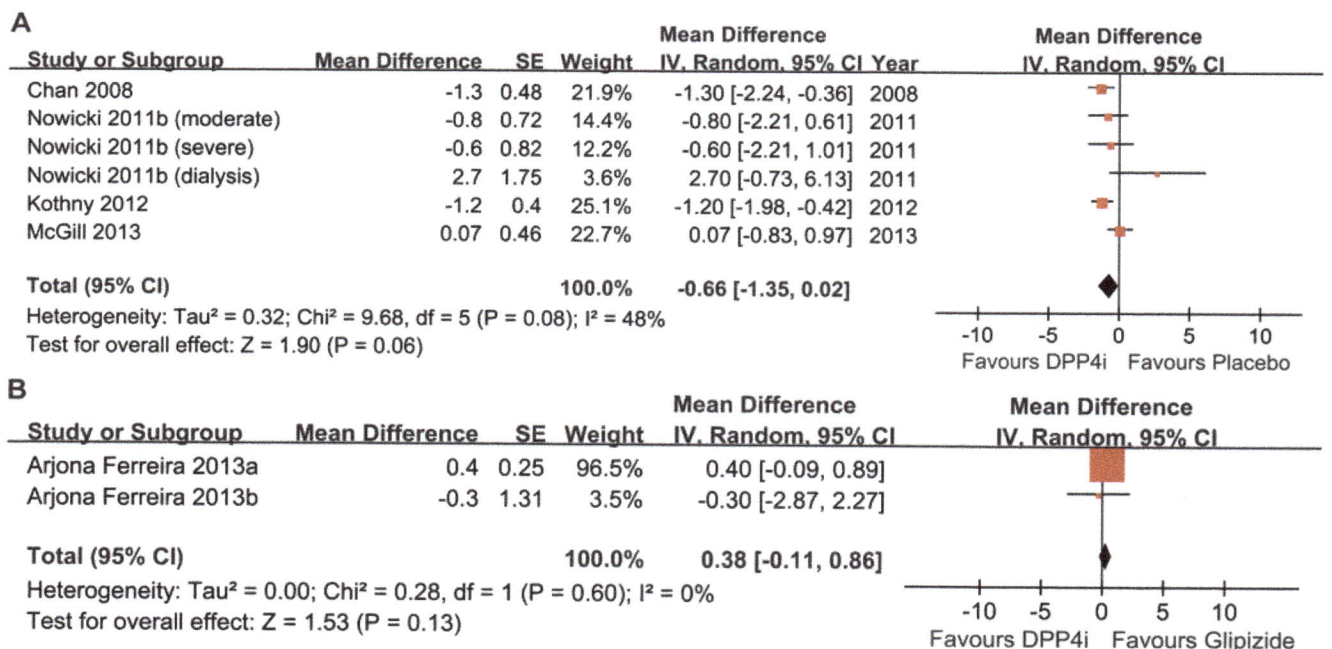

A

Study or Subgroup	Mean Difference	SE	Weight	Mean Difference IV, Random, 95% CI	Year
Chan 2008	-1.3	0.48	21.9%	-1.30 [-2.24, -0.36]	2008
Nowicki 2011b (moderate)	-0.8	0.72	14.4%	-0.80 [-2.21, 0.61]	2011
Nowicki 2011b (severe)	-0.6	0.82	12.2%	-0.60 [-2.21, 1.01]	2011
Nowicki 2011b (dialysis)	2.7	1.75	3.6%	2.70 [-0.73, 6.13]	2011
Kothny 2012	-1.2	0.4	25.1%	-1.20 [-1.98, -0.42]	2012
McGill 2013	0.07	0.46	22.7%	0.07 [-0.83, 0.97]	2013
Total (95% CI)			100.0%	-0.66 [-1.35, 0.02]	

Heterogeneity: Tau² = 0.32; Chi² = 9.68, df = 5 (P = 0.08); I² = 48%
Test for overall effect: Z = 1.90 (P = 0.06)

Mean Difference IV, Random, 95% CI — -10 -5 0 5 10 — Favours DPP4i Favours Placebo

B

Study or Subgroup	Mean Difference	SE	Weight	Mean Difference IV, Random, 95% CI
Arjona Ferreira 2013a	0.4	0.25	96.5%	0.40 [-0.09, 0.89]
Arjona Ferreira 2013b	-0.3	1.31	3.5%	-0.30 [-2.87, 2.27]
Total (95% CI)			100.0%	0.38 [-0.11, 0.86]

Heterogeneity: Tau² = 0.00; Chi² = 0.28, df = 1 (P = 0.60); I² = 0%
Test for overall effect: Z = 1.53 (P = 0.13)

Mean Difference IV, Random, 95% CI — -10 -5 0 5 10 — Favours DPP4i Favours Glipizide

Figure 6. Meta-analysis for the change in fasting blood glucose. A, DPP-4 inhibitor vs. placebo. B, DPP-4 inhibitor vs. glipizide.

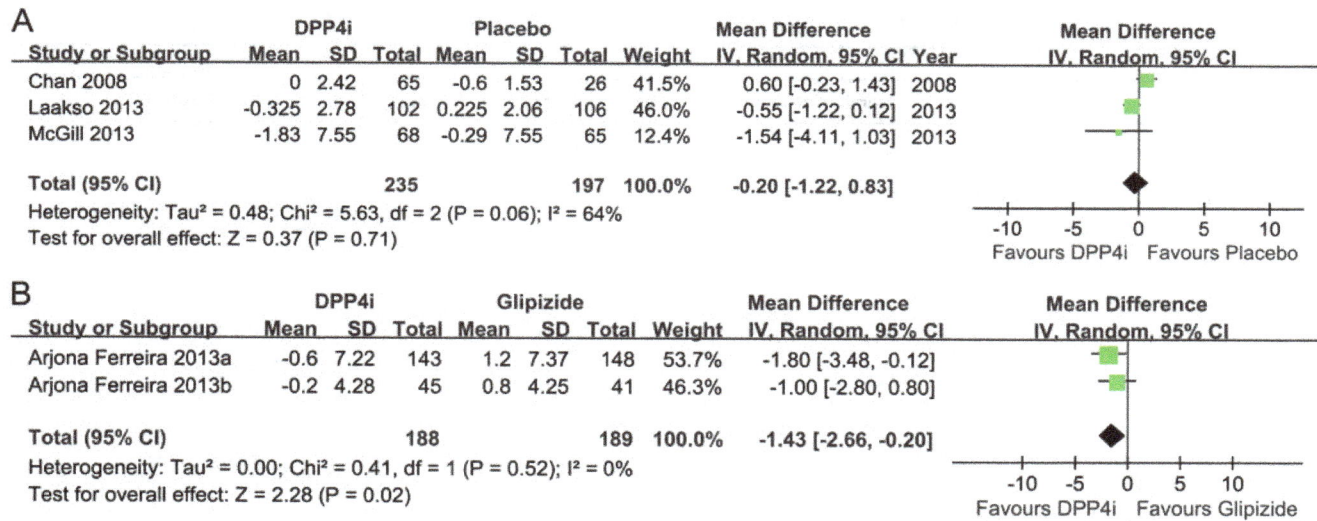

Figure 7. Meta-analysis for changes in bodyweight. A, DPP-4 inhibitor vs. placebo. B, DPP-4 inhibitor vs. glipizide.

study), and the progression of renal status (two studies). Although four of the studies focused on a change in eGFR, a reliable pooled estimate could not be performed due to the varied objects used for comparison and a lack of accurate standard deviation values. Nevertheless, the individual studies showed no obvious effect of DPP-4 inhibitors on renal function.

Five studies (1,137 participants) reported cardiovascular disease (CVD) events. However, because different definitions of CVD events were used, a pooled estimate was not available. Table S3 shows the number of participants who experienced CVD events in each trial. There was no difference in CVD incidence between the DPP-4 inhibitor and control groups.

Total mortality and adverse events. Most studies reported total mortality and the incidence of adverse events, as summarized in Table 2. There was no obvious difference in mortality, the incidence of adverse events (any AE, SAE, drug-related AE, and drug-related SAE), and discontinuation rate.

Discussion

The current study used a complete search, integration, and analysis of data to perform a systematic assessment regarding the efficacy and safety of DPP-4 inhibitors in T2DM patients with moderate to severe renal impairment. In contrast to the placebo

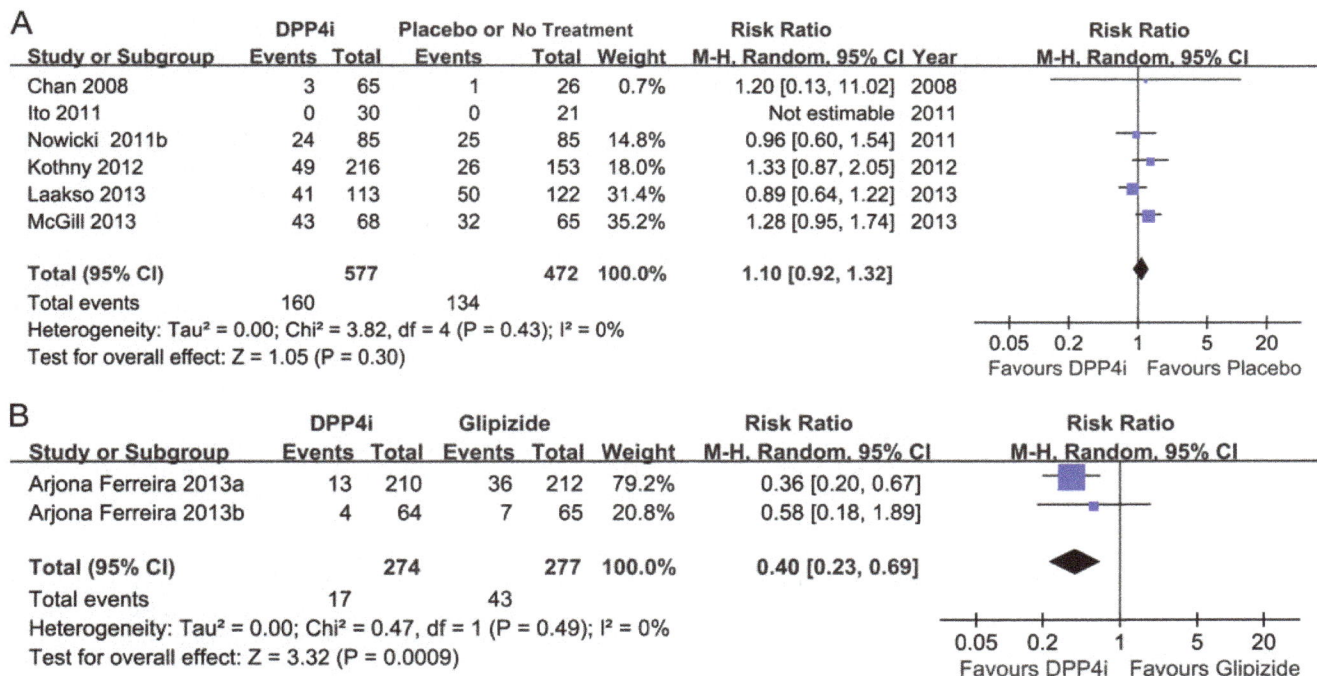

Figure 8. Meta-analysis for the risk of hypoglycemia. A, DPP-4 inhibitor vs. placebo. B, DPP-4 inhibitor vs. glipizide.

Table 2. Summary of safety outcomes for DPP-4 Inhibitors compared to comparators.

Outcome	Number of studies	Total number	Events	RR (95%CI)
Death				
PP-4 inhibitor vs. placebo	5	512/446	10/8	1.12 (0.44–2.85)
PP-4 inhibitor vs. glipizide	2	274/277	7/13	0.54 (0.22–1.33)
ildagliptin vs. sitagliptin	1	46/38	0/0	NA
Discontinuation				
PP-4 inhibitor vs. placebo	4	512/446	38/33	1.02 (0.65–1.60)
PP-4 inhibitor vs. glipizide	2	274/277	23/25	0.93 (0.54–1.60)
ildagliptin vs. sitagliptin	1	46/38	6/4	1.24 (0.38–4.07)
Any AE				
PP-4 inhibitor vs. placebo	4	482/425	397/342	1.01 (0.95–1.08)
PP-4 inhibitor vs. glipizide	2	274/277	196/205	0.97 (0.87–1.07)
SAE				
PP-4 inhibitor vs. placebo	4	482/425	105/94	0.97 (0.76–1.23)
PP-4 inhibitor vs. glipizide	2	274/277	57/58	0.99 (0.72–1.37)
ildagliptin vs. sitagliptin	1	46/38	15/10	1.24 (0.63–2.43)
Drug-related AE				
PP-4 inhibitor vs. placebo	3	397/350	113/105	0.96 (0.77–1.20)
PP-4 inhibitor vs. glipizide	2	274/277	37/52	0.72 (0.49–1.06)
Drug-related SAE				
PP-4 inhibitor vs. placebo	2	198/207	8/7	1.16 (0.43–3.10)
PP-4 inhibitor vs. glipizide	2	274/277	2/1	2.02(0.18–22.10)

AE, adverse event; SAE, serious adverse event; NA, not applicable.

and no treatment groups, the DPP-4 inhibitor groups typically had lower HbA1c levels, and a higher proportion of subjects that achieved the HbA1c goal of <7%; dialysis status did not affect these results. Sensitivity analysis indicated that the results were robust. There was no significant difference between the capacity of DPP-4 inhibitors and other active drugs such as sulfonylureas to reduce HbA1c levels. In contrast, DPP-4 inhibitors did not exhibit an FBG lowering effect, probably due to heterogeneity among the studies and an insufficient number of the samples. These results are consistent with those obtained in T2DM patients in similar studies [30–31]. It was reported previously that GLP-1 reduced HbA1c levels to a greater extent than did DPP-4 inhibitors [32–33], yet data in this article showed no difference between DPP-4 inhibitors and GLP-1 in severe renal dysfunction while a relatively poorer reducing effect of DPP-4 inhibitors was indeed observed in moderate renal dysfunction. The results might become more consistent with the previous reports if there was a larger sample size.

Regarding safety, data revealed that there was no change in the incidence of hypoglycemia with DPP-4 inhibitor treatment. The results remained consistent with dialysis patients with severe hypoglycemia. Moreover, there was no increase in weight gain, incidence of severe adverse effects, and total mortality. Although the definition of CVD was different among the trials included in this systematic review, no studies reported an increase in the incidence of CVD events as a result of DPP-4 inhibitor therapy. This is consistent with recent evidence showing that DPP-4 inhibitors did not increase CVD events in T2DM patients [34–35].

Although individual studies indicated that there was no deterioration in renal status during DPP-4 inhibitor administra-

tion, this conclusion could be strengthened by a pooled estimation on renal function. However, this could not be accomplished in the current study due to variations in the comparison objects and a lack of accurate standard deviation values. In addition, the effect of DDP-4 inhibitors on renal function in CKD patients remains unclear. Previous reports found either the progression of renal status or no affect on renal deterioration in patients treated with these agents [36–37]. Recently, studies assessing the attenuation of renal dysfunction in an ischemia-reperfusion injury model and remnant kidneys revealed that there might be a potential nephroprotective effect of DPP-4 inhibitors [38–39]. The mechanism for this might be associated with a reduction in apoptosis and inflammation and an increase in antioxidant production. Although a large number of ongoing trials have assessed the proteinuria-lowering effect of DPP-4 inhibitors [40–41], few primary articles have investigated the effect of these agents on renal status, particularly in individuals at an early stage of renal impairment. Therefore, there is little evidence that DPP-4 inhibitors could help delay the progression of renal status.

This is the first meta-analysis to assess the safety and efficacy of DPP-4 inhibitors in T2DM patients with moderate to severe renal impairment. The strength of this article is that it reports a comprehensive search that enrolled almost all the published and unpublished articles, including conferences abstracts, clinical trials registries, company websites, and FDA and EMA websites. In addition, a transparent GRADE approach provided an accurate assessment of the quality of evidence for each outcome.

However, the study also has some limitations. Notably, no studies at a low risk of bias were found, which could be attributed to several factors. For example, some studies might have inadequate random sequence generation and allocation sequence concealment. Moreover, the included open label study might have affected the results due to the lack of blinding. Articles with incomplete outcome data might have overestimated the efficacy of DPP-4 inhibitors on lowering HbA1c. In addition, all the above studies were sponsored by pharmaceutical companies, which might increase the risk of bias. A summary of the findings and the quality of evidence for this review are shown in Files S2 and S3. Although GRADE analysis indicated that the quality of evidence for each outcome was mostly low, 'any adverse events' were graded moderate. Due to insufficient data, our subgroup analyses were based on dialysis status rather than CKD stages. In addition, the dialysis group focused mainly on hemodialysis patients, with few data on peritoneal dialysis. However, it is quite necessary and difficult to establish good glycemic control for peritoneal dialysis patients due to the clinical use of glucose-containing dialysis solution [42]. Therefore, it is important to conduct further testing on the efficacy and safety of DPP-4 inhibitors in patients at various CKD stages and peritoneal dialysis. In addition, more attention should be paid to glycated albumin, which is a new and potentially better indicator of glycemic control, particularly in ESRD patients [43–44].

There are several different types of DPP-4 inhibitors, and each lacks sufficient testing. Therefore, we were unable to perform a detailed meta-analysis. The same problem exists for assessing the difference between DPP-4 inhibitors and other active agents, and for subgroup analyses based on different antidiabetic backgrounds.

Funnel plot asymmetry was observed and confirmed using Egger's and Begg's tests. This is recognized as a sign of potential publication bias. However, several alternative factors might also lead to asymmetry [45], including selection bias, poor methodological design, inadequate analysis in smaller studies, and true heterogeneity induced by factors such as different durations of intervention [46]. As shown in Figure 4, three studies in the lower left quadrant contributed to the asymmetry because of a long follow-up period and a high risk of bias (due to the inclusion of incomplete outcome data in two studies). Therefore, the asymmetry in our analysis might be attributed to true heterogeneity caused by clinical and methodological heterogeneity, even though no statistical heterogeneity was detected. Finally, it is inevitable that some unpublished articles might have been missed from the search.

This comprehensive analysis revealed that DPP-4 inhibitors lowered HbA1c, and did not increase the incidence of adverse events. Therefore, they represent a feasible treatment option for T2DM patients with moderate to severe renal impairment. However, considering the overall low quality of the data in this study, as judged by GRADE, DPP-4 inhibitors should be tested further in better-designed randomized trials. Additional attention should be paid to a comparison between DPP-4 inhibitors and other active drugs in patients at different stages of CKD, particularly including dialysis patients.

Conclusions

DPP-4 inhibitors are effective at lowering HbA1c in T2DM patients with moderate to severe renal impairment, and might lower the risk of adverse events. Further well-designed randomized trials focusing on the safety and efficacy of DPP-4 inhibitors in patients at different CKD stages are needed urgently because of the low quality of evidence in the current meta-analysis.

Supporting Information

Figure S1   Risk of bias graph of all included studies.

Figure S2   Subgroup analysis for change in HbA1c (DPP-4 inhibitor vs placebo or no treatment).

Table S1   PRISMA Checklist.

Table S2   Sensitivity analyses comparing DPP-4 inhibitors with placebo on HbA1c.

Table S3   Findings of comparing DPP-4 inhibitors with comparators on CVD.

File S1   Search strategies.

File S2   Summary of findings: Efficacy of DPP-4 inhibitors in type 2 diabetes mellitus patients with moderate to severe renal impairment.

File S3   Summary of findings: Safety of DPP-4 inhibitors in type 2 diabetes mellitus patients with moderate to severe renal impairment.

Acknowledgments

We thank all the members of our study team for their cooperation and the authors of the included trials for their wonderful work. We thank LetPub (www.letpub.com) for its linguistic assistance during the preparation of this manuscript.

Author Contributions

Conceived and designed the experiments: DC YF YL JL YC XW NW. Performed the experiments: DC YL JL YC XW NW. Analyzed the data: DC YF YL. Contributed reagents/materials/analysis tools: DC YL. Wrote the paper: DC YF NW.

References

1. National Kidney Foundation (2012) KDOQI Clinical Practice Guideline for Diabetes and CKD: 2012 update. Am J Kidney Dis 60:850–886.
2. Perkovic V, Heerspink HL, Chalmers J, Woodward M, Jun M, et al. (2013) Intensive glucose control improves kidney outcomes in patients with type 2 diabetes. Kidney Int 83:517–523.
3. Kidney Disease: Improving Global Outcomes (KDIGO) CKD Work Group (2013) KDIGO Clinical Practice Guideline for the Evaluation and Management of Chronic Kidney Disease. Kidney Int Suppl 3: 1–150.
4. Inzucchi SE (2002) Oral antihyperglycemic therapy for type 2 diabetes: scientific review. JAMA 287:360–372.
5. Nesto RW, Bell D, Bonow RO, Fonseca V, Grundy SM, et al. (2004) Thiazolidinedione use, fluid retention, and congestive heart failure: a consensus statement from the American Heart Association and American Diabetes Association. Diabetes Care 27:256–263.
6. Iglesias P, Diez JJ (2008) Insulin therapy in renal disease. Diabetes Obes Metab 10:811–823.
7. Drucker DJ, Nauck MA (2006) The incretin system: glucagon-like peptide-1 receptor agonists and dipeptidyl peptidase-4 inhibitors in type 2 diabetes. Lancet 368:1696–1705.
8. Park H, Park C, Kim Y, Rascati KL (2012) Efficacy and safety of dipeptidyl peptidase-4 inhibitors in type 2 diabetes: meta-analysis. Ann Pharmacother 46:1453–1469.
9. Giorda CB, Nada E, Tartaglino B (2014) Pharmacokinetics, safety, and efficacy of DPP-4 inhibitors and GLP-1 receptor agonists in patients with type 2 diabetes mellitus and renal or hepatic impairment. A systematic review of the literature. Endocrine DOI 10.1007/s12020-014-0179-0.

10. Ramirez G, Morrison AD, Bittle PA (2013) Clinical practice considerations and review of the literature for the Use of DPP-4 inhibitors in patients with type 2 diabetes and chronic kidney disease. Endocr Pract 19:1025–1034.

11. Liberati A, Altman DG, Tetzlaff J, Mulrow C, Gøtzsche PC, et al. (2009) The PRISMA statement for reporting systematic reviews and meta-analyses of studies that evaluate health care interventions: explanation and elaboration. Ann Intern Med 151:W65–W94.

12. Higgins JP, Altman DG, Gotzsche PC, Juni P, Moher D, et al. (2011) The Cochrane Collaboration's tool for assessing risk of bias in randomised trials. BMJ 343:d5928.

13. Guyatt G, Oxman AD, Akl EA, Kunz R, Vist G, et al. (2011) GRADE guidelines: 1. Introduction-GRADE evidence profiles and summary of findings tables. J Clin Epidemiol 64:383–394.

14. Deeks JJ, Higgins JPT, Altman DG (2011) Analysing data and undertaking meta-analyses. In: Higgins JPT, Green S, eds. Cochrane handbook for systematic reviews of interventions. Version 5.1.0. Oxford, UK:Cochrane Collaboration.

15. Higgins JP, Thompson SG, Deeks JJ, Altman DG (2003) Measuring inconsistency in meta-analyses. BMJ 327:557–560.

16. Chan JC, Scott R, Arjona Ferreira JC, Sheng D, Gonzalez E, et al. (2008) Safety and efficacy of sitagliptin in patients with type 2 diabetes and chronic renal insufficiency. Diabetes Obes Metab 10:545–555.

17. Ito M, Abe M, Okada K, Sasaki H, Maruyama N, et al. (2011) The dipeptidyl peptidase-4 (DPP-4) inhibitor vildagliptin improves glycemic control in type 2 diabetic patients undergoing hemodialysis. Endocr J 58:979–987.

18. Nowicki M, Rychlik I, Haller H, Warren ML, Suchower L, et al. (2011) Saxagliptin improves glycaemic control and is well tolerated in patients with type 2 diabetes mellitus and renal impairment. Diabetes Obes Metab 13:523–532.

19. Nowicki M, Rychlik I, Haller H, Warren M, Suchower L, et al. (2011) Long-term treatment with the dipeptidyl peptidase-4 inhibitor saxagliptin in patients with type 2 diabetes mellitus and renal impairment: a randomised controlled 52-week efficacy and safety study. Int J Clin Pract 65:1230–1239.

20. Lukashevich V, Schweizer A, Shao Q, Groop PH, Kothny W (2011) Safety and efficacy of vildagliptin versus placebo in patients with type 2 diabetes and moderate or severe renal impairment: a prospective 24-week randomized placebo-controlled trial. Diabetes Obes Metab 13:947–954.

21. Kothny W, Shao Q, Groop PH, Lukashevich V (2012) One-year safety, tolerability and efficacy of vildagliptin in patients with type 2 diabetes and moderate or severe renal impairment. Diabetes Obes Metab 14:1032–1039.

22. McGill JB, Sloan L, Newman J, Patel S, Sauce C, et al. (2013) Long-term efficacy and safety of linagliptin in patients with type 2 diabetes and severe renal impairment: a 1-year, randomized, double-blind, placebo-controlled study. Diabetes Care 36:237–244.

23. Laakso M, Rosenstock J, Groop PH, Hehnke U, Tamminen I, et al.(2013) Linagliptin vs placebo followed by glimepiride in Type 2 Diabetes patients with moderate to severe renal impairment. American Diabetes Association (ADA) 73rd Scientific Sessions, Chicago, USA.

24. Arjona Ferreira JC, Marre M, Barzilai N, Guo H, Golm GT, et al. (2013) Efficacy and safety of sitagliptin versus glipizide in patients with type 2 diabetes and moderate-to-severe chronic renal insufficiency. Diabetes Care 36:1067–1073.

25. Arjona Ferreira JC, Corry D, Mogensen CE, Sloan L, Xu L, et al. (2013) Efficacy and safety of sitagliptin in patients with type 2 diabetes and ESRD receiving dialysis: a 54-week randomized trial. Am J Kidney Dis 61:579–587.

26. Leiter L, Carr MC, Stewart M, Jones-Leone A, Yang F, et al. (2013) HARMONY 8: once-weekly glucagon-like peptide 1 receptor agonist albiglutide vs sitagliptin for patients with type 2 diabetes with renal impairment: week 26 results. European Association for the Study of Diabetes (EASD) 49th Annual Meeting, Barcelona, Spain.

27. Novartis Clinical Trial Results Database website. Available: http://www.novctrd.com/ctrdWebApp/clinicaltrialrepository/displayFile.do?trialResult=5924. Accessed: 2014 Jun 20.

28. Novartis Clinical Trial Results Database website. Available: http://www.novctrd.com/ctrdWebApp/clinicaltrialrepository/displayFile.do?trialResult=5923. Accessed: 2014 Jun 20.

29. Clinicaltrials.gov website. Available: http://www.clinicaltrials.gov./ct2/show/NCT01968044. Accessed: 2014 Jun 20.

30. Karagiannis T, Paschos P, Paletas K, Matthews DR, Tsapas A (2012) Dipeptidyl peptidase-4 inhibitors for treatment of type 2 diabetes mellitus in the clinical setting: systematic review and meta-analysis. BMJ 344:e1369.

31. Monami M, Iacomelli I, Marchionni N, Mannucci E (2009) Dipeptydil peptidase-4 inhibitors in type 2 diabetes: a meta-analysis of randomized clinical trials. Nutr Metab Cardiovasc Dis 20:224–235.

32. Pratley RE, Nauck M, Bailey T, Montanya E, Cuddihy R, et al. (2010) Liraglutide versus sitagliptin for patients with type 2 diabetes who did not have adequate glycaemic control with metformin: a 26-week, randomised, parallel-group, open-label trial. Lancet 375:1447–1456.

33. Wang T, Gou Z, Wang F, Ma M, Zhai SD (2014) Comparison of GLP-1 Analogues versus Sitagliptin in the Management of Type 2 Diabetes: Systematic Review and Meta-Analysis of Head-to-Head Studies. PLoS One 9:e103798.

34. White WB, Cannon CP, Heller SR, Nissen SE, Bergenstal RM, et al. (2013) EXAMINE Investigators. Alogliptin after acute coronary syndrome in patients with type 2 diabetes. N Engl J Med 369:1327–1335.

35. Scirica BM, Bhatt DL, Braunwald E, Steg PG, Davidson J, et al. (2013) SAVOR-TIMI 53 Steering Committee and Investigators.Saxagliptin and cardiovascular outcomes in patients with type 2 diabetes mellitus. N Engl J Med 369:1317–1326.

36. Kao DP, Kohrt HE, Kugler J (2008) Renal failure and rhabdomyolysis associated with sitagliptin and simvastatin use. Diabet Med 25:1229–1230.

37. Pendergrass M, Fenton C, Haffner SM, Chen W (2012) Exenatide and sitagliptin are not associated with increased risk of acute renal failure: a retrospective claims analysis. Diabetes Obes Metab 14:596–600.

38. Glorie LL, Verhulst A, Matheeussen V, Baerts L, Magielse J, et al. (2012) DPP4 inhibition improves functional outcome after renal ischemia-reperfusion injury, associated with antiapoptotic, immunological, and antioxidative changes. Am J Physiol Renal Physiol 303:F681–F688.

39. Joo KW, Kim S, Ahn SY, Chin HJ, Chae DW, et al. (2013) Dipeptidyl peptidase IV inhibitor attenuates kidney injury in rat remnant kidney. BMC Nephrol 14:98

40. Clinicaltrials.gov website. Available: http://www.clinicaltrials.gov./ct2/show/NCT01792518. Accessed: 2014 Jun 20.

41. Clinicaltrials.gov website. Available: http://www.clinicaltrials.gov./ct2/show/NCT02048904. Accessed: 2014 Jun 20.

42. Mehrotra R, de Boer IH, Himmelfarb J (2013) Adverse effects of systemic glucose absorption with peritoneal dialysis: how good is the evidence? Curr Opin Nephrol Hypertens 22:663–668.

43. Inaba M, Okuno S, Kumeda Y, Yamada S, Imanishi Y, et al. (2007) Glycated albumin is a better glycemic indicator than glycated hemoglobin values in hemodialysis patients with diabetes: effect of anemia and erythropoietin injection. J Am Soc Nephrol 18:896–903.

44. Freedman BI, Andries L, Shihabi ZK, Rocco MV, Byers JR, et al. (2011) Glycated albumin and risk of death and hospitalizations in diabetic dialysis patients. J Am Soc Nephrol 6:1635–1643.

45. Deeks JJ, Higgins JPT, Altman DG (2011) Addressing reporting biases. In: Higgins JPT, Green S, eds. Cochrane handbook for systematic reviews of interventions.Version 5.1.0. Oxford, UK: Cochrane Collaboration.

46. Egger M, Davey Smith G, Schneider M, Minder C (1997) Bias in meta-analysis detected by a simple, graphical test. BMJ 315: 629–634.

19

Decrease in Urinary Creatinine Excretion in Early Stage Chronic Kidney Disease

Elena Tynkevich[1,2]*, **Martin Flamant**[3], **Jean-Philippe Haymann**[4,5,6], **Marie Metzger**[1,2], **Eric Thervet**[7,8], **Jean-Jacques Boffa**[5,6,9], **François Vrtovsnik**[10], **Pascal Houillier**[11,12], **Marc Froissart**[1], **Bénédicte Stengel**[1,2] **and on behalf of the NephroTest Study Group**[¶]

1 CESP, Centre for Epidemiology and Population Health, INSERM Unit 1018, Villejuif, France, **2** University Paris-Sud 11, UMRS 1018, Villejuif, France, **3** AP-HP, Hôpital Bichat, Department of Physiology, Paris, France, **4** AP-HP, Hôpital Tenon, Department of Physiology, Paris, France, **5** INSERM UNIT 702, Paris, France, **6** University Pierre et Marie Curie-Paris 6, UMRS 702, Paris, France, **7** AP-HP, Hôpital Européen Georges Pompidou, Department of Nephrology, Paris, France, **8** AP-HP, Hôpital Européen Georges Pompidou, DHU Common and Rare Arterial Diseases, Paris, France, **9** AP-HP, Hôpital Tenon, Department of Nephrology, Paris, France, **10** AP-HP, Hôpital Bichat, Department of Nephrology, Paris, France, **11** University Paris Descartes-Paris 5, UMRS 775, Paris, France, **12** AP-HP, Hôpital Européen Georges Pompidou, Department of Physiology, Paris, France

Abstract

Background: Little is known about muscle mass loss in early stage chronic kidney disease (CKD). We used 24-hour urinary creatinine excretion rate to assess determinants of muscle mass and its evolution with kidney function decline. We also described the range of urinary creatinine concentration in this population.

Methods: We included 1072 men and 537 women with non-dialysis CKD stages 1 to 5, all of them with repeated measurements of glomerular filtration rate (mGFR) by ^{51}Cr-EDTA renal clearance and several nutritional markers. In those with stage 1 to 4 at baseline, we used a mixed model to study factors associated with urinary creatinine excretion rate and its change over time.

Results: Baseline mean urinary creatinine excretion decreased from 15.3±3.1 to 12.1±3.3 mmol/24 h (0.20±0.03 to 0.15±0.04 mmol/kg/24 h) in men, with mGFR falling from ≥60 to <15 mL/min/1.73 m^2, and from 9.6±1.9 to 7.6±2.5 (0.16±0.03 to 0.12±0.03) in women. In addition to mGFR, an older age, diabetes, and lower levels of body mass index, proteinuria, and protein intake assessed by urinary urea were associated with lower mean urinary creatinine excretion at baseline. Mean annual decline in mGFR was 1.53±0.12 mL/min/1.73 m^2 per year and that of urinary creatinine excretion rate, 0.28±0.02 mmol/24 h per year. Patients with fast annual decline in mGFR of 5 mL/min/1.73 m^2 had a decrease in urinary creatinine excretion more than twice as big as in those with stable mGFR, independent of changes in urinary urea as well as of other determinants of low muscle mass.

Conclusions: Decrease in 24-hour urinary creatinine excretion rate may appear early in CKD patients, and is greater the more mGFR declines independent of lowering protein intake assessed by 24-hour urinary urea. Normalizing urine analytes for creatininuria may overestimate their concentration in patients with reduced kidney function and low muscle mass.

Editor: Jaap A. Joles, University Medical Center Utrecht, Netherlands

Funding: The NephroTest CKD cohort study is supported by the following grants: INSERM GIS-IReSP AO 8113LS TGIR (B.S.), French Ministry of Health AOM 09114 (M.Fr.), INSERM AO 8022LS (B.S.), Agence de la Biomédecine R0 8156LL (B.S.), AURA (M.Fr.), and Roche 2009-152-447G (M.Fr.). The funders had no role in study design, data collection and analysis, decision to publish, or preparation of the manuscript.

Competing Interests: The authors have the following interests. This study was partly supported by Roche. B.S. has received consulting or lecture fees from AbbVie, Amgen, Fresenius, and MSD; M.F. has received research funds from Hoffmann-La Roche; M.F. has been employed by Amgen since January 1, 2011, but was a full-time academic associate professor during the time of study conception and data collection. There are no patents, products in development, or marketed products to declare.

* Email: elena.tynkevich@inserm.fr

¶ Membership of the NephroTest study group is provided in the Acknowledgments.

Introduction

Protein-energy wasting (PEW) is a state of decreased body stores of protein and energy fuels, assessed by biochemical and clinical measures [1–4]. Nutritional disorders are common in patients with end-stage chronic kidney disease (CKD) [1,5–8] and are often associated with inflammation [7,9–12]. Both conditions are known to be associated with high cardiovascular [10,11,13] and all-cause [5,10,14–17] mortality. While nutritional disorders have previously been studied in patients with end-stage CKD [1,6,14,16,18–24] or coronary heart disease [13,25], and in the general population [26–29], little is known about the timing of PEW in non-end-stage CKD [17,30].

Muscle wasting is one of the most valid markers of PEW [2,8,14]. Loss of muscle mass results from an imbalance between protein synthesis and degradation and is worsened by inactivity [22,31] and loss of appetite [9,32,33]. A variety of conditions, including diabetes mellitus [21,24], metabolic acidosis [34,35], and inflammation [19,31,36,37], may promote an increase in protein breakdown. Muscle mass may be assessed by biochemical [2,3,38,39], anthropometric [2,3], or bioelectrical measurements [40,41]. In steady state, urinary creatinine excretion is one of the most specific indexes of total body muscle mass, because creatine originates almost exclusively (98%) from skeletal muscle[39,42]. The amount of both filtered and secreted creatinine excreted in the urine represents the difference between creatinine generation and its extrarenal elimination. The former is proportional to muscle mass but also affected by meat intake [3,39,42], and the latter is known to increase in patients with severely reduced kidney function [42,43]. Several studies reported the normal range and determinants of urinary creatinine concentration in the general population[27]. Very few, however, have investigated its relation to kidney function decline, while taking into account the determinants of muscle mass, including reduced protein intake [17,30]. Moreover, most studies which investigated the association between urinary excretion of creatinine and renal function were based on glomerular filtration rate (GFR) estimated from plasma creatinine concentration, which is itself determined by muscular production of creatinine (and hence its urinary excretion). Thus, using a gold standard GFR measurement method, which is independent of plasma creatinine concentration, is methodologically crucial to study the correlation between urinary creatinine excretion and renal function decline.

We therefore studied the determinants of low urinary creatinine excretion as well as of the evolution of its rate over time, in a large cohort of patients with all stages of CKD and measured glomerular filtration rate (mGFR) from the NephroTest study. In addition, we document the range of urinary creatinine concentrations by age, gender, ethnicity and mGFR level.

Methods

Ethics statement

All patients signed written informed consents before inclusion in the cohort. The NephroTest study design was approved by an ethics committee (Direction générale pour la recherche et l'innovation. Comité consultatif sur le traitement de l'information en matière de recherche dans le domaine de la santé (CCTIRS). Ref: DGRI CCTIRS MG/CP09.503, 9th July 2009).

Patients and study design

The NephroTest study is a prospective hospital-based cohort that began in 2000; by the end of 2010, it had enrolled 1827 adult patients with all stages of CKD and all nephropathy types referred by nephrologists to any of three departments of physiology for annual extensive workups. Eligible patients were ≥18 years of age at inclusion and had neither started dialysis nor received a kidney transplant. Pregnant women were excluded.

Information

Data were recorded during a 5-hour in-person visit for a complete nephrological workup comprising a large set of clinical and laboratory measurements, including blood pressure, body mass index (BMI), and treatments received. Diabetes was defined as either fasting glycemia ≥7 mmol/L or HbA1c ≥6.5% or antidiabetic treatment, hypertension by either a systolic or diastolic blood pressure >140/90 mm Hg or antihypertensive treatment, metabolic acidosis as venous CO_2 <22 mmol/L or alkaline treatment.

Laboratory measurements

At each visit, mGFR was measured concurrently for all patients by ^{51}Cr-EDTA renal clearance and fractional creatinine clearance. Subjects also provided 24-hour urine collection, which enabled us to measure 24-hour creatinine clearance as well as creatininuria with the Jaffe method. Because 24-hour urine collection may be inaccurate, we primarily used 24-hour urinary creatinine extrapolated from fractional creatinine clearance in this study, on the assumption that creatinine excretion is stable over the 24-hour period. Moreover, the analysis of consistency between the two measures of creatinine clearance and that of mGFR enabled us to exclude outliers and to assess the completeness of the 24-hour urine collection. Thus, in addition to 84 patients with missing urinary creatinine, we excluded 78 patients with missing data for fractional creatinine clearance and 56 outliers for mGFR or for fractional or 24-hour creatinine clearance or both, leaving 1609 patients for the analysis of baseline data (Figure 1).

Gender-specific thresholds for low urinary creatinine excretion were defined as values <10th percentile of the distribution in patients with mGFR ≥60 mL/min/1.73 m², i.e., 11.4 mmol/24 h in men and 7.2 in women. Several markers of inflammation-malnutrition were also measured and studied, with the following cutoffs to define abnormal values: serum albumin <35 g/L, prealbumin <0.30 g/L, total cholesterol <5.5 mmol/L, triglycerides ≥1.7 mmol/L, transferrin <2 g/L, white blood cells (WBC) ≥7.5×10³/mm³, C-reactive protein (CRP) ≥10 mg/L, haptoglobin ≥90th percentile, orosomucoid ≥90th percentile, and plasma fibrinogen ≥5 g/L. Gender-specific thresholds were used to define high-density lipoprotein (HDL) cholesterol cutoff points: 1.0 mmol/L in men and 1.3 mmol/L in women. Urinary urea (mmol/24-hour), reflecting protein intake, and 24-hour proteinuria, were analyzed in quartiles.

Missing values accounted for less than 5% of most indicators. Mean imputation was used for those included in the multivariate analysis. A missing category was created for the indicators with > 5% of values missing, including prealbumin (24%), orosomucoid (37%), and haptoglobin (21%).

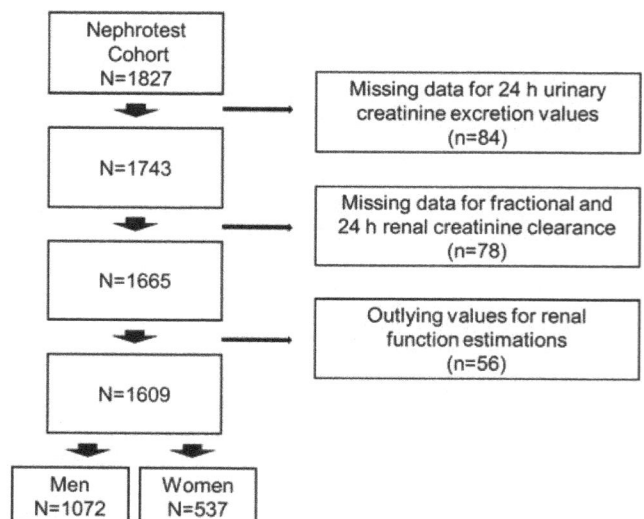

Figure 1. Flowchart of study sample.

Table 1. Patient characteristics according to mGFR level in 1609 patients.

	mGFR (ml/min per1.73 m^2)					p Value
	≥60	45–60	30–44	15–29	<15	
	(n = 282)	(n = 321)	(n = 472)	(n = 435)	(n = 99)	
Demographic parameters						
Men	188 (66.7)	233 (72.6)	321 (68.0)	274 (63.0)	56 (56.6)	0.01
Age (years)	52.0±15.1	58.7±14.4	61.0±15.0	61.0±15.0	60.9±15.2	<0.0001
African origin	53 (18.8)	48 (15.0)	56 (11.9)	44 (10.1)	8 (8.1)	<0.0001
Body mass index (kg/m^2)	25.9±4.9	26.3±4.9	26.6±4.8	26.6±5.0	27.0±6.0	0.19
Diabetes[a]	62 (22.0)	83 (25.9)	150 (31.8)	136 (31.3)	25 (25.3)	0.02
Metabolic acidosis[b]	6 (2.1)	11 (3.4)	47 (10.0)	100 (23.0)	46 (46.5)	<0.0001
Hypertension[c]	225 (79.8)	284 (88.5)	447 (94.7)	415 (95.4)	98 (99.0)	<0.0001
Any antihypertensive treatment	216 (76.6)	272 (84.7)	435 (92.2)	408 (93.8)	96 (97.0)	<0.0001
Laboratory parameters						
eGFR	75.9±19.6	54.3±12.1	39.5±9.8	25.4±8.5	13.7±5.6	<0.0001
HDL cholesterol (mmol/L)	1.36±0.40	1.35±0.42	1.30±0.44	1.24±0.39	1.29±0.50	0.001
Triglycerides (mmol/L)	1.1 (0.82–1.6)	1.2 (0.87–1.6)	1.4 (0.94–2.0)	1.4 (1.0–2.1)	1.5 (1.1–2.3)	<0.0001
Serum albumin (g/L)	40.2±3.7	40.3±3.9	39.3±4.5	38.8±4.6	38.9±5.0	<0.0001
Prealbumin (g/L)	0.29±0.07	0.30±0.06	0.30±0.07	0.33±0.0.8	0.34±0.08	<0.0001
Transferrin (g/L)	2.4±0.42	2.3±0.37	2.3±0.41	2.2±0.40	2.13±0.36	<0.0001
Homocysteine (umol/L)	13.5±4.3	16.9±6.1	19.1±6.3	21.7±7.6	24.0±7.8	<0.0001
Urinary urea (mmol/24h)	405.6±118.9	381.2±110.7	373.3±124.7	354.4±113.7	297.4±100.8	<0.0001
WBC count (10^3/mm^3)	6.1±1.8	6.2±2.0	6.5±2.3	6.8±2.2	6.7±1.9	0.0001
Plasma fibrinogen (g/L)	3.4±0.81	3.5±0.88	3.8±0.93	4.2±1.00	4.4±0.99	<0.0001
CRP>10 mg/L	15 (5.3)	23 (7.2)	43 (9.1)	50 (11.5)	8 (8.1)	0.20
Orosomucoid (g/L)	0.79±0.21	0.85±0.22	0.92±0.25	1.0±0.31	1.1±0.23	<0.0001
Haptoglobin (g/L)	1.2±0.58	1.2±0.58	1.4±0.61	1.5±0.67	1.5±0.69	<0.0001
Proteinuria (g/24h)	0.16 (0.10–0.50)	0.17 (0.11–0.40)	0.26 (0.13–0.93)	0.65 (0.23–1.8)	1.3 (0.55–2.3)	<0.0001

Abbreviations: BP, blood pressure; mGFR, measured glomerular filtration rate; HDL, high-density lipoprotein; WBC, white blood cells; CRP, C-reactive protein.
Values are reported as %, mean ± SD or median (interquartile range).
[a] Fasting glucose ≥7 mmol/L or HbA1c ≥6.5 or antidiabetic treatment or reported diabetes.
[b] Venous CO2 <22 mmol/L or alkaline treatment.
[c] Any antihypertensive treatment or systolic BP>140 or diastolic BP>90 mm Hg.

Statistical analyses

Variables were expressed as percentages, means ± SD, or medians (IQR: interquartile range), as appropriate. We first described patients' characteristics according to mGFR classes defined as follows: ≥ 0, 45-59, 30–44, 15–29, and <15 mL/min/1.73 m^2. Differences across mGFR classes were tested with ANOVA for continuous variables and with Chi-square test for categorical variables. We also provided urinary creatinine mean values and 10th, 25th, 75th, and 90th percentiles expressed in both mmol/24-h and mmol/kg/24-h, according to mGFR classes, overall and by age (< or ≥60 years), gender, and ethnicity (non-African vs African origin).

Crude and adjusted odds ratios (ORs) and 95% confidence intervals (95% CI) for low baseline urinary creatinine excretion according to clinical and laboratory parameters were estimated by logistic regression. To be included in the multivariate analysis, factors had to be significantly associated with low urinary creatinine excretion in the crude analysis with p<0.20 and uncorrelated with each other (−0.50<r<0.50). Well-established risk factors for muscle mass loss, such as diabetes, were also included regardless of their statistical significance in the crude

analysis. We studied three models: one crude, one adjusted only for age (treated continuously), gender, ethnicity, center, and mGFR, and another fully adjusted. These analyses were also carried out by replacing mGFR by estimated GFR (eGFR) using the CKD-EPI equation[44], and by sub-group defined by diabetes status.

Finally, we used a linear mixed model with random intercepts and slopes to estimate mean differences in urinary creatinine excretion rate according to covariates shown to be statistically significant in the logistic regression, as well as its annual slope associated with changes in mGFR and 24-hour urinary urea. In this analysis, we excluded 99 patients with CKD stage 5 at baseline and 37 with missing urinary urea, leaving 1473 patients with a median follow-up of 1.43 years (0–3.34, maximum 5 years). Median interval between visits was 1.12 year (1.00–1.69) for the 855 patients with at least two visits. This analysis was based on a total of 3268 observations. Interactions with time were tested for all covariates. In the final mixed model, we only included interaction terms which were statistically significant using Wald test and improved the model according to Akaike information criteria (AIC).

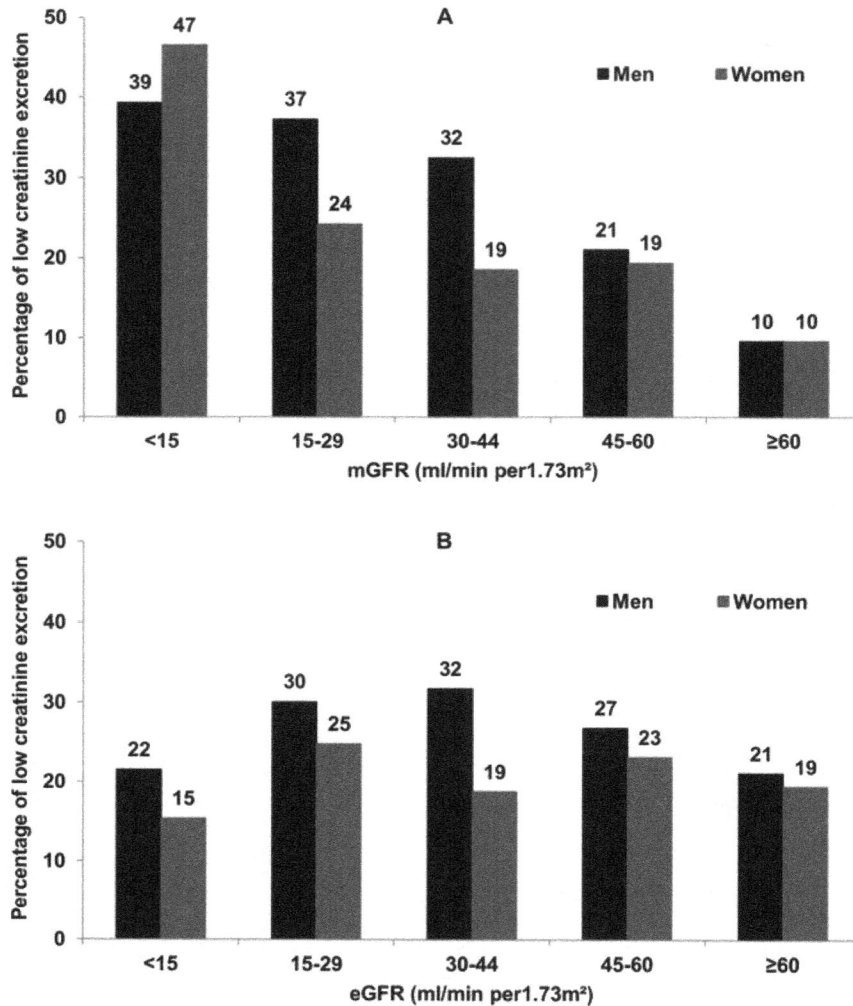

Figure 2. Percentages of low urinary creatinine excretion according to mGFR and eGFR level, by gender. Figure shows the percentage of patients with low creatinine excretion rates according to both measured (2A) and estimated (2B) glomerular filtration rate classes in men and women. Gender-specific thresholds were defined as the 10th percentile of the urinary creatinine distribution in patients with mGFR $\geq$60 mL/min/ 1.73 m^2.

A two-sided P-value <0.05 indicated statistical significance. Statistical analyses were performed with SAS software, version 9.3 (SAS institute, Cary, NC).

Results

Patient characteristics according to mGFR level

Patients' age increased and the percentage of those from sub-Saharan Africa or the French West Indies decreased with decreasing mGFR (Table 1). The level of all nutritional factors, except prealbumin, significantly decreased with mGFR decline, while that of inflammation factors (except CRP) as well as the prevalence of metabolic acidosis significantly increased.

Urinary creatinine excretion rate according to GFR level, by gender, age, and ethnicity

Urinary creatinine excretion was normally distributed. Mean urinary creatinine excretion rate decreased as mGFR decreased from $\geq$60 to <15 mL/min/1.73 m^2 in all categories defined by age, gender, and ethnicity (Table 2). It was higher in men and women with than without African origin. The percentage of patients with low creatinine excretion rates increased as mGFR decreased, reaching about four times the level of the reference category in those with mGFR less than 15 mL/min/1.73 m^2 in both genders (Figure 2A). Of note, this percentage was twice as high in patients with GFR $\geq$ 0 mL/min/1.73 m^2 when using eGFR instead of mGFR, and did not increase with decreasing eGFR (Figure 2B).

Factors associated with low urinary creatinine excretion rate at baseline

Odds ratios of low urinary creatinine excretion significantly and gradually increased as BMI decreased, both before and after adjusting for demographic variables and mGFR (Table 3). Urinary creatinine excretion was not significantly associated with diabetes and metabolic acidosis. Lower prealbumin and urinary urea levels were significantly associated with higher ORs of low urinary creatinine excretion. In contrast, there was no significant association with serum albumin. Triglycerides were inversely and significantly associated with urinary creatinine excretion. Inflam-

Table 2. Urinary creatinine excretion rate according to mGFR level, by gender, age, and ethnicity.

Ethnic origin, age, mGFR (mL/min per 1.73m²)	Men (n=1072)											Women (n=537)										
	Urinary creatinine excretion rate											Urinary creatinine excretion rate										
	mmol/kg/24h						mmol/24h					mmol/kg/24h						mmol/24h				
	N	m±sd	10th	25th	75th	90th	m±sd	10th	25th	75th	90th	N	m±sd	10th	25th	75th	90th	m±sd	10th	25th	75th	90th
Total																						
≥60	188	0.20±0.03	0.15	0.17	0.22	0.24	15.3±3.1	11.4	13.0	17.0	19.4	94	0.16±0.03	0.12	0.14	0.17	0.19	9.6±1.9	7.2	8.3	10.8	12.2
45–60	233	0.18±0.03	0.14	0.15	0.20	0.22	13.9±3.0	10.6	11.8	15.5	17.9	88	0.15±0.03	0.11	0.13	0.16	0.18	9.2±2.1	6.8	7.7	10.6	11.7
30–44	321	0.17±0.03	0.13	0.14	0.19	0.21	13.2±3.2	9.3	11.0	15.2	17.3	151	0.15±0.03	0.10	0.12	0.17	0.19	9.3±2.2	6.8	7.5	10.6	12.3
15–29	274	0.17±0.04	0.12	0.14	0.19	0.22	12.7±3.2	9.0	10.5	14.6	17.0	161	0.13±0.03	0.09	0.11	0.15	0.18	8.8±2.1	6.1	7.3	10.6	11.5
<15	56	0.15±0.04	0.11	0.13	0.18	0.20	12.1±3.3	7.7	9.2	14.0	16.8	43	0.12±0.03	0.08	0.09	0.14	0.15	7.6±2.5	5.0	5.5	8.9	10.8
Non-African origin																						
<60 years																						
≥60	92	0.20±0.03	0.16	0.18	0.22	0.24	15.3±2.9	11.7	13.0	16.9	19.1	45	0.16±0.03	0.12	0.14	0.19	0.22	9.7±1.8	7.6	8.9	10.8	11.9
45–60	78	0.18±0.03	0.15	0.17	0.20	0.22	14.5±3.0	11.4	12.5	16.0	18.5	35	0.16±0.03	0.13	0.13	0.18	0.20	9.4±2.3	6.8	7.8	10.8	11.9
30–44	96	0.19±0.03	0.15	0.17	0.21	0.22	14.6±3.4	11.0	12.3	16.8	18.6	61	0.16±0.04	0.12	0.13	0.18	0.22	9.7±2.4	7.0	8.1	11.0	12.8
15–29	91	0.17±0.03	0.13	0.15	0.19	0.22	13.2±2.6	10.3	11.4	14.8	16.7	61	0.14±0.03	0.10	0.11	0.16	0.19	8.9±2.3	6.0	7.4	10.9	12.0
<15	20	0.17±0.03	0.13	0.14	0.20	0.21	13.8±3.0	9.2	12.4	15.1	17.5	17	0.13±0.03	0.09	0.11	0.13	0.15	7.9±2.5	5.3	6.1	8.9	11.6
≥60 years																						
≥60	50	0.18±0.03	0.14	0.15	0.20	0.21	14.3±2.7	10.7	12.5	15.8	17.4	27	0.15±0.02	0.13	0.14	0.15	0.18	8.6±1.4	6.4	7.7	9.5	10.3
45–60	113	0.17±0.03	0.13	0.15	0.18	0.20	12.9±2.7	10.1	11.2	14.4	16.6	41	0.14±0.02	0.11	0.12	0.15	0.16	8.5±1.7	6.7	7.1	9.6	10.6
30–44	186	0.16±0.03	0.12	0.14	0.18	0.20	12.2±2.6	8.9	10.3	13.9	15.4	60	0.13±0.03	0.09	0.11	0.15	0.16	8.3±1.7	6.4	7.0	9.2	10.5
15–29	147	0.15±0.04	0.11	0.13	0.18	0.20	11.9±3.2	8.3	9.8	13.8	15.7	73	0.13±0.03	0.09	0.10	0.14	0.16	8.6±1.8	6.2	7.3	9.8	11.0
<15	28	0.14±0.03	0.11	0.12	0.15	0.18	10.9±2.6	7.5	8.5	13.4	14.4	14	0.10±0.03	0.07	0.08	0.14	0.15	6.7±2.3	4.0	4.8	8.4	10.0
African origin																						
<60 years																						
≥60	35	0.21±0.08	0.18	0.19	0.24	0.25	17.4±3.1	13.0	15.7	19.7	20.8	11	0.15±0.02	0.12	0.13	0.17	0.17	11.7±1.6	9.8	10.6	12.9	13.1
45–60	28	0.21±0.04	0.16	0.19	0.23	0.27	16.1±3.2	11.8	14.1	18.3	20.0	3	0.17±0.01	0.16	0.16	0.18	0.18	11.6±1.1	10.8	10.8	12.9	12.9
30–44	23	0.20±0.03	0.16	0.18	0.22	0.24	15.6±3.8	10.5	12.9	18.6	19.8	14	0.16±0.03	0.13	0.14	0.18	0.20	10.5±1.7	8.0	9.1	11.7	13.3
15–29	23	0.22±0.04	0.16	0.19	0.24	0.27	16.4±3.2	12.4	13.2	18.9	19.9	12	0.16±0.04	0.10	0.12	0.19	0.20	10.6±1.6	9.8	10.2	11.4	11.5
<15	3	0.18±0.03	0.09	0.09	0.24	0.24	14.1±8.0	5.1	5.1	20.0	20.0	3	0.12±0.02	0.11	0.11	0.14	0.14	10.1±3.8	7.2	7.2	14.4	14.4
≥60 years																						
≥60	6	0.19±0.02	0.16	0.16	0.20	0.22	14.3±0.42	10.8	11.5	17.9	18.6	1	–	–	–	–	–	–	–	–	–	–
45–60	11	0.17±0.04	0.15	0.15	0.19	0.21	13.4±1.7	10.4	11.0	14.8	16.6	6	0.14±0.02	0.12	0.12	0.15	0.17	10.0±1.3	8.4	9.1	11.4	11.5
30–44	13	0.16±0.03	0.13	0.14	0.17	0.20	12.9±1.8	11.7	11.8	13.8	15.2	6	0.14±0.03	0.10	0.13	0.17	0.20	10.1±3.6	7.4	7.6	10.3	17.0

Table . Cont.

Ethnic origin, age, mGFR (mL/min per1.73m²)	Men (n=1072)											Women (n=537)										
	Urinary creatinine excretion rate											Urinary creatinine excretion rate										
	mmol/kg/24h						mmol/24h					mmol/kg/24h						mmol/24h				
	N	m±sd	10th	25th	75th	90th	m±sd	10th	25th	75th	90th	N	m±sd	10th	25th	75th	90th	m±sd	10th	25th	75th	90th
15–29	5	0.16±0.01	0.15	0.16	0.16	0.17	10.9±2.6	8.8	9.8	12.2	13.1	4	0.16±0.04	0.11	0.13	0.19	0.20	10.3±2.3	7.8	8.4	12.3	12.5
<15	2	0.14±0.02	0.13	0.13	0.15	0.15	10.8±3.4	10.6	10.6	11.2	11.2	0	-	-	-	-	-	-	-	-	-	-

Abbreviations: mGFR, measured glomerular filtration rate.

mation, reflected by either higher WBC, plasma fibrinogen or haptoglobin levels, was also inversely and significantly associated with low urinary creatinine excretion after adjusting for confounders, but no such association was observed with CRP and orosomucoid. The higher the quartile of 24-hour proteinuria, the lower the ORs of low urinary creatinine excretion rate.

Fully adjusted ORs for low urinary creatinine excretion increased significantly as mGFR decreased (Table 4), but did not with eGFR: ORs were 0.95 (0.59–1.5), 0.90 (0.57–1.4), 0.94 (0.57–1.5), and 0.62 (0.29–1.3) for eGFR of 45–60, 30–44, 15–29, and <15 as compared with ≥60 mL/min/1.73 m². Other factors significantly associated with low creatinine excretion in the multivariate model were age, gender, ethnicity, BMI, 24-hour urinary urea and proteinuria. While the association with metabolic acidosis remained nonsignificant (data not shown), it is noteworthy that diabetes became strongly associated with low urinary creatinine excretion after adjustment for the other risk factors. Similar associations were observed in patients with and without diabetes except for pre-albumin, which was related to low urinary creatinine excretion only in those with diabetes.

Factors associated with baseline rate and annual change in urinary creatinine excretion

As expected, factors associated with lower mean creatinine excretion rate at baseline were similar to those found above with the logistic model. Each 10 mL/min/1.73 m² decrease in mGFR was associated with 0.23±0.03 mmol/24 h decrease in urinary creatinine excretion rate, and each 10 mmol/24h decrease in urinary urea with 0.09±0.00 mmol/24 h (Table 5). Patients with proteinuria in the highest quartile had a higher rate of 0.80±0.16 mmol/24 h than those in the lowest quartile.

Mean annual decline in mGFR was 1.53±0.12 mL/min/1.73 m² and mean annual decrease in urinary urea was 7.42±1.22 mmol/24 h. Mean change in urinary creatinine excretion rate was 0.28±0.02 mmol/24 h per year and did not differ according to baseline characteristics except gender: women had slower mean annual decrease than men. Patients with a fast annual decline in mGFR of 5 mL/min/1.73 m² (about 3 times the mean level) had a decrease in urinary creatinine excretion more than twice as big than those with stable mGFR, independent of changes in protein intake assessed by urinary urea as well as of other determinants.

Discussion

This study showed that decrease in urinary creatinine excretion may occur early in CKD independent of nutritional factors and protein intake. As expected, the study confirmed the impact of age, ethnicity and nutritional factors on urinary creatinine excretion, but also found a graded relationship with proteinuria and no significant association with inflammation. Together with the range of urinary creatinine excretion provided by age, gender, ethnicity as well as by mGFR, these findings have important clinical implications regarding management of muscle mass loss and validation of urine collection in CKD patients.

Very few studies have investigated the relation between muscle loss and kidney function decline. Foley et al. [28] reported a high prevalence (27.2%) of reduced muscle mass assessed by bioimpedance in community-dwelling adults. Although its prevalence increased as estimated glomerular filtration rate (eGFR) decreased, the association was no longer significant after adjustment for age and comorbidity. Nevertheless, these results are difficult to compare with ours, because bioimpedance measures not only muscle mass but also body water [38,45]. In the Modification of

Table 3. Factors associated with low urinary creatinine excretion rate at baseline, n = 1609.

	Crude OR (95% CI)	Age, gender, ethnicity, centre and mGFR-adjusted OR (95% CI)
BMI group (kg/m²)		
<18.5	4.0 (2.1-7.8)	7.5 (3.5–16.3)
18.5–25	1	1
25–30	0.53 (0.41–0.69)	0.29 (0.21–0.39)
30–35	0.45 (0.31–0.65)	0.22 (0.15–0.34)
≥35	0.20 (0.09–0.44)	0.11 (0.05–0.26)
Diabetes[a] (yes vs no)	1.3 (0.98–1.6)	0.84 (0.65–1.1)
Metabolic acidosis[b] (yes vs no)	1.3 (0.96–1.8)	0.91 (0.63–1.3)
Nutritional markers		
HDL cholesterol <vs ≥ 1.3/1.0 mmol/L*	0.73 (0.57–0.93)	0.62 (0.48–0.81)
Triglycerides ≥ vs <1.7 mmol/L	0.91 (0.71–1.2)	0.68 (0.52–0.89)
Serum albumin <vs ≥ 35 g/L	1.1 (0.79–1.5)	0.90 (0.62–1.3)
Prealbumin <vs ≥ 0.30 g/L	1.3 (1.03–1.7)	1.5 (1.1–1.9)
Urinary urea by quartiles (mmol/24h)		
lower	14.0 (9.2–21.2)	16.4 (10.5–25.7)
2nd	4.4 (2.9–6.8)	5.0 (3.2–7.9)
3nd	1.9 (1.2–3.0)	2.2 (1.4–3.5)
upper	1	1
Inflammation markers		
WBC count ≥ vs <7.5 10³/mm³	0.97 (0.75–1.3)	0.74 (0.56–0.98)
Plasma fibrinogen ≥ vs <5 g/L	1.1 (0.80–1.6)	0.68 (0.47–0.99)
Haptoglobin ≥ vs <90th percentile	0.91 (0.60–1.4)	0.60 (0.38–0.95)
Orosomucoid ≥ vs <90th percentile	1.6 (1.0–2.4)	1.1 (0.72–1.8)
CRP ≥ vs <10 mg/L	1.3 (0.89–1.9)	0.96 (0.63–1.4)
Proteinuria by quartiles (g/24h)		
lower	1	1
2nd	0.65 (0.48–0.89)	0.50 (0.35–0.71)
3nd	0.74 (0.54–1.0)	0.46 (0.32–0.66)
upper	0.56 (0.40–0.77)	0.29 (0.19–0.43)

Abbreviations: OR (95% CI), odds-ratios and 95% confidence interval; mGFR, measured glomerular filtration rate; BMI, body mass index; HDL, high-density lipoprotein; WBC, white blood cells; CRP, C-reactive protein.
Cut-off points of urinary urea were: <312.8 mmol/24h, 312.8–382.5 mmol/24h, 382.5–456.3 mmol/24h,>456.3 mmol/24 in men; <252.0 mmol/24h, 252.0–302.1 mmol/24h, 302.1–375.0 mmol/24h,>375.0 mmol/24h in women. Cut-off points of proteinuria urea were: <0.14 g/24h, 0.14–0.35 g/24,>1.1 g/24h in men; <0.12 g/24g, 0.12–0.21 g/24h, 0.21–0.89 g/24h,>0.89 g/24h in women.
*Gender-specific thresholds were used to define high-density lipoprotein cholesterol cut-off points: 1.0 mmol/L in men and 1.3 mmol/L in women.
[a] Fasting glucose ≥ 7 mmol/L or HbA1c ≥6.5 or antidiabetic treatment or reported diabetes.
[b] Venous CO2 <22 mmol/L or alkaline treatment.

Diet in Renal Disease (MDRD) study [30], several nutritional parameters, including urinary creatinine, showed lower values for patients with mGFR <21 ml/min/1.73 m² than for those with mGFR>37 ml/min/1.73 m². The associations, however, were strongly attenuated after controlling for protein and energy intakes leading the authors to conclude that they were mediated by the lower dietary intake associated with kidney function decline. In contrast, *Micco et al* [17] showed an inverse cross-sectional association between urinary creatinine excretion and CKD stages from 3 to 5 independent of nutritional factors as well as a decrease over time in urinary creatinine excretion independent of eGFR decline. The NephroTest study extends these findings to earlier CKD stages, showing that low creatinine excretion rate was indeed twice as common in stage 3a (GFR within 45–60 mL/min/1.73 m²) than in stages 1–2 (GFR ≥60 mL/min/1.73 m²), independent of both nutritional parameters and protein intake

assessed by urinary urea. Although an increase in extrarenal excretion of creatinine, including its conversion to other metabolites and its breakdown by gut bacteria [39,43] cannot be ruled out as an explanation of the above association, this is unlikely because it is usually significant in the latest stage of CKD. Similarly, while it is well-known that the relative participation of tubular secretion in creatinine excretion increases with kidney function decline, this has definitely no impact on the overall urinary creatinine excretion in steady state such as that of patients with CKD.

As expected and in line with other studies[13,18,26–28,30,39] age, gender and ethnicity were major determinants of urinary creatinine excretion rate. Moreover, the large sample size of the NephroTest study enabled for the first time to document the range of urinary creatinine excretion rate not only according to these variables as previously reported, but also according to mGFR

Table 4. Multivariate analysis of factors associated with low urinary creatinine excretion rate at baseline, by diabetes status.

OR (95% CI)

	Overall population	Without diabetes	With diabetes
	(n = 1609)	(n = 1153)	(n = 456)
Age, year	1.05 (1.04–1.06)	1.05 (1.04–1.07)	1.05 (1.02–1.07)
Gender (men vs women)	2.1 (1.5–2.9)	1.9 (1.3–2.9)	2.1 (1.1–3.9)
African vs non-African origin	0.28 (0.16–0.49)	0.42 (0.22–0.80)	0.15 (0.05–0.44)
mGFR (ml/min per1.73m2)			
≥60	1	1	1
45–60	2.4 (1.3–4.2)	2.1 (1.1–4.2)	2.5 (0.79–7.9)
30–44	3.6 (2.1–6.2)	3.2 (1.7–6.2)	3.8 (1.3–11.0)
15–29	5.2 (2.9–9.2)	5.0 (2.5–10.0)	4.7 (1.6–14.5)
<15	9.2 (4.3–19.6)	8.2 (3.3–20.5)	11.9 (2.6–55.4)
Diabetes mellitus			
no	1	-	-
yes	1.8 (1.3-2.6)	-	-
BMI group (kg/m²)			
<18.5	9.6 (4.2–21.9)	9.7 (4.1–22.9)	
18.5–25	1	1	5.0 (2.4–10.4)
25–30	0.29 (0.20–0.41)	0.32 (0.21–0.48)	1
30–35	0.24 (0.15–0.39)	0.12 (0.06–0.26)	1.6 (0.81–3.0)
≥35	0.12 (0.05–0.32)	0.12 (0.03–0.53)	0.51 (0.15–1.8)
Prealbumin (g/L)			
>0.30	1	1	1
<0.30	1.2 (0.84–1.7)	0.83 (0.54–1.3)	2.3 (1.3–4.2)
Urinary urea (mmol/24h)			
lowest	13.6 (8.3–22.1)	17.8 (9.0–35.5)	10.6 (4.8–23.4)
2nd	4.2 (2.6–6.9)	5.1 (2.5–10.2)	3.7 (1.7–7.8)
3rd	2.0 (1.2–3.4)	2.5 (1.2–5.2)	1.6 (0.75–3.5)
highest	1	1	1
Proteinuria (g/24h)			
lowest	1	1	1
2nd	0.63 (0.42–0.94)	0.65 (0.40–1.0)	0.58 (0.25–1.4)
3rd	0.52 (0.34–0.81)	0.51 (0.30–0.86)	0.63 (0.27–1.4)
highest	0.37 (0.23–0.60)	0.38 (0.21–0.69)	0.37 (0.16–0.86)

Abbreviations: OR (95% CI), odds-ratios and 95% confidence interval; mGFR, measured glomerular filtration rate; BMI, body mass index.
Cut-off points of urinary urea were: <312.8 mmol/24h, 312.8–382.5 mmol/24h, 382.5–456.3 mmol/24h,>456.3 mmol/24 in men; <252.0 mmol/24h, 252.0–302.1 mmol/24h, 302.1–375.0 mmol/24h,>375.0 mmol/24h in women. Cut-off points of proteinuria urea were: <0.14 g/24h, 0.14–0.35 g/24h, 0.35–1.1 g/24,>1.1 g/24h in men; <0.12 g/24g, 0.12–0.21 g/24h, 0.21–0.89 g/24h,>0.89 g/24h in women.
*Multivariate adjustment, including center.

level. These values could thus be used by clinicians to validate 24-hour urine collection in patients with reduced kidney function.

A large set of nutritional measures were available in this study. BMI has been reported to be significantly associated with muscle mass in both transplanted [20] and dialysis patients [14,19]. In line with other studies of CKD [13,17,18,25] and non CKD populations [26,27], we observed that urinary creatinine excretion was significantly lower with lower BMI. Prealbumin is also considered as an important nutritional marker [1,2,6,9,14,37,46]. We found that lower urinary creatinine levels were significantly associated with a low prealbumin level in patients with diabetes, but not in those without. The number of missing data for prealbumin, however, may have weakened the latter association.

In contrast, serum albumin was not associated with urinary creatinine excretion. Although it has been shown to be positively associated with total muscle mass estimated from X-ray absorptiometry [29], its usefulness as a nutritional marker has been challenged in end-stage renal disease (ESRD) patients[3,47,48]. Similarly, we failed to find that urinary creatinine excretion was significantly associated with transferrin, homocysteine, total and HDL cholesterol or triglycerides. As expected, urinary urea was significantly and positively associated with creatininuria in our study. Indeed, protein intake is an important determinant of muscle mass [28,39]. Our finding that the decrease in urinary creatinine excretion over time is associated with mGFR decline independent of both nutritional measurements and lowering

Table 5. Linear mixed model analysis of factors associated with mean differences in the level (in mmol/24h) and change over time (in mmol/24h per year) in urinary creatinine excretion rate.

	Mean difference in urinary creatinine excretion (95% Confidence Interval)
Intercept, mmol/24h *	12.68(12.39,12.98)
Factors associated with baseline urinary creatinine	
Age, year	−0.06(−0.07,−0.05)
Women vs men	−3.57(−3.83,−3.32)
African vs non African origin	1.87(1.57,2.18)
mGFR, per each 10 ml/min/1.73 m² decrease	−0.23(−0.29,−0.17)
Diabetes	−0.38(−0.63,−0.13)
BMI, kg/m²	
<18.5	−1.54(−2.21,−0.88)
18.5–25	0 (ref)
25–30	1.11(0.87,1.34)
30–35	1.71(1.39,2.02)
>35	1.91(1.41,2.42)
Urinary urea, per each 10 mmol/day decrease	−0.09(−0.10,−0.08)
Proteinuria	
lowest	0 (ref)
2ⁿᵈ	0.42(0.13,0.71)
3ʳᵈ	0.66(0.36,0.96)
highest	0.80(0.48,1.12)
Slope, mmol/24h per year**	−0.19(−0.24,−0.14)
Factors associated with changes in urinary creatinine	
Women vs Men	0.16(0.08,0.25)
mGFR, per each 5 ml/min/1.73m² per yr decrease†	−0.29(−0.34,−0.25)
Urinary urea, per each 25 mmol/24h per yr decrease†	−0.15(−0.17,−0.14)

*mean predicted level in urinary creatinine excretion rate in mmol/24h for 60-yr old non-African and non-diabetic men, with normal BMI (within 18.5 to 25 kg/m²), baseline mGFR of 40 ml/min/1.73 m², urinary urea of 400 mmol/d and proteinuria in the lowest quartiles.
** mean predicted change in urinary creatinine excretion rate in mmol/24h per year in men with stable mGFR and urinary urea, i.e., with no change in level from baseline.
† 5 ml/min/1.73 m² per yr decrease in mGFR and 25 mmol/24h per yr decrease in urinary urea correspond to about three times the mean annual decrease for each variable.

protein intake suggests that other mechanisms than reduced dietary intakes may explain muscle wasting in CKD.

Only sparse data are available about the potential impact of diabetes on muscle mass loss. *Cano et al.* [24] reports lower lean body mass estimated from creatinine generation in diabetic *vs* nondiabetic patients on hemodialysis. *Pupim et al.* [21] also showed that the loss of lean body mass accelerates in dialysis patients with diabetes. Mechanisms related to diabetes mellitus [32,37] have been suggested to explain this relation. *Siew et al.* [33] demonstrated a significant association between skeletal muscle protein breakdown and insulin resistance in nondiabetic chronic hemodialysis patients. In agreement with other studies [18,27], we found significantly lower urinary creatinine excretion in CKD patients with than without diabetes mellitus. Metabolic acidosis has also been shown to be associated with malnutrition-inflammation in end-stage CKD [35]. Its occurrence in the very late stages of CKD[49] may explain why we found no relation between low muscle mass and acidosis.

Although inflammation frequently accompanies poor nutritional status [1,7,14,31,36,48,50] and plays an important role in the pathophysiology of muscle wasting [36,50], there are conflicting results about the association of inflammatory status with muscle mass loss [36]. The elevated CRP levels often observed in CKD patients [7,8,11,12] reflect the generation of proinflammatory cytokines, which may contribute to muscle wasting by stimulating protein catabolism. In disagreement with some [14,19], but not all studies [18,28], inflammation defined by CRP ≥10 mg/L was not significantly associated with urinary creatinine excretion rate after adjusting for nutritional factors in this study. Importantly, there was no association with either of the other available inflammatory markers, including orosomucoid, haptoglobin, plasma fibrinogen, or WBC after multivariate adjustment. In contrast, there was a graded and independent relationship with 24-hour proteinuria which, to our knowledge, has not been described before. The complex associations of proteinuria with protein wasting and inflammation may explain the observed association. Further studies are needed to elucidate whether muscle wasting is related to inflammation in non-end-stage CKD or whether it depends on the type of malnutrition, as suggested in dialysis patients [48].

The strengths of this study include the use of a gold-standard method to measure renal function (mGFR), the ability to assess urinary creatinine excretion based on both carefully collected urine during a 5-hour visit and 24-hour urine collection as well as the availability of repeated measurements of these markers as well as of several potential determinants of muscle wasting that may have confounded the association of interest. It is worth noting that we found no association of urinary creatinine excretion with GFR estimated from the CKD-EPI equation, which is explained by the impact of creatinine generation on both serum and urinary creatinine resulting in overestimation of eGFR as compared with mGFR in patients with low urinary creatinine, and conversely, underestimation in those with high urinary creatinine. This study also has limitations. First, we had no information about physical activity [22,28,31], which might have explained some of our findings. Second, although no direct measure of muscle mass exists, it might be considered a limitation that we used urinary creatinine excretion as a measure of muscle mass instead of reference methods such as computerized tomography (CT) or magnetic resonance imaging (MRI) [40,41]. However, the time and money required for these methods make them impractical in large-scale clinical studies. Finally, demographic- and anthropo-metric parameter-based equations [51–53] used to estimate muscle mass in individuals with normal kidney function are inappropriate in the CKD population because they do not take into account the decrease in urinary creatinine excretion with reduced kidney function.

Conclusions

Our findings suggest that decrease in urinary creatinine excretion rate may appear early in CKD patients, independent of decreased protein intake assessed by urinary urea excretion, as well as of other determinants of muscle mass loss including gender,

an older age, non-African origin, diabetes, lower BMI and 24-h proteinuria levels. Urinary creatinine concentration is a useful tool, easy to apply routinely. Reference values provided by age, gender, and GFR level might help clinicians to identify individuals who may need both special interventions, including nutritional or exercise advice, and monitoring of their response to these interventions. The decrease of urinary creatinine excretion with GFR decline also questions the accuracy of normalizing for creatininuria when estimating urine analytes concentration which may be overestimated in CKD patients with reduced muscle mass.

Acknowledgments

We thank Jo-Ann Cahn for the English revision of this manuscript.

The NephroTest study group: Bichat Univ Hospital (Paris): François Vrtovsnik, Eric Daugas (Nephrology) and Martin Flamant, Emmanuelle Vidal-Petiot (Physiology); European Georges Pompidou Univ Hospital (Paris): Christian Jacquot, Alexandre Karras, Eric Thervet, Christian d'Auzac (Nephrology) and P. Houillier, M. Courbebaisse, D. Eladari et G. Maruani (Physiology); Tenon Univ Hospital (Paris): Jean-Jacques Boffa, Pierre Ronco, H. Fessi, Eric Rondeau (Nephrology) and Emmanuel Letavernier, Jean Philippe Haymann (Physiology); Landy Clinic (Saint-Ouen): P. Urena-Torres (Nephrology); Bordeaux Univ Hospital: Christian Combe (Nephrology), and Inserm (Villejuif): M. Metzger, B. Stengel, France.

Author Contributions

Analyzed the data: E. Tynkevich M. Flamant MM M. Froissart BS. Wrote the paper: E. Tynkevich M. Flamant M. Froissart BS. Contributed to concept and design of the work, interpretation of data, and the critical revision and final approval of the version to be published: E. Tynkevich M. Flamant JH MM E. Thervet JB FV PH M. Froissart BS.

References

1. Kalantar-Zadeh K, Ikizler TA, Block G, Avram MM, Kopple JD (2003) Malnutrition-inflammation complex syndrome in dialysis patients: causes and consequences. Am J Kidney Dis Off J Natl Kidney Found 42: 864–881.
2. Fouque D, Kalantar-Zadeh K, Kopple J, Cano N, Chauveau P, et al. (2008) A proposed nomenclature and diagnostic criteria for protein-energy wasting in acute and chronic kidney disease. Kidney Int 73: 391–398. doi: 10.1038/sj.ki.5002585.
3. Blumenkrantz MJ, Kopple JD, Gutman RA, Chan YK, Barbour GL, et al. (1980) Methods for assessing nutritional status of patients with renal failure. Am J Clin Nutr 33: 1567–1585.
4. Mak RH, Ikizler AT, Kovesdy CP, Raj DS, Stenvinkel P, et al. (2011) Wasting in chronic kidney disease. J Cachexia Sarcopenia Muscle 2: 9–25. doi: 10.1007/s13539-011-0019-5.
5. Kalantar-Zadeh K, Kopple JD (2001) Relative contributions of nutrition and inflammation to clinical outcome in dialysis patients. Am J Kidney Dis Off J Natl Kidney Found 38: 1343–1350. doi: 10.1053/ajkd.2001.29250.
6. Aparicio M, Cano N, Chauveau P, Azar R, Canaud B, et al. (1999) Nutritional status of haemodialysis patients: a French national cooperative study. French Study Group for Nutrition in Dialysis. Nephrol Dial Transplant 14: 1679–1686. doi: 10.1093/ndt/14.7.1679.
7. Stenvinkel P, Heimbürger O, Paultre F, Diczfalusy U, Wang T, et al. (1999) Strong association between malnutrition, inflammation, and atherosclerosis in chronic renal failure. Kidney Int 55: 1899–1911. doi: 10.1046/j.1523-1755.1999.00422.x.
8. Qureshi AR, Alvestrand A, Danielsson A, Divino-Filho JC, Gutierrez A, et al. (1998) Factors predicting malnutrition in hemodialysis patients: A cross-sectional study. Kidney Int 53: 773–782. doi: 10.1046/j.1523-1755.1998.00812.x.
9. Fouque D, Pelletier S, Mafra D, Chauveau P (2011) Nutrition and chronic kidney disease. Kidney Int 80: 348–357. doi: 10.1038/ki.2011.118.
10. Qureshi AR, Alvestrand A, Divino-Filho JC, Gutierrez A, Heimbürger O, et al. (2002) Inflammation, Malnutrition, and Cardiac Disease as Predictors of Mortality in Hemodialysis Patients. J Am Soc Nephrol 13: S28–S36.
11. Zimmermann J, Herrlinger S, Pruy A, Metzger T, Wanner C (1999) Inflammation enhances cardiovascular risk and mortality in hemodialysis patients. Kidney Int 55: 648–658. doi: 10.1046/j.1523-1755.1999.00273.x.
12. Ortega O, Rodriguez I, Gallar P, Carreño A, Ortiz M, et al. (2002) Significance of high C-reactive protein levels in pre-dialysis patients. Nephrol Dial Transplant Off Publ Eur Dial Transpl Assoc - Eur Ren Assoc 17: 1105–1109.
13. Ix JH, de Boer IH, Wassel CL, Criqui MH, Shlipak MG, et al. (2010) Urinary creatinine excretion rate and mortality in persons with coronary artery disease:

the Heart and Soul Study. Circulation 121: 1295–1303. doi: 10.1161/CIRCULATIONAHA.109.924266.
14. Honda H, Qureshi AR, Axelsson J, Heimburger O, Suliman ME, et al. (2007) Obese sarcopenia in patients with end-stage renal disease is associated with inflammation and increased mortality. Am J Clin Nutr 86: 633–638.
15. Kovesdy CP, George SM, Anderson JE, Kalantar-Zadeh K (2009) Outcome predictability of biomarkers of protein-energy wasting and inflammation in moderate and advanced chronic kidney disease. Am J Clin Nutr 90: 407–414. doi: 10.3945/ajcn.2008.27390.
16. Noori N, Kopple JD, Kovesdy CP, Feroze U, Sim JJ, et al. (2010) Mid-Arm Muscle Circumference and Quality of Life and Survival in Maintenance Hemodialysis Patients. Clin J Am Soc Nephrol 5: 2258–2268. doi: 10.2215/CJN.02080310.
17. Micco LD, Quinn RR, Ronksley PE, Bellizzi V, Lewin AM, et al. (2013) Urine Creatinine Excretion and Clinical Outcomes in CKD. Clin J Am Soc Nephrol: CJN.01350213d oi: 10.2215/CJN.01350213.
18. Oterdoom LH, van Ree RM, de Vries APJ, Gansevoort RT, Schouten JP, et al. (2008) Urinary creatinine excretion reflecting muscle mass is a predictor of mortality and graft loss in renal transplant recipients. Transplantation 86: 391–398. doi: 10.1097/TP.0b013e3181788aea.
19. Carrero JJ, Chmielewski M, Axelsson J, Snaedal S, Heimbürger O, et al. (2008) Muscle atrophy, inflammation and clinical outcome in incident and prevalent dialysis patients. Clin Nutr Edinb Scotl 27: 557–564. doi: 10.1016/j.clnu.2008.04.007.
20. Molnar MZ, Streja E, Kovesdy CP, Bunnapradist S, Sampaio MS, et al. (2011) Associations of body mass index and weight loss with mortality in transplant-waitlisted maintenance hemodialysis patients. Am J Transplant Off J Am Soc Transplant Am Soc Transpl Surg 11: 725–736. doi: 10.1111/j.1600-6143.2011.03468.x.
21. Pupim LB, Heimbürger O, Qureshi AR, Ikizler TA, Stenvinkel P (2005) Accelerated lean body mass loss in incident chronic dialysis patients with diabetes mellitus. Kidney Int 68: 2368–2374. doi: 10.1111/j.1523-1755.2005.00699.x.
22. Anand S, Chertow GM, Johansen KL, Grimes B, Kurella Tamura M, et al. (2011) Association of self-reported physical activity with laboratory markers of nutrition and inflammation: the Comprehensive Dialysis Study. J Ren Nutr Off J Counc Ren Nutr Natl Kidney Found 21: 429–437. doi: 10.1053/j.jrn.2010.09.007.

23. Kovesdy CP, Shinaberger CS, Kalantar-Zadeh K (2010) Epidemiology of dietary nutrient intake in ESRD. Semin Dial 23: 353–358. doi: 10.1111/j.1525-139X.2010.00745.x.

24. Cano NJM, Roth H, Aparicio M, Azar R, Canaud B, et al. (2002) Malnutrition in hemodialysis diabetic patients: evaluation and prognostic influence. Kidney Int 62: 593–601. doi: 10.1046/j.1523-1755.2002.00457.x.

25. Bansal N, Hsu C, Zhao S, Whooley MA, Ix JH (2011) Relation of body mass index to urinary creatinine excretion rate in patients with coronary heart disease. Am J Cardiol 108: 179–184. doi: 10.1016/j.amjcard.2011.03.020.

26. Oterdoom LH, Gansevoort RT, Schouten JP, de Jong PE, Gans ROB, et al. (2009) Urinary creatinine excretion, an indirect measure of muscle mass, is an independent predictor of cardiovascular disease and mortality in the general population. Atherosclerosis 207: 534–540. doi: 10.1016/j.atherosclerosis.2009.05.010.

27. Barr DB, Wilder LC, Caudill SP, Gonzalez AJ, Needham LL, et al. (2005) Urinary Creatinine Concentrations in the U.S. Population: Implications for Urinary Biologic Monitoring Measurements. Environ Health Perspect 113: 192–200. doi: 10.1289/ehp.7337.

28. Foley RN, Wang C, Ishani A, Collins AJ, Murray AM (2007) Kidney Function and Sarcopenia in the United States General Population: NHANES III. Am J Nephrol 27: 279–286. doi: 10.1159/000101827.

29. Baumgartner RN, Koehler KM, Romero L, Garry PJ (1996) Serum albumin is associated with skeletal muscle in elderly men and women. Am J Clin Nutr 64: 552–558.

30. Kopple JD, Greene T, Chumlea WC, Hollinger D, Maroni BJ, et al. (2000) Relationship between nutritional status and the glomerular filtration rate: results from the MDRD study. Kidney Int 57: 1688–1703. doi: 10.1046/j.1523-1755.2000.00014.x.

31. Evans WJ (2010) Skeletal muscle loss: cachexia, sarcopenia, and inactivity. Am J Clin Nutr 91: 1123S–1127S. doi: 10.3945/ajcn.2010.28608A.

32. Workeneh BT, Mitch WE (2010) Review of muscle wasting associated with chronic kidney disease. Am J Clin Nutr 91: 1128S–1132S. doi: 10.3945/ajcn.2010.28608B.

33. Siew ED, Pupim LB, Majchrzak KM, Shintani A, Flakoll PJ, et al. (2007) Insulin resistance is associated with skeletal muscle protein breakdown in non-diabetic chronic hemodialysis patients. Kidney Int 71: 146–152. doi: 10.1038/sj.ki.5001984.

34. Bailey JL, Wang X, England BK, Price SR, Ding X, et al. (1996) The acidosis of chronic renal failure activates muscle proteolysis in rats by augmenting transcription of genes encoding proteins of the ATP-dependent ubiquitin-proteasome pathway. J Clin Invest 97: 1447–1453. doi: 10.1172/JCI118566.

35. Kalantar-Zadeh K, Mehrotra R, Fouque D, Kopple JD (2004) Poor Nutritional Status and Inflammation: Metabolic Acidosis and Malnutrition-Inflammation Complex Syndrome in Chronic Renal Failure. Semin Dial 17: 455–465. doi: 10.1111/j.0894-0959.2004.17606.x.

36. Avesani CM, Carrero JJ, Axelsson J, Qureshi AR, Lindholm B, et al. (2006) Inflammation and wasting in chronic kidney disease: Partners in crime. Kidney Int 70: S8–S13. doi: 10.1038/sj.ki.5001969.

37. Mak RH, Ikizler TA, Kovesdy CP, Raj DS, Stenvinkel P, et al. (2011) Erratum to: Wasting in chronic kidney disease. J Cachexia Sarcopenia Muscle 2: 119. doi: 10.1007/s13539-011-0026-6.

38. Bhatla B, Moore H, Emerson P, Keshaviah P, Prowant B, et al. (1995) Lean body mass estimation by creatinine kinetics, bioimpedance, and dual energy x-ray absorptiometry in patients on continuous ambulatory peritoneal dialysis. ASAIO J Am Soc Artif Intern Organs 1992 41: M442–446.

39. Heymsfield SB, Arteaga C, McManus C, Smith J, Moffitt S (1983) Measurement of muscle mass in humans: validity of the 24-hour urinary creatinine method. Am J Clin Nutr 37: 478–494.

40. Mitsiopoulos N, Baumgartner RN, Heymsfield SB, Lyons W, Gallagher D, et al. (1998) Cadaver validation of skeletal muscle measurement by magnetic resonance imaging and computerized tomography. J Appl Physiol 85: 115–122.

41. Kaysen GA, Zhu F, Sarkar S, Heymsfield SB, Wong J, et al. (2005) Estimation of total-body and limb muscle mass in hemodialysis patients by using multifrequency bioimpedance spectroscopy. Am J Clin Nutr 82: 988–995.

42. Wyss M, Kaddurah-Daouk R (2000) Creatine and Creatinine Metabolism. Physiol Rev 80: 1107–1213.

43. Jones JD, Burnett PC (1974) Creatinine Metabolism in Humans with Decreased Renal Function: Creatinine Deficit. Clin Chem 20: 1204–1212.

44. Levey AS, Stevens LA, Schmid CH, Zhang YL, Castro AF, et al. (2009) A New Equation to Estimate Glomerular Filtration Rate. Ann Intern Med 150: 604.

45. Proctor DN, O'Brien PC, Atkinson EJ, Nair KS (1999) Comparison of techniques to estimate total body skeletal muscle mass in people of different age groups. Am J Physiol 277: E489–495.

46. Chertow GM, Ackert K, Lew NL, Lazarus JM, Lowrie EG (2000) Prealbumin is as important as albumin in the nutritional assessment of hemodialysis patients. Kidney Int 58: 2512–2517. doi: 10.1046/j.1523-1755.2000.00435.x.

47. Gama-Axelsson T, Heimbürger O, Stenvinkel P, Bárány P, Lindholm B, et al. (2012) Serum albumin as predictor of nutritional status in patients with ESRD. Clin J Am Soc Nephrol CJASN 7: 1446–1453. doi: 10.2215/CJN.10251011.

48. Stenvinkel P, Heimbürger O, Lindholm B, Kaysen GA, Bergström J (2000) Are there two types of malnutrition in chronic renal failure? Evidence for relationships between malnutrition, inflammation and atherosclerosis (MIA syndrome). Nephrol Dial Transplant 15: 953–960. doi: 10.1093/ndt/15.7.953.

49. Moranne O, Froissart M, Rossert J, Gauci C, Boffa JJ, et al. (2009) Timing of Onset of CKD-Related Metabolic Complications. J Am Soc Nephrol 20: 164–171. doi: 10.1681/ASN.2008020159.

50. Carrero JJ, Stenvinkel P (2009) Persistent inflammation as a catalyst for other risk factors in chronic kidney disease: a hypothesis proposal. Clin J Am Soc Nephrol CJASN 4 Suppl 1: S49–55. doi: 10.2215/CJN.02720409.

51. Ix JH, Wassel CL, Stevens LA, Beck GJ, Froissart M, et al. (2011) Equations to Estimate Creatinine Excretion Rate: The CKD Epidemiology Collaboration. Clin J Am Soc Nephrol 6: 184–191. doi: 10.2215/CJN.05030610.

52. De Keyzer W, Huybrechts I, Dekkers ALM, Geelen A, Crispim S, et al. (2012) Predicting urinary creatinine excretion and its usefulness to identify incomplete 24 h urine collections. Br J Nutr 108: 1118–1125. doi: 10.1017/S0007114511006295.

53. Rule AD, Bailey KR, Schwartz GL, Khosla S, Lieske JC, et al. (2009) For estimating creatinine clearance measuring muscle mass gives better results than those based on demographics. Kidney Int 75: 1071–1078. doi: 10.1038/ki.2008.698.

20

Fluid Overload, Pulse Wave Velocity, and Ratio of Brachial Pre-Ejection Period to Ejection Time in Diabetic and Non-Diabetic Chronic Kidney Disease

Yi-Chun Tsai[1,2,4], Yi-Wen Chiu[2,4], Hung-Tien Kuo[2,4], Szu-Chia Chen[4,5], Shang-Jyh Hwang[1,2,4,6], Tzu-Hui Chen[3], Mei-Chuan Kuo[1,2,4]*, Hung-Chun Chen[2,4]

1 Graduate Institute of Clinical Medicine, Kaohsiung Medical University, Kaohsiung, Taiwan, 2 Division of Nephrology, Kaohsiung Medical University Hospital, Kaohsiung, Taiwan, 3 Department of Nursing, Kaohsiung Medical University Hospital, Kaohsiung, Taiwan, 4 Faculty of Renal Care, Kaohsiung Medical University, Kaohsiung, Taiwan, 5 Department of Internal Medicine, Kaohsiung Municipal Hsiao-Kang Hospital, Kaohsiung, Taiwan, 6 Institute of Population Sciences, National Health Research Institutes, Miaoli, Taiwan

Abstract

Fluid overload is one of the characteristics in chronic kidney disease (CKD). Changes in extracellular fluid volume are associated with progression of diabetic nephropathy. Not only diabetes but also fluid overload is associated with cardiovascular risk factors The aim of the study was to assess the interaction between fluid overload, diabetes, and cardiovascular risk factors, including arterial stiffness and left ventricular function in 480 patients with stages 4–5 CKD. Fluid status was determined by bioimpedance spectroscopy method, Body Composition Monitor. Brachial-ankle pulse wave velocity (baPWV), as a good parameter of arterial stiffness, and brachial pre-ejection period (bPEP)/brachial ejection time (bET), correlated with impaired left ventricular function were measured by ankle-brachial index (ABI)-form device. Of all patients, 207 (43.9%) were diabetic and 240 (50%) had fluid overload. For non-diabetic CKD, fluid overload was associated with being female ($\beta = -2.87$, $P = 0.003$), heart disease ($\beta = 2.69$, $P = 0.04$), high baPWV ($\beta = 0.27$, $P = 0.04$), low hemoglobin ($\beta = -1.10$, $P < 0.001$), and low serum albumin ($\beta = -5.21$, $P < 0.001$) in multivariate analysis. For diabetic CKD, fluid overload was associated with diuretics use ($\beta = 3.69$, $P = 0.003$), high mean arterial pressure ($\beta = 0.14$, $P = 0.01$), low bPEP/ET ($\beta = -0.19$, $P = 0.03$), low hemoglobin ($\beta = -1.55$, $P = 0.001$), and low serum albumin ($\beta = -9.46$, $P < 0.001$). In conclusion, baPWV is associated with fluid overload in non-diabetic CKD and bPEP/bET is associated with fluid overload in diabetic CKD. Early and accurate assessment of these associated cardiovascular risk factors may improve the effects of entire care in late CKD.

Editor: Giuseppe Remuzzi, Mario Negri Institute for Pharmacological Research and Azienda Ospedaliera Ospedali Riuniti di Bergamo, Italy

Funding: Dr. Tsai's research was supported by the Kaohsiung Medical University Faculty of Renal Care and a grant from the Kaohsiung Medical University Research Foundation (KMU-Q103011). The author(s) received no specific funding for this work. The funders had no role in study design, data collection and analysis, decision to publish, or preparation of the manuscript.

Competing Interests: The authors have declared that no competing interests exist.

* Email: mechku@cc.kmu.edu.tw

Introduction

Cardiovascular disease (CVD) is the major cause of morbidity and mortality in patients with chronic kidney disease (CKD). The presentation of fluid overload is often noticed in patients with CKD, and excess fluid status induces elevated arterial pressure, left ventricular hypertrophy, and associated cardiovascular sequelae [1,2]. Hung et al. indicated a significant association of fluid overload with cardiovascular risk factors, such as diabetes, systolic blood pressure, and arterial stiffness in CKD patients not on dialysis [3]. Previous studies reported that fluid overload was a predictor of cardiovascular mortality in patients on dialysis [4–7]. Fluid overload is not only a characteristic but also a clinical indicator of cardiovascular burden.

On the other hand, diabetic CKD patients have a greater risk of commencing dialysis, and higher all-cause and cardiovascular mortality than non-diabetic CKD patients [8]. This is probably the result that more advanced atherosclerotic change of vascular or cardiac level in diabetic CKD or vascular disease in non-diabetic CKD is not necessarily atherosclerotic. Additionally, diabetics are more likely to have fluid overload than non-diabetics [9], and progression of diabetic nephropathy would contribute to the increase in extracellular fluid volume [10]. An interaction between fluid overload, diabetes, and vascular injury or cardiac dysfunction might exist in CKD. Accumulating evidence shows that pulse wave velocity (PWV), which can be easily measured by a clinical device, the ankle-brachial index (ABI)-form, has been regarded as a clinical indicator of arterial stiffness [11,12]. Cardiac dysfunction is frequently evaluated by echocardiography; however, its application in predicting cardiovascular events is limited because echocardiography is time-consuming and operator-dependent [13]. The ratio of brachial pre-ejection period (bPEP) and brachial ejection time (bET), measured easily by ABI device, was reported to have a significant correlation with impaired left ventricular systolic function [14]. Chen et al. found that bPEP/bET was an independent predictor for all-cause and cardiovascular mortality in CKD patients on or not on dialysis [13,15]. Hence, the aim of this study is to evaluate the relationship between fluid overload, diabetes, and baPWV or bPEP/bET and whether baPWV or bPEP/bET could be used as simple clinically available measures for risk stratification in late CKD.

Materials and Methods

Study Participants

All 612 of CKD stages 4–5 patients were invited to participate in the study from January 2011 to December 2011 at one hospital in Southern Taiwan. The study protocol was approved by the Institutional Review Board of the Kaohsiung Medical University Hospital. All patients had been enrolled in our integrated CKD program for more than 3 months (30.9±27.0 months). CKD was staged according to K/DOQI definitions and the estimated glomerular filtration rate (eGFR) was calculated using the equation of the 4-variable Modification of Diet in Renal Disease (MDRD) Study (CKD stage 3, eGFR: 30~59 ml/min/1.73 m²; CKD stage 4, eGFR: 15~29 ml/min/1.73 m²; CKD stage 5, eGFR<15 ml/min/1.73 m²) [16]. Of all patients, we excluded 115 with disabilities, 12 with impaired skin integrity, and 5 with pacemaker implantation. Four hundred and eighty patients were enrolled and scheduled for a study interview after informed consent.

Ethics Statement

The study protocol was approved by the Institutional Review Board of the Kaohsiung Medical University Hospital (KMUH-IRB-990125). Informed consents were obtained in written form from patients and all clinical investigations were conducted according to the principles expressed in the Declaration of Helsinki. The patients gave consent for the publication of the clinical details.

Measurement of fluid status

Fluid status was measured once by a bioimpedance spectroscopy method, Body Composition Monitor (BCM, Fresenius Medical Care) at enrollment. BCM has been validated extensively against all available gold-standard methods in the general and dialysis populations [17–20]. The information of normohydrated lean tissue, normohydrated adipose tissue, and extracellular fluid overload in whole body based on the difference of impedance in each tissue is provided by BCM. Fluid overload can be calculated from the difference between the normal expected and measured extracellular water (ECW) [21]. Fluid overload value, ECW, intracellular water (ICW) and total body water (TBW) were determined from the measured impedance data based on the model of Moissl et al [22,23]. The relative hydration status (ΔHS = fluid overload/ECW) has been used as an indicator of fluid status in a previous study [5]. In the present study, "Fluid overload" was defined as ΔHS of 7% or more corresponding to the value of 90th percentile for the normal reference population when the fluid status was measured with the same technology [3,22,23].

Assessment of baPWV, bPEP, and bET

Brachial-ankle pulse wave velocity (baPWV), as a good parameter of arterial stiffness, was measured by the ABI-form device, which automatically and simultaneously measured blood pressures in both arms and ankles using an oscillometric method [11,12], at the same time of fluid measurement for each patient. For measuring PWV, pulse waves obtained from the brachial and tibial arteries were recorded simultaneously, and the transmission time (ΔTba), which was defined as the time interval between the

initial increase in brachial and ankle waveforms, was determined. The transmission distance from the brachium to ankle was calculated according to body height. The path length from the suprasternal notch to the brachium(Lb) was obtained using the following equation: Lb = 0.2195×height of the patient (in cm)– 2.0734. The path length from the suprasternal notch to the ankle(La) was obtained using the following equation: La = (0.8129×height of the patient [in cm]+12.328). Finally, the following equation was used to automatically obtain baPWV: baPWV = (La–Lb)/ΔTba [24]. After obtaining bilateral PWV values, the higher one was used as representative for each subject. Additionally, bPEP, and bET was also measured by the ABI-form device.

The bET was automatically measured from the foot to the dicrotic notch (equivalent to the incisura on the downstroke of the aortic pressure wave contour produced by the closure of aortic valve) of the pulse volume waveform. The total electromechanical systolic interval (QS2) was measured from the onset of the QRS complex on the electrocardiogram to the first high-frequency vibration of the aortic component of the second heart sound on the phonocardiogram. The bPEP was also automatically calculated by subtracting the bET from the QS2 [13,15,25].

Data Collection

Demographic and clinical data of patients were obtained from interviews and medical records at enrollment. Blood and urine samples were obtained at the same time of fluid status measurement. Patients were asked to fast for at least 12 hours before blood sample collection for the biochemistry study. Protein in urine was measured using an immediate semiquantitative urine protein dipstick test and graded as negative, trace, 1+, 2+, 3+, or 4+. The body mass index was calculated as the ratio of weight in kilograms divided by square of height in meters. Blood pressure was recorded as the mean of two consecutive measurements with 5-minute intervals, using one single calibrated device. Mean arterial pressure was calculated as 2/3 diastolic blood pressure plus 1/3 systolic blood pressure. Diabetes was defined as those with a medical history through chart review. Cardiovascular disease was defined as a history of heart failure, acute or chronic ischemic heart disease, and myocardial infarction. Information regarding patient's medications including diuretics, HMG-CoA reductase inhibitors (statins), anti-hypertensive drugs, including calcium channel blocker, β-blocker, and angiotensin converting enzyme inhibitor, and angiotensin II receptor blocker within 3 months before enrollment was obtained from medical records.

Statistical Analysis

The study population was further classified into two groups according to the presence or absence of diabetes. Continuous variables were expressed as mean ± SD or median (25th, 75th percentile), as appropriate, and categorical variables were expressed as percentages. Skewed distribution continuous variables were log-transformed to attain normal distribution. The significance of differences in continuous variables between groups was tested using independent t-test or the Mann-Whitney U analysis, as appropriate. The difference in the distribution of categorical variables was tested using the Chi-square test. Linear regression models were utilized to evaluate the determinants of fluid overload in diabetes and non-diabetes. All the variables in Table 1 tested by univariate analysis and those variables with P-value less than 0.05 were selected in multivariate analysis. Statistical analyses were conducted using SPSS 18.0 for Windows (SPSS Inc., Chicago, Illinois) and some graphs were made by GraphPad Prism 5.0 (GraphPad Software Inc., San Diego CA,

Table 1. The clinical characteristics of study subjects stratified by Diabetes Mellitus.

	Entire Cohort (n = 480)	Non-diabetes (n = 269)	Diabetes (n = 211)	P-value
Demographic variables				
Age, year	65.4±12.7	65.6±13.9	65.0±10.9	0.57
Sex (male), %	54.6	50.9	59.2	0.07
Smoke, %	20.4	16.0	26.1	0.002
Alcohol, %	9.8	9.8	8.5	0.49
Cardiovascular disease, %	18.5	14.1	24.2	0.01
Hypertension, %	84.8	75.8	96.2	<0.001
Hyperlipidemia, %	52.7	42.0	66.4	<0.001
CKD stage 4, %	49.2	49.1	49.3	0.96
5	50.8	50.9	50.7	
Body Mass Index, kg/m^2	24.4±3.8	23.4±3.2	25.6±4.1	<0.001
Mean arterial pressure, mmHg	96.9±11.9	95.4±11.6	98.8±12.0	0.002
baPWV (cm/s)	1863.7±393.1	1782.6±365.1	1963.7±403.2	<0.001
bPEP/bET	0.4±0.1	0.4±0.1	0.3±0.1	0.01
Body Composition				
Lean tissue Index (kg/m^2)	13.7±2.6	13.7±2.6	13.8±2.7	0.56
Fat tissue Index (kg/m^2)	9.9±4.2	9.2±3.8	10.7±4.5	<0.001
Total body water (L)	32.6±6.6	31.7±6.0	34.1±7.2	<0.001
Intracellular water (L)	17.1±3.6	16.9±3.6	17.4±3.7	0.12
Extracellular water (L)	15.6±3.5	14.8±2.9	16.7±4.1	<0.001
ECW/ICW	0.9±0.1	0.9±0.1	1.0±0.2	<0.001
ECW/TBW (%)	47.7±3.5	46.9±3.2	48.9±3.5	<0.001
OH (L)	1.0(2)	0.9(1)	1.7(3)	<0.001
Relative hydration status[a] (%)	50	41.2	61.1	<0.001
Medications				
Diuretics, %	29.4	16.0	46.4	<0.001
Statin, %	31.0	23.4	40.8	<0.001
Hypertension medication, %	79.6	69.5	92.4	<0.001
Laboratory parameters				
eGFR, ml/min/1.73 m^2	15.3±7.5	15.3±7.6	15.4±7.5	0.89
Hemoglobin, g/dl	10.4±1.7	10.4±1.8	10.5±1.7	0.53
Albumin, g/dl	4.0±0.5	4.1±0.4	3.9±0.5	<0.001
Calcium-Phosphate product, mg^2/dl^2	38.5(34.2,44.0)	38.3(33.6,43.3)	39.2(34.8,45.4)	0.09
Uric acid, mg/dl	7.7±1.7	7.4±1.7	8.0±1.7	<0.001
Cholesterol, mg/dl	180(153,210)	179(153,210)	181(153,209)	0.91
Triglyceride, mg/dl	116(80,166)	104(75,151)	136(90,191)	<0.001
C-reactive protein, mg/L	1.3(0.6,3.6)	1.2(0.6,3.2)	1.8(0.7,4.4)	0.05
Urine protein[b] >1+, %	49.8	36.8	67.0	<0.001

Notes: Data are expressed as number (percentage) for categorical variables and mean ± SD or median (25th, 75th percentile) for continuous variables, as appropriate. Abbreviations: CKD, chronic kidney disease; baPWV, brachial-ankle pulse wave velocity; bPEP/bET, brachial prolonged pre-ejection period/brachial shorted ejection time; ECW, extracellular water; ICW, intracellular water; TBW, total body water; ACEI, angiotensin converting enzyme inhibitors; ARB, angiotensin II receptor blockers; eGFR, estimated glomerular filtration rate.
[a]Relative hydration status (△HS) was defined as OH/extracellular water.
[b]Urine protein was measured using dipstick test.

USA). Statistical significance was set at a two-sided p-value of less than 0.05.

Results

Characteristics of Entire Cohort

The comparison of clinical characteristics between groups based on the presence or absence of diabetes is shown in Table 1. A total of 211 (44.0%) had diabetes. The mean age was 65.4±12.7 years.

The median of OH (overhydration) value was 1.0 L. Diabetic patients had higher prevalence of cardiovascular disease (24.2%), hypertension (96.2%), and hyperlipidemia (66.4%) than non-diabetes. Diabetic patients had higher body mass index (25.6±4.1 kg/m²), mean arterial pressure (98.8±12.0 mmHg), fat tissue index (10.7±4.5 kg/m²), TBW (34.1±7.2 L), ECW (16.7±4.1 L), ECW/TBW (48.9±3.5%), and OH (1.7 L) than non-diabetic patients. Diabetic patients with fluid overload received more diuretics, statin, and anti-hypertension treatment. Higher baPWV, and lower bPEP/bET were found in diabetic patients than non-diabetic patients. Uric acid levels and the degree of proteinuria were higher and serum albumin was lower in diabetic patients than in non-diabetic patients.

Different zones can be identified in the plot of mean arterial pressure (Y-axis) versus relative hydration status (ΔHS) (X-axis), of normovolemic and normotensive patients (40.9%, zone A), fluid-overloaded and hypertensive patients (14.0%, zone B), fluid-overloaded but normo- or hypotensive patients (36.0%, zone C), hypertensive and normovolemic patients (9.1%, zone D), in Figure 1. Figure 1A shows a substantial scatter of baPWV quartiles, and the proportion of baPWV quartile 4 was the highest in zone B (36.4%) than other zones (P<0.001). Figure 1B shows that the proportion of diabetes was higher in zone B (59.7%) and C (51.7%) than other zones (P<0.001). There was no significant difference of gender distribution among zones (Figure 1C).

Determinants of fluid overload (relative hydration status, ΔHS) in non-diabetic CKD

Figure 2 shows a positive association of baPWV and fluid overload in non-diabetic CKD (r = 0.488, P<0.001). The determinants of fluid overload in non-diabetic patients are reported in Table 2. ΔHS correlated positively with age, heart disease, diuretics use, anti-hypertension drug use, baPWV, and urine protein, but negatively with the male gender, body mass index, eGFR, serum albumin, cholesterol, and hemoglobin levels in univariate linear regression analysis. Further multivariate analysis showed that increased ΔHS was associated with being female (β = −2.87, P = 0.003), heart disease (β = 2.69, P = 0.04), high baPWV (β = 0.27, P = 0.04), low hemoglobin (β = −1.10, P< 0.001), and low serum albumin (β = −5.21, P<0.001).

Determinants of fluid overload (relative hydration status, ΔHS) in diabetic CKD

Figure 3 shows a negative association of bPEP/bET and fluid overload in diabetic CKD (r = −0.251, P = 0.01). The determinants of fluid overload in diabetic patients are reported in Table 3. ΔHS correlated positively with diuretics use, anti-hypertensive drug use, mean arterial pressure, and urine protein, but negatively with age, male, body mass index, bPEP/bET, eGFR, serum albumin, and hemoglobin levels in univariate linear regression analysis. Further multivariate analysis showed that increased ΔHS was associated with diuretics use (β = 3.69, P = 0.003), high mean arterial pressure (β = 0.14, P = 0.01), low bPEP/bET (β = −0.19, P = 0.03), low hemoglobin (β = −1.55, P = 0.001), and low serum albumin (β = − 9.46, P<0.001).

Discussion

The aim of this study was to evaluate the relationship between fluid overload, diabetes and baPWV or bPEP/bET in patients with stages 4–5 CKD. Fluid overload was associated with baPWV, a clinical indicator of arterial stiffness, in non-diabetic CKD. Conversely, instead of baPWV, fluid overload was associated with

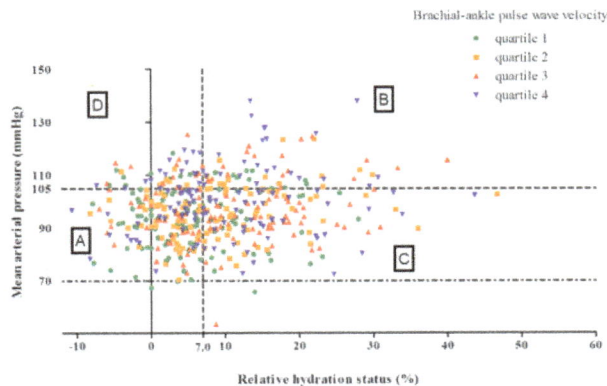
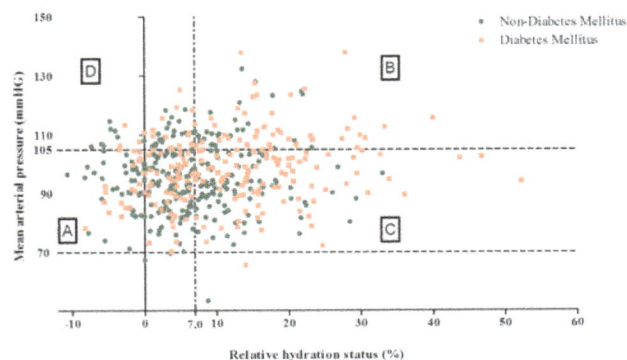
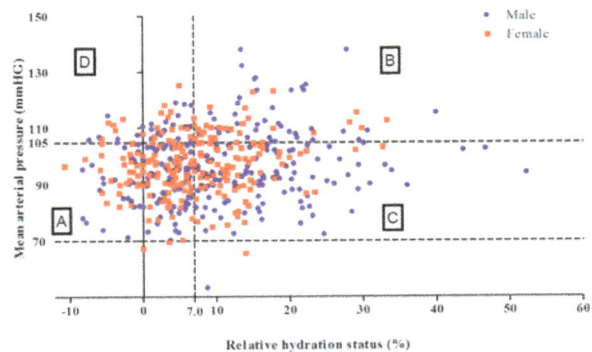

Figure 1. Scatter plot of brachial-ankle pulse wave velocity (1A), diabetes (1B), and gender (1C) between relative hydration status (%) in the X-axis and mean arterial pressure (mmHg) in the Y-axis in all study subjects.

bPEP/bET, a marker of left ventricular systolic function, in diabetic CKD.

Fluid overload may have an influence on vasculature and lead to vascular remodeling, characterized by dilatation of muscular and elastic type arteries and increased wall thickness, thereby inducing arterial stiffness and consequent cardiovascular sequelae [26]. Previous reports demonstrated that baPWV was associated with fluid overload in CKD [3,27]. On the other hand, diabetes has profound effects on vasculature, and baPWV appears to be associated with clinical variants of diabetes and microvascular and macrovascular complications [28–30]. There might be an interaction between fluid overload, baPWV, and diabetes. In the

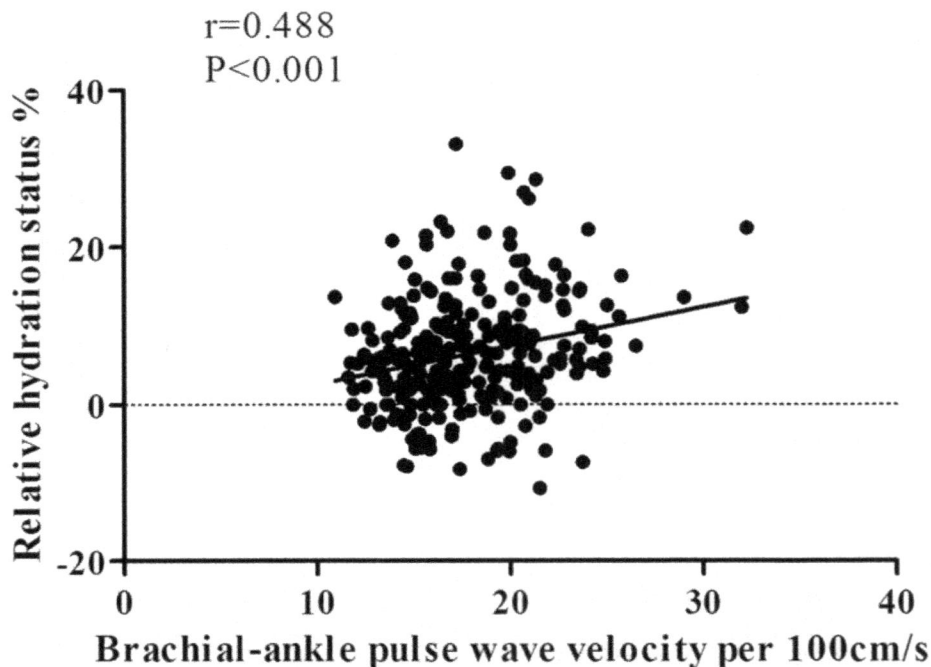

Figure 2. Relative hydration status was positively correlated with ratio of pulse wave velocity in non-diabetic chronic kidney disease.

Table 2. The determinants of relative hydration status in non-diabetic chronic kidney disease patients.

	Univariate		Multivariate	
	β (95%CI)	P-value	β (95%CI)	P-value
Clinical characteristics				
Age, year	0.12(0.06,0.18)	<0.001	0.01(−0.07,0.09)	0.7
Sex (male), %	−2.24(−3.97,−0.52)	0.01	−2.87(−4.76,−0.98)	0.003
Heart disease, %	4.43(1.99,6.86)	<0.001	2.69(0.13,5.25)	0.04
Diuretics, %	4.26(1.94,6.58)	<0.001	1.63(−0.69,3.96)	0.1
Anti-Hypertension drug, %	1.96(0.07,3.85)	0.04	0.64(−1.20,2.49)	0.5
Bady mass index, kg/m²	−0.29(−0.56,−0.02)	0.03	−0.19(−0.46,0.08)	0.2
Mean arterial pressure, mmHg	0.02(−0.05,0.10)	0.5	–	–
baPWV, per100 cm/s	0.49(0.25,0.72)	<0.001	0.27(0.01,0.54)	0.04
bPEP/bET, ×100	0.05(−0.09,0.19)	0.48	–	–
Laboratory parameters				
eGFR, ml/min/1.73 m²	−0.15(−0.26,−0.03)	0.01	−0.07(−0.21,0.07)	0.3
Hemoglobin, g/dl	−1.17(−1.65,−0.69)	<0.001	−1.10(−1.66,−0.53)	<0.001
Albumin, g/dl	−8.49(−10.63,−6.35)	<0.001	−5.21(−7.74,−2.68)	<0.001
Log Calcium-phosphate product, mg²/dl²	0.96(−9.27,11.20)	0.8	–	–
Uric acid, mg/dl	0.53(−0.01,1.06)	0.05	–	–
Log Cholesterol, mg/dl	−13.24(−22.34,4.14)	0.005	−3.32(−12.38,5.75)	0.4
C-reactive protein, mg/L	0.06(−0.02,0.14)	0.1	–	–
Urine protein >1+, %	1.004(1.001,1.007)	0.023	1.28(−0.64,3.20)	0.2

Abbreviations: baPWV, brachial-ankle pulse wave velocity; bPEP/bET, brachial prolonged pre-ejection period/brachial shorted ejection time; eGFR, estimated glomerular filtration rate.

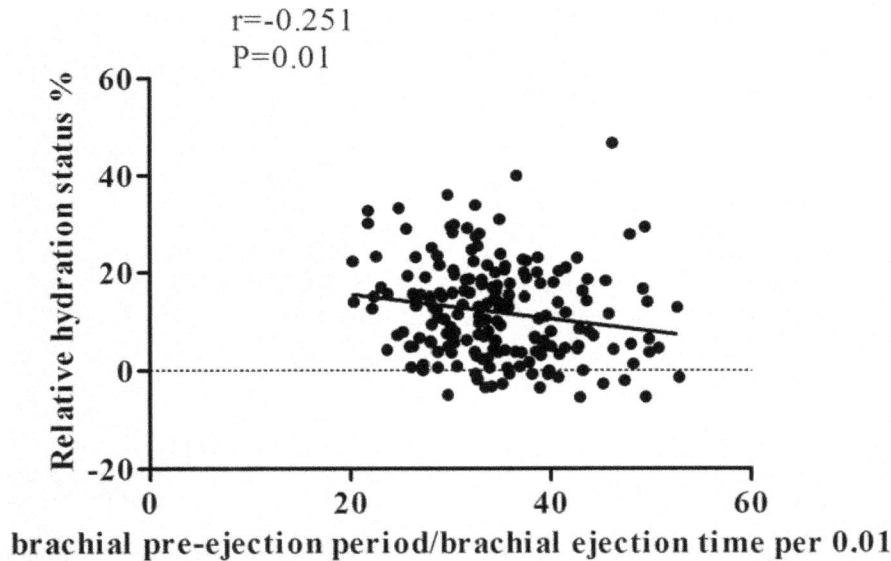

r=-0.251
P=0.01

Figure 3. Relative hydration status was negatively correlated with ratio of brachial pre-ejection period to ejection time in diabetic chronic kidney disease.

present study, a positive correlation between fluid overload and baPWV was found in multivariate analysis of all subjects ($\beta = 0.30$, $P = 0.02$). However, there was no interaction between diabetes and baPWV in the analysis of the determinants of fluid overload.

Hence, we divided all subjects into non-diabetes and diabetes groups to analyze the relationship between fluid overload and baPWV respectively and found a significant association between

Table 3. The determinants of relative hydration status in diabetic chronic kidney disease patients.

	Univariate		Multivariate	
	β (95%CI)	P-value	β (95%CI)	P-value
Clinical characteristics				
Age, year	−0.21(−0.34,−0.08)	0.001	−0.08(−0.20,0.04)	0.2
Sex (male), %	−3.26(−6.13,−0.40)	0.02	−2.06(−4.62,0.48)	0.1
Heart disease, %	0.42(−2.91,3.75)	0.8	–	–
Diuretics, %	4.45(1.66,7.24)	0.002	3.69(1.23,6.14)	0.003
Hypertension medication, %	5.98(0.66,11.30)	0.03	1.94(−2.43,6.32)	0.3
Body mass index, kg/m²	−0.46(−0.81,−0.12)	0.009	−0.01(−0.32,0.31)	0.9
Mean arterial pressure, mmHg	0.16(0.05,0.28)	0.006	0.14(0.03,0.24)	0.01
baPWV, per100 cm/s	0.23(−0.12,0.57)	0.2	–	–
bPEP/bET, ×100	−0.25(−0.45,−0.05)	0.01	−0.19(−0.37,−0.02)	0.03
Laboratory parameters				
eGFR, ml/min/1.73 m²	−0.24(−0.42,−0.05)	0.01	0.09(−0.10,0.27)	0.4
Hemoglobin, g/dl	−1.88(−2.68,−1.07)	<0.001	−1.55(−2.41,−0.68)	0.001
Albumin, g/dl	−12.88(−15.38,−10.37)	<0.001	−9.46(−12.21,−6.71)	<0.001
Log Calcium-phosphate product, mg²/dl²	0.08(−17.99,18.16)	0.9	–	–
Uric acid, mg/dl	0.28(−0.61,1.17)	0.5	–	–
Log Cholesterol, mg/dl	−9.73(−22.86,3.40)	0.1	–	–
C-reactive protein, mg/L	0.02(−0.23,0.27)	0.8	–	–
Urine protein >1+, %	1.004(1.001,1.007)	0.023	1.59(−1.35,4.53)	0.2

Abbreviations: baPWV, brachial-ankle pulse wave velocity; bPEP/bET, brachial prolonged pre-ejection period/brachial shorted ejection time; eGFR, estimated glomerular filtration rate.

fluid overload and baPWV in non-diabetic CKD, not in diabetic CKD.

Interestingly, instead of baPWV, low bPEP/bET, which has a significant correlation with impaired left ventricular ejection fraction [14], is correlated with fluid overload in diabetic CKD patients. This study also used the echocardiographic examination to evaluate cardiac function in 184 subjects and found that left ventricular ejection fraction was significantly correlated with fluid overload in diabetic CKD ($\beta = -0.21$, $P = 0.002$), not in non-diabetic CKD ($\beta = -0.02$, $P = 0.4$). These findings suggest that fluid overload may have different levels of influences on CKD patients depending on the presence or absence of diabetes. Fluid overload is correlated with vascular level alterations in non-diabetic CKD, and with cardiac level modifications in diabetic CKD.

Cardiovascular dysfunction progresses with arterial-cardiac interactions [31]. The arterial-cardiac compensatory adaptations maintain cardiac performance with enhanced contractility [32]. Fluid overload alters and blunts the arterial-cardiac response, leading to hemodynamic instability [32]. The difference of rates of progression of dysfunction between the heart and the vasculature may explain our results. Probably, the phenomenon of fluid overload directly affecting cardiac function beyond vasculature in diabetic CKD exists. Arterial stiffness may occur in early diabetic CKD and then fluid overload may subsequently have effect on left ventricular systolic dysfunction in late diabetic CKD. Further study is needed to evaluate the mechanisms between fluid overload, arterial stiffness and cardiac dysfunction in diabetic CKD.

Due to the strong association of fluid overload and adverse outcomes [27], precise measurement of fluid status is important in clinical practice of CKD patients. Traditional physical examination is not enough to detect slight variations of fluid status. Accumulating evidence suggests that multifrequency spectroscopic bioimpedance can provides information of increases in fluid status and associated body composition. Besides, using a non-invasive ABI-form device, clinicians can easily obtain the value of baPWV, a reliable marker of arterial stiffness, and bPEP/bET, a surrogate of left ventricular systolic function. These inexpensive and convenient tools might assist clinicians in assessing the risk of

renal progression and cardiovascular morbidity and mortality earlier.

The present study has some limitations that must be considered. This study was conducted at a single center. Fluid status, baPWV, bPEP/bET, clinical parameters, and the use of drugs were measured only once at enrollment. The association of time-varying baPWV, bPEP/bET, clinical parameters, and the use of drugs with time-varying fluid status could not be estimated. Additionally, our findings show the relative weak correlation between bPEP/bET and fluid overload in diabetic CKD. The weak correlation between fluid overload and bPEP/bET is probably related to the relatively small sample size of diabetic patients. Based on the association of bPEP/bET with cardiac function, we performed subgroup analysis to analyze the relationship between bPEP/bET and fluid overload in the heart disease group and the result was consistent ($\beta = -0.46$, $P = 0.03$). However, there was no significant correlation between bPEP/bET and fluid overload in the non-heart disease group. We need a large population study to evaluate the interaction between bPEP/bET, cardiac function and diabetes in a CKD cohort.

In conclusion, our study evaluates a relationship between fluid overload, diabetes, and arterial stiffness or cardiac function in late CKD patients. Fluid overload is correlated with arterial stiffness in non-diabetic CKD, and with left ventricular dysfunction in diabetic CKD. Fluid overload probably has distinct arterial-cardiac influences on CKD patients in the presence or absence of diabetes. Early and accurate assessment of these associated cardiovascular risk factors may improve the effects of entire care in late CKD patients.

Acknowledgments

The authors thank the from the staff of the Statistical Analysis Laboratory, Department of Medical Research, Kaohsiung Medical University Hospital, Kaohsiung Medical University for their assistance.

Author Contributions

Conceived and designed the experiments: YCT MCK. Performed the experiments: YCT THC. Analyzed the data: YCT YWC. Contributed reagents/materials/analysis tools: YWC HTK SCC SJH HCC. Contributed to the writing of the manuscript: YCT MCK.

References

1. Wizemann V, Schilling M (1995) Dilemma of assessing volume state–the use and the limitations of a clinical score. Nephrol Dial Transplant 10: 2114–2117.
2. Wizemann V, Leibinger A, Mueller K, Nilson A (1995) Influence of hydration state on plasma volume changes during ultrafiltration. Artif Organs 19: 416–419.
3. Hung SC, Kuo KL, Peng CH, Wu CH, Lien YC, et al. (2014) Volume overload correlates with cardiovascular risk factors in patients with chronic kidney disease. Kidney Int 85: 703–9.
4. Saran R, Bragg-Gresham JL, Levin NW, Twardowski ZJ, Wizemann V, et al. (2006) Longer treatment time and slower ultrafiltration in hemodialysis: associations with reduced mortality in the DOPPS. Kidney Int 69: 1222–1228.
5. Wizemann V, Wabel P, Chamney P, Zaluska W, Moissl U, et al. (2009) The mortality risk of overhydration in haemodialysis patients. Nephrol Dial Transplant 24: 1574–1579.
6. Paniagua R, Ventura MD, Avila-Diaz M, Hinojosa-Heredia H, Mendez-Duran A, et al. (2010) NT-proBNP, fluid volume overload and dialysis modality are independent predictors of mortality in ESRD patients. Nephrol Dial Transplant 25: 551–557.
7. Movilli E, Gaggia P, Zubani R, Camerini C, Vizzardi V, et al. (2007) Association between high ultrafiltration rates and mortality in uraemic patients on regular haemodialysis. A 5-year prospective observational multicentre study. Nephrol Dial Transplant 22: 3547–3552.
8. Fox CS, Matsushita K, Woodward M, Bilo HJ, Chalmers J, et al. (2012) Chronic Kidney Disease Prognosis Consortium: Associations of kidney disease measures with mortality and end-stage renal disease in individuals with and without diabetes: a meta-analysis. Lancet 380: 1662–1673.

9. Tsai YC, Tsai JC, Chiu YW, Kuo HT, Chen SC, et al. (2013) Is fluid overload more important than diabetes in renal progression in late chronic kidney disease? PLoS One 8: e82566.
10. Tucker BJ, Collins RC, Ziegler MG, Blantz RC(1991) Disassociation between glomerular hyperfiltration and extracellular volume in diabetic rats. Kidney Int 39: 1176–1183.
11. Yokoyama H, Shoji T, Kimoto E, Shinohara K, Tanaka S, et al. (2003) Pulse wave velocity in lower-limb arteries among diabetic patients with peripheral arterial disease. J Atheroscler Thromb 10: 253–258.
12. Yamashina A, Tomiyama H, Takeda K, Tsuda H, Arai T, et al. (2002) Validity, reproducibility, and clinical significance of noninvasive brachial-ankle pulse wave velocity measurement. Hypertens Res 25: 359–364.
13. Chen SC, Chang JM, Tsai JC, Lin TH, Hsu PC, et al. (2010) A systolic parameter defined as the ratio of brachial pre-ejection period to brachial ejection time predicts cardiovascular events in patients with chronic kidney disease. Circ J 74: 2206–2210.
14. Su HM, Lin TH, Lee CS, Lee HC, Chu CY, et al. (2009) Myocardial performance index derived from brachial-ankle pulse wave velocity: A novel and feasible parameter in evaluation of cardiac performance. Am J Hypertens 22: 871–876.
15. Chen SC, Chang JM, Tsai JC, Hsu PC, Lin TH, et al. (2010) A new systolic parameter defined as the ratio of brachial pre-ejection period to brachial ejection time predicts overall and cardiovascular mortality in hemodialysis patients. Hypertens Res 33: 492–498.
16. Levey AS, Bosch JP, Lewis JB, Greene T, Rogers N, et al. (1999) A more accurate.

17. Wabel P, Chamney P, Moissl U, Jirka T (2009) Importance of whole-body bioimpedance spectroscopy for the management of fluid balance. Blood Purif 27: 75–80.

18. Crepaldi C, Soni S, Chionh CY, Wabel P, Cruz DN, et al. (2009) Application of body composition monitoring to peritoneal dialysis patients. Contrib Nephrol 163: 1–6.

19. Wizemann V, Rode C, Wabel P (2008) Whole-body spectroscopy (BCM) in the.

20. Moissl UM, Wabel P, Chamney PW, Bosaeus I, Levin NW, et al. (2006) Body fluid volume determination via body composition spectroscopy in health and disease. Physiol Meas 27: 921–933.

21. Hur E, Usta M, Toz H, Asci G, Wabel P, et al. (2013) Effect of fluid management guided by bioimpedance spectroscopy on cardiovascular parameters in hemodialysis patients: a randomized controlled trial. Am J Kidney Dis 61: 957–965.

22. Wieskotten S, Heinke S, Wabel P, Moissl U, Becker J, et al. (2008) Bioimpedance-based identification of malnutrition using fuzzy logic. Physiol Meas 29: 639–654.

23. Van Biesen W, Williams JD, Covic AC, Fan S, Claes K, et al. (2011) Fluid status in peritoneal dialysis patients: the European Body Composition Monitoring (EuroBCM) study cohort. PLoS One. 6: e17148.

24. Chen SC, Chang JM, Liu WC, Huang JC, Chen YY, et al. (2012) Decrease in ankle-brachial index over time and cardiovascular outcomes in patients with hemodialysis. Am J Med Sci 344: 457–461.

25. Chen SC, Chang JM, Liu WC, Tsai JC, Chen LI, et al. (2011) Significant correlation between ratio of brachial pre-ejection period to ejection time and left ventricular ejection fraction and mass index in patients with chronic kidney disease. Nephrol Dial Transplant 26: 1895–1902.

26. Zheng D, Cheng LT, Zhuang Z, Gu Y, Tang LJ, et al. (2009) Correlation between.

27. Tsai YC, Tsai JC, Chen SC, Chiu YW, Hwang SJ, et al. (2014) Association of Fluid Overload With Kidney Disease Progression in Advanced CKD: A Prospective Cohort Study. Am J Kidney Dis 63: 68–75.

28. Kimoto E, Shoji T, Shinohara K, Inaba M, Okuno Y, et al. (2003) Preferential stiffening of central over peripheral arteries in type 2 diabetes. Diabetes 52: 448–52.

29. Tsuchikura S, Shoji T, Kimoto E, Shinohara K, Hatsuda S, et al. (2010) Central versus peripheral arterial stiffness in association with coronary, cerebral and peripheral arterial disease. Atherosclerosis 211: 480–5.

30. Kim WJ, Park CY, Park SE, Rhee EJ, Lee WY, et al. (2012) The association between regional arterial stiffness and diabetic retinopathy in type 2 diabetes. Atherosclerosis 225: 237–241.

31. Moody WE, Edwards NC, Chue CD, Ferro CJ, Townend JN (2013) Arterial disease in chronic kidney disease. Heart 99: 365–372.

32. Chen CH, Nakayama M, Nevo E, Fetics BJ, Maughan WL, et al. (1998) Coupled systolic-ventricular and vascular stiffening with age: implications for pressure regulation and cardiac reserve in the elderly. J Am Coll Cardiol 32: 1221–7.

21

Recipient-Related Risk Factors for Graft Failure and Death in Elderly Kidney Transplant Recipients

Xingqiang Lai[ȿ], **Guodong Chen**[ȿ], **Jiang Qiu, Changxi Wang, Lizhong Chen***

Organ Transplant Center, The First Affiliated Hospital, Sun Yat-sen University, Guangzhou, China

Abstract

Background: Elderly patients with end-stage renal disease have become the fastest growing population of kidney transplant candidates in recent years. However, the risk factors associated with long-term outcomes in these patients remain unclear.

Methods: We retrospectively analyzed 166 recipients aged 60 years or older who underwent primary deceased kidney transplantation between 2002 and 2013 in our center. The main outcomes included 1-, 3- and 5-year patient survival as well as overall and death-censored graft survival. The independent risk factors affecting graft and patient survival were analyzed using Cox regression analysis.

Results: The 1-, 3-, 5-year death-censored graft survival rates were 93.6%, 89.4% and 83.6%, respectively. Based on the Cox multivariate analysis, panel reactive antibody (PRA)>5% [hazard ratio (HR) 4.295, 95% confidence interval (CI) 1.321–13.97], delayed graft function (HR 4.744, 95% CI 1.611–13.973) and acute rejection (HR 4.971, 95% CI 1.516–16.301) were independent risk factors for graft failure. The 1-, 3-, 5-year patient survival rates were 84.8%, 82.1% and 77.1%, respectively. Longer dialysis time (HR 1.011 for 1-month increase, 95% CI 1.002–1.020), graft loss (HR 3.501, 95% CI 1.559–7.865) and low-dose ganciclovir prophylaxis (1.5 g/d for 3 months) (HR 3.173, 95% CI 1.063–9.473) were risk factors associated with patient death.

Conclusions: The five-year results show an excellent graft and patient survival in elderly kidney transplant recipients aged ≥ 60 years. PRA>5%, delayed graft function, and acute rejection are risk factors for graft failure, while longer duration of dialysis, graft loss and low-dose ganciclovir prophylaxis are risk factors for mortality in elderly recipients. These factors represent potential targets for interventions aimed at improving graft and patient survival in elderly recipients.

Editor: Stanislaw Stepkowski, University of Toledo, United States of America

Funding: This study was supported by the 5010 Clinical Research Project of Sun Yat-sen University (2007003) and the National Natural Science Fund Youth Science project (81302549). The funders had no role in study design, data collection and analysis, decision to publish, or preparation of the manuscript.

Competing Interests: The authors have declared that no competing interests exist.

* Email: clz@medmail.com.cn

ȿ These authors contributed equally to this work.

Introduction

Kidney transplantation is considered to be the best treatment option for patients with end-stage renal disease (ESRD), regardless of their age. Currently, the mean age of patients undergoing renal transplantation has increased. This trend is observed not only in western countries such as America but also in Asian countries. Patients ≥60 years with ESRD have become the fastest growing population of wait-listed individuals and kidney transplant candidates [1,2]. Over the last decade, both the absolute number and percent of transplants performed in patients aged ≥65 years have approximately doubled [1]. Previous studies have reported that elderly ESRD patients after kidney transplantation have lower mortality rates and improved quality of life compared with those who remain on dialysis treatment [3,4,5].

However, despite the known benefits of kidney transplantation over dialysis in the elderly patients, long-term outcomes of the recipients and their grafts are still limited [6]. Given the rapid increase in the number of senior renal transplant candidates combined with a growing shortage of donor kidneys, it is increasingly important to optimize the long-term outcomes in the elderly recipients. The characteristics of the elderly patients at transplantation may have an important impact on graft and patient survival. Published studies regarding the recipient factors that predict outcomes in elderly recipients are limited, especially in China. Accurately determining the possible predictors involved in graft and patient survival is crucial for improving long-term outcomes in elderly recipients.

Therefore, the aim of this study was to evaluate graft and patient survival in kidney transplant recipients aged ≥60 years and to determine the possible recipient-related risk factors associated with clinical outcome.

Patients and Methods

This retrospective cohort study was approved by the Institutional Review Board/Ethics Committee of The First Affiliated Hospital of Sun Yat-sen University, and all aspects of the study complied with the Helsinki Declaration of 1975. The Ethics Committee of The First Affiliated Hospital of Sun Yat-sen University specifically approved that not informed consent was required because all data were going to be analyzed anonymously. All of the organs were from donation after brain death (DBD) or donation after cardiac death (DCD), and all of the organ donors had provided informed written consent. No prisoner organs were used in this study.

All patients aged 60 years or older who underwent first-time kidney transplantation from deceased donors in our center between January 2002 and June 2013 were collected. We excluded patients who had received another organ besides the kidney. The recipient characteristics included age, gender, causes of ESRD, pre-transplant comorbidities [including diabetes mellitus, hypertension, coronary artery disease (CAD)], type and time on dialysis, and panel reactive antibody (PRA) level at transplantation. The induction agents, basic maintained immunosuppressive regimens, and regimens for cytomegalovirus (CMV) prophylaxis were also recorded. After surgery, the number and frequency of adverse events including delayed graft function (DGF), acute rejection (AR) and chronic rejection (CR) at any time, leucopenia, infectious events, graft loss and patient death, malignancy and other new onset diseases were recorded. The causes of graft failure and mortality were also recorded.

Patients received IL-2 receptor antagonist (IL2RA, including basiliximab or daclizumab) or rabbit anti-thymocyte globulin (rATG) as induction agents. The maintained immunosuppressive regimens consisted of cyclosporine or tacrolimus, mycophenolate mofetil (MMF) and prednisone. From 2002 to 2006, most of the recipients received a low-dose ganciclovir (1.5 g/d for 3 months) for CMV prophylaxis, whereas patients mainly received a high-dose ganciclovir (3.0 g/d for 3 months) since 2007. Sulfamethoxazole was administered orally for 3 months for Pneumocystis jirovecii pneumonia prophylaxis.

DGF was defined as the need for dialysis in the first week after transplantation. AR was diagnosed based on clinical manifestations such as fever, oliguria, and serum creatinine elevation of > 25% from the baseline value and was confirmed by a subsequent renal allograft biopsy. Biopsy-proven acute rejections (BPAR) included all acute rejections which were graded borderline or higher by Banff'97 criteria. CR was diagnosed by clinical findings with a decrease in kidney function and developing a gradual rise in serum creatinine, and was confirmed by renal allograft biopsy with histological features including thickening of the intima of arterioles and arteries, sclerosis of glomeruli, and tabular atrophy.

Statistical analysis

All data were analyzed by SPSS for Windows Version 19.0 (SPSS, Chicago, Illinois, USA). Continuous variables are expressed as counts and percentages, and categorical variables are expressed as the means with standard deviations (mean ± SD). Actuarial graft and patient survival were calculated using Kaplan–Meier analysis. To assess variables associated with transplant outcome, univariate and multivariate Cox proportional hazards regression models were employed. The association between outcomes and all co-variables were tested separately in univariate Cox analyses. To evaluate the potential independent risk factors for transplant outcomes, all variables associated with graft loss or patient death at a $P<0.2$ level in the univariate Cox analysis were

included in the final multivariate model. A P-value <0.05 was considered to indicate statistical significance.

Results

Patient characteristics

We collected data from 166 primary deceased kidney transplant recipients aged 60 or older between January 2002 and June 2013. The demographic and baseline characteristics of these elderly patients are shown in Table 1. The mean recipient age was 64.6 ± 3.8 years, and 109 (65.7%) recipients were male. The main cause of ESRD was chronic glomerulonephritis, followed by diabetes mellitus. Hypertension was the most prevalent comorbidity in these aged recipients. The mean duration of dialysis was 18.6 ± 22.1 months. Initial immunosuppressive induction therapy based on IL2RA was 68.1% and that based on rATG was 31.9%. At baseline, 56.6% and 43.4% of patients were on cyclosporine-based and tacrolimus-based immunosuppression, respectively; for CMV prophylaxis, 101 (60.8%) recipients received low-dose ganciclovir (1.5 g/d for 3 months), and 65 (39.2%) received high-dose ganciclovir (3.0 g/d for 3 months).

Graft and patient survival

The adverse events during the 5-year follow-up are shown in Table 2. The incidence of DGF, AR and chronic rejection (CR) was 9%, 16.9% and 8.3%, respectively. Infection was the most common adverse event in the elderly patients, with an incidence of 55.4%. The incidence of CMV infection was 17.5%, and most of which occurred in the first year post-transplantation. A total of 36 patients experienced graft loss and 29 patients died within 5-year follow-up. Overall and death-censored graft survival and patient survival are shown in Figure 1. The 1-, 3-, 5-year overall graft survival was 84.3%, 78% and 70.6%, respectively. However, when patient death was not considered as graft loss (death-censored), the 1-, 3-, 5-year graft survival reached 93.6%, 89.4% and 83.6%, respectively. Patient survival was 84.8% at 1 year, 82.1% at 3 year and 77.1% at 5 year. The causes of graft loss and patient death are shown in Table 3. The main causes of graft loss were patient death (52.8%) and AR (16.7%). Most of the patients died of infection (55.2%) and CAD (17.2%). In addition, among the infectious mortality, there were 11 deaths due to severe CMV disease.

Risk factors for graft loss

During a 5-year follow-up, there were 36 cases of graft loss in the cohort. More than half of the graft losses (52.8%) were due to patient death. Univariate analysis showed that longer dialysis time, PRA>5%, DGF and AR were risk factors for death-censored graft loss. Based on the Cox multivariate models, a PRA>5% [hazard ratio (HR) 4.295, 95% confidence interval (CI) 1.321–13.97], DGF (HR 4.744, 95% CI 1.611–13.973) and AR (HR 4.971, 95% CI 1.516–16.301) remained independent risk factors for death-censored graft loss, except for longer dialysis time (Table 4). The status of comorbidities, including diabetes mellitus, hypertension and CAD were not associated with shorter graft survival.

Risk factors for patient death

There were 29 deaths during the 5-year follow-up. The risk factors for patient death were shown in Table 5. Univariate analysis showed that longer dialysis time, AR, graft loss and low-dose ganciclovir prophylaxis were risk factors for patient death. However, when data was analysis by final Cox multivariate model, we found that longer dialysis time (HR 1.011 for 1-month increase, 95% CI 1.002–1.020), graft loss (HR 3.501, 95% CI 1.559–7.865) and low-dose ganciclovir prophylaxis (HR 3.173,

Table 1. Recipient baseline characteristics (N = 166).

Recipient age, yr (mean±SD)	64.6±3.8	Dialysis, n (%)	
Male recipients, n (%)	109 (65.7)	Nondialysis	46 (27.7)
Cause of ESRD, n (%)		Hemodialysis	87 (52.4)
Chronic glomerulonephritis	73 (44)	Peritoneal dialysis	33 (19.9)
Diabetes mellitus	51 (30.7)	Time on dialysis, months (mean±SD)	18.6±22.1
Hypertension	19 (11.4)	PRA>5%, n (%)	16 (9.6)
Obstructive nephropathy	7 (4.2)	IL2RA, n (%)	113 (68.1)
Polycystic kidney	6 (3.6)	rATG, n (%)	53 (31.9)
Others or unknown	10 (6)	Cyclosporine, n (%)	94 (56.6)
Comorbidities, n (%)		Tacrolimus, n (%)	72 (43.4)
Diabetes mellitus	70 (42.1)	Low-dose ganciclovir (1.5 g/d), n (%)	101 (60.8)
Hypertension	120 (72.3)	High-dose ganciclovir (3.0 g/d), n (%)	65 (39.2)
Coronary artery disease (CAD)	24 (14.5)		

95% CI 1.063–9.473) remained significant independent risk factors for mortality. AR, diabetes mellitus, hypertension, CAD, and DGF were not significantly associated with patient death.

Discussion

The rapid increase in elderly patients with ESRD has raised an important issue regarding the optimization of long-term outcomes in this population. Despite a higher percentage of cadaveric kidney donors being allocated to older patients, the short-term graft survival is excellent in the majority of these patients. However, longer-term graft survival in the elderly recipients is less than expected due to death with a functioning graft, which is the major cause of graft loss. Elderly renal transplant recipients are at

increased risk of graft loss and death compared with younger cohorts [7,8]. Considering the rapid growth of an aging ESRD population and the shortage of donor kidneys, identifying the possible risk factors of graft and patient survival in elderly recipients is crucial for improving their long-term outcome.

In this study, we retrospectively analyzed 166 cases of renal transplantation from deceased donors in recipients aged ≥60 years and identified the possible risk factors predicting poor clinical outcome. Consistent with previous studies, death with a functioning graft is the leading cause of graft loss in elderly patients, with a percentage of more than 50% [9]. When patient death was not considered as the cause of graft loss, the 1-, 3-, 5-year graft survival reached 93.6%, 89.4% and 83.6%, respectively. Similar to previous studies, a PRA>5% at the time of transplantation was

Table 2. Adverse events in 5-year follow-up.

Adverse events	n (%)
DGF	15 (9)
AR	28 (16.9)
CR	3 (8.3)
Leukopenia	9 (5.4)
All infections	92 (55.4)
Urinary tract	7 (4.2)
Probable bacterial or other	35 (21.1)
Confirmed bacterial	64 (38.6)
CMV	29 (17.5)
BK polyoma virus	1 (0.6)
Fungal	10 (6)
Liver impairment	39 (23.5)
New onset diabetes mellitus	18 (10.8)
Congestive heart failure	8 (4.8)
Cerebrovascular accident	4 (2.4)
Malignancy	9 (5.4)
Graft loss	36 (21.7)
Death	29 (17.5)

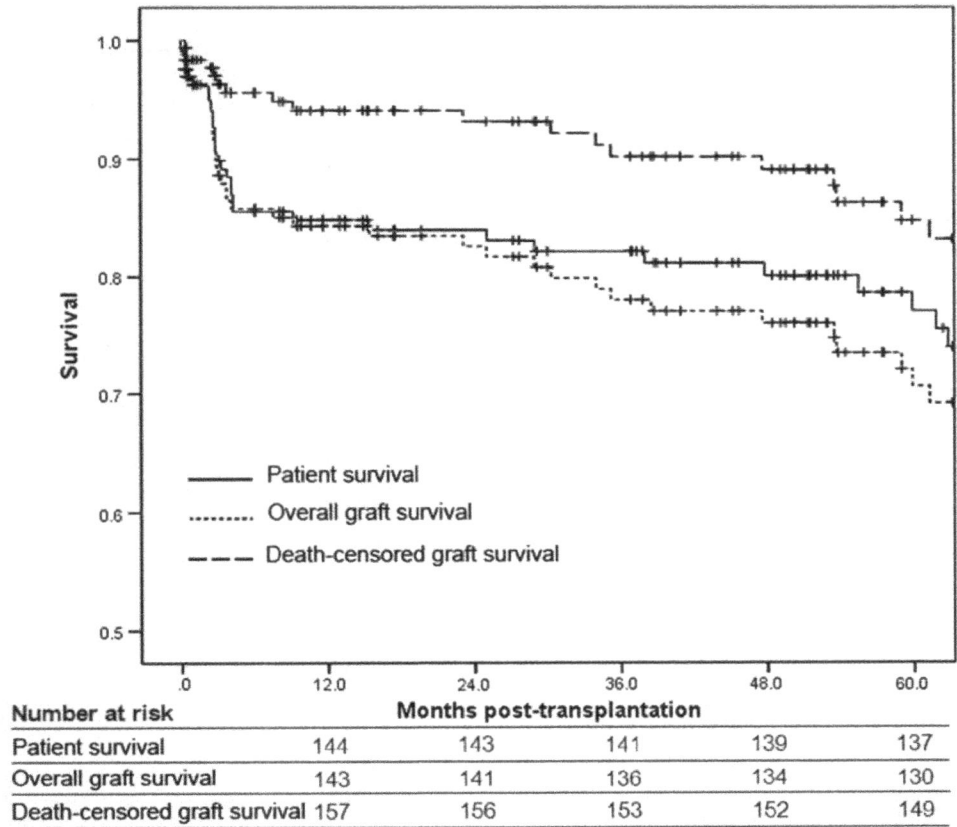

Figure 1. Patient survival, overall and death-censored graft survival.

Number at risk					
Patient survival	144	143	141	139	137
Overall graft survival	143	141	136	134	130
Death-censored graft survival	157	156	153	152	149

a significant independent risk factor for graft loss in recipients aged ≥60 years. Heldal et al. [10] reported a PRA>5% as a risk factor for graft loss in patients aged ≥70 years, whereas Faravardeh et al. [11] demonstrated that a PRA>10% was a risk factor for graft failure in recipients aged ≥65 years.

In our study, we found that patients aged ≥60 years experienced a low incidence of AR episodes, which were similar to previous findings [12]. Although the incidence of AR was lower in the elderly transplant recipients, the impact of AR episodes was far more severe than in the young recipients [13]. We found that both DGF and AR were risk factors for graft loss in recipients aged

≥60 years. Heldal et al. [10] reported that DGF was an independent predictor for death-censored graft loss in the elderly recipients aged 60 years or older. Similarly, in the study by Faravardeh et al. [11], DGF and AR were risk factors for graft failure not only in younger recipients but also in elderly cohorts aged ≥65 years. In a multicenter case-control study in Spain, Moreso et al. [14] also confirmed that AR was an independent predictor of death-censored graft failure in adult renal transplant recipients. However, in another prospective multicenter study performed in Spain, the authors did not find any significant association between AR and allograft loss in neither recipients

Table 3. Causes of graft loss and mortality (5 years).

Graft loss (N = 36)	n (%)	Mortality (N = 29)	n (%)
Patient death	19 (52.8)	Infection	16 (55.2)
AR	6 (16.7)	CAD	5 (17.2)
CR	3 (8.3)	Cerebrovascular accident	2 (6.9)
Chronic allograft nephropathy	4 (11.1)	Malignancy	3 (10.3)
Recurrence	1 (2.8)	Liver disease	1 (3.5)
ARF	1 (2.8)	Hemorrhage	1 (3.5)
PNF	1 (2.8)	Unknown	1 (3.5)
Technical failure	1 (2.8)		

ARF, acute renal failure; PNF, primary no function.

Table 4. Risk factors for death-censored graft loss (5 years).

Variables	Univariate analysis			Cox multivariate analysis		
	HR	95% CI	P value	HR	95% CI	P value
Age (1-year increase)	1.059	0.95–1.179	0.3	—	—	—
Gender (male vs female)	1.255	0.464–3.397	0.655	—	—	—
Dialysis time (1-month increase)	1.013	1.001–1.026	0.028	1.014	0.999–1.029	0.061
Diabetes mellitus	0.624	0.231–1.691	0.354	—	—	—
Hypertension	2.016	0.458–8.866	0.353	—	—	—
CAD	0.638	0.146–2.795	0.551	—	—	—
PRA>5%	10.503	4.037–27.325	<0.001	4.295	1.321–13.97	0.015
Induction (IL2RA vs rATG)	0.553	0.156–1.959	0.359	—	—	—
Cyclosporin vs tacrolimus	2.05	0.778–5.396	0.146	1.322	0.495–3.534	0.577
DGF	5.908	2.059–16.954	0.001	4.744	1.611–13.973	0.005
AR	6.782	2.612–17.609	<0.001	4.971	1.516–16.301	0.008

HR, hazard ratio; CI, confidence interval.

aged ≥60 years nor in younger recipients [15]. Nevertheless, AR and DGF can result in functional and structural damage to the graft, which leads to late poor graft outcomes. Therefore, a decrease in the incidence of AR or DGF may result in an improvement of late graft outcome.

The literature on the association between duration of dialysis and transplant outcome is rich and at times inconsistent. Most of the studies reported that longer duration of dialysis was associated with poorer patient and graft outcome in kidney transplant recipients [16,17,18], whereas some other studies didn't find any association between dialysis duration and patient or graft survival [15]. In addition, there are also some studies reported that longer time on dialysis was independent risk factor only for patient death, but not for graft loss [9,19]. In the study by Faravardeh et al. [11], the authors reported that longer dialysis time was a risk factor for graft loss and mortality in recipients aged <50 years, but not in those aged ≥50 years. Therefore, the risk of transplant outcome associated with increased dialysis duration time may differ

between various countries and populations. In this retrospective study, we demonstrated that increased time on dialysis was an independent risk factor for patient death. Since the maintenance of dialysis status may accelerate cardiovascular changes, including vascular calcification, left ventricular hypertrophy and congestive heart failure [20], longer time on dialysis may result in an increased risk of death, especially in the elderly with a higher incidence of vascular complications. In the current study, we did not find longer duration of dialysis to be a significant independent risk factor for graft failure in multivariate Cox regression model. This finding may be explained by the fact that the elderly may differ somewhat from the younger population, since the incidence of acute rejection appears to steadily reduce with increased age [1]. In addition, the mean duration of pretransplant dialysis in our cohort is 18.6 months, which is relatively short compared to previous studies. Furthermore, the relatively small sample may somewhat weaken the impact of dialysis time on graft survival.

Table 5. Risk factors for patient death (5 years).

Variables	Univariate analysis			Cox multivariate analysis		
	HR	95% CI	P value	HR	95% CI	P value
Age (1-year increase)	1.068	0.974–1.171	0.16	1.081	0.985–1.186	0.1
Gender (male vs female)	1.243	0.577–2.675	0.579	—	—	—
Dialysis time (1-month increase)	1.013	1.004–1.022	0.004	1.011	1.002–1.020	0.02
Diabetes mellitus	0.713	0.336–1.51	0.377	—	—	—
Hypertension	0.924	0.393–2.171	0.856	—	—	—
CAD	1.412	0.574–3.47	0.452	—	—	—
Induction (IL2RA vs rATG)	0.438	0.166–1.155	0.095	1.627	0.38–6.966	0.512
CsA vs FK506	1.627	0.777–3.407	0.197	1.554	0.735–3.289	0.249
DGF	2.345	0.889–6.185	0.085	2.303	0.856–6.196	0.098
AR	3.595	1.697–7.617	0.001	1.91	0.715–5.101	0.197
Graft loss	4.571	2.073–10.081	<0.001	3.501	1.559–7.865	0.002
Ganciclovir (1.5 g/d vs 3 g/d)	3.947	1.366–11.401	0.011	3.173	1.063–9.473	0.039

Graft failure was a significant risk factor for mortality for patients aged ≥60 years in our study, which was confirmed in previous studies [11]. The increased death rate was partly due to the potential immediate complications of graft loss and longer-term worse survival of returning to dialysis.

CMV infection is a common problem in immunocompromised hosts and an important cause of morbidity and mortality in kidney transplant recipients [21]. Previous studies had demonstrated that CMV infection was associated with acute and chronic graft rejection [22], increased incidence of opportunistic infection [23], graft loss and decreased recipient survival [24]. Universal prophylaxis with effective antiviral agents is one of the possible approaches for prevention of CMV infection. In China, ganciclovir remains the preferred agent for prophylaxis and treatment of CMV infection due to its effectiveness and affordable price to most patients. The study by Ahmed and colleagues demonstrated that low-dose ganciclovir (1.0 g/d for 3 months) was as effective at decreasing the incidence of clinical CMV disease as high-dose ganciclovir (3.0 g/d for 3–6 months) in renal transplant recipients [25]. However, in the present study, we found that a low-dose ganciclovir (1.5 g/d for 3 months) was significantly associated with shorter patient survival in elderly recipients. This difference could be explained by the fact that the mean age of Ahmed's recipients was 46.1±2.2 years, which was much lower than those in our study. Elderly patients are thought to generate a less robust immune response due to a decreased immunogenicity with increased age [26] combined with more pre-transplant comorbidities, which may increase the overall risk of infectious death in elderly transplant recipients [27,28]. Low-dose ganciclovir may be not as effective as high-dose ganciclovir for CMV prophylaxis in elderly recipients. Therefore, it is important to widely use a high-dose ganciclovir to decrease the incidence of CMV infection in the more susceptible population such as the elderly renal transplant recipients.

CAD was one of the most common comorbidities and causes of death in elderly recipients. Faravardeh et al. [11] reported that CAD was a risk factor for mortality in both recipients aged ≥65 years and the younger cohort aged <50 years, while Heldal et al. [10] found that CAD increased mortality in transplant recipients up to 70 years but not in older recipients. However, in our study, we did not find CAD to be a risk factor for mortality in patients aged ≥60 years at transplantation, which was consistent with Doyle's finding [29]. The lower prevalence of CAD in the elderly recipients may be a likely explanation for our finding because

there were fewer patients with CAD in our cohort and this likely led to a loss of some power to detect the significance of this factor. This is not surprising, as China is known traditionally for low incidence of CAD and low plasma cholesterol levels due to the Chinese diet and lifestyle [30,31]. Although the incidence of CAD has increased in the last 2 decades, the incidence attained is still significantly lower than that in the Western countries [32]. Furthermore, the morbidity and mortality of CAD is much lower in south China compared with in the north [30]. Since all of the patients included were from south of China, it is reasonable that the number and proportion of CAD was low in our study. Similar to previous studies, we did not find an association between diabetes and patient survival [9,29,33]. We also did not find hypertension as a significant risk factor for graft failure or patient death.

Our study has certain limitations inherent in its retrospective nature because data were collected from patients transplanted from 2002 to June 2013. There were certain patients missing in the follow-up (10.5% of the overall cohort), which may reduce potential adverse effects of various risk factors that would be observed over a longer-term. In addition, the relatively small sample size might have less power to detect the effect of variables that have a smaller impact on the poor clinical outcome.

In conclusion, the transplant outcomes are excellent among recipients aged 60 years or older. We found that PRA>5%, DGF and AR were risk factors for graft failure, while longer time on dialysis, failed grafts and low-dose ganciclovir prophylaxis were risk factors for mortality in recipients aged ≥60 years. These factors represent potential targets for interventions aimed at improving graft and patient survival in elderly recipients. Therefore, reducing PRA level and decreasing the incidence of DGF and AR may result in longer graft survival, while shortening the duration of dialysis may lead to longer patient survival. In addition, high-dose ganciclovir prophylaxis should be widely used in elderly recipient to decrease the incidence of CMV infection. Nevertheless, further prospective, randomized and multicenter studies are needed to confirm these findings.

Author Contributions

Conceived and designed the experiments: XQL GDC. Performed the experiments: XQL GDC. Analyzed the data: XQL GDC. Contributed reagents/materials/analysis tools: GDC JQ CXW LZC. Wrote the paper: XQL GDC. Finalized the manuscript: XQL GDC. Read and approved the final manuscript: LZC.

References

1. Danovitch GM, Gill J, Bunnapradist S (2007) Immunosuppression of the elderly kidney transplant recipient. Transplantation 84: 285–291.
2. McCullough KP, Keith DS, Meyer KH, Stock PG, Brayman KL, et al. (2009) Kidney and pancreas transplantation in the United States, 1998–2007: access for patients with diabetes and end-stage renal disease. Am J Transplant 9: 894–906.
3. Wolfe RA, Ashby VB, Milford EL, Ojo AO, Ettenger RE, et al. (1999) Comparison of mortality in all patients on dialysis, patients on dialysis awaiting transplantation, and recipients of a first cadaveric transplant. N Engl J Med 341: 1725–1730.
4. Johnson DW, Herzig K, Purdie D, Brown AM, Rigby RJ, et al. (2000) A comparison of the effects of dialysis and renal transplantation on the survival of older uremic patients. Transplantation 69: 794–799.
5. Oniscu GC, Brown H, Forsythe JL (2004) How great is the survival advantage of transplantation over dialysis in elderly patients? Nephrol Dial Transplant 19: 945–951.
6. Meier-Kriesche HU, Schold JD, Srinivas TR, Kaplan B (2004) Lack of improvement in renal allograft survival despite a marked decrease in acute rejection rates over the most recent era. Am J Transplant 4: 378–383.
7. Roodnat JI, Zietse R, Mulder PG, Rischen-Vos J, van Gelder T, et al. (1999) The vanishing importance of age in renal transplantation. Transplantation 67: 576–580.
8. Meier-Kriesche H, Ojo AO, Arndorfer JA, Port FK, Magee JC, et al. (2001) Recipient age as an independent risk factor for chronic renal allograft failure. Transplant Proc 33: 1113–1114.
9. Cardinal H, Hebert MJ, Rahme E, Houde I, Baran D, et al. (2005) Modifiable factors predicting patient survival in elderly kidney transplant recipients. Kidney Int 68: 345–351.
10. Heldal K, Hartmann A, Leivestad T, Svendsen MV, Foss A, et al. (2009) Clinical outcomes in elderly kidney transplant recipients are related to acute rejection episodes rather than pretransplant comorbidity. Transplantation 87: 1045–1051.
11. Faravardeh A, Eickhoff M, Jackson S, Spong R, Kukla A, et al. (2013) Predictors of graft failure and death in elderly kidney transplant recipients. Transplantation 96: 1089–1096.
12. Patel SJ, Knight RJ, Suki WN, Abdellatif A, Duhart BJ, et al. (2011) Rabbit antithymocyte induction and dosing in deceased donor renal transplant recipients over 60 yr of age. Clin Transplant 25: E250–E256.
13. Meier-Kriesche HU, Srinivas TR, Kaplan B (2001) Interaction between acute rejection and recipient age on long-term renal allograft survival. Transplant Proc 33: 3425–3426.
14. Moreso F, Alonso A, Gentil MA, Gonzalez-Molina M, Capdevila L, et al. (2010) Improvement in late renal allograft survival between 1990 and 2002 in Spain: results from a multicentre case-control study. Transpl Int 23: 907–913.

15. Morales JM, Marcen R, Del CD, Andres A, Gonzalez-Molina M, et al. (2012) Risk factors for graft loss and mortality after renal transplantation according to recipient age: a prospective multicentre study. Nephrol Dial Transplant 27 Suppl 4: v39–v46.

16. Meier-Kriesche HU, Port FK, Ojo AO, Rudich SM, Hanson JA, et al. (2000) Effect of waiting time on renal transplant outcome. Kidney Int 58: 1311–1317.

17. Goldfarb-Rumyantzev A, Hurdle JF, Scandling J, Wang Z, Baird B, et al. (2005) Duration of end-stage renal disease and kidney transplant outcome. Nephrol Dial Transplant 20: 167–175.

18. Remport A, Keszei A, Vamos EP, Novak M, Jaray J, et al. (2011) Association of pre-transplant dialysis duration with outcome in kidney transplant recipients: a prevalent cohort study. Int Urol Nephrol 43: 215–224.

19. Helantera I, Salmela K, Kyllonen L, Koskinen P, Gronhagen-Riska C, et al. (2014) Pretransplant dialysis duration and risk of death after kidney transplantation in the current era. Transplantation 98: 458–464.

20. Himmelfarb J, Ikizler TA (2010) Hemodialysis. N Engl J Med 363: 1833–1845.

21. Brennan DC (2001) Cytomegalovirus in renal transplantation. J Am Soc Nephrol 12: 848–855.

22. Cainelli F, Vento S (2002) Infections and solid organ transplant rejection: a cause-and-effect relationship? Lancet Infect Dis 2: 539–549.

23. George MJ, Snydman DR, Werner BG, Griffith J, Falagas ME, et al. (1997) The independent role of cytomegalovirus as a risk factor for invasive fungal disease in orthotopic liver transplant recipients. Boston Center for Liver Transplantation CMVIG-Study Group. Cytogam, MedImmune, Inc. Gaithersburg, Maryland. Am J Med 103: 106–113.

24. De Keyzer K, Van Laecke S, Peeters P, Vanholder R (2011) Human cytomegalovirus and kidney transplantation: a clinician's update. Am J Kidney Dis 58: 118–126.

25. Ahmed J, Velarde C, Ramos M, Ismail K, Serpa J, et al. (2004) Outcome of low-dose ganciclovir for cytomegalovirus disease prophylaxis in renal-transplant recipients. Transplantation 78: 1689–1692.

26. Martins PN, Pratschke J, Pascher A, Fritsche L, Frei U, et al. (2005) Age and immune response in organ transplantation. Transplantation 79: 127–132.

27. Meier-Kriesche HU, Ojo AO, Hanson JA, Kaplan B (2001) Exponentially increased risk of infectious death in older renal transplant recipients. Kidney Int 59: 1539–1543.

28. Kauffman HM, McBride MA, Cors CS, Roza AM, Wynn JJ (2007) Early mortality rates in older kidney recipients with comorbid risk factors. Transplantation 83: 404–410.

29. Doyle SE, Matas AJ, Gillingham K, Rosenberg ME (2000) Predicting clinical outcome in the elderly renal transplant recipient. Kidney Int 57: 2144–2150.

30. Tao SC, Huang ZD, Wu XG, Zhou BF, Xiao ZK, et al. (1989) CHD and its risk factors in the People's Republic of China. Int J Epidemiol 18: S159–S163.

31. Campbell TC, Parpia B, Chen J (1998) Diet, lifestyle, and the etiology of coronary artery disease: the Cornell China study. Am J Cardiol 82: 18T–21T.

32. Ueshima H, Sekikawa A, Miura K, Turin TC, Takashima N, et al. (2008) Cardiovascular disease and risk factors in Asia: a selected review. Circulation 118: 2702–2709.

33. Fabrizii V, Winkelmayer WC, Klauser R, Kletzmayr J, Saemann MD, et al. (2004) Patient and graft survival in older kidney transplant recipients: does age matter? J Am Soc Nephrol 15: 1052–1060.

22

Mimicking Hypoxia to Treat Anemia: HIF-Stabilizer BAY 85-3934 (Molidustat) Stimulates Erythropoietin Production without Hypertensive Effects

Ingo Flamme[1]*, **Felix Oehme**[2], **Peter Ellinghaus**[3], **Mario Jeske**[4], **Jörg Keldenich**[5], **Uwe Thuss**[5]

1 Cardiology/Hematology, Acute Care Research, Global Drug Discovery, Bayer Pharma AG, Wuppertal, Germany, 2 Biotech Development, Global Biologics, Bayer Pharma AG, Wuppertal, Germany, 3 Clinical Science, Global Biomarkers, Bayer Pharma AG, Wuppertal, Germany, 4 Global Chemical Product Development, Bayer Pharma AG, Wuppertal, Germany, 5 Drug Metabolism and Pharmacokinetics, Global Early Development, Bayer Pharma AG, Wuppertal, Germany

Abstract

Oxygen sensing by hypoxia-inducible factor prolyl hydroxylases (HIF-PHs) is the dominant regulatory mechanism of erythropoietin (EPO) expression. In chronic kidney disease (CKD), impaired EPO expression causes anemia, which can be treated by supplementation with recombinant human EPO (rhEPO). However, treatment can result in rhEPO levels greatly exceeding the normal physiological range for endogenous EPO, and there is evidence that this contributes to hypertension in patients with CKD. Mimicking hypoxia by inhibiting HIF-PHs, thereby stabilizing HIF, is a novel treatment concept for restoring endogenous EPO production. HIF stabilization by oral administration of the HIF-PH inhibitor BAY 85-3934 (molidustat) resulted in dose-dependent production of EPO in healthy Wistar rats and cynomolgus monkeys. In repeat oral dosing of BAY 85-3934, hemoglobin levels were increased compared with animals that received vehicle, while endogenous EPO remained within the normal physiological range. BAY 85-3934 therapy was also effective in the treatment of renal anemia in rats with impaired kidney function and, unlike treatment with rhEPO, resulted in normalization of hypertensive blood pressure in a rat model of CKD. Notably, unlike treatment with the antihypertensive enalapril, the blood pressure normalization was achieved without a compensatory activation of the renin–angiotensin system. Thus, BAY 85-3934 may provide an approach to the treatment of anemia in patients with CKD, without the increased risk of adverse cardiovascular effects seen for patients treated with rhEPO. Clinical studies are ongoing to investigate the effects of BAY 85-3934 therapy in patients with renal anemia.

Editor: Benedetta Bussolati, Center for Molecular Biotechnology, Italy

Funding: This study was funded by Bayer Pharma AG. All the authors are employees of Bayer Pharma AG. The funder provided support in the form of salaries for all authors, but did not have any additional role in the study design, data collection and analysis, decision to publish, or preparation of the manuscript. The specific roles of the authors are articulated in the 'author contributions' section.

Competing Interests: Dr. Flamme has read the journal's policy and the authors of this manuscript have the following competing interests: All the authors are employees of Bayer Pharma AG, the funding organization for this study.

* Email: ingo.flamme@bayer.com

Introduction

The glycoprotein erythropoietin (EPO) is an indispensable growth factor for the production of red blood cells in the bone marrow. EPO is mainly secreted by the kidney but also, to a small degree in adults, by the liver. Anemia is a frequent complication of chronic kidney disease (CKD) because failing kidneys produce insufficient EPO to maintain normal red blood cell levels and hepatic EPO production cannot compensate [1]. Since its introduction into clinical use in 1989, recombinant human EPO (rhEPO) has become the standard therapy for anemia associated with renal failure [2]. However, treatment with rhEPO may be associated with an increased risk of cardiovascular events [3]. The chronic, intermittent treatment regimen can result in rhEPO levels that greatly exceed the normal physiological range for endogenous EPO. This could contribute to the increased blood pressure observed in patients with CKD treated with rhEPO because EPO has been found to directly induce endothelial dysfunction in resistance arteries in patients with CKD [4–6]. Therefore, it is highly desirable to develop alternative therapies to rhEPO that have equivalent efficacy in the treatment of anemia while avoiding excessive plasma EPO levels.

The expression of EPO in response to hypoxia is the accepted paradigm of oxygen-regulated gene expression. Systematic analysis of EPO gene regulatory elements led to the discovery of the hypoxia-inducible factors (HIFs), HIF-1 and HIF-2, which are constituents of the common oxygen-sensing pathway that enables higher organisms to cope with changes in oxygen supply [7,8]. HIFs are the transcriptional activators of a plethora of hypoxia-inducible genes. The pattern of target gene response facilitates the homeostasis of oxygen supply by adjusting the levels of oxygen-carrying erythrocytes and regulating angiogenesis, thereby enabling metabolic adaptation to changing oxygen levels.

HIFs are heterodimers consisting of an α- and a β-subunit, which bind to distinct hypoxia-responsive elements in the regulatory sequences of hypoxia-inducible genes. Whereas HIF-β

is constitutively expressed, the availability of HIF-α is under the control of a family of three enzymes, the HIF prolyl hydroxylases (also known as prolyl hydroxylase domain-containing protein 1–3, PHD1–3 or C. elegans EGL9 homolog 1–3, EGLN1–3) [9,10]. HIF-PHs are oxygen-dependent and 2-oxoglutarate-consuming dioxygenases that, in the presence of oxygen, hydroxylate the HIF-α subunits at two distinct proline residues, thereby tagging them for polyubiquitination and proteasomal degradation [11,12]. An E3 ubiquitin ligase protein complex consisting of the von Hippel–Lindau protein and elongin B and C (VBC complex) recognizes the hydroxylated HIF-α subunits and is required for the degradation of HIFs under normoxia [13]. Human genetic data suggest that renal EPO gene expression is under the non-redundant control of the PHD2–HIF-2α axis. A mutation in von Hippel–Lindau protein (Arg200Trp) that affects the interaction with hydroxylated HIFs, and loss- and gain-of-function mutations of the PHD2 and HIF-2α genes, respectively, have been identified as the underlying causes for rare forms of benign polycythemia at inappropriately high EPO levels. In contrast to patients with other forms of polycythemia, there is no tendency to develop arterial hypertension [14,15]. The phenotype has been reproduced in transgenic mice and is in support of earlier observations that the increase in EPO transcription *in vivo* is by far the most sensitive response to hypoxia in the kidney [16–20].

Conversely, small increases in the availability of oxygen to EPO-producing cells (located in the peritubular interstitium) may be followed by critically reduced EPO transcription. This is the case in renal failure, when a reduced glomerular filtration rate and tubular reabsorption result in decreased oxygen utilization [21]. In concert with pro-inflammatory cytokines and insufficient clearance of uremic toxins, the reduced EPO production provides the basis for renal anemia [1,22]. However, although patients with CKD and anemia present with low serum EPO levels, their kidneys are still able to produce EPO in response to a hypoxic stimulus [23]. This has also been shown in rats with gentamicin-induced renal anemia [24]. Compared with controls, higher oxygen tension in failing kidneys has been directly demonstrated in the rat remnant kidney (subtotal nephrectomy) model, which is commonly used as a model for CKD that comprises proteinuria, uremia, reduced EPO production with anemia, and increased blood pressure [25].

Data from epidemiological studies also support the hypothesis that hypoxia can overcome the EPO arrest in failing kidneys. Patients with end-stage renal disease (ESRD) living at altitude (above 6,000 feet) and undergoing hemodialysis required less rhEPO, but had higher hematocrit levels, than patients with ESRD living at sea level and undergoing hemodialysis [26]. Similarly, patients with ESRD showing poor treatment response at baseline who moved to a dialysis center at altitude showed increases in hematocrit and decreases in rhEPO requirements relative to a control group [27].

HIF-PH inhibitors provide a novel therapeutic approach to the treatment of anemia that is based on mimicking the hypoxia-driven expression of endogenous EPO in the kidney [28,29]. Here, we present for the first time a comprehensive pharmacological characterization of a novel HIF-PH inhibitor (BAY 85-3934, molidustat), ranging from its activity *in vitro* to its effects in healthy rats and monkeys and in models of impaired kidney function. Our preclinical data confirm that, by pharmacological inhibition of HIF-PH, the failing kidney can be stimulated to produce sufficient EPO to correct for renal anemia, and that in contrast to treatment with rhEPO, adverse hypertensive effects are not only avoided, but CKD-associated hypertension may be ameliorated by this new therapeutic approach.

Materials and Methods

Compounds and reagents

BAY 85-3934, 2-[6-(morpholin-4-yl)pyrimidin-4-yl]-4-(1H-1,2,3-triazol-1-yl)-1,2-dihydro-3H-pyrazol-3-one, was synthesized as described previously [30]. For *in vitro* experiments, BAY 85-3934 was prepared as a stock solution of 10 mM in DMSO. For oral administration in rats, BAY 85-3934 was prepared as a solution in ethanol:Solutol HS 15:water (10:20:70), and for oral administration in cynomolgus monkeys as a solution in 0.5% tylose. The compound was administered in a volume of 2–5 ml/kg body weight and control animals received equal volumes of the vehicle. Before administration, the formulation was freshly prepared in water from a stock solution in ethanol/Solutol HS 15 stored at −20°C. Human recombinant EPO (Ortho Biotech) was administered via s.c. injection twice weekly at a dose of 100 IU/kg body weight, with saline (0.9% NaCl) as vehicle control.

In the chronic disease models of subtotal nephrectomy and inflammation, the sodium salt of BAY 85-3934 was used. For administration in drinking water, BAY 85-3934 sodium and enalapril were prepared as 100 mM sodium bicarbonate saline solutions (adjusted to pH 7) at final concentrations of 80 ppm and 30 ppm, respectively. Sham and vehicle control animals received saline only. Unless otherwise stated, chemicals and reagents were purchased from Sigma-Aldrich.

Protein expression and purification

Recombinant human HIF-PHs were purified from Sf9 insect cell lysates. After infection with the recombinant virus stocks, generated via cloning of the respective cDNAs into pBacPAC transfer vectors (Clontech Laboratories), Sf9 cells were incubated for 48 h at 27°C with continuous shaking. Expression of the recombinant protein was confirmed by SDS-PAGE and western blot analysis of the expressed proteins. The lysate was centrifuged at 75,000 g at 4°C for 30 min and the supernatant containing the soluble HIF-PHs was incubated for 1 h at 2–8°C with CM Sepharose. After several wash steps, bound proteins were eluted from Sepharose using a linear NaCl gradient. Fractions containing HIF-PH activity were pooled, dialyzed against 100 mM Tris, 1.5 mM $MgCl_2$, 2 mM DTT, 0.01% Tween-20, supplemented with 1% BSA and complete protease inhibitor cocktail without EDTA (Roche Diagnostics), and stored at −80°C. The VBC complex was expressed in *Escherichia coli* BL21(DE3) pLysS cells using the plasmid pST39-HisTrxNVHL-elongin B-elongin C. Protein expression and purification were performed as described previously [31]. DELFIA labeling reagent (PerkinElmer) was used to label purified VBC complex with europium according to the manufacturer's instructions.

Prolyl hydroxylase assay

The prolyl hydroxylase assay was performed as described previously [32] with minor modifications. Biotinylated HIF-1α 556–574 (biotinyl-DLDLEMLAPYIPMDDDFQL) was bound to white 96-well NeutrAvidin high binding capacity plates (Pierce Biotechnology), which were pre-blocked with Blocker Casein (Pierce Biotechnology) and subsequently blocked with 1 mM biotin. The immobilized peptide substrate was incubated with the appropriate amount of HIF-PH in buffer containing 20 mM Tris (pH 7.5), 5 mM KCl, 1.5 mM $MgCl_2$, 20 μM 2-oxoglutarate, 10 μM $FeSO_4$, 2 mM ascorbate, 4% protease inhibitors without EDTA (Roche Diagnostics) in a final volume of 100 μl, with or without test compound added at appropriate concentrations. The reaction time was 60 min. To stop the reaction, plates were washed three times with wash buffer.

Hydroxylated biotinyl-HIF-1α 556–574 was incubated with Eu-VBC in 100 µl binding buffer (50 mM Tris [pH 7.5], 120 mM NaCl) for 60 min at room temperature. After washing six times with DELFIA wash buffer (PerkinElmer) and adding 100 µl enhancer solution (PerkinElmer), the amount of bound VBC was determined by measuring time-resolved fluorescence with a Tecan infinite M200 plate reader. Measurements were taken in triplicate or more, and results were expressed as means ± SEM. IC$_{50}$ values were determined after curve fitting using GraphPad Prism software (GraphPad Software, La Jolla, CA, USA) applying the four-parameter logistic equation to the data sets. When adjustment of the concentration of free Fe^{2+} was necessary, the reaction buffer was supplemented with appropriate amounts of ammonium iron(II) sulfate ((NH$_4$)$_2$Fe(SO$_4$)$_2$.6H$_2$O, Mohr's salt).

Cell lines, cell culture media, and luciferase reporter assay

A549 and HeLa carcinoma cell lines (American Type Culture Collection) were cultured in DMEM/F-12 (Gibco), and Hep3B cells in RPMI medium, both supplemented with antibiotics, L-glutamine and 10% fetal calf serum. A549 cells stably transfected with the HIF-RE2-luc HIF reporter construct (constructed in pGL3, Promega GmbH) were seeded on 384-well plates (Greiner) at a density of 2500 cells/well in a volume of 25 µl complete cell culture medium, and re-incubated for 16–24 h before the test [33]. Test compounds were added at appropriate dilutions in a volume of 10 µl, and cells were re-incubated for 6 h before measurement. Luciferase activity was determined in a luminometer after addition of cell lysis/luciferase buffer. Cell line identities were verified by STR DNA typing (DSMZ GmbH).

Western blot analysis

For western blot analysis, cell lysates were separated on 4–12% SDS polyacrylamide gradient gels (Invitrogen). Proteins were blotted onto polyvinylidene difluoride (PVDF) membranes (Amersham Biosciences). HIF-1α protein was detected using a HIF-1α specific monoclonal antibody (BD Transduction Laboratories) at a dilution of 1:250. HIF-2α protein was detected using a HIF-2α specific polyclonal antibody (Novus Biologicals) at a dilution of 1:1000. Anti-β-actin antibody served as a loading control. Binding of the antibodies was visualized by binding of a horseradish peroxidase-conjugated anti-mouse IgG antibody (Amersham Pharmacia Biotech), and subsequently enhanced using chemiluminescence (Chemiluminescent Peroxidase Substrate), according to the manufacturers instructions. Novex Sharp Pre-stained Protein Standard (Invitrogen) was used as molecular weight marker.

Studies in animals

All procedures conformed to national legislation (dt. Tierschutzgesetz v. 18.05.2006) and EU directives (86/609) for the use of animals for scientific purposes and were approved by the institutional animal care office of Bayer AG and by the competent regional authority (LANUV Recklinghausen). All surgical procedures were performed under deep anesthesia (2% isoflurane) with immediate post-operative analgesia (ketamine/carprofen), and all efforts were made to minimize suffering. Rats were sacrificed by exposure to 10% isoflurane and consecutive cervical dislocation. Standard laboratory diet and tap water were available ad libitum. Rats were provided with wood sticks for chewing and gnawing, and monkeys were provided with appropriate toys such as balls and climbing bars. Animals were housed in temperature- and humidity-controlled cages with a 12 h light/dark cycle. In each experiment, the number of animals used was minimized. Animals were either randomly assigned to experimental groups or, if appropriate, were assigned based on hematocrit levels.

Studies in rats

Male Wistar rats (240–340 g in body weight) were housed with five animals per cage for at least 1 week before experimentation. Blood samples from rats were collected under anesthesia (2% isoflurane in air) by puncturing the retro-orbital vein plexus with a glass capillary. In a repeat-dose, 26-day experiment, animals were administered vehicle or BAY 85-3934 at doses of 0.5 mg/kg, 1.25 mg/kg, 2.5 mg/kg, and 5 mg/kg. PCV was determined at baseline and at weekly intervals after centrifugation in a hematocrit capillary tube (Brand) for 10 min at full speed in a Haemofuge centrifuge (Heraeus). The number of reticulocytes in 5 µl blood was counted after staining with thiazol orange (Becton Dickinson) according to the manufacturer's instructions by FACS analysis on a BD FACSCalibur system (Becton Dickinson). The efficacy of BAY 85-3934 (2.5 mg/kg, once-daily, oral) was also compared with that of rhEPO (25 IU/kg, 50 IU/kg, and 100 IU/kg, twice-weekly, s.c. injection). The time-course of induction of EPO mRNA expression and plasma EPO was determined at baseline and 0.5 h, 1 h, 2 h, 4 h, 6 h, and 8 h after oral administration of a single dose of BAY 85-3934 (5 mg/kg).

Studies in cynomolgus monkeys

Male and female cynomolgus monkeys (2.8–5.6 kg in body weight) were used, which were housed two per cage. Blood samples from conscious cynomolgus monkeys were taken by puncturing a superficial vein. In a 5-day, repeat-dose study of plasma EPO response, BAY 85-3934 was administered at doses of 0.5 mg/kg and 1.5 mg/kg at 0 h, 24 h, 48 h, 72 h, and 96 h. Blood samples were taken at 7 h, 31 h, 55 h, 79 h, 103 h, and 168 h. Erythropoietic parameters were also evaluated after a 2-week treatment period with s.c. administration of rhEPO (100 IU/kg twice weekly at days 1, 4, 8, and 11) and BAY 85-3934 (1.5 mg/kg) once daily.

Gentamicin-induced kidney failure model

Male Wistar rats were treated once daily with gentamicin (Gibco/Invitrogen) at a dose of 100 mg/kg body weight via i.p. injection on 14 consecutive days [34,35]. Control animals received injections of an equal volume of 0.9% saline. After gentamicin treatment, PCV was determined and animals were distributed to the vehicle or treatment groups with respect to equal mean PCV. On day 15, BAY 85-3934 was given orally once daily at doses of 1 mg/kg, 2.5 mg/kg, 5.0 mg/kg, and 10.0 mg/kg, five times weekly.

PG-PS-induced inflammatory anemia model

Female Lewis rats (Harlan Laboratories), with a body weight of 155–181 g were used. Body weight, ankle diameter, hematocrit, and blood cell count were determined at baseline and thereafter at regular intervals. PG-PS from *Streptococcus pyogenes* (Becton Dickinson) was dissolved in sterile saline and administered via i.p. injection at 15 mg/kg. Animals that did not show an inflammatory response were not studied further. Two weeks after injection, animals were distributed into treatment groups in equal proportions based on their hematocrit levels. On day 15, BAY 85-3934 was given orally once daily at doses of 2.5 mg/kg and 5.0 mg/kg. At the end of the study, animals were sacrificed and kidney and liver samples were processed for qRT-PCR analysis.

Subtotal nephrectomy model

Subtotal nephrectomy was conducted in adult male Wistar rats. Body weight, blood pressure, hematocrit, and blood cell counts were determined at baseline and thereafter at weekly intervals. At baseline, rats were randomly distributed into two groups: those that underwent subtotal nephrectomy and those that underwent a sham procedure without reduction of renal mass. Surgery was performed in deeply anesthetized (2% isoflurane in air) animals. Kidneys were accessed via a dorsolateral incision of the body wall of about 2 cm in length. The right kidney was removed after ligature of the renal peduncle, and subsequently the upper and lower pole of the left kidney were removed, followed by careful hemostasis. Approximately one third of the initial kidney mass remained (removed tissue was weighed to check this was achieved). In the sham-treated animals, both kidneys were exposed before closure of the wound. Three weeks after surgery, animals were allocated to each group in equal proportions with respect to systolic blood pressure and hematocrit values. For 5 weeks, animals were treated twice weekly with rhEPO (100 IU/kg), or once daily with BAY 85–3936 sodium (2.5 mg/kg or 5.0 mg/kg) or vehicle. In experiments using enalapril or a combination of BAY 85-3934 sodium and enalapril, study drugs were administered with drinking water. BAY 85-3934 sodium and enalapril were administered in drinking water at concentrations of 80 ppm and 30 ppm, respectively. This was equivalent to approximately 2 mg/kg/day for enalapril and 5 mg/kg/day for BAY 85-3934. Systolic blood pressure and heart rate were determined using the tail-cuff method (a semi-automatic, non-invasive blood pressure monitor; TSE Systems), with three repeated measurements per animal.

Blood analytics

EPO was measured in plasma samples taken from rodents using a commercial ELISA kit (R&D Systems), according to the manufacturer's instructions. Relative plasma EPO levels were given in picograms per milliliter. In cynomolgus monkeys, EPO was measured using a combination anti-human EPO ELISAs (R&D Systems and Roche Diagnostics), with human EPO as a standard [36]. Values were given as units per liter. For determination of plasma prorenin from rats, a commercial ELISA (Oxford Biomedical Research) was used according to the manufacturer's instructions. Hemoglobin in rodent blood samples was determined on a Cell-Dyn 3700 apparatus (Abbott Diagnostics). BAY 85-3934 plasma concentrations were determined after protein precipitation with acetonitrile/ammonium acetate using an internal standard, followed by separation using HPLC/mass spectrometry.

RNA extraction and qRT-PCR

Total RNA was extracted from shock-frozen cell or tissue samples using the TRIzol method. Integrity of obtained RNA was checked on a Bioanalyzer (Agilent Technologies). For reverse transcription, 1 µg of total RNA was digested with RNase-free DNase I (Gibco) for 15 min at room temperature, and then reverse-transcribed using Promiscript (Promega GmbH) in a total reaction volume of 40 µl according to the standard protocol of the supplier. After inactivation of the enzyme by heating to 65 °C for 15 min, the obtained cDNA was diluted to a final volume of 150 µl with double-distilled water, and 4 µl used per PCR reaction. qRT-PCR, including normalization of raw data to cytosolic β-actin, was carried out as described previously [37]. The resulting expression is given in arbitrary units. The sequences of the oligonucleotide primers and probes used are given in Table 1.

Statistical analysis

Data are presented as the mean ± SEM. In dose–response experiments, statistical significance was evaluated by sequential application of a two-tailed t-test comparing compound-treated groups with corresponding controls. For inter-group comparisons, one-way ANOVA followed by Dunnett's or Bonferroni's multiple comparison was applied. A P value of <0.05 was considered statistically significant.

Results

Characterization of BAY 85-3934 in vitro

BAY 85-3934 resulted from the optimization of a compound identified by high-throughput screening. To measure the activity of HIF-PH inhibitors quantitatively, a microplate assay was developed that employed the interaction of the VBC complex with the peptide HIF-1α 556–574 after being hydroxylated at proline 564 by recombinant HIF-PH. Activity of the recombinant enzyme was dependent on the concentrations of several cofactors, 2-oxoglutarate, Fe^{2+}, and ascorbate, in the reaction mixture. These concentrations were optimized to give a robust and highly reproducible assay [32].

Under standard assay conditions, in the presence of 20 µM 2-oxoglutarate, 10 µM Fe^{2+}, and 2 mM ascorbate, the mean IC_{50} values of BAY 85-3934 for PHD1, PHD2, and PHD3 were 480 nM, 280 nM, and 450 nM, respectively. The IC_{50} values were found to be dependent on the concentration of 2-oxoglutarate in the reaction buffer. By lowering the 2-oxoglutarate concentration from 20 µM to 0.3 µM, the potency of the test compound increased up to 10-fold (Fig. 1A). Variation of the concentrations of Fe^{2+} and ascorbate in the reaction buffer by factors of 30 and 200, respectively, did not alter the potency of the inhibitor by more than 2-fold (Fig. 1B, C). The IC_{50} values were always well below the concentration of Fe^{2+}.

It was further explored whether inhibition of HIF-PHs would result in the stabilization of HIFs. Exposure of three different human cell lines (HeLa, A549, and Hep3B) to concentrations of BAY 85-3934 up to 10 µM for 2 h led to dose-dependent increases in both HIF-1α and HIF-2α. Within the individual cell lines, there was no difference between the HIF isoforms with regard to the threshold concentration of BAY 85-3934 that was necessary for the induction of detectable amounts of HIF. However, HeLa cells, which had an induction threshold of 0.25 µM of BAY 85-3934, appeared to be more sensitive than Hep3B and A549 cells, which had induction thresholds of 0.5 µM and 2.5 µM, respectively (Fig. 1D). Exposure of HeLa cells to 5 µM BAY 85-3934 for 20 min was sufficient to induce detectable concentrations of HIF-1α (Fig. 1E). After exposure of A549 cells to 20 µM BAY 85-3934 for 120 min, with subsequent withdrawal of the culture medium and replacement with medium containing 100 µM cycloheximide (an inhibitor of protein synthesis), induction of HIF-1α was no longer detectable after 30 min (Fig. 1F). Therefore, it can be ruled out that disappearance of HIF-1α was the result of de novo synthesis of HIF-PH.

In a cellular reporter assay, BAY 85-3934 induced the expression of the firefly luciferase reporter gene under the control of a hypoxia responsive element promoter at a mean (± SD) EC_{50} of 8.4± 0.7 µM ($n = 4$). As in the enzymatic assay, and in contrast to experiments with iron-chelating agents (data not shown), luciferase activity was not altered by a high concentration of Fe^{2+} (50 µM) in the culture medium (Fig. 1G). The high IC_{50} value observed corresponds well to the low sensitivity of A549 cells shown by western blot analysis.

Table 1. Oligonucleotide primers and probes used for quantitative RT-PCR analysis of samples from rat tissues, and human cell lines (in italics).

Symbol	Gene name	Forward primer	Probe	Reverse primer
ADM	Adrenomedullin	CGCAGTTCCGAAAGAAGTGG	TAAGTGGGCGCTAAGTCGTGGGAAGAG	CCCGTAGGGTAGCTGCTGGA
		CGCCAGAGCATGAACAACTTC	*TGGCACACCAGATCTACCAGTTCAC*	*GCGACGTTGTCCTTGTCCTT*
ANGPTL-4	Angiopoietin-like 4	CTGGGTGCCACCAATGTTTC	CCCAATGGCCTTTCCCTGCCCT	CGTGGTCTTGGTCCCAGGTA
		GGCCTCTCCGTACCCTTCTC	*TCACGACCTCCGCAGGGACAA*	*AGAGGCTCTTGGCGCAGTT*
Beta-actin	Beta-actin	ACCTTCAACACCCCAGCCA	ACGTAGCCATCCAGGCTGTGTTGTCC	CAGTGGTACGACCAGAGGCA
		TCCACCTTCCAGCAGATGTG	*ATCAGCAAGCAGGAGTATGACGAGTCCG*	*CTAGAAGCATTTGCGGTGGAC*
CAIX	carbonic anhydrase IX	TCGTCTGGAGCTCACCTCATT	CCGCACTCTGCAACCCCTGGAAC	CGGGAGAGACTGGAGCTCAT
		ACCTGGTGACTCTCGGCTACA	*TGAACTTCCGAGCGACGCAGCCT*	*CCTCAATCACTCGCCCATTC*
eNOS	Endothelial nitric oxide synthase	CACACTGCTAGAGGTGCTGGAA	AATTTCCATCCGTGGCACTGCCTG	GGGTGAGGATCAGCGGG
EPO	Erythropoietin	CCGCTCCACTCCGAACAC	AGCGGATACTTTCTGCAAGCTCTTCCG	CCCGGAGGAAGTTGGAGTAGA
		CCCCTCCAGATGCGGC	*TCAGCTGCTCCACTCCGAACAATCAC*	*GAGTTTGCGGAAAGTGTCAGC*
GLUT-1	Glucose transporter-1	CAGCCTGTGTATGCCACCAT	TCGGGTATCGTCAACACGGCC	GACGAACAGCGACACCACAGT
		AGCCTGTGTATGCCACCATTG	*CCGGTATCGTCAACACGGCCT*	*GCTCGCTCCACCACAAACA*
HMOX-1	Heme oxygenase-1	TATCGTGCTCGCATGAACACT	TGGAGATGACCCCCGAGGTCAAGC	GGCGGTCTTAGCCTCTTCTGT
IGFBP-1	Insulin-like growth factor binding protein-1	CTGCCAAACTGCAACAAGAA	TCACAGCAAACAGTGCGAGACATCTC	AGAGCCCAGCTTCTCCATC
IGFBP-3	Insulin-like growth factor binding protein-3	TCCCAAACTGTGACAAGAAGG	AGAAACAGTGTCGCCCTTCCAAAGG	GTCCACGCACCAGCAGAA
		CCACCCCCTCCATTCAAAG	*TAATCATCATCAAGAAAGGGCATGCT*	*CTTTGTAGCGCTGGCTGTCTT*
LDH-A	Lactate dehydrogenase-A	ATTCGGCTCGGTTCCGTTA	CTGATGGGAGAAAGGCTGGGAGTTCA	CCACCCGTGACAGCTCAGT
PDK-1	Pyruvate dehydrogenase lipoamide kinase-1	CACCATGCAGACAAAGGCG	TCCCCCGATTCAAGTTCACGTCACA	AGTCAAATCCTCCTCCCCCA
PHD1	Prolyl hydroxylase domain-containing protein-1	TCTTTGACCGGTTGCTCATTT	TGGTCTGACCGACGGAATCCAC	GTGGCATAGGCTGGCTTCA
PHD2	Prolyl hydroxylase domain-containing protein-2	AAGCCCAGTTTGCTGACATTG	CCCAAGTTTGATAGATTGCTGTTTT	GAGGGTTACGCCGGTCAGA
PHD3	Prolyl hydroxylase domain-containing protein-3	CCCTCCTATGCCACCAGGTA	CATGACTGTCTGGTACTTCGATGCT	TCTTTTTGGCTTCTGCCCTTT
VEGF-A	Vascular endothelial growth factor-A	CGCAAGAAATCCCGGTTTAA	CTGGAGCGTTCACTGTGAGCCT	CAAATGCTTTCTCCGCTCTGA
		AGCGGAGAAAGCATTTGTTTG	*CAAGATCCGCAGACGTGTAAATGTTCCTG*	*CTTGCAACGCGAGTCTGTGT*

Finally, we investigated whether BAY 85-3934 induced the transcription of hypoxia-sensitive genes in HeLa, A549, and Hep3B cells. The mRNA expression levels of a panel of HIF target genes were analyzed by quantitative RT-PCR (qRT-PCR) in the three cell lines 4 h after exposure to concentrations of BAY 85-3934 up to 10 μM. mRNA levels were found to be induced by BAY 85-3934 in a dose-dependent manner. The basal level of expression and the factor of induction varied considerably between cell lines. The highest induction factors (up to 20-fold) were observed for carbonic anhydrase IX (CA-IX) in HeLa cells, CA-IX and angiopoietin-like 4 (ANGPTL-4) in A549 cells, and EPO and ANGPTL-4 in Hep3B cells (Fig. 1H). The other genes examined were induced between 2- and 5-fold. The mRNA expression level of ANGPTL-4 was not increased by BAY 85-3934 in HeLa cells. EPO mRNA was not detectable at baseline and not induced in HeLa or A549 cells. The threshold concentration for

induction of CA-IX expression was 500 nM in HeLa cells, and greater than 1 μM for all other genes that showed a response.

The selectivity of BAY 85-3934 was examined via a broad panel of radio-ligand binding assays ($n = 67$), and by examining the activity of BAY 85-3934 against related enzymes (matrix metalloproteinases and other peptidases, $n = 8$). At a concentration of 10 μM, no significant ($> 50\%$) activity in any of these assays was detected (data not shown). BAY 85-3934 was found to have pharmacokinetic properties suitable for oral dosing studies in rats and monkeys.

Induction of EPO and erythropoiesis in male Wistar rats

Experiments were conducted in male Wistar rats to assess the threshold doses for EPO induction and the erythropoietic activity of BAY 85-3934. Following a single oral administration of BAY 85-3934, EPO was statistically significantly induced at doses of

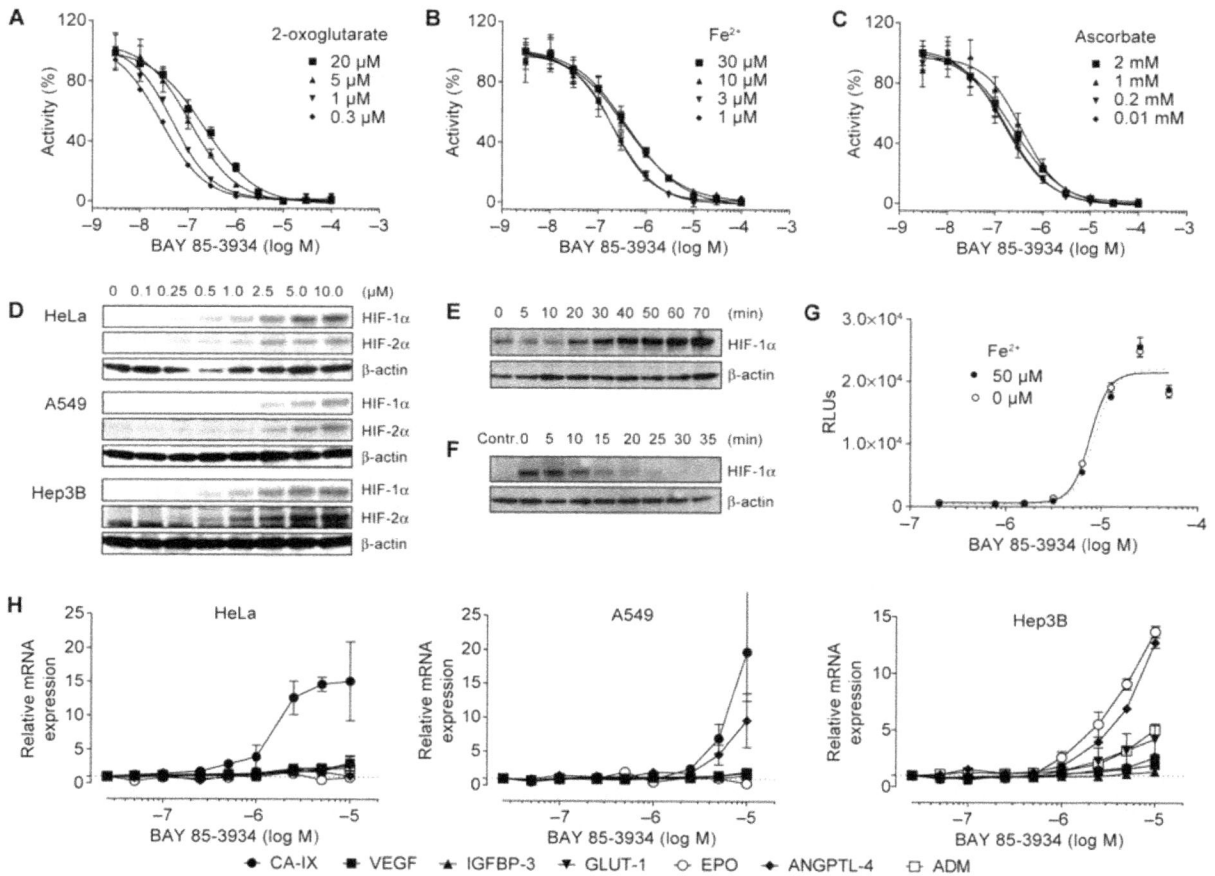

Figure 1. Characterization of the *in vitro* activity of BAY 85-3934. (A)–(C) Concentration–response curves of hypoxia-inducible factor prolyl hydroxylase (PHD2) activity for BAY 85--934 after the addition of increasing concentrations of 2-oxoglutarate, Fe^{2+}, and ascorbate. Data, presented as means $\pm$ SEM of 4 replicates, were normalized to basal activity without BAY 85-3934 (100%) and residual activity (0%). (D) Detection of HIF-1α and HIF-2α in HeLa, A549, and Hep3B cells by western blot analysis. (E) Time-course of induction of HIF-1α in HeLa cells after addition of serum-free medium containing BAY 85-3934 (5 μM). β-actin levels were measured as a loading control. (F) Time-course of disappearance of HIF-1α in A549 cells after induction with BAY 85-3934 (20 μM). Culture medium was withdrawn and replaced with medium containing cycloheximide (100 μM). β-actin levels were measured as a loading control (D–F show representative data of 3 independent experiments). (G) Concentration–response curve for luciferase activity of A549 HIF-RE2 reporter cells (relative luciferase units [RLUs]) after addition of BAY 85-3934 in the presence or absence of additional Fe^{2+}. Data are presented as means $\pm$ SEM of 4 replicates. (H) Relative mRNA expression levels (means $\pm$ SD of 2 replicates) of a panel of HIF target genes (shown as fold-increase from baseline levels) after exposure to BAY 85-3934 in HeLa, A549, and Hep3B cells. For definition of gene symbols, see Table 1.

1.25 mg/kg and above (Fig. 2A). EPO induction was maximal at doses of 500 mg/kg and above, and these plasma concentrations were maintained for over 48 h following administration (data not shown). Induction of EPO after single-dose administration was followed by a dose-dependent increase in the proportion of reticulocytes at doses of 1.25 mg/kg and above (Fig. 2B).

In a 26-day, repeat-dose experiment, treatment with BAY 85-3934 resulted in a dose-dependent increase in mean packed cell volume (PCV; i.e. hematocrit) (Fig. 2C). A significant elevation of mean PCV from that in the vehicle control was observed from a dose of 1.25 mg/kg, which resulted in a gain of approximately 3% in mean PCV by day 26. At the highest dose (5 mg/kg), a mean PCV gain of 17% from baseline was observed. BAY 85-3934 was well tolerated, and body weight increased normally in animals in all dose groups.

The efficacy of oral treatment with BAY 85-3934 was compared with that of standard rhEPO treatment in male Wistar rats. All treatments resulted in a significant increase in hematocrit compared with the control group ($p<0.001$) (Fig. 2D). Over time,

the mean gains in hematocrit and hemoglobin were very similar for the BAY 85-3934 treated group and for rats that received the highest dose of EPO. Therefore, in this model, the once-daily dose of BAY 85-3934 (2.5 mg/kg) can be considered equivalent to a twice-weekly dose of rhEPO (100 IU/kg).

The time-course of BAY 85-3934 plasma levels, induction of EPO mRNA expression, and plasma EPO was examined. In male Wistar rats, BAY 85-3934 (5 mg/kg) was rapidly absorbed, with a plasma maximum concentration (C_{max}) of 30 min (Fig. 2E). The half-life was 3.4 h, and oral bioavailability was approximately 38%. The peak level of EPO mRNA expression was reached 2 h after administration (Fig. 2E). EPO plasma concentration reached a maximum at 6 h, at which point almost 90% of BAY 85-3934 had been eliminated from the plasma, and expression of EPO mRNA was approaching baseline levels (Fig. 2E).

The time-course of gene expression was further examined in the kidney for EPO and a panel of other HIF target genes following a single-dose administration of BAY 85-3934 (5 mg/kg). EPO mRNA expression was induced to about 50-fold over baseline,

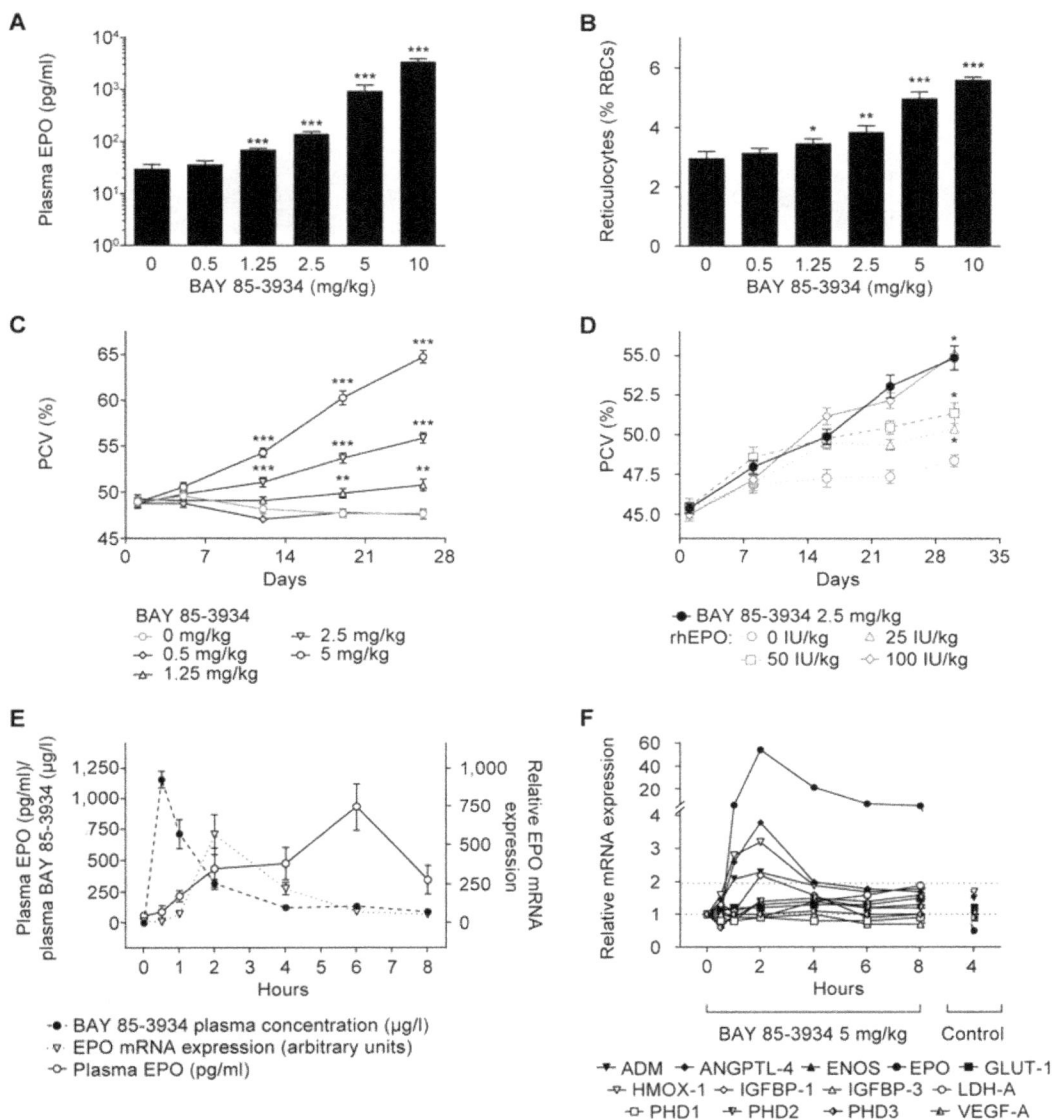

Figure 2. Characterization of the *in vivo* activity of BAY 85-3934 (in male Wistar rats). Data are presented as means ± SEM. (A) Increase in plasma erythropoietin (EPO) at 4 h and (B) reticulocytes (as a proportion of red blood cells [RBCs]) at 72 h following single oral dosing of BAY 85-3934. Data were pooled from two sequential experiments (n = 2×5 animals per group). *$p<0.05$, **$p<0.01$, and ***$p<0.001$; unpaired t-test, sequentially pairwise-applied to dose groups and corresponding vehicle group. (C) Change in packed cell volume (PCV) during once-daily dosing with BAY 85-3934 (n = 12 animals per group). **$p<0.01$ and ***$p<0.001$; two-way ANOVA with Dunnett's multiple comparison test versus vehicle group. (D) Induction of erythropoiesis after subcutaneous administration of recombinant human EPO (rhEPO) twice weekly or BAY 85-3934 (2.5 mg/kg) once daily (n = 10 animals per group). *$p<0.001$ compared with control (t-test) at day 30. (E) BAY 85-3934 plasma levels, kidney EPO relative mRNA expression, and plasma EPO levels after oral administration of BAY 85-3934 (5 mg/kg) (n = 5 animals per group). (F) Relative mRNA expression levels of HIF target genes in rat kidney after administration of BAY 85-3934 (5 mg/kg). Baseline expression was set at 1 (n = 5 animals per group; error bars not show for clarity of presentation). For definition of gene symbols, see Table 1.

with a peak 2 h after administration (Fig. 2F). Of the other genes investigated, only heme oxygenase-1 (HMOX-1), insulin-like growth factor binding protein-1, adrenomedullin, and ANGPTL-4 showed significant induction of mRNA expression of more than 2-fold over baseline, with induction factors of 3.2-, 2.2-, 2.3-, and 3.8-fold, respectively ($p<0.01$). Peak levels were seen 2 h after administration. Induction of mRNA expression was moderate (less than 2-fold) or absent for the other genes examined.

Repeat-dose studies in cynomolgus monkeys

A multiple-dose study in cynomolgus monkeys was conducted to evaluate whether repeat administration of BAY 85-3934 would result in EPO accumulation and/or adaptation of the EPO response. EPO was significantly induced 7 h after administration of BAY 85-3934 (1.5 mg/kg) in all animals, and showed a clear increase after the 0.5 mg/kg dose in females (Fig. 3A). In all groups, EPO concentrations had returned to baseline concentrations 24 h after administration of the study drug. Notably, there was no adaptation of the EPO response after repeated dosing in

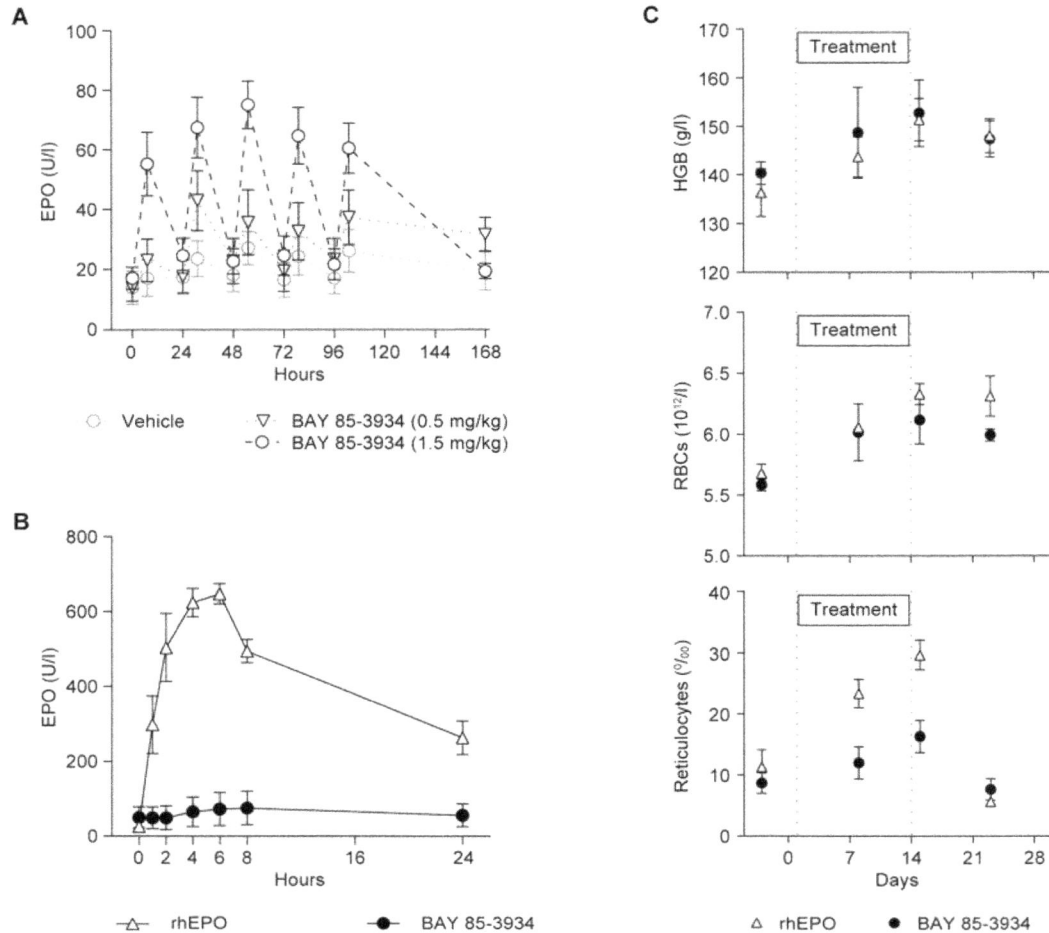

Figure 3. Effects of BAY 85-3934 or recombinant human erythropoietin (rhEPO) on erythropoietic parameters in cynomolgus monkeys. Data are presented as means ± SEM. (A) Plasma erythropoietin (EPO) concentrations after repeat oral administration of BAY 85-3934 (*n* = 6 animals per group). (B) Plasma EPO concentrations after a single s.c. administration of rhEPO (100 IU/kg) or a single oral dose of BAY 85-3934 (1.5 mg/kg) (*n* = 3 animals per group). (C) Erythropoietic parameters (hemoglobin [HGB], red blood cells [RBCs], and reticulocytes) after s.c. administration of rhEPO twice weekly (100 IU/kg) for 2 weeks or BAY 85-3934 (1.5 mg/kg) once daily for 2 weeks (*n* = 3 animals per group).

any of the treated animals. Platelet and white blood cell counts were unchanged. With respect to EPO induction, the 0.5 mg/kg dose was determined as the minimal effective dose in this study, although statistical significance versus control animals was not reached in this small and heterogeneous animal cohort.

In a further study, the efficacy of oral treatment with BAY 85-3934 was evaluated in comparison with rhEPO. Animals were administered a single dose of rhEPO (100 IU/kg) by s.c. injection or BAY 85-3934 (1.5 mg/kg, oral). After administration of rhEPO, plasma concentrations of rhEPO were more than 8-fold higher than the endogenous EPO levels induced by treatment with BAY 85-3934 (Fig. 3B). The area under the curve (AUC) of rhEPO was more than 6-fold higher than the AUC of endogenous EPO. However, in a 14-day repeat-dose study, both treatments resulted in mean gains of hemoglobin and red blood cells that were almost completely congruent over time (Fig. 3C). Mean reticulocyte counts were 2-fold higher after treatment with rhEPO than after treatment with BAY 85-3934, but returned to baseline values 8 days after treatment cessation.

Erythropoietic efficacy of BAY 85-3934 in rats with gentamicin-induced renal anemia

The effect of BAY 85-3934 on the induction of endogenous EPO production was evaluated in an animal model of impaired kidney function, the gentamicin-induced kidney failure model. A mean creatinine clearance of 30% of that of untreated animals and high expression levels of several markers of acute and chronic kidney injury were indicative of substantial renal impairment in these animals. Treatment with BAY 85-3934 significantly and dose-dependently induced plasma EPO levels (Fig. 4A). Accordingly, EPO mRNA expression increased dose-dependently in kidney samples taken from these animals (Fig. 4B). The mean absolute levels of induction were lower in the gentamicin-treated animals than in the controls.

Significant induction of EPO mRNA expression was detected in liver samples, in the control group at BAY 85-3934 doses of 2.5 mg/kg and above, and in gentamicin-treated animals at BAY 85-3934 doses of 5 mg/kg and above (Fig. 4C). As expected, the expression of EPO mRNA was considerably lower in liver samples than in kidney samples. Unlike the expression in the kidney, hepatic mRNA concentrations of EPO were slightly, but

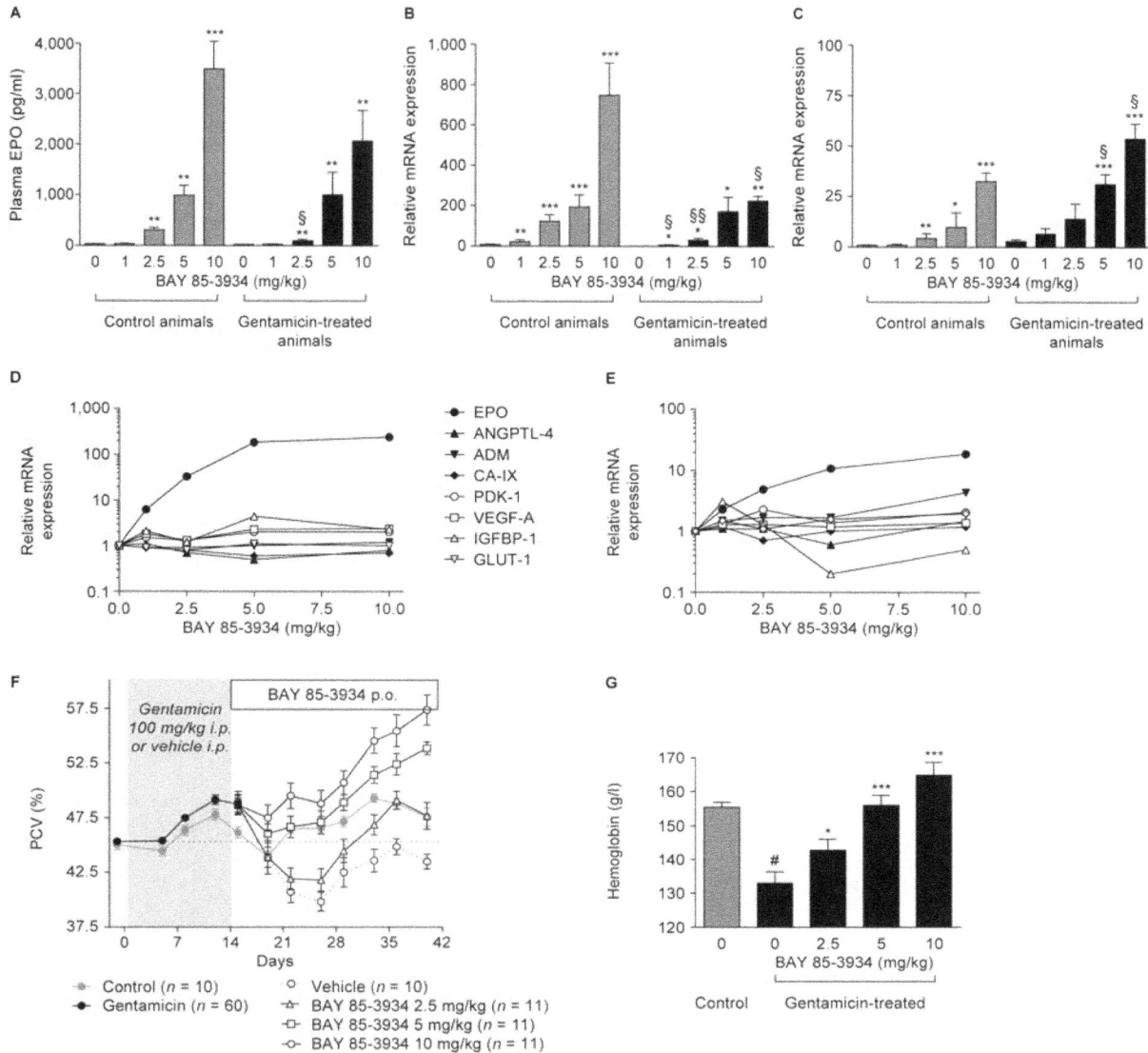

Figure 4. Effects of BAY 85-3934 administration in male Wistar rats treated with gentamicin to induce renal anemia. Data are presented as means ± SEM. (A) Plasma EPO levels, and (B) kidney and (C) liver relative expression of erythropoietin (EPO) mRNA 4 h after oral administration of BAY 85-3934. Before administration, rats had been treated with vehicle or gentamicin. (n = 5 animals per group). *$p < 0.05$, **$p < 0.01$, and ***$p < 0.001$ compared with vehicle group, $^{§}p < 0.05$ and $^{§§}p < 0.001$ compared with control group, t-test. (D) Kidney and (E) liver mRNA expression levels of hypoxia-inducible factor target genes relative to mean of vehicle treated animals after oral administration of BAY 85-3934 (n = 4 to 5 animals per group, error bars not shown for clarity of presentation). For definition of gene symbols, see Table 1. (F) Time-course of changes in packed cell volume (PCV) following treatment with BAY 85-3934 or vehicle (once daily, five times per week, number of animals as indicated). (G) Hemoglobin levels 7 days after start of treatment with BAY 85-3934 or vehicle at day 22 of experiment shown in (F). *$p < 0.05$, **$p < 0.01$, and ***$p < 0.001$ compared with vehicle group; $^{#}p < 0.05$ compared with sham group; t-test.

significantly, higher in gentamicin-treated animals than in hepatic samples from healthy (control) animals. In rats with renal impairment, it cannot be ruled out that the liver contributes significantly to plasma EPO concentrations after treatment with BAY 85-3934. However, in the absence of BAY 85-3934 treatment, the liver does not compensate for reduced renal EPO production.

In this study, the expression of other HIF target genes may also have been affected, although the magnitude of response was considerably lower than that seen for EPO mRNA expression in kidney and liver samples (Fig. 4D, 4E). Furthermore, unlike EPO

mRNA expression, no dose-response was observed after administration of BAY 85-3934.

Treatment with BAY 85-3934 prevented the development of gentamicin-induced renal anemia. At the end of the study, rats treated with gentamicin and vehicle showed a lower mean PCV than control animals (Fig. 4F). However, treatment with BAY 85-3934 (5 mg/kg and 10 mg/kg) 5 days per week prevented the decline in mean PCV, with final values significantly higher than in control animals ($p < 0.001$). Rats administered BAY 85-3934 (2.5 mg/kg) showed mean PCV levels similar to those in control animals, with mean PCV returning to baseline values within 2 weeks after onset of treatment with study drug. A significant dose-dependent increase in hemoglobin values was seen in animals treated with BAY 85-3934, as measured 7 days after the start of treatment (Fig. 4G). All doses led to an increase in reticulocyte counts, which were significantly higher than the increase associated with spontaneous recovery (data not shown).

Erythropoietic efficacy of BAY 85-3934 in rodents with inflammatory anemia induced by peptidoglycan-polysaccharide (PG-PS)

Renal anemia, particularly in patients with ESRD on dialysis, is often associated with systemic inflammation and EPO resistance. The potential for BAY 85-3934 to reverse anemia was evaluated in a rodent model of protracted inflammatory anemia associated with chronic polyarthritis, induced by challenge with PG-PS [38]. The severity of the inflammatory response after PG-PS challenge was underscored by the finding that there was elevated expression of a panel of cytokines and inflammatory marker genes, several of which are known to disturb iron utilization (interleukin-1, interleukin-6, tumor necrosis factor-α, and hepcidin) and to impair proliferation and differentiation of erythroid precursors (interleukin-1 and tumor necrosis factor-α) [39].

Daily treatment of rats with BAY 85-3934 (5 mg/kg) reversed mean PCV decline, and values returned to normal levels within 5 weeks of PG-PS challenge (Fig. 5A). The low dose of BAY 85-3934, 2.5 mg/kg, halted further decline of mean PCV levels, and by the end of the study, there was a trend for mean PCV values to be higher than in PG-PS-pretreated animals that received vehicle only. A small but significant increase in kidney EPO mRNA expression, interpreted as anemia-reactive, was not sufficient to counteract the inflammation-induced anemia in PG-PS-challenged animals. However, in response to treatment with BAY 85-3934, a significantly larger increase in EPO mRNA expression in the kidneys was observed. Among the inflammatory markers, the expression levels of monocyte chemotactic protein-1 and hepcidin were significantly reduced in animals in the 5 mg/kg dose group (Fig. 5B). Although treatment did not influence the course of polyarthritis, as monitored by hind limb ankle diameter and development of body weight gain, the initial increase in white blood cell count was attenuated (data not shown).

Efficacy of BAY 85-3934 in a disease model of subtotal nephrectomy

As well as anemia and inflammation, CKD is often accompanied by hypertension, upon which treatment with rhEPO may have an unfavorable impact. The effects of BAY 85-3934 were compared with rhEPO in the remnant kidney (subtotal nephrectomy) model in rats. This commonly used model of CKD displays the triad of renal impairment, anemia, and hypertension.

Subtotal nephrectomy resulted in a mild reduction in mean hematocrit, and an increase in mean systolic blood pressure as determined by tail cuff measurement (Fig. 6A, B). Treatment with rhEPO or BAY 85-3934 (2.5 mg/kg and 5 mg/kg) significantly increased mean PCV (Fig. 6A). In fact, 2 weeks after onset of treatment, animals in the 5 mg/kg group were switched to treatment with 2.5 mg/kg because their mean PCV had exceeded 50%.

After treatment with rhEPO, there was no difference in systolic blood pressure compared with untreated controls (Fig. 6B). In contrast, treatment with BAY 85-3934 led to a sustained reduction in mean systolic blood pressure, with almost normalized values in the 2.5 mg/kg group. Furthermore, systolic blood pressure was significantly lower in animals treated with BAY 85-3934 5 mg/kg than in control and rhEPO-treated animals. This was also

mirrored by complete prevention of cardiac hypertrophy, which manifested in control animals and rhEPO-treated animals, but was absent in animals treated with BAY 85-3934 (data not shown). The mean plasma levels of prorenin were about 4-fold reduced in nephrectomized rats compared with sham-operated animals, which was consistent with the increased blood pressure observed (Fig. 6C). Unexpectedly, and unlike the case for other hypertensive treatments, the decrease in blood pressure after treatment with BAY 85-3934 was not followed by the return of prorenin to normal levels.

The effect of treatment with BAY 85-3934 was also compared with that of a standard antihypertensive treatment, the angiotensin-converting enzyme inhibitor enalapril. As expected, treatment with enalapril (administered at 30 ppm via drinking water) resulted in a significant reduction in mean systolic blood pressure compared with control, while mean PCV remained unchanged (Fig. 6D, E). Treatment with BAY 85-3934 sodium (administered at 80 ppm via drinking water) significantly reduced mean systolic blood pressure compared with controls, while increasing mean PCV. In normotensive rats, treatment with BAY 85-3934 at the same dose for 3 days did not affect blood pressure (data not shown). A combination of both treatments resulted in a slight reduction of mean systolic blood pressure; however, the difference was not significant compared with treatment with either study drug alone. In contrast to treatment with BAY 85-3934, the decrease in blood pressure with enalapril was accompanied by reversion of plasma prorenin levels to normal values (Fig. 6F). Compared with animals treated with enalapril alone, a small decrease in plasma prorenin levels was seen for animals treated with a combination of the two drugs.

In all of the experiments reported, no significant adverse events related to treatment with BAY 85-3934 were observed.

Discussion

HIF-PH inhibitors are being evaluated in clinical studies as novel therapeutics for the treatment of anemia (e.g. FG-4592, AKB-6548, GSK1278863) [40]. They function as stabilizers of HIF, thereby mimicking the hypoxia-driven expression of endogenous EPO in the kidney [28]. To date, publications on pharmacological data for compounds under clinical development are still scant [29]. Here we present for the first time, a comprehensive pharmacological profile of a novel HIF-PH inhibitor under clinical development [41,42], from in vitro characterization to animal models of kidney disease. It was demonstrated that BAY 85-3934 was a reversible, 2-oxoglutarate-competitive, pan-HIF-PH inhibitor with high selectivity against related enzymes (matrix metalloproteinases and other peptidases) and a broad panel of radio-ligand binding assays. There is, however, a lack of validated assays for other 2-oxoglutarate dependent dioxygenases. A fourth, putative HIF-PH (PH-4, P4H–TM) has been identified, located in the membrane of the endoplasmic reticulum that we and others have previously described [33,43]. This enzyme is distantly related to PHDs, and evidence for its involvement in the hypoxia-dependent regulation of erythropoiesis in man is still elusive because, unlike for PHD2, no data from human genetics exists to help elucidate its role.

BAY 85-3934 consistently induced EPO and erythropoiesis after oral administration in rodent and non-rodent species. BAY 85-3934 was effective in animal models of renal and inflammatory anemia and, unlike rhEPO therapy, reduced blood pressure in a CKD model. Notably, the levels of endogenous EPO that were induced during treatment were close to the normal physiological range of EPO. This is in contrast to the standard therapy for renal

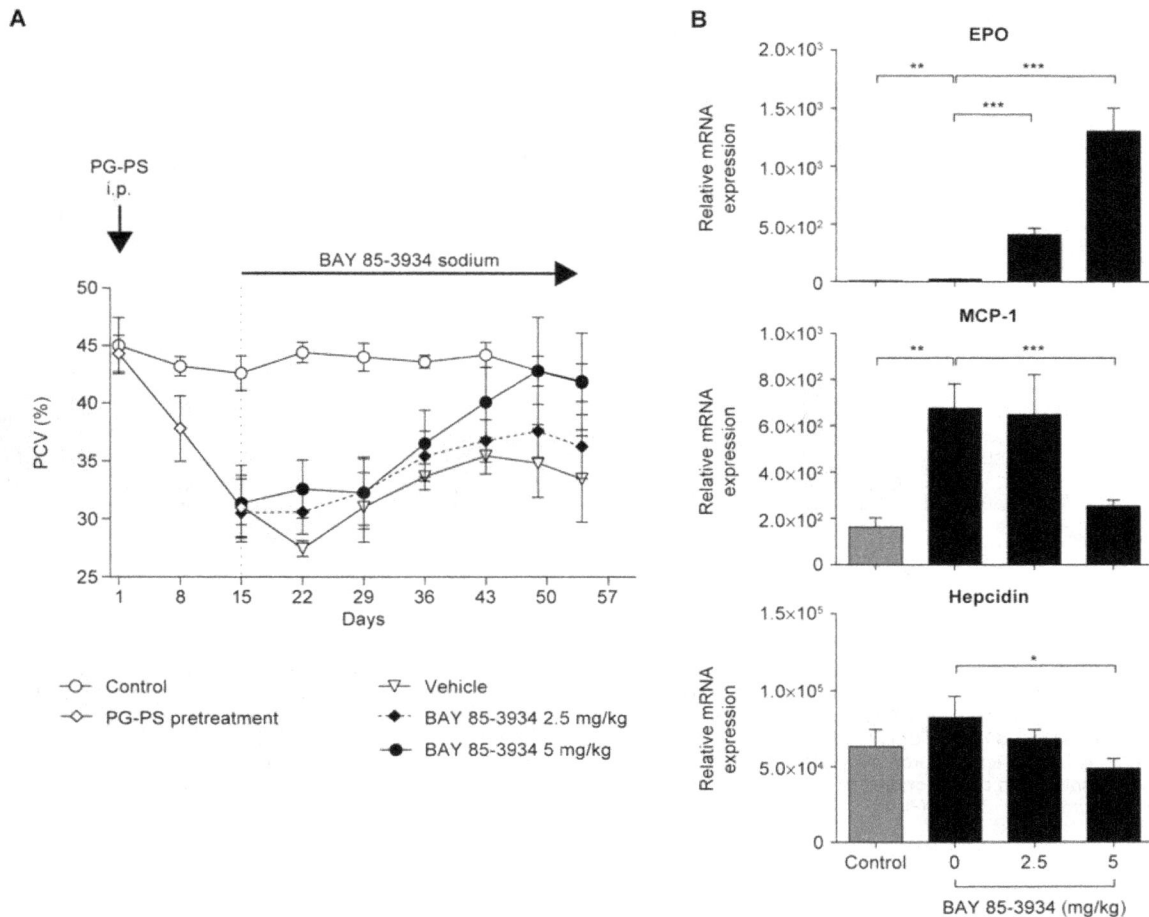

Figure 5. Effect of BAY 85-3934 administration on peptidoglycan-polysaccharide (PG-PS)-induced inflammatory anemia in female Lewis rats. Data are presented as means ± SEM. (A) Packed cell volume (PCV) in PG-PS-treated animals administered BAY 85-3934 or vehicle ($n = 11$–12 animals per group), compared with control animals treated with vehicle alone ($n = 5$ animals). (B) Relative expression of erythropoietin (EPO) and monocyte chemotactic protein-1 (MCP-1) mRNA in kidney, and hepcidin mRNA in liver at the end of the study. *$p < 0.05$, **$p < 0.01$, and ***$p < 0.001$; t-test.

anemia, whereby rhEPO levels exceed those normally seen for endogenous EPO.

BAY 85-3934 behaves as a hypoxia mimetic in the presence of oxygen both *in vitro* and *in vivo*, and HIF-1α and HIF-2α were dose-dependently and concordantly induced in human cell lines. With an induction threshold below 1 μM, BAY 85-3934 appears to be a potent cellular HIF stabilizer. These data compare favorably with those reported for other HIF-PH inhibitors [44–46]. The cellular effects are most likely to be due to direct modulation of HIF-PH, because BAY 85-3934 induced the stabilization of HIF-1α within 20 min after application. After withdrawal of the compound, stabilization of HIF-1α was completely reversed within 40 min. The kinetics of induction and disappearance of HIF-1α closely resemble those of HIF-1α in tonometer experiments after de-oxygenation and re-oxygenation [47]. Functionality of HIF stabilization was demonstrated in a hypoxia-sensitive luciferase reporter cell line, and by analysis of HIF target gene expression in human cell lines. Expression patterns were cell-line-specific, with a measurable response of EPO gene expression only in Hep3B cells. However, the drug concentrations needed to induce the transcriptional response *in vitro* were well above those that were effective for the induction of EPO *in vivo*. This could be the result of differences in cellular

uptake mechanisms or oxygen levels, or could mirror the high sensitivity of renal EPO gene expression to hypoxia [18,48].

In preclinical models and in a proof-of-concept study [41], oral administration of BAY 85-3934 was followed by a dose-dependent increase in EPO expression and subsequent erythropoiesis. EPO induction showed clear hysteresis with respect to plasma levels of the compound, and was transient. Accumulation of EPO or adaptation of the EPO response was not observed when administered once daily over 5 consecutive days to cynomolgus monkeys. This is in contrast to the rapid acclimatization of the EPO response that is observed at high altitude, which manifests as a decline in plasma EPO concentrations after 2 days [49].

Chronic, once-daily administration of BAY 85-3934 in cynomolgus monkeys led to increases in red blood cell production comparable to those achieved by chronic intermittent treatment with rhEPO. In contrast to this standard therapy, the EPO peak concentrations induced by BAY 85-3934 were within the normal physiological range of a factor of approximately 2-fold. Thus, the abnormally high peak concentrations typically associated with standard rhEPO therapy, which may impact on the long-term safety of treatment [3,50], might be avoided by therapy with BAY 85-3934. The fact that the reticulocyte count was 2-fold higher at days 8 and 15 in animals treated with rhEPO than in those treated

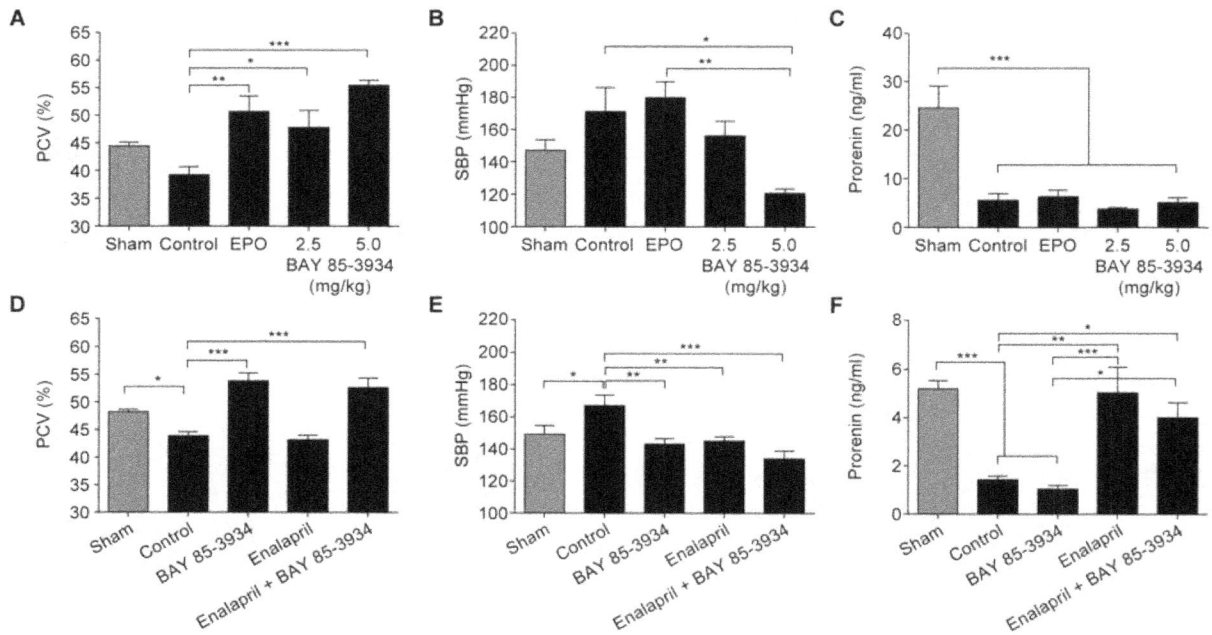

Figure 6. Effect of BAY 85-3934, erythropoietin (EPO), and enalapril in the rat subtotal nephrectomy model. Data are presented as means ± SEM. (A) Packed cell volume (PCV), (B) systolic blood pressure (SBP), and (C) prorenin following oral administration of BAY 85-3934 (2.5 mg/kg or 5 mg/kg once daily) or rhEPO (100 IU/kg s.c. twice weekly) for 5 weeks, compared with control and sham-operated animals ($n = 4$–6 animals per group). Efficacy of BAY 85-3934 sodium (80 ppm), enalapril (30 ppm), and a combination of both, administered in drinking water for 5 weeks, on (D) PCV, (E) SBP (at 4 weeks), and (F) prorenin ($n = 9$–10 animals per group). $*p < 0.05$, $**p < 0.01$, $***p < 0.001$; one-way ANOVA followed by Dunnett's multiple comparison test to corresponding sham or control group for (A), (C), (D), and (E), and Bonferroni's multiple comparison test to corresponding sham or control group for (B) and (F).

with BAY 85-3934 may be due to the timing of measurement, because reticulocyte counts usually reach peak levels 4 days after administration of rhEPO.

BAY 85-3934 was effective in ameliorating and preventing renal anemia in rats after treatment with the nephrotoxic antibiotic gentamicin. This shows that in failing kidneys, responsiveness of the EPO gene to HIF-PH inhibition is preserved, a finding that is in line with previous reports [23,24,51]. EPO mRNA expression was induced in failing kidneys by a similar degree, and with comparable sensitivity, to that in healthy control animals. However, the absolute mean expression levels were remarkably reduced, possibly as a consequence of loss of kidney parenchyma. The reduction of EPO expression is believed to be responsible for the occurrence of anemia in the gentamicin model, and in this respect the model resembles the renal anemia observed in patients with CKD [34]. In view of the rapid drop in reticulocyte counts, additional toxic effects of gentamicin on erythropoiesis in the bone marrow are also likely. The data from the expression analyses indicate that hepatic EPO production may significantly contribute to the EPO plasma pool under treatment with BAY 85-3934. Distinct hypoxia-sensitive elements on the EPO gene have been identified as relevant for hepatic EPO expression [52]. However, the liver is not able to compensate for lost renal EPO production without pharmacological intervention. Treatment of patients without functioning kidneys with a HIF-PH-inhibitor has shown that the liver can fully compensate for the lack of renal EPO production [51]. Likewise, hepatic siRNA knock-down of all three HIF-PHs in mice with renal impairment was required to induce sufficient compensatory hepatic EPO production, a requirement that can be replicated by administration of a pan-HIF-PH inhibitor [53].

Systemic inflammation is common in patients with ESRD receiving chronic hemodialysis and may diminish responsiveness to EPO, ultimately presenting as EPO resistance [54,55]. BAY 85-3934 was effective in correcting inflammation-induced anemia in a rat model of polyarthritis. Whether reduction of monocyte chemotactic protein-1 and hepcidin mRNA expression are hematopoiesis-independent effects of HIF-PH inhibition or result from the correction of anemia cannot be determined based on the current data. Hepatic expression of hepcidin, which is an important pathogenic factor responsible for disturbed iron utilization in inflammatory anemia, is known to be reduced after stimulation of the bone marrow with EPO [56,57].

The rat model of subtotal nephrectomy shows the key features of CKD – renal impairment, anemia, and hypertension. Notably in this model, and in contrast to treatment with rhEPO, treatment with BAY 85-3934 not only effectively corrected anemia, but also reduced hypertension associated with kidney disease in a dose-dependent manner. The underlying mechanism of this is not clear, but may be related to transcriptional and structural changes in the diseased kidney. Anti-inflammatory and anti-fibrotic changes of transcriptional response were observed in animals of the high dose group but are considered secondary to blood-pressure-normalizing effects rather than a direct effect of BAY 85-3934 on inflammation; however, kidney-protective effects of activation of the HIF-signaling cascade have been postulated [58–60].

Antihypertensive therapy is often associated with compensatory increases in renin and activation of the renin–angiotensin–aldosterone system [61]. Paradoxically, following treatment with BAY 85-3934, plasma prorenin levels remained low despite normalization of blood pressure. This effect may provide an additional benefit in the treatment of patients with CKD and anemia. This was in contrast to treatment with enalapril, which showed the expected effect of increasing prorenin. This effect was slightly diminished in combination with BAY 85-3934. Various lines of evidence suggest a link between the up-regulation of HIF and a reduction of blood pressure. Several vasomotor-relevant genes are known members of the HIF target gene cluster [11]. Patients with Chuvash polycythemia, who constitutively express high HIF levels, have been found to have significantly lower blood pressure than matched controls [62]. Furthermore, in transgenic mice with stabilized HIFs, juxtaglomerular cells switch from a renin- to an EPO-secreting cell type [63].

In addition to efficacy in the treatment of anemia, the potential effects of HIF stabilization on long-term health must be considered. HIFs regulate a battery of genes that are important for hypoxia adaptation, and inhibition of HIF-PH may have effects on metabolism and angiogenesis. In the EPO-producing cells of the kidney, the transcriptional activation of EPO is mainly under the control of the PHD2-HIF-2α axis, while in the liver PHD1 and PHD3 also contribute to the oxygen-dependent transcriptional repression of EPO [53,64]. The rare gain-of-function mutations of HIF-2α and the loss-of-function mutations in the PHD2 gene are associated with benign erythrocytosis [15]. This phenotype can be reproduced in the corresponding transgenic animal models [16,19,20]. BAY 85-3934 is a pan-HIF-PH inhibitor, hence potential mode-of-action-dependent implications for safety may be best assessed in view of the phenotype associated with global HIF activation, which is known in patients suffering from Chuvash polycythemia [14]. In addition to severe polycythemia and lowered systemic blood pressure, these patients show changes in muscle metabolism, mild organomegaly, and increased basal tone and hypoxic vasoconstriction of pulmonary blood vessels compared with matched controls. Despite lifelong activation of the HIF system, no increase in the incidence of malignancies has been found. Furthermore, the manifestations of this phenotype would not be expected to arise to the same extent from intermittent activation of the HIF system, and the magnitude of the effect may be comparable to intermittent and moderate high altitude exposure [62,65,66].

To explore the transcriptional response after exposure to BAY 85-3934, a panel of HIF target genes was examined, identified in the scientific literature as hypoxia-responsive genes [11,67–69]. CAIX is known to be a reliable histochemical marker of hypoxia and, in our studies, was strongly induced in vitro, but was not induced in vivo [70]. The expression of HIF target genes was analyzed in kidney and liver samples from rats after exposure to BAY 85-3934 in several settings and at a range of doses. The kidney was chosen as the pharmacological target organ in which EPO response is triggered by the action of the compound. The liver was selected because it is the primary organ of metabolism of

this drug. With the exception of EPO, the induction of hypoxia-sensitive gene transcription was found to be absent or comparatively minor, with no fundamental difference between the organs from healthy rats and those from anemia-induced rats, even at doses at which EPO levels were increased by two orders of magnitude.

PHD2 and PHD3 are up-regulated under hypoxia, while PHD1 is hypoxia-insensitive. Interestingly, HIF-dependent transcriptional induction of HIF-PHs has been described as an important negative feedback mechanism that, under hypoxia, compensates for decreased oxygen levels, a mechanism possibly underlying the adaptive modulation of EPO response under prolonged hypoxia [71]. However, in the present studies, the expression of genes encoding HIF-PHs remained unchanged and no adaptive responses were observed after repeated dosing.

Whether the transcriptional changes observed in the preclinical studies translate into corresponding changes at the protein level that are of functional importance can only be answered for the EPO gene, which was the most sensitive gene to treatment with BAY 85-3934. This finding is in line with studies in rodents exposed to hypoxia in vivo [18,48].

In conclusion, the pan HIF-PH inhibitor BAY 85-3934 acts as a hypoxia mimetic in vivo, with effective reversion of anemia in animal models of renal and inflammatory anemia. BAY 85-3934 was found to be effective in raising hematocrit levels while stimulating endogenous EPO production within its normal physiological range. Furthermore, BAY 85-3934 can be administered as an oral therapy and, unlike rhEPO, showed antihypertensive effects in a model of CKD. Thus, BAY 85-3934 is an attractive new drug candidate for the treatment of EPO-sensitive anemia, in particular anemia associated with CKD.

Acknowledgments

We thank S. Tan, Pennsylvania State University, State College, PA, USA, for providing the plasmid pST39-HisTrxNVHL–elongin B–elongin C, J. Fandrey, University of Duisburg-Essen, Essen, Germany for providing Hep3B cells, H. Ehmke, University of Hamburg, Germany for critical reading of the manuscript and A. Kaiser, Bayer Pharma AG, for advice on statistical analysis. Medical writing assistance, funded by Bayer Pharma AG, was provided by W. Gattrell of Oxford PharmaGenesis Ltd, Oxford, UK.

Author Contributions

Conceived and designed the experiments: IF FO PE MJ JK UT. Performed the experiments: IF FO PE JK UT. Analyzed the data: IF FO PE MJ JK UT. Contributed reagents/materials/analysis tools: FO MJ. Contributed to the writing of the manuscript: IF FO PE MJ JK UT.

References

1. Nangaku M, Eckardt KU (2006) Pathogenesis of renal anemia. Semin Nephrol 26: 261–268.
2. Grabe DW (2007) Update on clinical practice recommendations and new therapeutic modalities for treating anemia in patients with chronic kidney disease. Am J Health Syst Pharm 64: S8–14.
3. Unger EF, Thompson AM, Blank MJ, Temple R (2010) Erythropoiesis-stimulating agents-time for a reevaluation. N Engl J Med 362: 189–192.
4. Briet M, Barhoumi T, Mian MO, Sierra C, Boutouyrie P, et al. (2013) Effects of recombinant human erythropoietin on resistance artery endothelial function in stage 4 chronic kidney disease. J Am Heart Assoc 2: e000128.
5. Krapf R, Hulter HN (2009) Arterial hypertension induced by erythropoietin and erythropoiesis-stimulating agents (ESA). Clin J Am Soc Nephrol 4: 470–480.
6. Maschio G (1995) Erythropoietin and systemic hypertension. Nephrol Dial Transplant 10 Suppl 2: 74–79.
7. Semenza GL (2011) Oxygen sensing, homeostasis, and disease. N Engl J Med 365: 537–547.
8. Wang GL, Semenza GL (1996) Molecular basis of hypoxia-induced erythropoietin expression. Curr Opin Hematol 3: 156–162.
9. Bruick RK, McKnight SL (2001) A conserved family of prolyl-4-hydroxylases that modify HIF. Science 294: 1337–1340.
10. Epstein AC, Gleadle JM, McNeill LA, Hewitson KS, O'Rourke J, et al. (2001) C. elegans EGL-9 and mammalian homologs define a family of dioxygenases that regulate HIF by prolyl hydroxylation. Cell 107: 43–54.
11. Schofield CJ, Ratcliffe PJ (2004) Oxygen sensing by HIF hydroxylases. Nat Rev Mol Cell Biol 5: 343–354.
12. Wenger RH, Hoogewijs D (2010) Regulated oxygen sensing by protein hydroxylation in renal erythropoietin-producing cells. Am J Physiol Renal Physiol 298: F1287–1296.
13. Min JH, Yang H, Ivan M, Gertler F, Kaelin WG, Jr., et al. (2002) Structure of an HIF-1alpha -pVHL complex: hydroxyproline recognition in signaling. Science 296: 1886–1889.
14. Gordeuk VR, Sergueeva AI, Miasnikova GY, Okhotin D, Voloshin Y, et al. (2004) Congenital disorder of oxygen sensing: association of the homozygous Chuvash polycythemia VHL mutation with thrombosis and vascular abnormalities but not tumors. Blood 103: 3924–3932.

15. Lee FS, Percy MJ (2011) The HIF pathway and erythrocytosis. Annu Rev Pathol 6: 165–192.

16. Arsenault PR, Pei F, Lee R, Kerestes H, Percy MJ, et al. (2013) A knock-in mouse model of human PHD2 gene-associated erythrocytosis establishes a haploinsufficiency mechanism. J Biol Chem 288: 33571–33584.

17. Hickey MM, Lam JC, Bezman NA, Rathmell WK, Simon MC (2007) von Hippel-Lindau mutation in mice recapitulates Chuvash polycythemia via hypoxia-inducible factor-2alpha signaling and splenic erythropoiesis. J Clin Invest 117: 3879–3889.

18. Kramer BK, Bucher M, Sandner P, Ittner KP, Riegger GA, et al. (1997) Effects of hypoxia on growth factor expression in the rat kidney in vivo. Kidney Int 51: 444–447.

19. Minamishima YA, Moslehi J, Bardeesy N, Cullen D, Bronson RT, et al. (2008) Somatic inactivation of the PHD2 prolyl hydroxylase causes polycythemia and congestive heart failure. Blood 111: 3236–3244.

20. Takeda K, Aguila HL, Parikh NS, Li X, Lamothe K, et al. (2008) Regulation of adult erythropoiesis by prolyl hydroxylase domain proteins. Blood 111: 3229–3235.

21. Eckardt KU, Kurtz A, Bauer C (1989) Regulation of erythropoietin production is related to proximal tubular function. Am J Physiol 256: F942–947.

22. Dunn A, Lo V, Donnelly S (2007) The role of the kidney in blood volume regulation: the kidney as a regulator of the hematocrit. Am J Med Sci 334: 65–71.

23. Kato A, Hishida A, Kumagai H, Furuya R, Nakajima T, et al. (1994) Erythropoietin production in patients with chronic renal failure. Ren Fail 16: 645–651.

24. Shimizu S, Enoki Y, Sakata S, Kohzuki H, Ohga Y, et al. (1994) Erythropoietin response to acute hypobaric or anaemic hypoxia in gentamicin-administered rats. Acta Physiol Scand 151: 225–231.

25. Priyadarshi A, Periyasamy S, Burke TJ, Britton SL, Malhotra D, et al. (2002) Effects of reduction of renal mass on renal oxygen tension and erythropoietin production in the rat. Kidney Int 61: 542–546.

26. Brookhart MA, Schneeweiss S, Avorn J, Bradbury BD, Rothman KJ, et al. (2008) The effect of altitude on dosing and response to erythropoietin in ESRD. J Am Soc Nephrol 19: 1389–1395.

27. Brookhart MA, Bradbury BD, Avorn J, Schneeweiss S, Winkelmayer WC (2011) The effect of altitude change on anemia treatment response in hemodialysis patients. Am J Epidemiol 173: 768–777.

28. Muchnik E, Kaplan J (2011) HIF prolyl hydroxylase inhibitors for anemia. Expert Opin Investig Drugs 20: 645–656.

29. Rabinowitz MH (2013) Inhibition of hypoxia-inducible factor prolyl hydroxylase domain oxygen sensors: tricking the body into mounting orchestrated survival and repair responses. J Med Chem 56: 9369–9402.

30. Thede K, Flamme I, Oehme F, Ergüden J, Stoll F, et al. (2008) Substituted Dihydropyrazolones for treating cardiovascular and hematological diseases. United States patent application WO 2008/067871.

31. Tan S (2001) A modular polycistronic expression system for overexpressing protein complexes in Escherichia coli. Protein Expr Purif 21: 224–234.

32. Oehme F, Jonghaus W, Narouz-Ott L, Huetter J, Flamme I (2004) A nonradioactive 96-well plate assay for the detection of hypoxia-inducible factor prolyl hydroxylase activity. Anal Biochem 330: 74–80.

33. Oehme F, Ellinghaus P, Kolkhof P, Smith TJ, Ramakrishnan S, et al. (2002) Overexpression of PH-4, a novel putative proline 4-hydroxylase, modulates activity of hypoxia-inducible transcription factors. Biochem Biophys Res Commun 296: 343–349.

34. Nagano N, Koumegawa J, Arai H, Wada M, Kusaka M (1990) Effect of recombinant human erythropoietin on new anaemic model rats induced by gentamicin. J Pharm Pharmacol 42: 758–762.

35. Suzuki S, Takamura S, Yoshida J, Shinzawa Y, Niwa O, et al. (1995) Comparison of gentamicin nephrotoxicity between rats and mice. Comp Biochem Physiol C Pharmacol Toxicol Endocrinol 112: 15–28.

36. Rinaudo D, Toniatti C (2000) Sensitive ELISA for mouse erythropoietin. Biotechniques 29: 218–220.

37. Ellinghaus P, Scheubel RJ, Dobrev D, Ravens U, Holtz J, et al. (2005) Comparing the global mRNA expression profile of human atrial and ventricular myocardium with high-density oligonucleotide arrays. J Thorac Cardiovasc Surg 129: 1383–1390.

38. Sartor RB, Anderle SK, Rifai N, Goo DA, Cromartie WJ, et al. (1989) Protracted anemia associated with chronic, relapsing systemic inflammation induced by arthropathic peptidoglycan-polysaccharide polymers in rats. Infect Immun 57: 1177–1185.

39. Weiss G, Goodnough LT (2005) Anemia of chronic disease. N Engl J Med 352: 1011–1023.

40. Denny WA (2012) Giving anemia a boost with inhibitors of prolyl hydroxylase. J Med Chem 55: 2943–2944.

41. Boettcher M, Lentini S, Kaiser A, Flamme I, Kubitza D, et al. (2013) First-in-man study with BAY 85-3934 – A new oral selective HIF-PH inhibitor for the treatment of renal anemia. J Am Soc Nephrol 24: 347A.

42. Macdougall IC, Berns JS, Akizawa T, Fishbane S, Bernhardt T (2013) DIALOGUE Phase 2 program for BAY85-3934 a HIF-PH inhibitor with daily oral treatment in anemic patients suffering from CKD/ESRD. J Am Soc Nephrol 24: 413A.

43. Laitala A, Aro E, Walkinshaw G, Maki JM, Rossi M, et al. (2012) Transmembrane prolyl 4-hydroxylase is a fourth prolyl 4-hydroxylase regulating EPO production and erythropoiesis. Blood 120: 3336–3344.

44. Asikainen TM, Ahmad A, Schneider BK, Ho WB, Arend M, et al. (2005) Stimulation of HIF-1alpha, HIF-2alpha, and VEGF by prolyl 4-hydroxylase inhibition in human lung endothelial and epithelial cells. Free Radic Biol Med 38: 1002–1013.

45. Bao W, Qin P, Needle S, Erickson-Miller CL, Duffy KJ, et al. (2010) Chronic inhibition of hypoxia-inducible factor prolyl 4-hydroxylase improves ventricular performance, remodeling, and vascularity after myocardial infarction in the rat. J Cardiovasc Pharmacol 56: 147–155.

46. Ivan M, Haberberger T, Gervasi DC, Michelson KS, Gunzler V, et al. (2002) Biochemical purification and pharmacological inhibition of a mammalian prolyl hydroxylase acting on hypoxia-inducible factor. Proc Natl Acad Sci U S A 99: 13459–13464.

47. Jewell UR, Kvietikova I, Scheid A, Bauer C, Wenger RH, et al. (2001) Induction of HIF-1alpha in response to hypoxia is instantaneous. FASEB J 15: 1312–1314.

48. Sandner P, Gess B, Wolf K, Kurtz A (1996) Divergent regulation of vascular endothelial growth factor and of erythropoietin gene expression in vivo. Pflugers Arch 431: 905–912.

49. Abbrecht PH, Littell JK (1972) Plasma erythropoietin in men and mice during acclimatization to different altitudes. J Appl Physiol 32: 54–58.

50. Koulouridis I, Alfayez M, Trikalinos TA, Balk EM, Jaber BL (2013) Dose of erythropoiesis-stimulating agents and adverse outcomes in CKD: a metaregression analysis. Am J Kidney Dis 61: 44–56.

51. Bernhardt WM, Wiesener MS, Scigalla P, Chou J, Schmieder RE, et al. (2010) Inhibition of prolyl hydroxylases increases erythropoietin production in ESRD. J Am Soc Nephrol 21: 2151–2156.

52. Fandrey J (2004) Oxygen-dependent and tissue-specific regulation of erythropoietin gene expression. Am J Physiol Regul Integr Comp Physiol 286: R977–988.

53. Querbes W, Bogorad RL, Moslehi J, Wong J, Chan AY, et al. (2012) Treatment of erythropoietin deficiency in mice with systemically administered siRNA. Blood 120: 1916–1922.

54. Elliott J, Mishler D, Agarwal R (2009) Hyporesponsiveness to erythropoietin: causes and management. Adv Chronic Kidney Dis 16: 94–100.

55. Johnson DW, Pollock CA, Macdougall IC (2007) Erythropoiesis-stimulating agent hyporesponsiveness. Nephrology (Carlton) 12: 321–330.

56. Ganz T, Nemeth E (2011) Hepcidin and disorders of iron metabolism. Annu Rev Med 62: 347–360.

57. Tanno T, Bhanu NV, Oneal PA, Goh SH, Staker P, et al. (2007) High levels of GDF15 in thalassemia suppress expression of the iron regulatory protein hepcidin. Nat Med 13: 1096–1101.

58. Deng A, Arndt MA, Satriano J, Singh P, Rieg T, et al. (2010) Renal protection in chronic kidney disease: hypoxia-inducible factor activation vs. angiotensin II blockade. Am J Physiol Renal Physiol 299: F1365–1373.

59. Song YR, You SJ, Lee YM, Chin HJ, Chae DW, et al. (2010) Activation of hypoxia-inducible factor attenuates renal injury in rat remnant kidney. Nephrol Dial Transplant 25: 77–85.

60. Yu X, Fang Y, Ding X, Liu H, Zhu J, et al. (2012) Transient hypoxia-inducible factor activation in rat renal ablation and reduced fibrosis with L-mimosine. Nephrology (Carlton) 17: 58–67.

61. Neutel JM, Smith DH (2013) Hypertension management: rationale for triple therapy based on mechanisms of action. Cardiovasc Ther 31: 251–258.

62. Yoon D, Okhotin DV, Kim B, Okhotina Y, Okhotin DJ, et al. (2010) Increased size of solid organs in patients with Chuvash polycythemia and in mice with altered expression of HIF-1alpha and HIF-2alpha. J Mol Med (Berl) 88: 523–530.

63. Kurt B, Paliege A, Willam C, Schwarzensteiner I, Schucht K, et al. (2013) Deletion of von Hippel-Lindau protein converts renin-producing cells into erythropoietin-producing cells. J Am Soc Nephrol 24: 433–444.

64. Minamishima YA, Kaelin WG Jr (2010) Reactivation of hepatic EPO synthesis in mice after PHD loss. Science 329: 407.

65. Formenti F, Constantin-Teodosiu D, Emmanuel Y, Cheeseman J, Dorrington KL, et al. (2010) Regulation of human metabolism by hypoxia-inducible factor. Proc Natl Acad Sci U S A 107: 12722–12727.

66. Smith TG, Brooks JT, Balanos GM, Lappin TR, Layton DM, et al. (2006) Mutation of von Hippel-Lindau tumour suppressor and human cardiopulmonary physiology. PLoS Med 3: e290. doi:10.1371/journal.pmed.0030290.

67. Greijer AE, van der Groep P, Kemming D, Shvarts A, Semenza GL, et al. (2005) Up-regulation of gene expression by hypoxia is mediated predominantly by hypoxia-inducible factor 1 (HIF-1). J Pathol 206: 291–304.

68. Warnecke C, Weidemann A, Volke M, Schietke R, Wu X, et al. (2008) The specific contribution of hypoxia-inducible factor-2alpha to hypoxic gene expression in vitro is limited and modulated by cell type-specific and exogenous factors. Exp Cell Res 314: 2016–2027.

69. Wenger RH, Stiehl DP, Camenisch G (2005) Integration of oxygen signaling at the consensus HRE. Sci STKE 2005: re12.

70. Potter C, Harris AL (2004) Hypoxia inducible carbonic anhydrase IX, marker of tumour hypoxia, survival pathway and therapy target. Cell Cycle 3: 164–167.

71. Stiehl DP, Wirthner R, Koditz J, Spielmann P, Camenisch G, et al. (2006) Increased prolyl 4-hydroxylase domain proteins compensate for decreased oxygen levels. Evidence for an autoregulatory oxygen-sensing system. J Biol Chem 281: 23482–23491.

23

Correlation between Renal Function and Common Risk Factors for Chronic Kidney Disease in a Healthy Middle-Aged Population: A Prospective Observational 2-Year Study

Michiya Ohno[1]*, Fumiko Deguchi[2], Kumiko Izumi[1], Hirotoshi Ishigaki[1], Hiroshi Sarui[3], Akihiko Sasaki[3], Tomonori Segawa[4], Takahiko Yamaki[4], Takao Kojima[2], Hiroshige Ohashi[1]

1 Division of Nephrology, Murakami Memorial Hospital, Asahi University School of Dentistry, Gifu City, Gifu, Japan, 2 Division of Health Center, Murakami Memorial Hospital, Asahi University School of Dentistry, Gifu City, Gifu, Japan, 3 Division of Diabetes and Endocrinology, Murakami Memorial Hospital, Asahi University School of Dentistry, Gifu City, Gifu, Japan, 4 Division of Cardiology, Murakami Memorial Hospital, Asahi University School of Dentistry, Gifu City, Gifu, Japan

Abstract

Background/Aims: Age, proteinuria, metabolic syndrome, and hyperuricemia are the reported risk factors for chronic kidney disease (CKD) and cardiovascular disease (CVD). However, the best predictor of changes in renal function in the early stages of renal disease in a healthy middle-aged population is still unknown. Our study evaluated the correlation between changes in renal function and common risk factors to determine such a predictor.

Methods: In total, 2,853 healthy persons aged ≤50 years participated in the study. They had no proteinuria and were not on medications for hypertension, diabetes mellitus, hyperlipidemia, or hyperuricemia. Over 2 years, participants underwent annual health screening. The relationship between changes in estimated glomerular filtration rate (eGFR) and changes in risk factors for CKD was evaluated using univariate and multivariate linear regression analyses.

Results: Over 2 years, eGFR showed a significant decrease. Univariate regression analysis revealed that changes in fasting plasma glucose (FPG), total cholesterol, LDL-cholesterol, serum uric acid levels, and hemoglobin showed a significant negative correlation with changes in eGFR. Multiple regression analysis confirmed that changes in FPG, serum uric acid levels, in particular, and hemoglobin had a significant negative correlation with changes in eGFR.

Conclusion: The changes in eGFR and other variables over 2 years were small and could be within expected biologic variation. A longer observational study is needed to elucidate whether FPG, serum uric acid and hemoglobin represent the earliest markers of eGFR decline.

Editor: Giuseppe Remuzzi, Mario Negri Institute for Pharmacological Research and Azienda Ospedaliera Ospedali Riuniti di Bergamo, Italy

Funding: The authors have no support or funding to report.

Competing Interests: The authors have declared that no competing interests exist.

* Email: mohno@murakami.asahi-u.ac.jp

Introduction

Chronic kidney disease (CKD) increases the risk of end-stage renal disease and cardiovascular disease (CVD) [1–3]. In Japan, the prevalence of CKD is approximately 13% of the adult population [4]. CKD is classified into stages 1 to 5 based on the levels of proteinuria and estimated glomerular filtration rate (eGFR), which is calculated from the age and serum creatinine level [5]. As CKD progresses through these 5 stages, the risk of CVD increases; CVD associated with CKD is known as the cardiorenal syndrome [1–3]. CKD and CVD also share common risk factors, such as hypertension, diabetes mellitus, and dyslipidemia [6]. Recently, lifestyle-related metabolic syndrome and hyperuricemia have also been reported as risk factors for CKD [7–10].

The most significant factor contributing to renal function decline in healthy persons is aging; however, significant individual variation in age-related GFR reduction is observed. The prevalence of high blood pressure and disorders of glucose and lipid metabolism also increases with age. These complications lead to a vicious circle that promotes renal function decline. Age-related decline in the rate of renal function is reportedly more rapid when GFR decreases at a younger age [11].

The prevalence of metabolic syndrome among adults in the USA is positively correlated with serum uric acid levels [7]. Metabolic syndrome, characterized by truncal obesity, hyperglycemia, elevated blood pressure, and insulin resistance, is recognized as a risk factor for kidney disease [8]. If obesity and metabolic syndrome have been caused at a younger age because of lifestyle factors such as poor dietary and exercise habits, lifestyle improvement may suppress renal function deterioration. However, the relationship between changes in renal function and various common risk factors including elevated blood pressure and abnormal blood glucose, lipid, and uric acid levels has not been studied in young and middle-aged persons.

Therefore, we performed the present study to evaluate the relationship between changes in renal function and common risk factors for CKD. Various confounding clinical factors influence changes in eGFR. To minimize the effect of such confounding factors, this study was limited to healthy middle-aged subjects aged ≤ 50 years who were not on medications for hypertension, diabetes mellitus, hyperlipidemia, or hyperuricemia and who had no proteinuria with ≥ 60 mL/min/1.73 m^2 of eGFR.

Subjects and Methods

This study was performed in accordance with the principles of the Declaration of Helsinki and was approved by the ethics committee of Murakami Memorial hospital. All subjects gave written informed consent for participation prior to the initiation of the study.

Subjects and study design

This prospective observational study investigated the relationship between changes in renal function in healthy subjects aged $\leq$ 50 years and common risk factors for CKD. Apparently healthy persons who participated in a health screening program at our hospital from April 2009 to March 2010 were assessed for eligibility for this study (n = 5,728). We found a total of 3,188 participants aged ≤ 50 years with an eGFR of ≥ 60 mL/min/ 1.73 m^2. The screening program (an interview regarding health status, routine physical examination, chest radiographic examination, electrocardiography, and laboratory tests for cardiovascular risk factors) revealed that 335 subjects among them had proteinuria or were on treatment for hypertension, diabetes, dyslipidemia, or hyperuricemia. Consequently, 2,853 subjects were enrolled in this study. The endpoint was the relationship between changes in eGFR and changes in body mass index (BMI), blood pressure, fasting plasma glucose (FPG), hemoglobin A$_{1c}$ (HbA$_{1c}$), lipids (including total cholesterol, LDL-cholesterol, HDL-cholesterol, and triglycerides), uric acid levels, and hemoglobin over 2 years. During the 2-year period, health screenings that included urine and blood tests on early morning specimens were conducted annually. CKD was defined as persistence of <60 mL/ min/1.73 m^2 eGFR for longer than 3 months. CKD was not evaluated by annual screening. The relationship between changes in eGFR, BMI, blood pressure, FPG, HbA$_{1c}$, cholesterol, triglycerides, uric acid levels, and hemoglobin from baseline to 2-year follow-up was evaluated. The change in eGFR was set as a dependent variable, and changes in BMI, blood pressure, FPG, HbA$_{1c}$, cholesterol, triglycerides, uric acid levels, and hemoglobin were used as independent variables for univariate analysis. In addition, the impact of longitudinal changes in each variable on the change in eGFR was assessed using multivariate analysis. HbA$_{1c}$ was calculated as per the National Glycohemoglobin Standardization Program (NGSP) value according to the Japan Diabetes Society (JDS) guidelines: HbA$_{1c}$ (NGSP) = 1.02×HbA$_{1c}$ (JDS)+0.25 [12]. In the text and tables, HbA$_{1c}$ (NGSP) values have been provided. Changes in variables (Δ) were calculated as the difference between the baseline value and the value at 2 years.

Blood pressure was measured after participants were seated in a chair for 5 min with their arms supported at heart level. Systolic and diastolic blood pressures were respectively recorded as the first and fifth Korotkoff sounds using a mercury sphygmomanometer.

Three consecutive blood pressure measurements were taken, allowing 2 min between each measurement; the mean of the second and third measurements was recorded as blood pressure. eGFR was calculated using the Japanese Society of Nephrology formula [5].

Statistical analysis

Data in the text and tables are expressed as mean ± SD. The normality of the distribution of variables was confirmed by checking a bell-shaped histogram. Subsequently, the differences between two variables with a normal distribution were compared using the paired t-test. The differences between two variables without a normal distribution were compared using the Wilcoxon signed rank tests. Nominal variables were compared using the McNemar's test. Simple and multiple linear regression analyses were performed to examine the relationship between changes in eGFR and changes in other variables over 2 years using the values at baseline and 2 years. P values of <0.05 were considered statistically significant.

Results

Changes in variables

During 2-year follow-up, all except 81 subjects were assessed annually (Figure 1). No subject developed proteinuria or had to be started on medications for hypertension, diabetes, hyperlipidemia, or hyperuricemia.

During the study period, eGFR showed a significant decrease from 77.7±11.3 mL/min/1.73 m^2 to 76.4±11.2 mL/min/ 1.73 m^2 (Δ -1.25 ± 8.56 mL/min/1.73 m^2). BMI, systolic and diastolic blood pressure, FPG, HbA$_{1c}$, total cholesterol, and HDL-cholesterol all showed a slight but significant increase (Table 1). Figure 2 shows changes in eGFR according to CKD classification between baseline and 2 years. eGFR did not always decline and was elevated in some subjects (Figure 2).

Results of linear regression analysis

Univariate analysis revealed that changes in FPG, total cholesterol, LDL-cholesterol, uric acid levels, and hemoglobin had a significant negative correlation with changes in eGFR (Table 2). To determine the independent contribution of each factor to the change in eGFR, a series of multivariate models based on risk factors for CKD were constructed. Model 1 included all factors, Model 3 was based on the significant factors in the univariate regression analysis, and Models 2 and 4 excluded total cholesterol because of multicolinearity in Models 1 and 3. Multivariate analyses using Model 3 revealed that changes in FPG, uric acid levels, and hemoglobin had a significant negative correlation with changes in eGFR, while BMI showed a positive correlation. The standardized regression coefficient (β) for changes in uric acid levels was the most negative among the significant variables (uric acid: -0.279; hemoglobin: -0.084; FPG: -0.080) (Table 3).

Prevalence of hyperuricemia

The influence of hyperuricemia on changes in eGFR was also analyzed. At baseline, hyperuricemia (serum uric acid levels $\geq$ 7 mg/dL in men and ≥ 6 mg/dL in women) was found in 12.6% of men and 1.0% of women. After 2 years, fewer subjects had hyperuricemia than at baseline (Table 4). Almost all changes in serum uric acid levels were within the normal range.

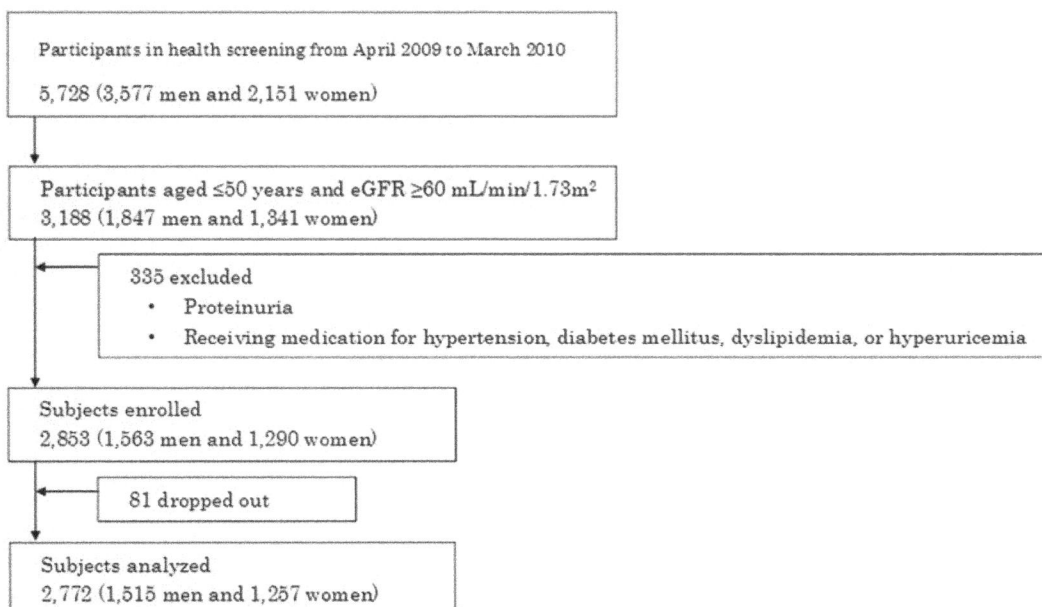

Figure 1. Disposition of the study population.

Discussion

This prospective observational study was the first to evaluate the relationship between changes in eGFR and changes in variables related to renal function over 2 years in healthy subjects aged ≤50 years. This study demonstrated that changes in the serum uric acid levels that were largely within the normal range were a sensitive indicator of changes in eGFR and thus changes in renal function in healthy middle-aged subjects. During the 2-year follow-up, eGFR did not always change unidirectionally (Figure 2). An increase in eGFR was associated with a decline in serum uric acid levels, while a decrease in eGFR was associated with elevation of serum uric acid levels. eGFR was calculated according to patient age and serum creatinine levels; it decreases with aging and an increase in serum creatinine levels. In this study, the changes in eGFR over only 2 years were more strongly influenced by the decrease in serum creatinine levels than the increase in age. Thus, decline in serum creatinine levels with age generally meant elevation of eGFR so that renal function was maintained. However, changes in eGFR in some of the present subjects may also represent physiological changes in renal function; the observation period was too short to determine the direction of change in eGFR in some cases. There was a significant association between changes in hemoglobin and those in eGFR (table 1, 2), although hemoglobin did not change significantly in this time frame. These results showed that subjects with positive changes in hemoglobin which were not significant had larger negative changes in eGFR in all subjects, and that a very slight hemoglobin decline within the normal range was associated with elevation of eGFR. Elevation of eGFR may be related to a decrease in hemoglobin because of the alteration of fluid balance. Whether the change in serum uric acid levels within the normal range has any clinical importance has been unclear. Therefore, these changes in eGFR and other variables over 2 years are so small but statistically significant that they are clinically meaningless.

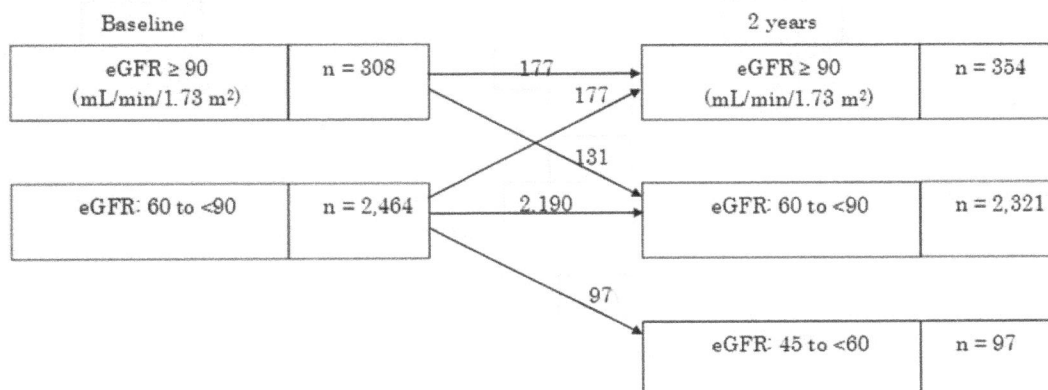

Figure 2. Change in eGFR over 2 years. eGFR was classified from stage 1 to stage 3a according to the CKD stage. Note that eGFR changed over 2 years.

Table 1. Characteristics of subjects at baseline and 2 years.

Characteristic	Baseline	2 years	Δ	95% CI	P value
Gender (male/female)	1515/1257				
Age (years)	42.6±5.1	44.6±5.2			
Metabolic syndrome (n, %)	103, 3.7	119, 4.3			0.130 b
BMI (kg/m²)	22.21±3.15	22.34±3.21	0.14±0.95	0.10, 0.17	<0.001 a
Systolic BP (mmHg)	114.0±15.1	114.8±14.8	0.80±9.54	0.45, 1.16	<0.001 a
Diastolic BP (mmHg)	72.1±10.6	72.6±10.7	0.48±6.20	0.25, 0.72	<0.001 a
FPG (mg/dL)	93.4±10.9	93.9±11.7	0.56±7.74	0.27, 0.85	<0.001 a
HbA$_{1c}$ (%)	4.89±0.37	4.94±0.37	0.04±0.22	0.04, 0.05	<0.001 a
Total cholesterol (mg/dL)	193.7±31.3	200.2±31.4	6.54±21.67	5.73, 7.36	<0.001 a
HDL-cholesterol (mg/dL)	57.0±13.5	59.6±16.0	2.56±8.25	2.25, 2.86	<0.001 a
LDL-cholesterol (mg/dL)	115.5±28.9	116.0±28.5	0.55±18.41	−0.13, 1.24	0.113 a
Triglycerides (mg/dL)	79.1±62.0	79.1±66.3	0.01±49.23	−1.82, 1.85	0.988 a
Uric acid (mg/dL)	4.84±1.38	4.88±1.35	0.04±0.65	0.02, 0.07	<0.001 a
Hb (g/dL)	13.84±1.76	13.82±1.72	−0.02±0.91	−0.06, 0.01	0.161 a
eGFR (mL/min/1.73 m²)	77.7±11.3	76.4±11.2	−1.25±8.57	−1.57, −0.93	<0.001 a

All values are expressed as mean ± SD. P values: a, paired t-test; b, McNemar's test comparing baseline with 2 years.
Abbreviations and symbols: Δ, change in the variable over 2 years; 95% CI, 95% confidence interval; BMI, body mass index; BP, blood pressure; FPG, fasting plasma glucose; HbA$_{1c}$, hemoglobin A$_{1c}$; eGFR, estimated glomerular filtration rate; HDL, high density lipoprotein; LDL, low density lipoprotein; Hb, hemoglobin.

A study by Bellomo et al. [13] in healthy normotensive individuals showed that serum uric acid levels were associated with the risk of eGFR decline over 5 years. They analyzed changes in eGFR as a continuous variable rather than as a variable in the incidence of stage 3 CKD. The adjusted hazard ratio for a decrease in eGFR by 10 mL/min/1.73 m² was 1.23 (95% confidence interval: 1.09, 1.39) for every 1.2 mg/dL increase in the serum uric acid level. Serum uric acid levels showed a slight, but significant, relationship with eGFR decline using multiple regression analysis (β, women: −0.17; β, men: −0.15). More

Table 2. Simple linear regression analysis of factors related to ΔeGFR.

Risk factors	ΔeGFR	
	β	P value
Baseline		
Male (vs. female)	−0.035	0.062
Age (years)	0.031	0.107
MetS (vs. no)	−0.006	0.770
Δ		
BMI (kg/m²)	0.002	0.934
Systolic BP (mmHg)	0.004	0.848
Diastolic BP (mmHg)	−0.036	0.061
FPG (mg/dL)	−0.080	<0.001
HbA$_{1c}$ (%)	−0.025	0.184
Total cholesterol (mg/dL)	−0.081	<0.001
HDL-cholesterol (mg/dL)	−0.018	0.349
LDL-cholesterol (mg/dL)	−0.081	<0.001
Triglycerides (mg/dL)	−0.006	0.734
Uric acid (mg/dL)	−0.287	<0.001
Hb (g/dL)	−0.148	<0.001

All values are expressed as mean ± SD.
Abbreviations and symbols: eGFR, estimated glomerular filtration rate; Δ, change in the variable over 2 years; β, standardized regression coefficient; MetS, metabolic syndrome; BMI, body mass index; BP, blood pressure; FPG, fasting plasma glucose; HbA$_{1c}$, hemoglobin A$_{1c}$; HDL, high density lipoprotein; LDL, low density lipoprotein; Hb, hemoglobin.

Table 3. Multiple regression models for factors related to ΔeGFR.

Risk factors	ΔeGFR							
	Model 1 ($R^2 = 0.105$)		Model 2 ($R^2 = 0.102$)		Model 3 ($R^2 = 0.097$)		Model 4 ($R^2 = 0.94$)	
	β	P value	β	P value	β	P value	β	P value
Δ								
BMI (kg/m²)	0.056	0.007	0.056	0.006				
Systolic BP (mmHg)	0.046	0.067	0.047	0.060				
Diastolic BP (mmHg)	−0.044	0.077	−0.046	0.068				
FPG (mg/dL)	−0.084	<0.001	−0.080	<0.001	−0.088	<0.001	−0.081	<0.001
HbA₁c (%)	−0.023	0.249	−0.021	0.290				
Total cholesterol (mg/dL)	0.142	0.014			0.111	0.007		
HDL-cholesterol (mg/dL)	−0.022	0.388	0.025	0.213				
LDL-cholesterol (mg/dL)	−0.147	0.006	−0.022	0.258	−0.110	0.006	−0.012	0.532
Triglycerides (mg/dL)	−0.012	0.625	0.022	0.255				
Uric acid (mg/dL)	−0.284	<0.001	−0.279	<0.001	−0.273	<0.001	−0.269	<0.001
Hb (g/dL)	−0.087	<0.001	−0.084	<0.001	−0.084	<0.001	−0.073	<0.001

Model 1: all variables, Model 2: all variables except total cholesterol, Model 3: significant variables in univariate analysis, Model 4: significant variables in univariate analysis except total cholesterol.
Abbreviations and symbols: eGFR, estimated glomerular filtration rate; Δ, change in the variable over 2 years; β, standardized regression coefficient; BMI, body mass index; BP, blood pressure; FPG, fasting plasma glucose; HbA₁c, hemoglobin A₁c; HDL, high density lipoprotein; LDL, low density lipoprotein; Hb, hemoglobin.

Table 4. Prevalence of hyperuricemia (male, n = 1,515; female, n = 1,257).

Gender	Baseline	2 years
Male, n (%)	191 (12.6)	194 (12.8)
Female, n (%)	12 (1.0)	12 (1.0)

Hyperuricemia: serum uric acid ≥7 mg/dL in males and ≥6 mg/dL in females.

recently, Iseki et al. [14] demonstrated that an increase in the serum uric acid level with or without hyperuricemia over a 10-year period was more closely related to eGFR decline than the baseline serum uric acid level or the presence of diabetes, and that an increase in uric acid levels within the normal range (N/N) was more closely associated with eGFR decline than the change in uric acid levels from normouricemia to hyperuricemia (N/H) or any variation within the hyperuricemic range (H/H) (decrease in eGFR per 1 mg/dL increase of serum uric acid levels was 4.19 mL/min/1.73 m^2 for N/N, 2.36 mL/min/1.73 m^2 for N/H, and 2.01 mL/min/1.73 m^2 for H/H). These results suggest that changes in eGFR related to the change in serum uric acid levels over several years may represent physiological variations, but it may also be an early indicator of renal dysfunction in a healthy middle-aged population.

Linear regression analysis revealed significant β values for changes in serum uric acid levels, hemoglobin, FPG, and BMI despite the relatively low coefficient of determination ($R^2 = 0.102$). As R^2 seemed to be relatively low because regression analysis included confounding variables for the change in eGFR, the change in serum uric acid levels (which showed the most negative β value of -0.279) was not sufficient to completely explain the change in eGFR. In other words, low R^2 values revealed that the change in eGFR was influenced by many confounding factors. However, this study demonstrated that the change in serum uric acid levels was the most sensitive factor for the change in eGFR among those evaluated in this population.

The association between elevated serum uric acid levels at baseline and progression of CKD has been reported previously [13,15–18]. A two-year study of Japanese residents of Okinawa revealed that a higher baseline serum uric acid level was associated with elevation of serum creatinine levels over 2 years [15]. Another Japanese study of healthy subjects with normal renal function and no proteinuria, who were not receiving medications for hypertension, diabetes, or hyperlipidemia, and who underwent annual health screening demonstrated that the baseline serum uric acid level was an independent predictor of future development of CKD (eGFR <60 mL/min/1.73 m^2) after a median of 4.6 years [16]. Moreover, an association has been reported between elevated serum uric acid levels and metabolic syndrome, which are known risk factors for CKD [7,9,10].

The current classification of hyperuricemia is based on the concept that this condition results from either overproduction of urate due to a metabolic disorder, underexcretion due to abnormal renal urate transport activity, or a combination of the two [19]. Underexcretion of urate was widely considered to be the main cause of elevation of the serum uric acid level associated with renal function decline; therefore, an elevated serum uric acid level has been found to be a marker for CKD rather than as a cause of CKD [20,21]. However, recent epidemiological studies have demonstrated that elevated serum uric acid levels are associated with the progression of renal disease in humans [13,15–18] and can accelerate renal disease in animals [22–24]. A 12-month

epidemiological study of general population without renal dysfunction revealed that serum uric acid levels were positively correlated with albuminuria, suggesting glomerular damage [25]. Animal studies have indicated that an elevated serum uric acid level may be directly toxic to the kidney [22–24]. Mild hyperuricemia may cause direct renal toxicity in rats, which was manifested by renal vasoconstriction, systemic hypertension, and tubulointerstitial injury via a crystal-independent mechanism [22]. Uric acid may have these effects through the inhibition of endothelial nitric oxide bioavailability, activation of the renin–angiotensin system, and/or a direct influence on endothelial and vascular smooth muscle cells [26–28]. This hypothesis was clinically supported by the report that elevation of uric acid levels was a risk factor for hypertension [29–31]. An ultrasonographic study of flow-mediated dilatation demonstrated that elevation of uric acid levels was an independent predictor of endothelial dysfunction in patients with CKD [32]. In addition, uric acid has been found to promote oxidative stress through the renin–angiotensin system in cultured human endothelial cells [33]. Two small, short-term, single-center studies have shown improved blood pressure control and the slowing of the progression of CKD after serum uric acid level reduction with allopurinol [34,35]. The association of uric acid with CKD in the above reports has suggested that uric acid may be directly toxic to the kidney, and that elevation of uric acid levels may exacerbate other factors that promote CKD such as hypertension. Uric acid may also be a risk factor for metabolic syndrome. Moreover, elevation of serum uric acid levels may be an independent risk factor for renal injury based on the above reports.

This study showed that elevation of BMI and FPG was associated with a decrease in eGFR. These have both been known as risk factors for CKD [2,6,36].

This study had some limitations. First, the subjects were limited to participants undergoing health screening at our center, suggesting that they may not be representative of the healthy Japanese population ≤50 years old. Second, the 2-year study period was too small to meaningfully assess changes in renal function because serum creatinine levels were only measured once a year. The impact of serum creatinine levels may be more than age on changes in eGFR (calculated from age and serum creatinine levels) over the 2-year period. Interpretation of serum creatinine levels can also be directly influenced by muscle mass, exercise, and fluid balance disorders such as dehydration. Third, the eGFR changed at a statistically significant level between baseline and 2-year follow-up values. Hemoglobin did not change significantly in this time frame. Nevertheless, there was a significant association between changes in hemoglobin and those in eGFR (table 1, 2). These changes could be within the respective biologic variation. A longer epidemiological study about changes in eGFR and other variables is needed for health screening. Fourth, some subjects had low eGFRs at baseline. A high serum creatinine level was previously reported to be >8.0% in a community-based study [37]. Finally, this study did not evaluate urate production or the influence of age on serum uric acid levels. In particular, dietary intake, including the amount and types of alcohol, should be evaluated as a confounding variable that can influence uric acid production. It has been reported that hyperuricemia was negatively correlated with age in men [38,39]. Thus, changes in the serum uric acid level may be somewhat augmented by age.

In conclusion, the changes in eGFR and other variables over 2 years were small and could be within expected biologic variation. A longer observational study is needed to elucidate whether FPG, serum uric acid and hemoglobin represent the earliest markers of eGFR decline.

References

1. Go AS, Chertow GM, Fan D, McCulloch CE, Hsu CY (2004) Chronic kidney disease and the risks of death, cardiovascular events, and hospitalization. N Engl J Med 351: 1296–1305.
2. Ninomiya T, Kiyohara Y, Kubo M, Tanizaki Y, Doi Y, et al. (2005) Chronic kidney disease and cardiovascular disease in a general Japanese population: the Hisayama Study. Kidney Int 68: 228–236.
3. Ryan TP, Fisher SG, Elder JL, Winters PC, Beckett W, et al. (2009) Increased cardiovascular risk associated with reduced kidney function. Am J Nephrol 29: 620–625.
4. Imai E, Horio M, Watanabe T, Iseki K, Yamagata K, et al. (2009) Prevalence of chronic kidney disease in the Japanese general population. Clin Exp Nephrol 13: 621–630.
5. Matsuo S, Imai E, Horio M, Yasuda Y, Tomita K, et al. (2009) Collaborators developing the Japanese equation for estimated GFR: Revised equations for estimated GFR from serum creatinine in Japan. Am J Kidney Dis 53: 982–992.
6. Yamagata K, Ishida K, Sairenchi T, Takahashi H, Ohba S, et al. (2007) Risk factors for chronic kidney disease in a community-based population: a 10-year follow-up study. Kidney Int 71: 159–166.
7. Choi HK, Ford ES (2007) Prevalence of the metabolic syndrome in individuals with hyperuricemia. Am J Med 120: 442–447.
8. Cirillo P, Sato W, Reungjui S, Heinig M, Gersch M, et al. (2006) Uric acid, the metabolic syndrome, and renal disease. J Am Soc Nephrol 17 (Suppl 3): S165–S168.
9. Ishizaka N, Ishizaka Y, Toda E, Nagai R, Yamakado M (2005) Association between serum uric acid, metabolic syndrome, and carotid atherosclerosis in Japanese individuals. Arterioscler Thromb Vasc Biol 25: 1038–1044.
10. Ford ES, Li C, Cook S, Choi HK (2007) Serum concentrations of uric acid and the metabolic syndrome among US children and adolescents. Circulation 115: 2526–2532.
11. Imai E, Horio M, Yamagata K, Iseki K, Hara S, et al. (2008) Slower decline of glomerular filtration rate in the Japanese general population: a longitudinal 10-year follow-up study. Hypertens Res 31: 433–441.
12. Kashiwagi A, Kasuga M, Araki E, Oka Y, Hanafusa T, et al. (2012) International clinical harmonization of glycated hemoglobin in Japan: From Japan Diabetes Society to National Glycohemoglobin Standardization Program values. J Diabetes Invest 3: 39–40.
13. Bellomo G, Venanzi S, Verdura C, Saronio P, Esposito A, et al. (2010) Association of uric acid with change in kidney function in healthy normotensive individuals. Am J Kidney Dis 56: 264–272.
14. Iseki K, Iseki C, Kinjo K (2013) Changes in serum uric acid have a reciprocal effect on eGFR change: a 10-year follow-up study of community-based screening in Okinawa, Japan. Hypertens Res 36: 650–654.
15. Iseki K, Oshiro S, Tozawa M, Iseki C, Ikemiya Y, et al. (2001) Significance of hyperuricemia on the early detection of renal failure in a cohort of screened subjects. Hypertens Res 24: 691–697.
16. Sonoda H, Takase H, Dohi Y, Kimura G (2011) Uric acid levels predict future development of chronic kidney disease. Am J Nephrol 33: 352–357.
17. Yamada T, Fukatsu M, Suzuki S, Wada T, Joh T (2011) Elevated serum uric acid predicts chronic kidney disease. Am J Med Sci 342: 461–466.
18. Weiner DE, Tighiouart H, Elsayed EF, Griffith JL, Salem DN, et al. (2008) Uric acid and incident kidney disease in the community. J Am Soc Nephrol 19: 1204–1211.
19. Ichida K, Matsuo H, Takada T, Nakayama A, Murakami K, et al. (2012) Decreased extra-renal urate excretion is a common cause of hyperuricemia. Nat Commun 764: 1–7.
20. Feig DI: Uric acid (2009) a novel mediator and marker of risk in chronic kidney disease? Curr Opin Nephrol Hypertens 18: 526–530.
21. Nashar K, Fried LF (2012) Hyperuricemia and the progression of chronic kidney disease: is uric acid a marker or an independent risk factor? Adv Chronic Kidney Dis 19: 386–391.
22. Mazzali M, Hughes J, Kim YG, Jefferson JA, Kang DH, et al. (2011): Elevated uric acid increases blood pressure in the rat by a novel crystal-independent mechanism. Hypertension 38: 1101–1106.
23. Mazzali M, Kanellis J, Han L, Feng L, Xia YY, et al. (2002) Hyperuricemia induces a primary renal arteriolopathy in rats by a blood pressure-independent mechanism. Am J Physiol Renal Physiol 282: F991–F997.
24. Sánchez-Lozada LG, Tapia E, Avila-Casado C, Soto V, Franco M, et al. (2002) Mild hyperuricemia induces glomerular hypertension in normal rats. Am J - Physiol Renal Physiol 283: F1105–F1110.
25. Suzuki K, Konta T, Kudo K, Sato H, Ikeda A, et al. (2013) The association between serum uric acid and renal damage in a community-based population: the Takahata study. Clin Exp Nephrol 17: 541–548.
26. Kang DH, Nakagawa T, Feng L, Watanabe S, Han L, et al. (2002) A role for uric acid in the progression of renal disease. J Am Soc Nephrol 13: 2888–2897.
27. Kang DH, Park SK, Lee IK, Johnson RJ (2005) Uric acid-induced C-reactive protein expression: implication on cell proliferation and nitric oxide production of human vascular cells. J Am Soc Nephrol 16: 3553–3562.
28. Khosla UM, Zharikov S, Finch JL, Nakagawa T, Roncal C, et al. (2005) Hyperuricemia induces endothelial dysfunction. Kidney Int 67: 1739–1742.
29. Nagahama K, Inoue T, Iseki K, Touma T, Kinjo K, et al. (2004) Hyperuricemia as a predictor of hypertension in a screened cohort in Okinawa, Japan. Hypertens Res 27: 835–841.
30. Sundström J, Sullivan L, D'Agostino RB, Levy D, Kannel WB, et al. (2005) Relations of serum uric acid to longitudinal blood pressure tracking and hypertension incidence. Hypertension 45: 28–33.
31. Forman JP, Choi H, Curhan GC (2007) Plasma uric acid level and risk for incident hypertension among men. J Am Soc Nephrol 18: 287–292.
32. Kanbay M, Yilmaz MI, Sonmez A, Turgut F, Saglam M, et al. (2011) Serum uric acid level and endothelial dysfunction in patients with nondiabetic chronic kidney disease. Am J Nephrol 33: 325–331.
33. Yu MA, Sánchez-Lozada LG, Johnson RJ, Kang DH (2010) Oxidative stress with activation of the renin-angiotensin system in human vascular endothelial cells as a novel mechanism of uric acid-induced endothelial dysfunction. J Hypertens 28: 1234–1242.
34. Siu YP, Leung KT, Tong MK, Kwan TH (2011) Use of allopurinol in slowing the progression of renal disease through its ability to lower serum uric acid level. Am J Kidney Dis 47: 51–59.
35. Badve SV, Brown F, Hawley CM, Johnson DW, Kanellis J, et al. (2011): Challenges of conducting a trial of uric-acid-lowering therapy in CKD. Nat Rev Nephrol 7: 295–300.
36. Ninomiya T, Kiyohara Y, Kubo M, Yonemoto K, Tanizaki Y, et al. (2006) Metabolic syndrome and CKD in a general Japanese population: the Hisayama Study. Am J Kidney Dis 48: 383–391.
37. Culleton BF, Larson MG, Evans JC, Wilson PW, Barrett BJ, et al. (1999) Prevalence and correlates of elevated serum creatinine levels: the Framingham Heart Study. Arch Intern Med 159: 1785–1790.
38. Nakanishi N, Tatara K, Nakamura K, Suzuki K (1999) Risk factors for the incidence of hyperuricaemia: a 6-year longitudinal study of middle-aged Japanese men. Int J Epidemiol 28: 888–893.
39. Nagahama K, Iseki K, Inoue T, Touma T, Ikemiya Y, et al. (2004) Hyperuricemia and cardiovascular risk factor clustering in a screened cohort in Okinawa, Japan. Hypertens Res 27: 227–233.

Acknowledgments

We would like to thank our Health Center staff for data collection, Hajime Yamakage (Satista Co., Ltd.) for the statistical support, and Enago for the English language review.

Author Contributions

Conceived and designed the experiments: MO HO. Performed the experiments: MO FD KI HI HS AS TS TY TK HO. Analyzed the data: MO FD AS. Wrote the paper: MO.

24

Hyponatremia as a Predictor of Mortality in Peritoneal Dialysis Patients

Tae Ik Chang[1], Yung Ly Kim[2], Hyungwoo Kim[2], Geun Woo Ryu[2], Ea Wha Kang[1], Jung Tak Park[2], Tae-Hyun Yoo[2], Sug Kyun Shin[1], Shin-Wook Kang[2,3], Kyu Hun Choi[2], Dae Suk Han[2], Seung Hyeok Han[2]*

[1] Department of Internal Medicine, NHIS Medical Center, Ilsan Hospital, Goyangshi, Gyeonggi-do, Republic of Korea, [2] Department of Internal Medicine, College of Medicine, Yonsei University, Seoul, Republic of Korea, [3] Brain Korea 21 for Medical Science, Severance Biomedical Science Institute, Yonsei University, Seoul, Republic of Korea

Abstract

Background and Aim: Hyponatremia is common in patients with chronic kidney disease and is associated with increased mortality in hemodialysis patients. However, few studies have addressed this issue in peritoneal dialysis (PD) patients.

Methods: This prospective observational study included a total of 441 incident patients who started PD between January 2000 and December 2005. Using time-averaged serum sodium (TA-Na) levels, we aimed to investigate whether hyponatremia can predict mortality in these patients.

Results: Among the baseline parameters, serum sodium level was positively associated with serum albumin ($\beta = 0.145$; $p = 0.003$) and residual renal function (RRF) ($\beta = 0.130$; $p = 0.018$) and inversely associated with PD ultrafiltration ($\beta = -0.114$; $p = 0.024$) in a multivariable linear regression analysis. During a median follow-up of 34.8 months, 149 deaths were recorded. All-cause death occurred in 81 (55.9%) patients in the lowest tertile compared to 37 (25.0%) and 31 (20.9%) patients in the middle and highest tertiles, respectively. After adjusting for multiple potentially confounding covariates, increased TA-Na level was associated with a significantly decreased risk of all-cause (HR per 1 mEq/L increase, 0.79; 95% CI, 0.73–0.86; $p < 0.001$) and infection-related (HR per 1 mEq/L increase, 0.77; 95% CI, 0.70–0.85; $p < 0.001$) deaths.

Conclusions: This study showed that hyponatremia is an independent predictor of mortality in PD patients. Nevertheless, whether correcting hyponatremia improves patient survival is unknown. Future interventional studies should address this question more appropriately.

Editor: Pasqual Barretti, Sao Paulo State University, Brazil

Funding: This work was supported by the Brain Korea 21 Project for Medical Science, Yonsei University, by a National Research Foundation of Korea (NRF) grant funded by the Korean government (MEST) (No. 2011-0030711), and by a grant of the Korea Healthcare Technology R&D Project, Ministry of Health and Welfare, Republic of Korea (A102065). The funders had no role in study design, data collection and analysis, decision to publish, or preparation of the manuscript.

Competing Interests: The authors have declared that no competing interests exist.

* Email: hansh@yuhs.ac

Introduction

Electrolyte handling is universally impaired in patients with chronic kidney disease (CKD) because of failing kidney function. Therefore, these patients are vulnerable to complications caused by electrolyte imbalance. Although this issue is partly resolved by dialysis treatment, patients with end-stage renal disease (ESRD) commonly suffer from electrolyte disturbances [1].

Hyponatremia, usually defined as a serum sodium concentration <135 mEq/L, is one of the most common electrolyte disorders and is believed to be an important risk factor for mortality in patients with many serious medical conditions including advanced heart failure or liver cirrhosis [2–5]. In these conditions, it is generally assumed that hyponatremia reflects the severity of the underlying disease rather than directly contributing to mortality. Hyponatremia is also common in CKD patients [1]. Moreover, recent studies have shown that lower serum sodium concentrations are associated with increased mortality in mainte-

nance hemodialysis (HD) patients and CKD patients prior to dialysis therapy [6–10]. However, the underlying mechanisms are complex and still need to be clarified. In addition, it is still uncertain whether hyponatremia itself can contribute to mortality or merely represents a surrogate marker for other unknown risk factors in chronic maintenance dialysis patients.

Although peritoneal dialysis (PD) is an established therapeutic modality in ESRD, characteristics of dialysis treatment clearly differ between PD and HD. In particular, serum levels of electrolytes fluctuate between dialysis sessions in patients receiving HD due to the intermittent nature of HD treatment, while these levels remain relatively stable in PD patients. This unique feature led us to investigate which factors are associated with hyponatremia and its clinical outcomes in patients chronic PD. To date, few studies have addressed this issue, in particular the relationship between serum sodium level and risk of death, in PD patients [11–15]. Therefore, the purpose of this study was to investigate whether hyponatremia can predict mortality in a large prospective cohort of incident patients undergoing PD.

Methods

Ethics statement

The study was carried out in accordance with the Declaration of Helsinki and approved by the Institutional Review Board of Ilsan Hospital Clinical Trial Center. We obtained informed written consent from all participants involved in our study.

Patients

The study population included 549 ESRD patients who started PD at Yonsei University Severance Hospital or NHIS Ilsan Hospital between January 2000 and December 2005. Exclusion criteria were 1) <18 years of age at initiation of PD, 2) follow-up duration less than 6 months, 3) prior history of HD or a kidney transplant before the initiation of PD, 4) recovery of kidney function, or 5) initiation of PD for other reasons such as acute renal failure or congestive heart failure. Therefore, this prospective observational study included a total of 441 incident patients (Figure 1).

Data collection

Demographic and clinical data were collected at the beginning of PD including age, gender, body mass index (BMI) calculated as weight/(height)^2, cause of ESRD, and presence of diabetes and coronary artery disease. Each subject was scored using the Charlson Comorbidity Index at the start of PD. This index is a scoring system that includes weight factors for important concomitant diseases [16,17]. All patients underwent urea kinetic studies within three months of PD initiation including Kt/V urea, normalized protein catabolic rate (nPCR), percentage of lean body mass (%LBM), PD ultrafiltration, and residual glomerular filtration rate (GFR). Residual GFR was calculated as the average urea and creatinine clearance from a 24-h urine collection [18]. nPCR was calculated by the methods described by Randerson et al. [19] and normalized to standard body weight (total body water/0.58). Total body water was estimated by Watson formula [20]. The %LBM was determined from creatinine kinetics according to Keshaviah et al. [21]. Laboratory data obtained at the time of dialysis adequacy measurement were considered baseline values and included serum sodium, potassium, and

bicarbonate concentrations, serum albumin, ferritin, and serum C-reactive protein (CRP) levels. All laboratory parameters were recorded longitudinally throughout the follow-up period, and were calculated as an average of the mean of measurements every 3-month period. Because dialysis adequacy is generally measured within the first month after starting dialysis therapy and every 6 month thereafter in our centers, time-averaged dialysis adequacy parameters were determined as an average of the mean of the measurements in every 6-month period. Serum sodium concentration was measured by an electrode-based method (UniCel DXC 800; Beckman Coulter, Inc., CA, USA) and was corrected for serum glucose level (in such a case of serum glucose above a normal of 100 mg/dL) using the following formula: Corrected sodium = measured sodium+0.016×(serum glucose−100) [22].

Study outcomes

Study participants were followed until December 31, 2011. The primary outcome parameters were all-cause, cardiovascular, and infection-related mortality.

Statistical analysis

All values are expressed as the mean ± standard deviation or percentages. Statistical analyses were performed using SPSS for Windows version 13.0 (SPSS, Inc., Chicago, IL, USA) and the software packages R version 3.0.2. Data were analyzed using Student's t–test and the Chi-square test, and ANOVA was used for multiple comparisons. The Kolmogorov-Smirnov test was used to determine the normality of the distribution of parameters. If data were not normally distributed, they were expressed as the median and interquartile range (or after log-transformation) and were compared using the Mann–Whitney test or Kruskal-Wallis test. Relationships between serum sodium and continuous variables were assessed using Pearson's correlation coefficient, and categorical variables were evaluated using Spearman's R test. Multiple linear regression analysis was performed to identify the determinants of serum sodium level.

Under conditions of competing risk, Kaplan-Meier analyses and traditional Cox regression models can produce misleading results, so corresponding competing risk methods were used [23–25]. The cumulative incidence of death was compared among 3 groups based on tertile of time-averaged serum sodium (TA-Na) levels (< 137, 137 to 139, and ≥139 mEq/L) using the K-sample test developed by Gray [23]. Data for switch to HD, kidney transplantation, and loss to follow-up were censored in the analysis. Patients who died within the first 3 months after converting to HD or receiving a kidney graft were considered deaths related to PD. To determine risk factors for mortality, multivariate Cox regression using methods of Fine and Gray [24] was performed, and four different models were constructed; Model 1 adjusted for epidemiologic parameters including age, sex, BMI, and Charlson Comorbidity Index score. Model 2 adjusted for all parameters in model 1 plus medication use including dose of furosemide, use of icodextrin, and use of high-glucose dialysate. Model 3 adjusted for all parameters in model 2 plus dialysis dose including PD ultrafiltration and total Kt/Vurea. Model 4 adjusted for all parameters in model 3 plus malnutrition-inflammatory parameters including serum potassium, serum bicarbonate, serum albumin, serum ferritin, CRP, residual GFR, nPCR, and %LBM. The results are expressed as a hazard ratio (HR) and 95% confidence interval (CI). First-order interaction terms between covariates were examined for all models, but there was no evidence of an interaction between those covariates. A p–value less than 0.05 was considered statistically significant.

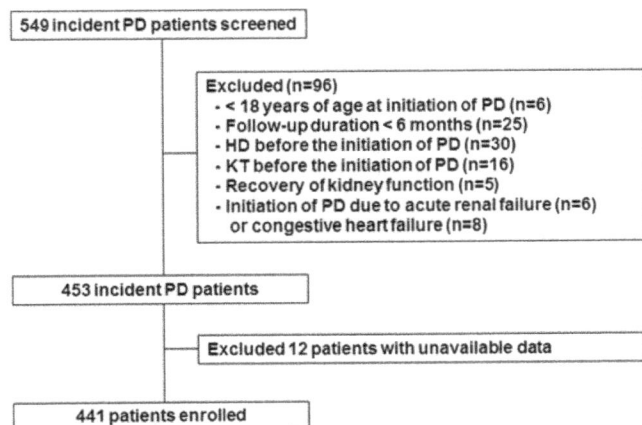

Figure 1. Flow chart of participants in the cohort. PD, peritoneal dialysis; HD, hemodialysis; KT, kidney transplant.

Table 1. Clinical characteristics of the study subjects stratified by time-averaged serum sodium level.

	Time-averaged serum sodium (mEq/L; number of subjects)				
	Total (n=441)	<137 (n=145)	137 to <139 (n=148)	≥139 (n=148)	p for trend
Age (years)	59.2±13.8	60.6±13.4	58.3±14.2	58.8±13.8	0.251
Gender (male)	240 (54.4)	76 (52.4)	79 (53.4)	85 (57.4)	0.388
Body mass index (kg/m²)	22.9±6.7	22.4±2.6	23.5±7.7	22.6±3.3	0.846
Presence of diabetes mellitus	227 (51.5)	73 (50.3)	73 (49.3)	81 (54.7)	0.446
Presence of coronary artery disease	70 (15.9)	27 (18.6)	24 (16.2)	19 (12.8)	0.176
Charlson Comorbidity Index score	3.0±1.0	3.2±1.0	3.0±1.1	3.0±0.9	0.065
Laboratory findings*					
Serum sodium (mEq/L)	137.7±2.7	134.5±2.1	138.0±0.6	140.3±0.9	<0.001
Serum potassium (mEq/L)	4.1±0.7	4.2±0.8	4.1±0.6	4.1±0.7	0.274
Serum bicarbonate (mEq/L)	25.9±2.4	25.7±2.3	26.1±2.3	26.0±2.5	0.206
Serum albumin (g/dL)	3.1±0.5	2.9±0.5	3.1±0.6	3.2±0.5	<0.001
Serum ferritin (ng/mL)	274.3 [52–521]	294.7 [52–509]	258.3 [59–521]	271.2 [56–514]	0.314
C-reactive protein (mg/dL)	0.7 [0.01–16.2]	0.8 [0.01–14.2]	0.4 [0.01–6.3]	0.8 [0.01–16.2]	0.623
Residual GFR (mL/min/1.73m²)*	4.0 [0.2–29.3]	3.9 [0.2–18.9]	4.0 [0.3–29.3]	4.4 [0.3–19.0]	0.004
Daily ultrafiltration (mL)*					
Peritoneal dialysis	731.6±569.3	811.2±601.6	751.2±563.1	634.1±531.4	0.008
Total	1827.6±691.4	1847.6±706.0	1794.2±700.2	1841.4±671.3	0.943
Automated peritoneal dialysis	5 (1.1)	1 (0.7)	2 (1.4)	2 (1.4)	0.594
Icodextrin use daily	35 (7.9)	25 (17.2)	10 (6.8)	0 (0.0)	<0.001
2.5% and/or 4.25% dialysate use daily	105 (23.8)	38 (26.2)	41 (27.7)	26 (17.6)	0.081
Total weekly Kt/V urea*	2.3±0.8	2.2±0.7	2.3±0.9	2.4±0.8	0.061
nPCR (g/Kg/day)*	0.9±0.3	0.9±0.3	0.9±0.3	1.0±0.2	0.012
Lean body mass (% body weight)*	66.4±12.4	61.4±11.9	66.8±13.8	67.4±14.2	<0.001
Anti-hypertensive medications					
ACE inhibitor or ARB	302 (68.5)	98 (67.6)	104 (70.3)	100 (67.6)	0.995
Alpha and/or beta blocker	217 (49.2)	72 (49.7)	78 (52.7)	67 (45.3)	0.450
Calcium channel blocker	265 (60.1)	86 (59.3)	91 (61.5)	88 (59.5)	0.981

Table 1. Cont.

	Time-averaged serum sodium (mEq/L; number of subjects)				
	Total (n = 441)	<137 (n = 145)	137 to <139 (n = 148)	≥139 (n = 148)	p for trend
Thiazide or thiazide-like diuretics	48 (10.9)	19 (13.1)	13 (8.8)	16 (10.8)	0.534
Lasix or other loop diuretics	200 (45.4)	64 (44.1)	71 (48.0)	65 (43.9)	0.966
Dose of furosemide (mg/day)	46.8±61.6	48.7±63.5	52.4±66.1	39.4±54.4	0.192

Values for categorical variables are given as number (percentage); values for continuous variables are given as mean ± standard deviation or median [interquartile range].

*Laboratory and dialysis-specific parameters are given as time-averaged values. GFR, glomerular filtration rate; nPCR, normalized protein catabolic rate; ACE, angiotensin converting enzyme; ARB, angiotensin receptor blocker.

Results

Patient characteristics

The mean age of the patients was 59.2 years (range, 22 to 85 years), 54.4% were males, and patients were on PD for a mean duration of 43.2 months (range, 6 to 142 months). The mean baseline and TA-Na levels were 138.2±3.7 mEq/L and 137.7±2.7 mEq/L (median, 138.1 mEq/L; range, 126.2 to 143.1 mEq/L) respectively. Table 1 details the baseline characteristics of the 441 patients categorized by tertile of TA-Na level. Serum albumin (p for trend <0.001), residual GFR (p for trend = 0.004), nPCR (p for trend = 0.012), and %LBM (p for trend <0.001) were higher at higher TA-Na level, whereas PD ultrafiltration (p for trend = 0.008) and use of icodextrin (p for trend <0.001) were lower at higher TA-Na level. However, we observed no significant differences in the types of antihypertensive agents, dosage of furosemide used, or use of high-glucose dialysate according to TA-Na level.

Factors associated with baseline serum sodium

Correlation analyses were performed to identify factors associated with baseline serum sodium level (Table 2). There was no correlation between age, gender, BMI, Charlson Comorbidity Index score, serum potassium, serum CRP, total Kt/V urea, nPCR and serum sodium. In contrast, baseline serum sodium level positively correlated with serum albumin ($\rho = 0.177$; $p<0.001$), residual GFR ($\rho = 0.211$; $p<0.001$), and %LBM ($\rho = 0.109$; $p = 0.022$), whereas it inversely correlated with serum ferritin level ($\rho = -0.133$; $p = 0.005$) and PD ultrafiltration ($\rho = -0.169$; $p<0.001$). A multivariate linear regression analysis that was adjusted for these factors revealed that serum albumin ($\beta = 0.145$; $p = 0.003$), residual GFR ($\beta = 0.130$; $p = 0.018$), and PD ultrafiltration ($\beta = -0.114$; $p = 0.024$) were independently associated with baseline serum sodium.

Hyponatremia as a predictor of mortality

During follow-up, 149 deaths were recorded, and the median survival period was 34.8 months (range, 6.0 to 142.2 months). Infection (37.6%) was the most common cause of death in this study, followed by cardiovascular disease (36.2%). All-cause death occurred in 81 (55.9%) patients in the lowest tertile compared with 37 (25.0%) and 31 (20.9%) patients in the middle and highest tertiles ($p<0.001$), respectively. Similar findings were observed for cardiovascular and infection-related deaths (data not shown).

Higher TA-Na was associated with lower mortality (Table 3). Even after adjusting for various parameters, the association between the two was significant and consistent. Using serum TA-Na as a continuous variable, the HR for all-cause mortality was 0.79 for every 1 mEq/L increase in TA-Na (95% CI, 0.73–0.86; $p<0.001$), indicating that higher TA-Na was significantly associated with decreased risk of mortality. Moreover, the increased mortality risk associated with lower TA-Na was similar for infection-related (HR, 0.77 per 1 mEq/L higher TA-Na; 95% CI, 0.70–0.85; $p<0.001$) death. In addition, patients with TA-Na<137 mEq/L conferred a 3.35- and 3.18-fold increased risk of all-cause and infection-related mortality, respectively, compared with patients with TA-Na≥139 mEq/L. However, the risk for cardiovascular death was not associated with TA-NA levels. The cumulative incidence of death was significantly lower in patients with higher TA-Na level compared to patients with a TA-Na level <137 mEq/L (Figure 2).

Discussion

In this study, we sought to delineate the relationship between serum sodium level and mortality in our ESRD cohort of patients with PD. We showed that serum sodium level exhibited a significant positive association with serum albumin and residual renal function (RRF), while it inversely correlated with PD ultrafiltration. In addition, low TA-Na level independently predicted all-cause mortality, suggesting that hyponatremia is a potential predictor of adverse outcomes in these patients.

Serum sodium concentration in humans is tightly regulated and the presence of hypotonic hyponatremia implies that the extracellular fluid compartment contains water in excess of sodium. Interestingly, the kidneys' ability to dilute urine, that is to elaborate urine with minimal osmolality, is generally preserved even in advanced CKD. However, its ability to concentrate is, indeed, severely limited in these patients [26]. Furthermore, in ESRD patients, water and sodium removal are almost exclusively determined by dialysis procedure, particularly when accompanied by complete loss of RRF. Therefore, dialysis-dependent patients are vulnerable to develop dysnatremia. However, the clinical impact of hyponatremia in these patients has been inadequately studied.

Table 2. Cross-sectional correlation analyses between baseline serum sodium level and patient characteristics.

		Serum Na	Age	BMI	CCI	K	Albumin	Ferritin*	CRP*	Residual GFR*	PD UF	Total Kt/Vurea	nPCR	LBM
Serum Na	ρ	1												
	p	-												
Age	ρ	−0.047	1											
	p	0.329	-											
BMI	ρ	0.072	−0.019	1										
	p	0.129	0.695	-										
CCI	ρ	−0.058	0.041	0.083	1									
	p	0.223	0.695	0.082	-									
K	ρ	0.022	−0.133	−0.007	0.021	1								
	p	0.640	0.005	0.880	0.659	-								
Albumin	ρ	0.177	−0.230	0.021	−0.058	0.031	1							
	p	<0.001	<0.001	0.661	0.226	0.510	-							
Ferritin*	ρ	−0.133	0.266	0.024	0.032	−0.140	−0.094	1						
	p	0.005	<0.001	0.609	0.508	0.003	0.048	-						
CRP*	ρ	0.006	0.261	−0.070	0.030	−0.070	−0.096	0.243	1					
	p	0.909	<0.001	0.161	0.542	0.162	0.053	<0.001	-					
Residual GFR*	ρ	0.211	−0.058	−0.039	−0.044	−0.003	0.145	−0.246	−0.070	1				
	p	<0.001	0.222	0.419	0.360	0.958	0.002	<0.001	0.158	-				
PD UF	ρ	−0.169	−0.026	0.026	0.126	0.121	−0.015	0.129	0.096	−0.365	1			
	p	<0.001	0.590	0.588	0.008	0.574	0.754	0.007	0.055	<0.001	-			
Total Kt/Vurea	ρ	0.068	0.033	−0.013	−0.019	−0.074	0.147	−0.088	0.047	0.533	0.065	1		
	p	0.156	0.489	0.780	0.697	<0.001	0.002	0.066	0.342	<0.001	0.171	-		
nPCR	ρ	0.054	−0.165	0.227	−0.020	0.152	0.271	−0.152	−0.114	0.238	0.067	0.451	1	
	p	0.260	<0.001	<0.001	0.675	0.001	<0.001	0.001	0.022	<0.001	0.067	0.157	-	
LBM	ρ	0.109	−0.458	−0.046	0.021	0.098	0.269	−0.218	−0.193	0.376	0.027	0.293	0.464	1
	p	0.022	<0.001	0.333	0.660	0.039	<0.001	<0.001	<0.001	<0.001	0.577	<0.001	<0.001	-

*Data for ferritin, CRP, and residual GFR were log-transformed.

BMI, body mass index; CCI, Charlson Comorbidity Index score; Na, sodium; K, serum potassium; tCO2, serum bicarbonate; CRP, C-reactive protein; GFR, glomerular filtration rate; PD UF, peritoneal dialysis ultrafiltration; nPCR, normalized protein, LBM, percentage of lean body mass.

Table 3. Multivariable Cox regression analyses for all-cause, cardiovascular, and infection-related mortality.

	Model 1			Model 2			Model 3			Model 4		
	HR	(95% CI)	p	HR	(95% CI)	p	HR	(95% CI)	p	HR	(95% CI)	p
Continuous model												
(per 1mEq/L TA-Na increase)												
All-cause mortality	0.78	(0.73–0.84)	<0.001	0.77	(0.72–0.83)	<0.001	0.78	(0.73–0.84)	<0.001	0.79	(0.73–0.86)	<0.001
Cardiovascular mortality	0.93	(0.84–1.02)	0.100	0.91	(0.82–1.00)	0.043	0.93	(0.84–1.02)	0.120	0.95	(0.84–1.08)	0.440
Infection-related mortality	0.78	(0.72–0.85)	<0.001	0.78	(0.72–0.85)	<0.001	0.78	(0.71–0.85)	<0.001	0.77	(0.70–0.85)	<0.001
Categorical (tertile) model												
All-cause mortality												
TA-Na<137 mEq/L	3.35	(2.15–5.24)	<0.001	3.70	(2.34–5.85)	<0.001	3.53	(2.23–5.60)	<0.001	3.35	(2.01–5.60)	<0.001
137 mEq/L≤TA-Na<139 mEq/L	1.13	(0.67–1.91)	0.640	1.16	(0.69–1.96)	0.570	1.12	(0.67–1.88)	0.660	1.17	(0.66–2.07)	0.600
TA-Na≥139 mEq/L	1.00	(reference)		1.00	(reference)		1.00	(reference)		1.00	(reference)	
Cardiovascular mortality												
TA-Na<137 mEq/L	1.82	(0.93–3.55)	0.079	2.09	(1.06–4.10)	0.033	1.90	(0.96–3.77)	0.067	1.70	(0.78–3.71)	0.180
137 mEq/L≤TA-Na<139 mEq/L	1.29	(0.64–2.61)	0.480	1.29	(0.63–2.61)	0.480	1.20	(0.59–2.45)	0.610	1.37	(0.64–2.92)	0.420
TA-Na≥139 mEq/L	1.00	(reference)		1.00	(reference)		1.00	(reference)		1.00	(reference)	
Infection-related mortality												
TA-Na<137 mEq/L	2.94	(1.65–5.26)	<0.001	3.05	(1.68–5.51)	<0.001	2.94	(1.60–5.41)	<0.001	3.18	(1.58–6.41)	0.0012
137 mEq/L≤TA-Na<139 mEq/L	0.79	(0.36–1.74)	0.560	0.81	(0.36–1.76)	0.570	0.79	(0.36–1.76)	0.570	0.78	(0.31–2.02)	0.610
TA-Na≥139 mEq/L	1.00	(reference)		1.00	(reference)		1.00	(reference)		1.00	(reference)	

TA-Na, time-averaged serum sodium; HR, hazard ratio; CI, confidence interval. Model 1 adjusted for epidemiologic parameters including age, sex, body mass index, and Charlson Comorbidity Index score. Model 2 adjusted for all model 1 parameters plus medication including dose of furosemide, use of icodextrin, and use of high glucose dialysate. Model 3 adjusted for all model 2 parameters plus dialysis dose including peritoneal dialysis ultrafiltration (PDUF) and total Kt/V urea. Model 4 adjusted for all model 3 parameters plus malnutrition-inflammatory parameters including serum potassium, serum bicarbonate, serum albumin, serum ferritin, C-reactive protein (CRP), residual glomerular filtration rate (GFR), normalized protein catabolic rate (nPCR), and percentage of lean body mass (%LBM). Laboratory (serum sodium, potassium, bicarbonate, albumin, ferritin, and CRP) and dialysis-specific (PDUF, Kt/V urea, residual GFR, nPCR, %LBM) parameters are given as time-averaged values.

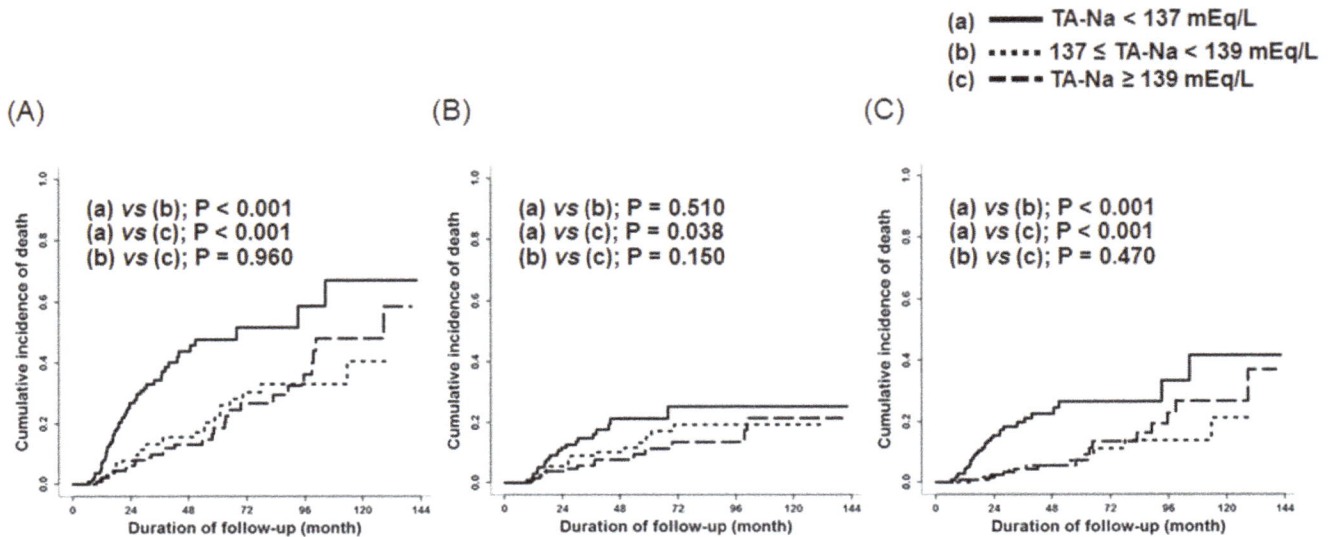

Figure 2. The Cumulative incidence of all-cause (A), cardiovascular (B), and infection-related (C) mortality based on the level of time-averaged serum sodium (TA-Na).

In our study, hyponatremia (defined as <135 mEq/L) was present in 58 patients (13.2%) at the initiation of PD. However, previous studies of PD patients have used a more strict definition of hyponatremia (defined as ≤130 mEq/L on 2 consecutive measurements) [13–15]. When we use this definition, 11 patients (2.5%) presented with hyponatremia at the start of PD. In addition, 21 patients (4.8%) developed hyponatremia during follow-up, which was comparable with the 5.2% of patients reported in a previous study by Zevallos et al. [13] but much lower than the 14.5% of patients observed in a recent study by Dimitriadis et al [14]. However, when we defined hyponatremia as <135 mEq/L, which is the threshold generally accepted in clinical practice, 115 patients (26.1%) developed hyponatremia during the follow-up period. These findings suggest that hyponatremia is common in PD patients, although the incidence may differ depending on the chosen definition.

The underlying mechanisms for hyponatremia in PD patients are complex and unclear. In general, as suggested by Edelman et al. [27], serum sodium concentration is determined by rapidly exchangeable body sodium, potassium, and total body water. Thus, hypotonic hyponatremia typically develops due to decrease in the fraction of body sodium and potassium over body water. Such reduction is potentially caused by various combinations of changes in body cations and water. In particular, the cation fraction can be often decreased in patients on dialysis because these patients are prone to fluid overload. In addition to this mechanism, dialysis-specific conditions should be taken into to explain hyponatremia in dialysis patients. Of note, therapeutic modality itself such as diffusive transport, convective transport, and ultrafiltration can induce the changes of body cations and water and thus results in altered serum sodium concentrations in PD patients [28]. Therefore, in patients on PD, alterations in serum sodium concentrations can occur as a result of the dialytic and nondialytic changes in the mass balance of body sodium, body potassium, and body water.

In addition, osmotic shift of water from the intracellular into the extracellular compartment and intracellular entry of sodium are putative mechanisms of PD-associated hyponatremia in certain clinical states, including potassium deficit, protein-energy wasting

(PEW) and use of icodextrin solutions as PD dialysate [13,29–31]. However, although there is evidence suggesting that entry of extracellular sodium into the cells causes hyponatremia in various settings [13,29–31], hyponatremia is unlikely to occur unless such a shift is accompanied by imbalances of monovalent cations and water that decrease the cation fraction as aforementioned.

The most important finding in this study is the strong and significant association between lower serum sodium concentration and mortality in PD patients. This association has previously been shown in maintenance dialysis patients and CKD patients prior to dialysis therapy [6–10,12,15]. In keeping with these, our robust finding supports evidence that hyponatremia portends a poor prognosis in these patients. In multivariate models with rigorous adjustments, low serum sodium concentration remained an independent predictor of mortality. In addition, patients with TA-Na level <137 mEq/L had adjusted HRs for all-cause, and infection-related mortality of 3.35 and 3.18, respectively, compared to the reference group with TA-Na level ≥139 mEq/L, indicating that higher serum sodium level is associated significantly with lower mortality risk. Relevant to our finding is a recent observation in HD patients based on data from the Dialysis Outcomes and Practice Pattern Study, showing that patients with mean serum sodium level <137 mEq/L had a 45% higher risk of death compared with patients with serum sodium ≥140 mEq/L [7].

The underlying mechanisms for increased mortality in advanced CKD patients with lower serum sodium level are also unclear. In severely ill patients without CKD, vasopressin is secreted in response to neurohormonal activation. Whether vasopressin contributes to the development of hyponatremia in patients with CKD is largely unknown. Possibly, vasopressin could explain the association between hyponatremia and mortality in this population if it acts in the same manner as in non-CKD patients with serious underlying conditions [32]. In addition, hyponatremia is related to other adverse features. In particular, reduced RRF may limit free water clearance, resulting in hyponatremia. Interestingly, RRF was identified as a significant factor associated with baseline serum sodium in this study; higher residual GFR was independently associated with a higher serum sodium concentration. This finding suggests that residual kidney function even in the advanced stage can contribute to sodium handling and prevent hyponatremia by excreting relatively more water than sodium. Conversely, loss of RRF in the end may result in inability to control excess water, leading to hyponatremia. Furthermore, PEW status may affect sodium level by depleting intracellular potassium and solutes [13,29]. In the present study, there were significant associations between serum sodium level and some nutritional markers such as serum albumin and %LBM. If this is the case, low sodium level can represent underlying unfavorable conditions. Finally, inflammatory response has recently been suggested as a cause of hyponatremia [33–35]. Among many inflammatory markers, interleukin-6 is reported to induce central vasopressin secretion [35]. Of note, loss of RRF, PEW, and inflammation are established predictors of mortality in patients on dialysis [36–38], and all of the aforementioned mechanisms together may account for the association between hyponatremia and mortality in these patients.

There are several limitations to the present study. This was an observational study with a relatively small sample size. Hence, causality of our findings needs further confirmation. In particular, there has been much concern about whether hyponatremia directly causes death or is merely a marker of disease severity. Furthermore, it is unknown whether correcting hyponatremia can improve clinical outcomes in CKD patients. A detailed discussion about these issues is beyond our scope. However, it is likely that hyponatremia can occur in severe underlying conditions and may itself further increase the risk of adverse outcomes. Lack of

information to further explain hyponatremia is another drawback. Because this was an observational study, we could not collect data describing the amount of sodium removed by PD or the amount being ingested in the diet. Other data representing overall volume status such as body weight changes, dietary water intake, and a bioelectrical impedance analysis were not available for analysis. Despite these limitations, this study showed that low TA-Na level independently predicted all-cause and infection-related mortality, even after extensive adjusting for demographic, clinical, laboratory, and dialysis-specific covariates. Our robust findings suggest that hyponatremia portends a poor prognosis, and thus physicians should be more meticulous in clinical practice with respect to correcting both this electrolyte imbalance and underlying disease.

Conclusion

This study showed that a low serum sodium concentration was an independent predictor of mortality in PD patients. The relationship between low serum sodium level and adverse outcomes may be attributed to loss of RRF and underlying conditions such as PEW. Whether correcting hyponatremia improves patient survival requires further investigations.

Author Contributions

Conceived and designed the experiments: TIC THY SKS SWK KHC DSH SHH. Performed the experiments: TIC YLK HWK GWR EWK JTP. Analyzed the data: TIC SHH. Contributed to the writing of the manuscript: TIC SHH.

References

1. Combs S, Berl T (2014) Dysnatremias in patients with kidney disease. Am J kidney Dis 63: 294–303.
2. Adrogue HJ, Madias NE (2000) Hyponatremia. N Engl J Med 342: 1581–1589.
3. Upadhyay A, Jaber BL, Madias NE (2006) Incidence and prevalence of hyponatremia. Am J Med 119 (suppl 1): S30–S35.
4. Arroyo V, Rodes J, Gutierrez-Lizarraga MA, Revert L (1976) Prognostic value of spontaneous hyponatremia in cirrhosis with ascites. Am J Dig Dis 21: 249–256.
5. Bettari L, Fiuzat M, Shaw LK, Wojdyla DM, Metra M, et al. (2012) Hyponatremia and long-term outcomes in chronic heart failure–an observational study from the Duke Databank for Cardiovascular Diseases. J Card Fail 18: 74–81.
6. Waikar SS, Curhan GC, Brunelli SM (2011) Mortality associated with low serum sodium concentration in maintenance hemodialysis. Am J Med 124: 77–84.
7. Hecking M, Karaboyas A, Saran R, Sen A, Hörl WH, et al. (2012) Predialysis serum sodium level, dialysate sodium, and mortality in maintenance hemodialysis patients: the Dialysis Outcomes and Practice Patterns Study (DOPPS). Am J Kidney Dis 59: 238–248.
8. Mc Causland FR, Brunelli SM, Waikar SS (2012) Dialysate sodium, serum sodium and mortality in maintenance hemodialysis. Nephrol Dial Transplant 27: 1613–1618.
9. Nigwekar SU, Wenger J, Thadhani R, Bhan I (2013) Hyponatremia, mineral metabolism, and mortality in incident maintenance hemodialysis patients: a cohort study. Am J Kidney Dis 62: 755–762.
10. Kovesdy CP, Lott EH, Lu JL, Malakauskas SM, Ma JZ, et al. (2012) Hyponatremia, hypernatremia, and mortality in patients with chronic kidney disease with and without congestive heart failure. Circulation 125: 677–684.
11. Lee HH, Choi SJ, Lee HN, Na SY, Chang JH, et al. (2010) De novo hyponatremia in patients undergoing peritoneal dialysis: A 12-month observational study. Korean J Nephrol 29: 31–37.
12. Kang SH, Cho KH, Park JW, Yoon KW, Do JY (2013) Characteristics and clinical outcomes of hyponatraemia in peritoneal dialysis patients. Nephrology (Carlton) 18: 132–137.
13. Zevallos G, Oreopoulos DG, Halperin ML (2001) Hyponatremia in patients undergoing CAPD: Role of water gain and/or malnutrition. Perit Dial Int 21: 72–76.
14. Dimitriadis C, Sekercioglu N, Pipili C, Oreopoulos DG, Bargman JM (2014) Hyponatraemia in peritoneal dialysis: Epidemiology in a single center and correlation with clinical and biochemical parameters. Perit Dial Int 34: 260–270.
15. Tseng MH, Cheng CJ, Sung CC, Chou YC, Chu P, et al. (2014) Hyponatremia is a surrogate marker of poor outcome in peritoneal dialysis-related peritonitis. BMC nephrol 15: 113.

16. Charlson ME, Pompei P, Ales KL, MacKenzie CR (1987) A new method of classifying prognostic comorbidity in longitudinal studies: development and validation. J Chronic Dis 40: 373–383.
17. Charlson M, Szatrowski TP, Peterson J, Gold J (1994) Validation of a combined comorbidity index. J Clin Epidemiol 47: 1245–1251.
18. Nolph KD, Moore HL, Prowant B, Meyer M, Twardowski ZJ, et al. (1993) Cross sectional assessment of weekly urea and creatinine clearances and indices of nutrition in continuous ambulatory peritoneal dialysis patients. Perit Dial Int 13: 178–183.
19. Randerson DH, Chapman GV, Farrell PC (1981) Amino acid and dietary status in CAPD patients, in Peritoneal Dialysis, edited by Atkins RC, Farrell PC, Thomson N, Edinburgh, Churchill- Livingstone. 180–191.
20. Watson PE, Watson ID, Batt RD (1980) Total body water volumes for adult males and females estimated from simple anthropometric measurements. Am J Clin Nutr 33: 27–39.
21. Keshaviah PR, Nolph KD, Moore HL, Prowant B, Emerson PF, et al. (1994) Lean body mass estimation by creatinine kinetics. J Am Soc Nephrol. 4: 1475–1485.
22. Katz MA (1973) Hyperglycemia-induced hyponatremia–calculation of expected serum sodium depression. N Engl J Med 289: 843–844.
23. Kim HT (2007) Cumulative incidence in competing risks data and competing risks regression analysis. Clin Cancer Res 13: 559–565.
24. Fine J, Gray R (1999) A proportional hazards model for the subdistribution of a competing risk. J Am Stat Assoc 94: 496–509.
25. Verduijn M1, Grootendorst DC, Dekker FW, Jager KJ, le Cessie S (2011) The analysis of competing events like cause-specific mortality–beware of the Kaplan-Meier method. Nephrol Dial Transplant 26: 56–61.
26. Hoorn EJ, Zietse R (2008) Hyponatremia revisited: translating physiology to practice Nephron Physiol 108: 46–59.
27. Edelman IS, Leibman J, O'Meara MP, Birkenfeld LW (1958) Interrelations between serum sodium concentration, serum osmolality and total exchangeable sodium, total exchangeable potassium and total body water. J Clin Invest 37: 1236–1256.
28. Nguyen MK, Kurtz I (2005) A new formula for predicting alterations in plasma sodium concentration in peritoneal dialysis. Am J Physiol Renal Physiol 288: F1113–F1117.
29. Cherney DZ, Zevallos G, Oreopoulos D, Halperin ML (2001) A physiological analysis of hyponatremia: implications for patients on peritoneal dialysis. Perit Dial Int 21: 7–13.
30. Posthuma N, ter Wee PM, Donker AJ, Oe PL, van Dorp W, et al. (1997) Serum disaccharides and osmolality in CCPD patients using icodextrin or glucose as daytime dwell. Perit Dial Int 17: 602–607.
31. Gokal R, Moberly J, Lindholm B, Mujais S (2002) Metabolic and laboratory effects of icodextrin. Kidney Int Suppl 81: S62–S71.

32. Hoorn EJ, Zietse R (2013) Hyponatremia and mortality: moving beyond associations. Am J Kidney Dis 62: 139–149.

33. Mandai S, Kuwahara M, Kasagi Y, Kusaka K, Tanaka T, et al. (2013) Lower serum sodium level predicts higher risk of infection-related hospitalization in maintenance hemodialysis patients: an observational cohort study. BMC Nephrol 14: 276.

34. Beukhof CM, Hoorn EJ, Lindemans J, Zietse R (2007) Novel risk factors for hospital-acquired hyponatraemia: a matched case-control study. Clin Endocrinol (Oxf) 66: 367–372.

35. Swart RM, Hoorn EJ, Betjes MG, Zietse R (2011) Hyponatremia and inflammation: the emerging role of interleukin-6 in osmoregulation. Nephron Physiol 118: 45–51.

36. Vilar E, Farrington K (2011) Emerging importance of residual renal function in end-stage renal failure. Semin Dial 24: 487–494.

37. Han SH, Han DS (2014) Nutrition in patients on peritoneal dialysis. Nat Rev Nephrol 8: 163–175.

38. Wang AY (2011) Consequences of chronic inflammation in peritoneal dialysis. Semin Nephrol 31: 159–171.

25

Sarcoidosis in Native and Transplanted Kidneys: Incidence, Pathologic Findings, and Clinical Course

Serena M. Bagnasco[1]*, Srinivas Gottipati[1], Edward Kraus[2], Nada Alachkar[2], Robert A. Montgomery[3], Lorraine C. Racusen[1], Lois J. Arend[1]

1 Department of Pathology, Johns Hopkins University, Baltimore, Maryland, United States of America, 2 Department of Medicine, Johns Hopkins University, Baltimore, Maryland, United States of America, 3 Department of Surgery, Johns Hopkins University, Baltimore, Maryland, United States of America

Abstract

Renal involvement by sarcoidosis in native and transplanted kidneys classically presents as non caseating granulomatous interstitial nephritis. However, the incidence of sarcoidosis in native and transplant kidney biopsies, its frequency as a cause of end stage renal disease and its recurrence in renal allograft are not well defined, which prompted this study. The electronic medical records and the pathology findings in native and transplant kidney biopsies reviewed at the Johns Hopkins Hospital from 1/1/2000 to 6/30/2011 were searched. A total of 51 patients with a diagnosis of sarcoidosis and renal abnormalities requiring a native kidney biopsy were identified. Granulomatous interstitial nephritis, consistent with renal sarcoidosis was identified in kidney biopsies from 19 of these subjects (37%). This is equivalent to a frequency of 0.18% of this diagnosis in a total of 10,023 biopsies from native kidney reviewed at our institution. Follow-up information was available in 10 patients with biopsy-proven renal sarcoidosis: 6 responded to treatment with prednisone, one progressed to end stage renal disease. Renal sarcoidosis was the primary cause of end stage renal disease in only 2 out of 2,331 transplants performed. Only one biopsy-proven recurrence of sarcoidosis granulomatous interstitial nephritis was identified.

Conclusions: Renal involvement by sarcoidosis in the form of granulomatous interstitial nephritis was a rare finding in biopsies from native kidneys reviewed at our center, and was found to be a rare cause of end stage renal disease. However, our observations indicate that recurrence of sarcoid granulomatous inflammation may occur in the transplanted kidney of patients with sarcoidosis as the original kidney disease.

Editor: Giovanni Camussi, University of Torino, Italy

Funding: The authors have no support or funding to report.

Competing Interests: The authors have declared that no competing interests exist.

* Email: sbagnas1@jhmi.edu

Introduction

Sarcoidosis is a systemic disorder of unclear etiology, which results from an abnormal cell-mediated immune reaction, and is characterized by non caseating granulomatous inflammation with epithelioid cells and multinucleated giant cells. Sarcoidosis affects individuals mostly in their third or fourth decades. Its incidence has been reported to be as high as 40 cases per 100,000 in Europe [1]. In the US population sarcoidosis is about three times more common in blacks than in white [2].

Sarcoidosis most commonly affects the lungs, but multiple organs such as the central nervous system, liver, heart, skin, and kidney can be involved.

Sarcoid involvement of the native kidney, in the form of granulomatous tubulointerstitial nephritis, is unusual, but its frequency is unclear, with estimates up to 30% of patients with this disorder in earlier studies [3] and as low as 0.7% in more recent reports [4,5]. It is also not clear how often renal sarcoidosis leads to end stage renal disease (ESRD).

Only a few cases of recurrent sarcoidosis with granulomatous inflammation in the transplanted kidney have been described [6,7,8,9]. A multicenter study from France [10], reported recurrence in the transplanted kidney of 3 recipients with sarcoidosis as the original disease.

The main objectives of this study were to evaluate the incidence of renal sarcoidosis in patients with diagnosis of systemic sarcoidosis and with kidney abnormalities requiring a kidney biopsies, its frequency as a cause of ESRD in transplant recipients, the incidence of recurrence of renal sarcoidosis in transplanted kidneys, and the overall frequency of interstitial granulomatous sarcoidosis in native kidney biopsies. To this end we searched the electronic medical records and the archives of the Department of Pathology at the Johns Hopkins Hospital over a period between 2000 and 2011. Our findings are described and discussed here.

The study was approved by the John Hopkins Institutional Review Board (protocol NA_00001141, which includes approval by Johns Hopkins IRB of a waiver of consent for subjects whose clinical information was used for studies covered by this protocol).

Methods

Patients

Computerized records were searched to identify kidney biopsies reviewed in the Department of Pathology at Johns Hopkins University from 1/1/2000 to 6/30/2011.

The demographic and clinical information provided at time of biopsy and afterwards were recorded, when available, for subjects with native kidney biopsies and for those with renal graft biopsies, and included: age at biopsy, gender, race, relevant past medical history, serum creatinine (mg/dL), urinalysis, pertinent serology tests, clinical course and follow up (when documented).

GFR was estimated according to the MDRD calculation [11].

Biopsies

Native kidney biopsies were processed for light microscopy, immunofluorescence and electron microscopy. Special stains of sections from paraffin embedded tissue such as Grocott methenamine silver, and stain for Acid Fast Bacilli were performed to rule out fungi and mycobacteria. Kidney allograft biopsies were stained for C4d as previously described [12,13] and graded for rejection according to the Banff classification [14,15].

Biopsies from patients with histologic findings of granulomatous inflammation were re-examined for this study by one nephropathologist (SMB).

Statistical analysis

Continuous variables with normal distribution were analyzed by un-paired, two-tailed Student's T test, with $P \leq 0.05$ as indicative of significant difference. Chi square test or Mann-Whitney test were used for categorical variables. Statistical analyses were performed with GraphPad Prism software, version 5 (GraphPad Software, Inc., San Diego, CA, USA).

Results

A total of 14,306 kidney biopsies were reviewed in the Department of Pathology at the Johns Hopkins Hospital between January 2000 to June 2011, of which 10,023 were from native kidneys, and 4,283 from kidney allografts.

A diagnosis of sarcoidosis was reported in the medical history of 52 patients who had renal/urinary abnormalities requiring native or allograft kidney biopsy, with a total of 57 kidney biopsies performed on these subjects. The demographic data in Table 1 show that age ranged from 20 to 80 years at time of kidney biopsy, there was a higher proportion of females (57%), and a higher number of black individuals (73%).

In 51 patients with a history of sarcoidosis a biopsy of the native kidney was performed, the pathologic findings in these biopsies are listed in Table 2.

Interstitial nephritis was the main diagnosis in approximately half of these patients (27 cases, granulomatous and non granulomatous), the remaining patients showed renal lesions without no obvious association with sarcoidosis. Granulomatous interstitial nephritis as the manifestation of renal sarcoidosis was identified in 19 of these biopsies, in which infections, drug reactions, and Wegener' granulomatosis could be ruled out. This is equivalent to a frequency of 0.18% of this diagnosis in a total of 10,023 biopsies from native kidney reviewed at our institution.

There were no distinct demographic or clinical features in those patients with granulomatous interstitial involvement by sarcoidosis, compared to those with a history of sarcoidosis but without renal granulomatous inflammation.

The 19 patients with a biopsy-proven granulomatous sarcoidosis in the native kidney had abnormal serum creatinine: 3.96 ± 2.35 mg/dl (average $\pm$ SD; range 1.9–9 mg/dl). Proteinuria was known to be present in 12 patients, ranging from trace to 2.5 g/24 hours, it was quantified in 8 patients with an average of 0.94 ± 0.65 g/24 hours. Hypercalcemia was present in 7 of 19 patients but only 3 had evidence of microcalcifications in the kidney biopsy.

Histologic evaluation of these 19 biopsies showed that the non caseating granulomatous inflammation was usually extensive, involving more than 50% of the kidney sample in 16 biopsies (figure 1). Most biopsies showed only rare eosinophils, and only 3 biopsies showed eosinophils present in more than one cluster with >4 eosinophils per high power field, usually embedded in the granulomatous inflammation. There was more than 50% global glomerulosclerosis in 7 biopsies. Tubulointerstitial scarring involving more than 50% of the sampled kidney was identified in 12 biopsies.

Only limited data on follow up were available in 10 patients with renal granulomatous sarcoidosis in the native kidney (Table 3). The patients with this lesion were treated with doses of prednisone ranging from 25 to 80 mg/day, tapered or suspended within one to three years, with general improvement of renal function, although in 4 patients with more than 50% tubulointerstitial scarring serum creatinine did not return to previous baseline level, and one patient progressed to ESRD requiring dialysis.

In order to estimate how often sarcoidosis appears as a primary cause of ESRD in our center we reviewed our transplant database and the electronic medical records of the transplant recipients searching for the original renal disease in the native kidney.

From 2000 to the end of 2010, a total of 2,331 patients received a kidney transplant at the Comprehensive Transplant Program at

Table 1. Characteristics of all patients with a diagnosis of sarcoidosis, in whom a biopsy from native or transplanted kidney was performed.

Patient number	52
Gender: Male/Female	22/30
Age at time of biopsy	50±13
Race: Black/White (N)	31/11 (42)
Hypertension	21
Diabetes	12

Values are presented as Mean ± SD. (N) indicates the number of patients for whom this information was available.

Table 2. Main histological diagnoses in 56 native kidney biopsies from 51 patients carrying a diagnosis of sarcoidosis.

Diagnosis	N
Granulomatous interstitial nephritis*	19
Interstitial nephritis without granuloma	8
Diabetic nephropathy	7
Focal Segmental Glomerulosclerosis	6
Chronic/Advanced sclerosing changes**	6
Immune complex mediated glomerulonephritis	3
Acute tubular injury	3
Amyloid	1
Membranous glomerulopathy	1
Thin glomerular basement membrane disease	1
Non specific changes	1

*A diagnosis of granulomatous interstitial nephritis consistent with renal sarcoidosis was rendered when other potential differential diagnoses (drug reactions, bacterial, mycobacterial and fungal infections, de novo or recurrent Wegener' granulomatosis, foreign body reaction) could be excluded.
**This category includes: Severe global glomerulosclerosis; Tubulointerstitial scarring; Hypertensive nephrosclerosis; Transplant glomerulopathy with tubulointerstitial scarring.

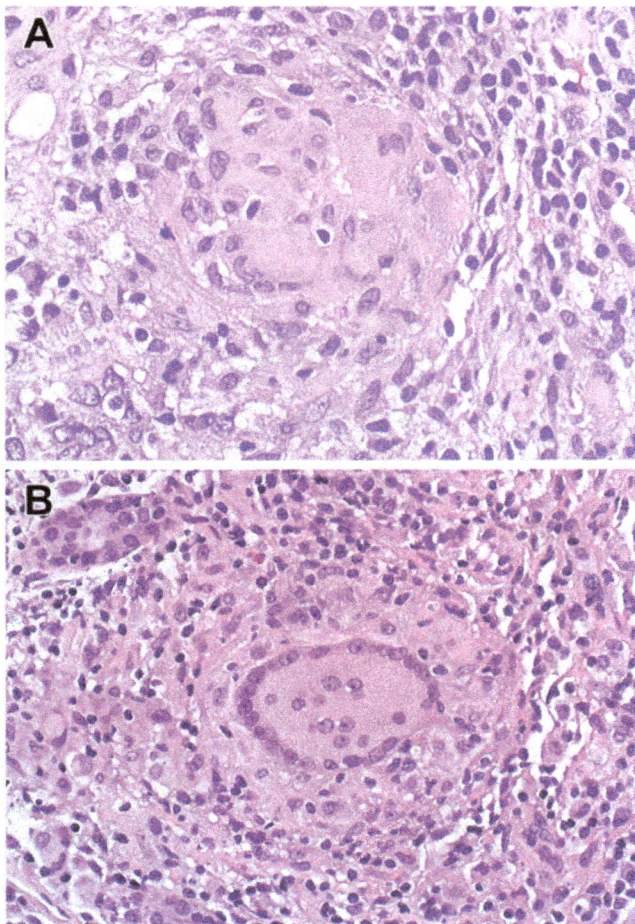

Figure 1. Moderate to severe interstitial inflammation with non caseating granuloma in renal sarcoidosis (A). Multinucleated cells in granulomatous inflammatory infiltrate in renal sarcoidosis (B).

the Johns Hopkins Hospital. The immunosuppressive regimen included induction with either daclizumab or ATG, tacrolimus, mycophenolate, and steroids. Episodes of cellular rejection (both clinical and subclinical) with Banff grades of 1A or 1B were treated with a 3-day pulse of dexamethasone 100 mg/day followed by a taper. If the Banff score was 2A, 2B, or 3 patients received a 7-day course of anti-thymocyte globulin. Both clinical and sub-clinical C4d positive AMR in the presence of DSA was treated with plasmapheresis/IVIg.

A clinical history of systemic sarcoidosis was recorded for 4 kidney transplant recipients. All had inactive disease at the time of transplantation. Two had previous history of lung sarcoidosis, but the cause of ESRD was hypertensive nephrosclerosis. Only two patients (one black female, and one white female) had sarcoidosis in lung and kidney, and lost their native kidneys due to renal sarcoidosis. This suggests that the frequency of sarcoidosis as primary cause of renal failure leading to ESRD could be estimated as less than 1 in 1000 in patients who received a transplanted kidney. Post-transplant, the maintenance immunosuppression may reduce the risk of recurrence of sarcoidosis in transplant recipients.

Review of the transplant outcome in these 4 patients revealed that one lost the graft to chronic changes unrelated to sarcoidosis after 12 years, requiring hemodialysis. Recurrent renal sarcoidosis was detected in a single patient, a 51 year old Caucasian female who had been diagnosed with sarcoidosis at the age of 47, with involvement of the lungs, CNS, and kidney (biopsy-proven) by granulomatous disease, treated with Prednisone 5 mg, and Azathioprine 75 mg daily, and quiescent at the time of transplantation. She received a pre-emptive, HLA-compatible live donor kidney, requiring no pre-transplant desensitization, and with immediate function, resulting in a stable serum creatinine of 1.2 mg/dL (eGFR 48 mL/min/1.73 m^2). Induction immunosuppression consisted of basiliximab, followed by post-transplant standard maintenance immunosuppressive regimen with Prednisone 5 mg once a day, Tacrolimus 0.5 mg twice a day and Mycophenolate 500 mg twice a day. Recurrence was discovered in an incidental kidney biopsy performed at 17 months post-transplant during a hernia surgical repair, with no evidence of active sarcoidosis, no urinary infections, and stable eGFR 47 mL/min/1.73 m^2. The biopsy showed tubulointerstitial granulomatous

Table 3. Follow up summary for patients with renal granulomatous sarcoidosis in the native kidney.

Patients	10
Gender F/M	5/5
Race B/W	7/3
Age years	49±14 (50)
Serum Creatinine, mg/dl	
Baseline	1.6±0.5 (1.4)
At biopsy	4.3±2.6 (3.0)
At last FU	2.4±1.6 (1.8)
Prednisone mg/day	50±17 (50)
Years of treatment	1.5±0.8 (1.0)
Total FU years	3.0±3.1 (1.7)
ESRD	1

Data are shown as Mean ± SD (Median).

inflammation, with negative C4d, and was interpreted as most consistent with recurrent sarcoidosis, although it was not possible to completely rule out a component of cell mediated rejection (Banff score: g0, i3, t3, v0, ah0, cg0, ci3, ct3, cv1, mm2, ptc undetermined, C4d0, ti3). She was treated for 5 days with Prednisone 80 mg per day, eventually tapered to a maintenance dose of 15 mg per day, while continuing Mycophenolate 500 mg three times per day, and Tacrolimus 1 mg two times per day. The increased immunosuppression was complicated by Herpes virus esophagiitis, and Cytomegalovirus infection, resolved with antiviral treatment, and resolution of infection (eGFR of 34 mL/min/1.73 m^2 six months later).

Discussion

The main objectives of this study were to evaluate the incidence of granulomatous tubulointerstitial nephritis in patients with a diagnosis of sarcoidosis; the overall frequency of this diagnosis in native kidney biopsies; the frequency of sarcoidosis as the primary kidney disease leading to ESRD; the incidence of recurrence of renal sarcoidosis in transplanted kidneys.

We found that among patients with a clinical history of sarcoidosis and evidence of renal disease requiring a native kidney biopsy 37% had granulomatous interstitial nephritis.

The demographic characteristics of our cohort of patients with a history of sarcoidosis showed a prevalence of female gender (57%) matching previously observed gender distribution [16], and a significantly higher proportion of black individuals (73%), reflecting estimates that in the US population sarcoidosis is three times more common in blacks (35.5 per 100,000) than in whites (10.0 per 100,000) [2].

Clinical information available on these patients shows that hypercalcemia was present in 7 (21%) of patients with a history of sarcoidosis, similar to previous estimates [17]. However only 3 of these individuals showed sparse microcalcifications in their kidney biopsies.

Granulomatous interstitial nephritis by itself is rare in biopsies from both native kidneys [18,19], and from transplanted kidneys [20], with an overall estimated occurrence of <1% biopsies. In our center the incidence of this pathologic finding is also very low 0.48% (unpublished observation), consistent with previous reports. In this study, the frequency of granulomatous inflammation ascribable to sarcoidosis in native kidney biopsies appears even lower: 0.18% of 10,023 diagnostic biopsies from native kidney reviewed at our institution.

Given the limited follow up information on the patients with biopsy-proven renal granulomatous sarcoidosis in the native kidney it is not possible to comment on specific characteristics that may influence the course of this renal lesion, except that tubulointerstitial scarring may indicate poor prognosis.

At time of diagnosis serum creatinine was noted to be abnormal in most of these patients, some presenting with acute kidney injury. In some, the possibility that a component of tubulointerstitial damage could be associated with pharmacologic treatment was entertained in the differential diagnosis. Such possibility should be considered in the therapeutic approach in these cases.

It is not clear how many patients with renal sarcoidosis progress to end stage renal disease. In this study, 3 or 5% of a total of 55 patients (including 51 patients with native kidney biopsies and 4 transplant recipients) with a diagnosis of systemic sarcoidosis progressed to ESRD, slightly higher but similar to an estimated 2% reported in a French cohort [21].

Recurrence of renal sarcoidosis post transplantation was documented in only one out of two transplant recipients with ESRD due to sarcoidosis at our center in the past ten years, and was detected 17 months after transplant as an asymptomatic lesion in an incidental biopsy.

Aside from few case reports, the recurrence of sarcoidosis in kidney transplant recipients was examined in a recent, retrospective, multicenter study from France, describing 10 patients with ESRD due to sarcoidosis, who received a kidney transplant [10]. Of these, 3 patients developed granulomatous tubulointerstitial nephritis in the renal graft, representing a 30% recurrence of renal sarcoidosis. The recurrence occurred within 18 months post-transplantation, while the patients were receiving a maintenance immunosuppression regimen including 5 mg prednisone per day. Treatment for recurrence consisted of increasing the corticosteroids dose from 0.3 to 0.5 mg/kg/day for 1 month, followed by a progressive tapering of the dose. The outcome was resolution with improved GFR for one patient, one patient progressed to renal graft failure, and the third patient died from a pulmonary embolism. Perhaps follow-up biopsies at one or two years post transplant may be indicated in to rule out "subclinical" recurrence in transplant recipient with renal granulomatous sarcoidosis as the original disease.

The clinical management and immunosuppression of these rare patients may be challenging. The available literature suggests that steroids should be maintained in the therapeutic regimen post-transplantation to prevent recurrence of disease [7,8,9]. Recently, monoclonal antibodies inhibiting interleukin 12, interleukin 23, and tumor necrosis factor alpha have been tested in patients with lung and/or skin sarcoidosis, however, the superiority of this treatment compared with steroids is unclear [22]. The recurrence in our patient was treated with an increased dose of steroids with subsequent decrease of her serum creatinine toward her baseline level. Over-immunosuppression should be avoided to reduce the risk of infection. Over-immunosuppression may have played a role in the lethal fungal infection of the pediatric patient reported by Vargas et al.[9]. The post-biopsy course of our index case suggests that development of CMV and HSV was temporally associated with the escalation in her steroids and other maintenance immunosuppression, and cause and effect relationship seems likely.

In summary, our study indicates that less than 1% of patients with renal abnormalities requiring a native kidney biopsy have a clinical history of sarcoidosis. Our observations on kidney biopsies suggest that in patients with history of sarcoidosis and renal dysfunction about one third shows pathologic manifestation of renal involvement by sarcoidosis as interstitial nephritis with granulomatous inflammation. Although renal involvement by sarcoid granulomatous interstitial nephritis is a rare primary cause of ESRD in transplant recipients, it can recur in the renal allograft.

Author Contributions

Conceived and designed the experiments: SB LJA. Analyzed the data: SB SG EK NA RAM LR LJA. Contributed to the writing of the manuscript: SB EK RAM LR.

References

1. Tekeste H, Latour F, Levitt RE (1984) Portal hypertension complicating sarcoid liver disease: case report and review of the literature. Am J Gastroenterol 79: 389–396.
2. Rybicki BA, Major M, Popovich J, Maliank MJ, Iannuzzi MC (1997) Racial Differences in Sarcoidosis Incidence: A 5-Year Study in a Health Maintenance Organization. American Journal of Epidemiology 145: 234–241.
3. Longcope WT, Freiman DG (1952) A study of sarcoidosis; based on a combined investigation of 160 cases including 30 autopsies from The Johns Hopkins Hospital and Massachusetts General Hospital. Medicine (Baltimore) 31: 1–132.
4. Baughman RP, Judson MA, Rossman MD, Yeager H Jr, Case Control Etiologic Study of Sarcoidosis (ACCESS) research group, et al. (2001) Clinical characteristics of patients in a case control study of sarcoidosis. Am J Respir Crit Care Med 164: 1885–1889.
5. Rossman KM (2007) Lesson learned from ACCESS (A Case Controlled Etiologic Study of Sarcoidosis). Proc Am Thorac Soc 4: 453–456.
6. Shen SY H-C, Posner JN, Shabazz B (1986) Recurrent sarcoid granulomatous nephritis and reactive tuberculin skin test in a renal transplant recipient. Am J Med 80: 699–702.
7. Brown JH, Newstead CG, Lawler W (1992) Sarcoid-like granulomata in a renal transplant. Nephrol Dial Transplant 7: 173–177.
8. Kukura S, Lácha J, Voska L, Honsová E, Teplan V (2004) Recurrence of sarcoidosis in renal allograft during pregnancy. Nephrol Dial Transplant 19: 1640–1642.
9. Vargas F, Craver RD, Matti Vehaskari V (2010) Recurrence of granulomatous interstitial nephritis in transplanted kidney. Pediatr Transplant 14: e54–e57.
10. Aouizerate J, Kamar N, Thervet E, Randoux C, Moulin B, et al. (2010) Renal transplantation in patients with sarcoidosis: a French multicenter study. Clin J Am Soc Nephrol 5: 2101–2108.
11. Levey AS, Bosch JP, Lewis JB, Greene T, Rogers N, et al. (1999) A More Accurate Method To Estimate Glomerular Filtration Rate from Serum Creatinine: A New Prediction Equation. Ann Intern Med 130: 461–470.
12. Bagnasco SM, Tsai W, Rahman MH, Kraus ES, Barisoni L, et al. (2007) CD20-Positive Infiltrates in Renal Allograft Biopsies with Acute Cellular Rejection Are Not Associated with Worse Graft Survival. American Journal of Transplantation 7: 1968–1973.
13. Bagnasco SM, Mani H, Gandolfo MT, Haas M, Racusen LC, et al. (2009) Oxalate deposits in biopsies from native and transplanted kidneys, and impact on graft function. Nephrol Dial Transplant 24: 1319–1325.
14. Solez K, Colvin RB, Racusen LC, Sis B, Halloran PF, et al. (2007) Banff '05 Meeting Report: Differential Diagnosis of Chronic Allograft Injury and Elimination of Chronic Allograft Nephropathy (CAN). American Journal of Transplantation 7: 518–526.
15. Racusen LC, Colvin RB, Solez K, Mihatsch MJ, Halloran PF, et al. (2003) Antibody-Mediated Rejection Criteria - an Addition to the Banff '97 Classification of Renal Allograft Rejection. Am J Transplant 3: 708–714.
16. Wirnsberger RM, Wouters EF, Drent M (1998) Clinical presentation of sarcoidosis in The Netherlands an epidemiological study. Neth J Med 53: 53–60.
17. Berliner AR, Choi MJ (2006) Sarcoidosis: the nephrologist's perspective. Am J Kidney Dis 48: 856–870.
18. Bijol V, Nosé V, Rennke HG (2006) Granulomatous interstitial nephritis: a clinicopathologic study of 46 cases from a single institution. Int J Surg Pathol 14: 57–63.
19. Joss N, Young B, Geddes C (2007) Granulomatous interstitial nephritis. Clin J Am Soc Nephrol 2: 222–230.
20. Meehan SM, Haas M (2000) Granulomatous tubulointerstitial nephritis in the renal allograft. Am J Kidney Dis 36: E27.
21. Mahévas M, Boffa JJ, Delastour V, Belenfant X, Chapelon C, et al. (2009) Renal sarcoidosis: clinical, laboratory, and histologic presentation and outcome in 47 patients. Medicine (Baltimore) 88.
22. Judson MA, Baughman RP, Costabel U, Drent M, Gibson KF, et al. (2014) Safety and efficacy of ustekinumab or golimumab in patients with chronic sarcoidosis. European Respiratory Journal.

26

Outcome of Patients with Primary Immune-Complex Type Mesangiocapillary Glomerulonephritis (MCGN) in Cape Town South Africa

Ikechi G. Okpechi[1]*, Thandiwe A. L. Dlamini[1], Maureen Duffield[2], Brian L. Rayner[1], George Moturi[3], Charles R. Swanepoel[1]

1 Division of Nephrology and Hypertension, Groote Schuur Hospital and University of Cape Town, South Africa, **2** Division of Anatomical Pathology, National Health and Laboratory Services (NHLS), University of Cape Town, South Africa, **3** Department of Medicine, Aga Khan University Hospital, Nairobi, Kenya

Abstract

Background and Aim: Mesangiocapillary glomerulonephritis (MCGN) is a common cause of chronic kidney disease in developing countries. Data on the renal outcome of patients with idiopathic MCGN is limited. The aim of this study is to investigate the outcome of patients with idiopathic MCGN presenting to the Groote Schuur Hospital (GSH) Renal Unit in Cape Town.

Materials and Methods: A retrospective study of patients with idiopathic MCGN followed up at our clinic. Seventy-nine patients with no identifiable cause of MCGN were included for analysis. A composite renal outcome of persistent doubling of serum creatinine or end stage renal disease (ESRD) was used. Kaplan Meier survival and Cox regression analysis were used to assess survival and identify factors predicting the outcome.

Results: The mean age at biopsy was 33.9±13.6 years and 41.8% were black. Mean duration of follow up was 13.5±18.8 months. Twenty-three patients (34.2%) reached the composite endpoint. Overall, median renal survival was 38.7±11.7 months (95% CI 15.7–61.8) with 2-year and 5-year renal survival of 61% and 40.3% respectively. No significant difference was found for renal survival between males and females, treatment or non-treatment with immunosuppression, presence or absence of crescents or histological type of MCGN ($p > 0.05$). On univariate Cox-regression analysis, factors found to be associated with the outcome were the estimated glomerular filtration rate at biopsy (OR 0.97 [95%CI: 0.95–0.99], $p < 0.0001$), black race (OR 3.03 [95%CI: 1.27–7.21], $p = 0.012$) and presence of interstitial fibrosis in the biopsy (OR 2.64 [95%CI: 1.07–6.48], $p = 0.034$). Age, systolic blood pressure and attaining complete or partial remission approached significant values with the endpoint.

Conclusions: The outcome of idiopathic MCGN in Cape Town is poor and requires further prospective studies to improve our understanding of this common disease.

Editor: Giuseppe Remuzzi, Mario Negri Institute for Pharmacological Research and Azienda Ospedaliera Ospedali Riuniti di Bergamo, Italy

Funding: The authors have no support or funding to report.

Competing Interests: The authors have declared that no competing interests exist.

* Email: Ikechi.Okpechi@uct.ac.za

Introduction

Mesangiocapillary glomerulonephritis (MCGN; also known as membranoproliferative GN [MPGN]) is a histological pattern of glomerular injury characterized by mesangial hypercellularity, increased mesangial matrix and thickening of glomerular capillary walls secondary to subendothelial deposition of immune complexes and/or complement factors, cellular entrapment, and new basement membrane formation [1,2]. MCGN has traditionally been divided into three distinct morphological types: type I (classical MCGN), is characterized by the presence of subendothelial deposits of immune complexes; type II MCGN (dense deposit disease), characterized by the presence of dense deposits in the basement membrane and type III MCGN, (considered as a variant of type I) and characterized by the presence of additional subepithelial deposits.

MCGN is a common cause of glomerulonephritis and the nephrotic syndrome in many low to middle income countries but especially in Africa [3–8]. In Romania, MCGN was the most frequent primary glomerulonephritis (GN) and was responsible for 29.4% of all primary glomerulonephritides reported from 1995 to 2004 [3]. In a previous study from our centre, we reported MCGN to account for 20.4% of all primary GN with 90.4% of cases being type I MCGN [6]. However, IgA nephropathy remains the most common primary glomerular disease reported from many developed countries where the occurrence of primary MCGN has steadily declined in recent decades [9–12]. Although the "hygiene hypothesis" [13,14] may explain some of the differences in prevalence of glomerular diseases seen in emerging and developed countries, results from recent research in this field has now made some authors to question the existence of idiopathic MCGN [15]. Their doubt is predominantly borne out of advances in methods of analysis of biopsy specimens and a more thorough and detailed evaluation of patients to identify possible causes of so-called idiopathic MCGN [15]. However, these studies have been published from high income countries where IgAN is still predominant. Sethi et al have therefore proposed a new classification for MCGN based on immune complex deposition (with or without complement) and sole complement deposition in the glomerulus denoting dysregulation of the alternative pathway of complement [16] (see Figure S1 and Figure 2).

The treatment recommendation of the KDIGO on the use of immunotherapies in idiopathic MCGN is only limited to cases in which crescents are present [17] and treatment of adults with the disease is often unrewarding as approximately 60% of patients will progress to end-stage renal disease (ESRD) within 10 years [18–20]. Given that so-called idiopathic MCGN is the most frequent primary GN seen in our population, the aim of this study is to report on the outcome of patients in Cape Town with idiopathic MCGN and to identify the factors that predict renal outcomes in such patients who are longitudinally followed up in our centre.

Materials and Methods

Ethics Statement

The study received approval from the Human Research Ethics Committee (HREC REF: 227/2012) of the University of Cape Town. All patient records/information was anonymized and de-identified prior to analysis.

Study population

Hospital records of patients who had a kidney biopsy performed between January 2000 to December 2011 and who were diagnosed with idiopathic MCGN and followed up at the renal clinic at Groote Schuur Hospital Cape Town were retrieved for retrospective collection of data. The written records and the electronic records of these patients were rigorously assessed in order to exclude patients with MCGN with possible secondary cause. All selected patients were proven to have tested negative for common viral infections (HIV, Hepatitis B and C), other commonly encountered infections (such as mycobacterium tuberculosis, syphilis) and autoimmune diseases (lupus and rheumatoid arthritis). As these patients were not acutely ill at presentation or showing evidence for any chronic infections, tests for malaria, schistosomiasis, leprosy among other possible infections that have been reported to be associated with MCGN were not performed; and although these infections are unusual in Cape Town, the patients never manifested any features of them during follow up. Serum protein electrophoresis, urine protein electrophoresis and bone marrow biopsy were not clinically indicated and were thus not performed in our patients. We identified 85 patients with complete records and with no known secondary causes of MCGN but excluded 6 patients whose biopsies only had C3 complement deposits alone.

Data Collection

Demographic, clinical and biochemical records of patients included in the study were obtained at the time of biopsy and during follow-up visits to the renal clinic. Data collected therefore included age at time of biopsy, gender, indication for biopsy, duration of follow up, serial recorded blood pressures (systolic and diastolic) and various laboratory measurements (serum albumin, creatinine, cholesterol, complements (C3 and C4 – expressed as normal or low) and proteinuria [g/24 hrs]. The racial grouping of our patient population was categorized as Black Africans and non-Black Africans (to include patients of mixed ancestry and Whites). The estimated glomerular filtration rate was calculated using the Modification of Diet in Renal Disease (MDRD) formula [21]. Treatment received by the patients was also recorded.

Histology

Light microscopic and immunohistochemical features of the renal biopsies were noted and recorded. Histological data collected included number of glomeruli per biopsy, percentage of sclerosed glomeruli reported, degree of interstitial fibrosis (none, mild, moderate or severe), presence of crescentic lesions and type of deposit present on immunohistochemical analysis (IgA, IgG, IgM or C3). All patients included had immune complex type MCGN (immune complex deposits were present with or without complement deposit) according to the newly proposed classification of Sethi et al [16]. Those with only C3 deposits were excluded in the analysis. Electron microscopic examination of all biopsy specimens was performed. All the histological specimens were reviewed by one pathologist (M.D.).

Definitions used in this study

Blood pressure. Hypertension was defined as systolic BP (SBP) persistently ≥140 mmHg and/or diastolic BP (DBP) ≥ 90 mmHg or if on treatment with anti-hypertensive medications [22]. Blood pressure at biopsy and average BP during follow up visits were recorded.

Remission. As there is no guideline for defining remission in MCGN, we used the following criteria and categorized patients into 3 groups: complete remission (CR), partial remission (PR) or no remission (NR) [23]:

- CR was defined as proteinuria of <0.2 g/day with stable eGFR if normal at baseline or increase in eGFR by 25% if abnormal at baseline.

- PR was defined as reduction in proteinuria (for proteinuria between 0.2 and 2.9 g) and stable eGFR if normal at baseline or increase in eGFR by 25% if abnormal at baseline.

- NR was defined as persistent proteinuria of ≥3 g/day or progressive or worsening renal impairment.

Study end-point

The composite end point of this study was persistent doubling of the serum creatinine over the baseline value or end-stage renal disease (ESRD). For patients who reached the end point, the period of follow-up was the interval between first renal biopsy and the time the end point was reached.

Statistics

The data were analyzed using IBM SPSS Statistics 21 software (SPSS, Chicago, IL). Categorical variables were presented as percentages and continuous variables as means ± SD. Comparison was made between those reaching the end-point and those not reaching the end-point using the Student's t-test, chi-square test or Fisher's exact test. Estimate of survival was done using the Kaplan–Meier survival method. Renal survival with time to ESRD was assessed using Kaplan–Meier estimates and log-rank test for comparison of survival estimates between groups. Univariate analysis was performed using Cox regression analysis to assess the association between relapse-free survival and explanatory variables. Significant P-value was taken as P<0.05.

Results

Baseline characteristics of the patients

There were a total of 79 patients eligible for inclusion in the study with renal biopsy diagnosis of MCGN and with no clinical or biochemical evidence for a secondary cause of MCGN. The mean age of all the patients was 33.9±13.6 years with 74.7% of the patients being males. Racial distribution of the subjects was 41.8%, 54.4% and 3.8% for blacks, patients of mixed ancestry and whites respectively. We observed that 20.3% of the patients were either actively abusing substance (predominantly methamphetamines – called "Tik" in Cape Town) or were referred to us from a correctional services department for treatment. Nephrotic syndrome was by far the most frequent indication for renal biopsy in 77.9%. Other features at time of biopsy are shown in Table 1.

Histological characteristics of the renal biopsies

Table 2 summarizes the histological features of the biopsies. The average number of glomeruli per biopsy was 16.5±10.5 with an average of 6.2% glomeruli reported as sclerosed. In 63.5% the interstitium was completely normal with no evidence of fibrosis at the time of biopsy; severe interstitial fibrosis was present in 4.1%. IgM deposits (59.4%) and C3 deposits (69.8%) were more frequently seen.

Comparison of the features of patients reaching or not reaching end-point

Twenty-three of 79 patients (34.2%) reached the end-point. There were more black African patients reaching end-point than non-black patients (60.9% vs 33.9%; p = 0.044). Average of all systolic and diastolic blood pressures during follow up visits were significantly higher in those who reached the end-point than in those who did not reach the end-point (p<0.05) (Table 3). However, SBP and DBP at initial presentation, although higher in those reaching the end-point were not significantly different. A significantly higher proportion of patients had attained a complete or partial remission at six months after diagnosis in those not reaching end-point than in those who did (36.2% vs 4.8%; p = 0.007).

The frequencies of immune (IgA, IgG and IgM) or complement (C3) deposits observed in the biopsies were not significantly different in both groups. Presence of any interstitial fibrosis (mild, moderate or severe) was significantly higher in the group reaching end-point (56.5% vs 30.4%; p = 0.041); although there were more patients in the group that reached end-point with crescentic lesion present on biopsy, this was not significantly different between the 2 groups. Of all the biochemical features, only serum creatinine (and estimated GFR) at presentation were significantly different between the 2 groups (Table 4). Those who reached the end-point had a significantly higher value of serum creatinine (p = 0.001) at the time of renal biopsy (which was usually the first presentation of the patient). There were more patients in the end-

Table 1. Demographic, clinical and biochemical features of all the patients.

Baseline characteristics (n = 79)	Value
Mean age (years)	33.9±13.6
Gender (Male) (%)	74.7
Ethnicity (%):	
- Blacks	41.8
- Mixed ancestry	54.4
- Whites	3.8
Mean duration of follow-up (months)	13.5±18.8
Hypertension at biopsy (%)	65.8
Oedema present at biopsy (%)	84.8
History of substance abuse or incarceration (%)	20.3
History of schizophrenia (%)	5.1
SBP at biopsy (mmHg)	159.9±30.1
DBP at biopsy (mmHg)	95.8±17.8
Indication for renal biopsy (%):	
- Nephrotic syndrome	77.9
- Nephrotic-nephritic syndrome	10.3
- AKI	5.9
Serum albumin at biopsy (g/L)	25.9±7.3
Serum cholesterol at biopsy (mmol/L)	6.7±2.3
Serum creatinine at biopsy (μmol/L)	180.6±166.8
Estimated MDRD GFR at biopsy (ml/min/1.73 m²)	65.1±35.2
Proteinuria at biopsy (g/24 hrs)	8.2±6.4
Low complement C3 at biopsy (%)	15.2
Low complement C4 at biopsy (%)	-

SBP – Systolic blood pressure, DBP – Diastolic blood pressure, AKI – Acute kidney injury, MDRD – Modification of diet in renal failure, GFR – Glomerular filtration rate.

Table 2. Histological features of the renal biopsies (n = 79).

Variable	Value
Number of glomeruli	16.5±10.5
Interstitial fibrosis (%):	
- No fibrosis	63.5
- Mild fibrosis	24.3
- Moderate fibrosis	8.1
- Severe fibrosis	4.1
Mean percentage of sclerosed glomeruli (%)	6.2
Crescentic lesions present (%)	17.1
Immunohistochemical features (%):	
- IgA deposit present	18.8
- IgG deposit present	43.8
- IgM deposit present	59.4
- C3 deposit present	69.8

Ig – Immunoglobulin, C3 – Complement 3.

point group with low serum complement; however, this was not significantly different from those not reaching the end-point.

As treatment often followed a conservative care approach, use of an angiotensin converting enzyme inhibitor (ACE-i) or angiotensin receptor blocker (ARB) was common but was not significantly different between the 2 groups (87.0% vs 92.9%; p = 0.409). There were more patients who reached endpoint that received immunosuppression therapy: prednisone: 52.2% vs 25.0%; p = 0.034, pulse cyclophosphamide: 26.1% vs 8.9%; p = 0.071, Azathioprine: 8.7% vs 3.6%; p = 0.635).

Survival Analysis

The cumulative renal survival curve is shown in Figure 1. Overall, the median renal survival was 38.7±11.7 months (95% confidence interval [95%CI]: 15.7–61.8) with 2-year and 5-year renal survival being 61.0% and 40.3% respectively. Kaplan-Meier

Table 3. Comparison of clinical and histological factors associated with outcome.

Factors	End-point		p
	NO (n = 56)	YES (n = 23)	
Age at biopsy (years)	33.0±12.6	36.1±16.0	0.364
Duration of follow-up (Months)	11.6±17.1	17.9±22.1	0.178
Gender (Male) (%)	71.4	82.6	0.398
Race (%):			**0.044**
- Blacks	33.9	60.9	
- Non-Blacks	66.1	39.1	
Hypertension at biopsy (%)	64.3	69.6	0.796
SBP at initial presentation (mmHg)	155.3±29.4	167.9±30.6	0.198
Average SBP at follow-up (mmHg)	141.7±19.8	168.1±30.1	**0.003**
DBP at initial presentation (mmHg)	93.4±18.5	100.0±16.3	0.257
Average DBP at follow-up (mmHg)	88.4±13.8	99.2±19.2	**0.018**
Complete or partial remission at 6 months:	36.2	4.8	**0.007**
Histological features (%):			
- IgA deposits present	22.7	21.1	1.000
- IgG deposits present	47.7	57.9	0.585
- IgM deposits present	68.2	68.4	1.000
- C3 deposits present	62.8	78.9	0.252
- Any interstitial fibrosis present (%)	30.4	56.5	**0.041**
- Any crescentic lesion present (%)	14.3	26.1	0.330

SBP – Systolic blood pressure, DBP – Diastolic blood pressure, Ig – Immunoglobulin, C3 – Complement 3.

Table 4. Comparison of biochemical and treatment factors associated with outcome.

Factors	End-point		p
	NO (n = 56)	YES (n = 23)	
Complement C3 at biopsy	1.05±0.41	1.23±0.62	0.311
Low complement C3 at biopsy (%)	14.3	17.4	0.706
Complement C4 at biopsy	0.36±0.33	0.37±0.19	0.891
Low complement C4 at biopsy (%)	-	-	-
Serum cholesterol (mmol/L)	6.1±1.4	7.9±3.2	0.079
Serum albumin at biopsy (g/L)	26.1±6.9	25.2±8.2	0.667
Serum creatinine at biopsy (μmol/L)	124.7±86.9	315.2±229.0	**0.001**
Estimated MDRD GFR at biopsy (ml/min)	75.3±30.6	40.5±34.0	**<0.0001**
Proteinuria at biopsy (g/day)	8.1±6.9	8.3±5.2	0.872
Treatment with ACE-i/ARB (%)	92.9	87.0	0.409
Treatment with prednisone (%)	25.0	52.2	**0.034**
Treatment with cyclophosphamide (%)	8.9	26.1	0.071
Treatment with Azathioprine (%)	3.6	8.7	0.635

MDRD – Modification of Diet in Renal Disease; GFR – Glomerular filtration rate; ACE-I – Angiotensin converting enzyme inhibitors; ARB – Angiotensin receptor blockers.

renal survival curves for differences in outcome based on race (log rank p = 0.009), gender (log rank p = 0.995), treatment with I/V cyclophosphamide (log rank p = 0.440) and presence or absence of interstitial fibrosis (log rank p = 0.028) are shown in figure 2. *Cox univariate regression analysis for predictors of end-point.*

Factors associated with the end-point, identified through Cox-regression analysis are shown in Table 5. Estimated GFR at biopsy (OR 0.97 [95%CI 0.95–0.99], p<0.0001), being of black African descent (OR 3.03 [95%CI 1.27–7.21], p = 0.012) and

presence of interstitial fibrosis at biopsy (OR 2.64 [95%CI 1.07–6.48], p = 0.034) were the factors identified to be associated with the end-point. Early complete or partial remission (at six months after renal biopsy) did not influence the renal outcome in these patients (OR: 0.17 [95%CI: 0.02–1.27]; p = 0.084).

Discussion

The analysis of our data of patients with idiopathic MCGN in Cape Town shows that a number of important demographic,

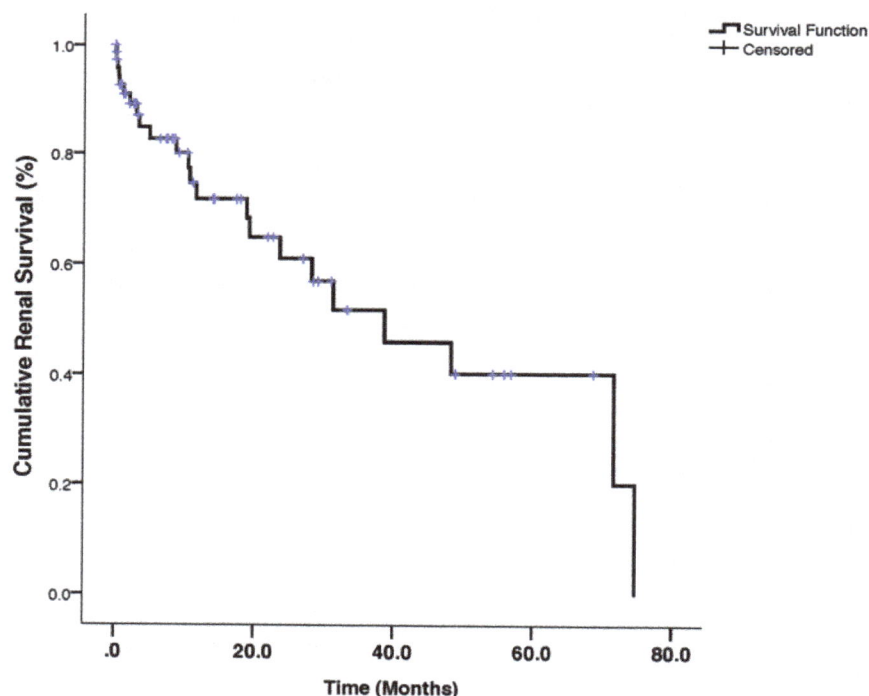

Figure 1. Kaplan-Meier curve for overall renal survival in the study population.

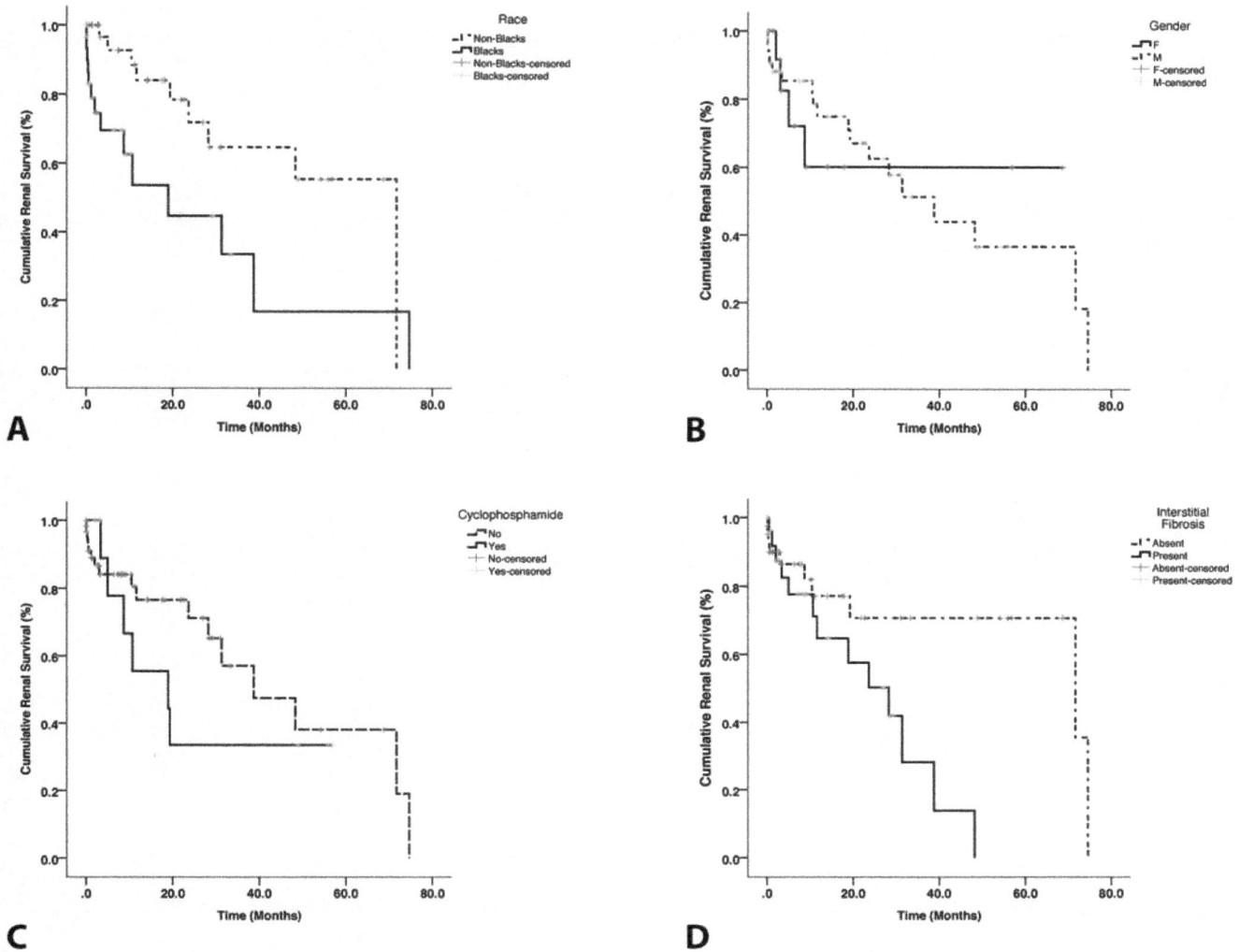

Figure 2. Kaplan-Meier curve for renal survival based on histological features of MCGN. (A) shows differences in outcome between Black Africans and non-Black Africans (log rank p = 0.009); (B) shows gender differences in outcome (log rank p = 0.995); (C) differences between patients who received treatment with cyclophosphamide and those who didn't receive treatment (log rank p = 0.440) and (D) shows differences in outcomes based on the presence of interstitial fibrosis in the biopsy (log rank p = 0.028).

Table 5. Cox univariate regression analysis for predictors of the end-point.

Variable	OR (95% CI)	P value
Age	1.03 (0.99–1.06)	0.089
Gender (Female)	0.99 (0.33–2.99)	0.995
Estimated GFR at biopsy	0.97 (0.95–0.99)	**<0.0001**
Average SBP during follow-up	1.01 (0.99–1.03)	0.082
Average DBP during follow-up	1.00 (0.98–1.03)	0.982
Remission status at 6 months (CR/PR)	0.17 (0.02–1.27)	0.084
Race (Blacks)	3.03 (1.27–7.21)	**0.012**
Interstitial fibrosis (Present)	2.64 (1.07–6.48)	**0.034**
Crescent (Present)	1.66 (0.64–4.29)	0.295
Cyclophosphamide (Yes)	1.45 (0.56–3.78)	0.443

GFR – Glomerular filtration rate; SBP – systolic blood pressure; DBP – diastolic blood pressure; CR – complete remission, PR – partial remission.

clinical and histological features may adversely predict the renal outcome in these patients. Given that there are no published recent outcome studies on idiopathic MCGN, this study has shown that in comparison with previous studies, the renal outcome of patients with idiopathic MCGN remains dismally low in comparison to outcomes in previously published studies (Table 6) [18–20,24–28]. Importantly, we have observed that lower estimated GFR at presentation (often a surrogate of late presentation), being of black African ethnicity and presence of interstitial fibrosis in the renal histology were the predicting factors of renal outcome in our patients. The 2-year and 5-year renal survival was found to be low in this study.

Late presentation of patients is common in many centres in Africa and is thought to be an important factor responsible for disease outcome [7,29,30]. Many late presenters will have markedly elevated serum creatinine (low eGFR) and may have features of ureamia or be in need of dialysis at first presentation. Late presenters may account for 36.5% of our patients having significant interstitial fibrosis on histology (Table 2). Reasons for late presentation are often tied to poverty (lack of transportation, long distances to health care facility, lack of health insurance, low level of education), cultural beliefs (visits to the traditional healer) or due to late referral. Although in this study we did not evaluate the duration of symptoms in our patients, many patients often report having been ill for many weeks and in some instances many months before presenting to hospital. In one study, late evaluation of patients with chronic kidney disease (CKD) was reported to be associated with greater burden and severity of comorbid disease, black ethnicity, lack of health insurance, and shorter duration of survival [31]. However, late presentation alone may not explain the elevated serum creatinine as the pathogenesis of MCGN itself (involving complement activation, capillary wall damage and reduction in filtration at the glomerulus) may have accounted for this. We did not exclude the possible effects of genetic factors relative to outcome in this study; hence our finding of the black race being associated with outcome may be put down to socio-economic factors rather than genetic as many of the black patients who use the public health care system in South Africa are indigent.

Although SBP and DBP during follow-up were not predictors of the endpoint on regression analysis, they were significantly higher in those patients reaching endpoint than those who didn't. Uncontrolled hypertension combined with impaired sieving function with consequent protein overload play a pathogenic role in the progression of CKD. The utility of adequate BP control to reduce progression of kidney disease in diabetic and non-diabetic CKD has been shown from various studies and is recommended by various guidelines [21,22,32,33]. One systematic review and meta-analysis of randomized controlled trials on the effects of intensive BP lowering on the progression of CKD has reported that in 5 trials that involved 1703 patients, intensive BP lowering reduced the risk of progressive kidney failure by 27% in people with proteinuria at baseline [34]. In one large population based study, the odds ratios to develop progression of urine albumin excretion during follow-up was 1.91 (95% CI 1.72 to 2.12) per 10-mmHg increase in BP during follow-up and this was independent of baseline BP and other biochemical and patient factors during follow-up [35]. In our study, several patients were receiving treatment with an agent that blocked the renin angiotensin aldosterone pathway. Previous studies from our centre have also highlighted inadequate control of BP as a factor for poor outcomes in patients with proliferative and non-proliferative glomerulonephritis [36,37]. Poor BP control may be related to the disease process or in some instances to poor adherence to therapy. Emphasis on BP control in patients with MCGN may therefore be

useful in improving renal outcomes since, unlike in many other glomerular diseases, immunosuppression has a limited role in the treatment of patients.

Renal survival in MCGN has often been reported to be low and with probably worse outcomes in comparison with other glomerular diseases, probably due to lack of specific therapy for MCGN. Recommendations from the KDIGO guideline for treatment of MCGN are limited to cases with abnormal renal function and are drawn mainly from small observational studies [17]. It was interesting that treatment with immunosuppression did not make any difference with regards to the outcome even though there were more patients in our study who reached endpoint that received immunosuppression (Table 4). Renal survival in this study was found to be 61% at 2 years and 40.3% at 5 years, much lower than for studies reported from developed countries. Although some older studies have found type of MCGN to predict outcome, we did not apply this to our study given the new approach to classifying patients with MCGN [16]. However, like some previous studies have reported, we found that any degree of interstitial fibrosis present at time of biopsy (mild/moderate/severe) is a poor prognostic factor for renal outcome.

Given recent publications on this subject, a major question that this study needed to address is whether everything was done to exclude all known secondary causes of MCGN before a labeling of the "idiopathic" diagnosis. The answer to that question is "yes – as far as was possible" given the clinical features of the patients at time of presentation and during follow up. All the patients included in this study had the immune-complex type of MCGN hence, secondary causes will include various chronic bacterial and viral infections, autoimmune diseases and monoclonal gammopathy (dysproteinaemia). All the patients included in this study tested negative for HIV, hepatitis B and C, syphilis and did not demonstrate serological or histological features of post-infectious glomerulonephritis. Our patients also tested negative for cryoglobulins and commonly occurring autoimmune diseases like SLE and rheumatoid arthritis. As it was not clinically indicated, no patient was tested for a dysproteinaemia and there were no features to suggest the disease being present at time of presentation or during the period of follow-up. Our patients typically present at a younger age (mean age in this study is 33.9 ± 13.9 years) compared to other studies where dysproteinaemias have been reported [38,39]. The lack of evidence for a secondary cause of MCGN is supported by the absence of clinical manifestation of any chronic infection or systemic disease during the period of follow up in our patients. However, the high frequency of patients with IgM deposits (59.4%) in their biopsy may be suggestive of a recent (maybe sub-clinical infection) at time of biopsy.

There still remains on our part a persistent and a renewed concern that there is a huge gap in our understanding of this common disease in Cape Town even though we continue to see many "healthy" patients presenting with nephrotic syndrome in whom renal histology show MCGN that is labeled as idiopathic after a detailed and thorough assessment. It could be that we have continued to miss a yet to be identified sub-clinical chronic antigenaemic process possibly resulting from an environmental exposure to drugs (substance abuse), tattoo ink or previous incarceration from one of the correctional services department in Cape Town all of which we have observed to be quite common amongst these patients. Further prospective studies are required to reprove this.

There were a number of limitations for this study. Firstly is our inability to assess for the monoclonality of the Ig deposits at time of biopsy. However, as our patients were young and never exhibited clinical features to suggest monoclonal gammopathy at any time

Table 6. Summary of some selected studies reporting outcomes in idiopathic MCGN.

Author (Year publication) [REF]	Sample size	Country of study	Study design	Mean duration of follow-up (years)	Study population	Renal survival	Predictors of outcome
Habib R (1973) [18]	105	France	Retrospective	5.75	Paediatric	Type I: 66% Type II: 45%	Crescents, Type II disease, nephrotic syndrome, macroscopic haematuria, impaired renal function at presentation
Swainson et al (1983) [24]	40	UK	Observational	5–22	Adult and Paediatric	5-year: 58% 10-year: 48%	Low complements, crescents, impaired renal function at presentation
Cameron et al (1983) [20]	104	UK	Observational	8	Adult and paediatric	Type I: 62% Type II: 51%	Glomerulosclerosis, crescents, nephrotic syndrome, Type II disease
McEnery (1990) [25]	76	USA	Retrospective	10.6	Paediatric	10-year: 82% 20-year: 56%	Not analyzed
Orlowski et al (1988) [26]	50	Poland	Observational	10	Adult	5-year: 90% 10-year: 82%	Hypertension
Schmitt et al (1990) [19]	220	Germany	Retrospective	5	Adult and Paediatric	5-year: 51% 10-year: 36%	Hypertension, crescents, interstitial fibrosis
Perdersen (1995) [27]	37	Denmark	Observational	2.7	Adult and Paediatric	5-year: 35% 10-year: 16%	Older age, hypertension
Little et al (2006) [28]	70	UK	Retrospective	13.8	Adult and paediatric	8.3–20 years: 30%*	Nephrotic range proteinuria, crescents, mesangial proliferation
This study	79	South Africa	Retrospective	1.1	Adult	2-year: 61.0% 5-year: 40.3%	Abnormal serum creatinine at presentation, black race, interstitial fibrosis, hypertension

UK – United Kingdom; USA – United States of America.
*Median time to ESRD.

during follow-up, this diagnosis was clinically excluded. Secondly, given the high number of patients with intravenous drug abuse and the common finding of IgM deposition in glomeruli, our study is also limited by the absence of routine testing for IgG/IgM mixed cryoglobulins. However, given that cryoprecipitates which can occasionally be observed as hyaline-like globules were not observed in the histological materials of these patients further makes this unlikely. Finally, the retrospective design of this study limited the type of data that can be collected and analyzed. This therefore warrants a prospective study of patients with "idiopathic" MCGN with emphasis on a more rigorous evaluation to exclude or identify possible secondary causes. For now however, patients identified with MCGN in whom we are unable to find a cause, efforts to reduce proteinuria and treat BP to target will be our major aim.

Conclusions

The outcome of idiopathic MCGN in Cape Town is poor and is related to socio-demographic as well as to some clinical and histological features at time of presentation. Being the most frequent primary glomerular disease reported in Cape Town, there is need for a prospectively designed study of idiopathic MCGN in order to increase our understanding of its pathogenesis and maybe find ways to its treatment.

References

1. D'Amico G, Ferrario F (1992) Mesangiocapillary glomerulonephritis. J Am Soc Nephrol. 2 (10 Suppl): S159–166.
2. Sethi S, Nester CM, Smith RJ (2012) Membranoproliferative glomerulonephritis and C3 glomerulopathy: resolving the confusion. Kidney Int. 81: 434–441.
3. Covic A, Schiller A, Volovat C, et al (2006) Epidemiology of renal disease in Romania: a 10 year review of two regional renal biopsy databases. Nephrol Dial Transplant 21: 419–424.
4. Barsoum RS, Francis MR (2000) Spectrum of glomerulonephritis in Egypt. Saudi J Kidney Dis Transpl 11: 421–429.
5. Khalifa EH, Kaballo BG, Suleiman SM, Khalil EA, El-Hassan AM (2004) Pattern of glomerulonephritis in Sudan: histopathological and immunofluorescence study. Saudi J Kidney Dis Transpl 15: 176–179.
6. Okpechi I, Swanepoel C, Duffield M, Mahala B, Wearne N, et al (2011) Patterns of renal disease in Cape Town South Africa: a 10-year review of a single-centre renal biopsy database. Nephrol Dial Transplant 26: 1853–1861.
7. Okpechi IG, Rayner BL, Swanepoel CR (2010) Nephrotic syndrome in adult black South Africans: HIV-associated nephropathy as the main culprit. J Natl Med Assoc. 102: 1193–1197.
8. Asinobi AO, Gbadegesin RA, Adeyemo AA, Akang EE, Arowolo FA, et al (1999) The predominance of membranoproliferative glomerulonephritis in childhood nephrotic syndrome in Ibadan, Nigeria. West Afr J Med. 18: 203–206.
9. Kawamura T, Usui J, Kaseda K, Takada K, Ebihara I, et al (2013) Primary membranoproliferative glomerulonephritis on the decline: decreased rate from the 1970s to the 2000s in Japan. Clin Exp Nephrol. 17: 248–254.
10. Hanko JB, Mullan RN, O'Rourke DM, McNamee PT, Maxwell AP, et al (2009) The changing pattern of adult primary glomerular disease. Nephrol Dial Transplant 24: 3050–3054.
11. Schena FP (1997) Survey of the Italian Registry of Renal Biopsies. Frequency of the renal diseases for 7 consecutive years. The Italian Group of Renal Immunopathology. Nephrol Dial Transplant 12: 418–426.
12. Rychlík I, Jancová E, Tesar V, Kolsky A, Lácha J, et al (2004) The Czech registry of renal biopsies. Occurrence of renal diseases in the years 1994–2000. Nephrol Dial Transplant 19: 3040–3049.
13. Strachan DP (1989) Hay fever, hygiene, and household size. BMJ 299: 1259–1260.
14. Johnson RJ, Hurtado A, Merszei J, Rodriguez-Iturbe B, Feng L (2003) Hypothesis: dysregulation of immunologic balance resulting from hygiene and socioeconomic factors may influence the epidemiology and cause of glomerulonephritis worldwide. Am J Kidney Dis 42: 575–581.
15. Fervenza FC, Sethi S, Glassock RJ (2012) Idiopathic membranoproliferative glomerulonephritis: does it exist? Nephrol Dial Transplant. 27: 4288–4294.
16. Sethi S, Fervenza FC (2011) Membranoproliferative Glomerulonephritis: Pathogenetic Heterogeneity and Proposal for a New Classification. Semin Nephrol 31: 341–348.
17. Kidney Disease: Improving Global Outcomes (KDIGO) Glomerulonephritis Work Group. KDIGO Clinical Practice Guideline for Glomerulonephritis (2012) Kidney int. 2(suppl): 139–274.
18. Habib R, Kleinknecht C, Gubler MC, Maiz HB (1973) Idiopathic membranoproliferative glomerulonephritis. Morphology and natural history. Perspect Nephrol Hypertens 1: 491–514.
19. Schmitt H, Bohle A, Reineke T, Mayer-Eichberger D, Vogl W (1990) Long-term prognosis of membranoproliferative glomerulonephritis type I. Significance of clinical and morphological parameters: an investigation of 220 cases. Nephron 55: 242–250.
20. Cameron JS, Turner DR, Heaton J, Williams DG, Ogg CS, et al (1983) Idiopathic mesangiocapillary glomerulonephritis. Comparison of types I and II in children and adults and long-term prognosis. Am J Med. 74: 175–192.
21. National Kidney Foundation K/DOQI clinical practice guidelines for chronic kidney disease; evaluation, classification and stratification (2002) Am J Kidney Dis 39(2 Suppl 1): S1–S266.
22. Mancia G, De Backer G, Dominiczak A, Cifkova R, Fagard R, et al (2007) 2007 Guidelines for the Management of Arterial Hypertension: The Task Force for the Management of Arterial Hypertension of the European Society of Hypertension (ESH) and of the European Society of Cardiology (ESC). J Hypertens 25: 1105–1187.
23. Renal Disease Subcommittee of the American College of Rheumatology Ad Hoc Committee on Systemic Lupus Erythematosus Response Criteria (2006) The American college of rheumatology response criteria for proliferative and membranous renal disease in systemic lupus erythematosus clinical trials. Arthritis Rheum 54: 421–432.
24. Swainson CP, Robson JS, Thomson D, MacDonald MK (1983) Mesangiocapillary glomerulonephritis: a long-term study of 40 cases. J Pathol 141: 449–468.
25. McEnery PT (1990) Membranoproliferative glomerulonephritis: the Cincinnati experience – cumulative renal survival from 1957 to 1989. J Pediatr 116: S109–S114.
26. Orlowski T, Rancewicz Z, Lao M, Juskowa J, Klepacka J, et al (1988) Long-term immunosuppressive therapy of idiopathic membranoproliferative glomerulonephritis. Klin Wochenschr 66: 1019–1023.
27. Pedersen RS (1995) Long-term prognosis in idiopathic membranoproliferative glomerulonephritis. Scand J Urol Nephrol 29: 265–272.
28. Little MA, Dorman A, Gill D, Walshe JJ (2000) Mesangioproliferative glomerulonephritis with IgM deposition: clinical characteristics and outcome. Ren Fail 22: 445–457.
29. Naicker S, Aboud O, Gharbi MB (2008) Epidemiology of acute kidney injury in Africa. Semin Nephrol. 28: 348–353.
30. Olowu WA (2003) Renal failure in Nigerian children: factors limiting access to dialysis. Pediatr Nephrol. 18: 1249–1254.
31. Kinchen KS, Sadler J, Fink N, Brookmeyer R, Klag MJ, et al (2002) The timing of specialist evaluation in chronic kidney disease and mortality. Ann Intern Med. 137: 479–486.
32. Jafar TH, Stark PC, Schmid CH, Landa M, Maschio G, et al (2003) Progression of chronic kidney disease: the role of blood pressure control, proteinuria, and angiotensin-converting enzyme inhibition: a patient-level meta-analysis. Ann Intern Med 139: 244–252.

Supporting Information

Figure S1 Glomerular features of one of our study patients identified with immune complex type MCGN. A – The H&E stain showing increased lobulation of the displayed glomerulus and increased mesangial matrix; B – silver stain showing double contours/splitting of the glomerular basement membrane; C – F shows positive immunohistochemical stains for C3, IgG, IgA and IgM respectively; G–I are the electron micrographs (x 30,000) showing sub-endothelial and intramembranous deposits. (Courtesy Dr M Duffield and Mr. D. Rademeyer – National Health and Laboratory Services [NHLS] Cape Town).

Acknowledgments

None

Author Contributions

Conceived and designed the experiments: IGO TALD MD BLR GM CRS. Performed the experiments: IGO TALD MD BLR GM CRS. Analyzed the data: IGO TALD MD BLR GM CRS. Contributed reagents/materials/analysis tools: IGO TALD MD BLR GM CRS. Wrote the paper: IGO TALD MD BLR GM CRS.

33. Chobanian AV, Bakris GL, Black HR, Cushman WC, Green LA, et al (2003) The seventh report of the Joint National Committee on Prevention, Detection, Evaluation, and Treatment of High Blood Pressure: the JNC7 report. JAMA 289: 2560–2572.

34. Lv J, Ehteshami P, Sarnak MJ, Tighiouart H, Jun M, et al (2013) Effects of intensive blood pressure lowering on the progression of chronic kidney disease: a systematic review and meta-analysis. CMAJ. 185: 949–957.

35. Brantsma AH, Atthobari J, Bakker SJ, de Zeeuw D, de Jong PE, et al (2007) What predicts progression and regression of urinary albumin excretion in the nondiabetic population? J Am Soc Nephrol. 18: 637–645.

36. Ayodele OE, Okpechi IG, Swanepoel CR (2013) Long-term renal outcome and complications in South Africans with proliferative lupus nephritis. Int Urol Nephrol. 45: 1289–1300.

37. Okpechi IG, Ayodele OE, Jones ES, Duffield M, Swanepoel CR (2012) Outcome of patients with membranous lupus nephritis in Cape Town South Africa. Nephrol Dial Transplant. 27: 3509–3515.

38. Zand L, Kattah A, Fervenza FC, Smith RJ, Nasr SH, et al (2013) C3 glomerulonephritis associated with monoclonal gammopathy: a case series. Am J Kidney Dis. 62: 506–514.

39. Sethi S, Zand L, Leung N, Smith RJ, Jevremonic D, et al (2010) Membranoproliferative glomerulonephritis secondary to monoclonal gammopathy. Clin J Am Soc Nephrol. 5: 770–782.

27

Efficacy of Short-Term High-Dose Statin Pretreatment in Prevention of Contrast-Induced Acute Kidney Injury: Updated Study-Level Meta-Analysis of 13 Randomized Controlled Trials

Joo Myung Lee[1]⊙, Jonghanne Park[1]⊙, Ki-Hyun Jeon[1], Ji-hyun Jung[1], Sang Eun Lee[1], Jung-Kyu Han[1], Hack-Lyoung Kim[2], Han-Mo Yang[1], Kyung Woo Park[1], Hyun-Jae Kang[1], Bon-Kwon Koo[1], Sang-Ho Jo[3], Hyo-Soo Kim[1,4]*

1 Department of Internal Medicine and Cardiovascular Center, Seoul National University Hospital, Seoul, Korea, 2 Cardiovascular Center, Seoul National University, Boramae Medical Center, Seoul, Korea, 3 Division of Cardiology, Department of Internal Medicine, Hallym University Sacred Heart Hospital, Anyang-si, Gyeonggi-do, Korea, 4 Department of Molecular Medicine and Biopharmaceutical Sciences, Graduate School of Convergence Science and Technology, Seoul National University, Seoul, Korea

Abstract

Background: There have been conflicting results across the trials that evaluated prophylactic efficacy of short-term high-dose statin pre-treatment for prevention of contrast-induced acute kidney injury (CIAKI) in patients undergoing coronary angiography (CAG). The aim of the study was to perform an up-to-date meta-analysis regarding the efficacy of high-dose statin pre-treatment in preventing CIAKI.

Methods and Results: Randomized-controlled trials comparing high-dose statin versus low-dose statin or placebo pre-treatment for prevention of CIAKI in patients undergoing CAG were included. The primary endpoint was the incidence of CIAKI within 2–5 days after CAG. The relative risk (RR) with 95% CI was the effect measure. This analysis included 13 RCTs with 5,825 total patients; about half of them (n = 2,889) were pre-treated with high-dose statin (at least 40 mg of atorvastatin) before CAG, and the remainders (n = 2,936) pretreated with low-dose statin or placebo. In random-effects model, high-dose statin pre-treatment significantly reduced the incidence of CIAKI (RR 0.45, 95% CI 0.35–0.57, $p < 0.001$, $I^2 = 8.2\%$, NNT 16), compared with low-dose statin or placebo. The benefit of high-dose statin was consistent in both comparisons with low-dose statin (RR 0.47, 95% CI 0.34–0.65, $p < 0.001$, $I^2 = 28.4\%$, NNT 19) or placebo (RR 0.34, 95% CI 0.21–0.58, $p < 0.001$, $I^2 = 0.0\%$, NNT 16). In addition, high-dose statin showed significant reduction of CIAKI across various subgroups of chronic kidney disease, acute coronary syndrome, and old age (≥60 years), regardless of osmolality of contrast or administration of N-acetylcystein.

Conclusions: High-dose statin pre-treatment significantly reduced overall incidence of CIAKI in patients undergoing CAG, and emerges as an effective prophylactic measure to prevent CIAKI.

Editor: Giuseppe Remuzzi, Mario Negri Institute for Pharmacological Research and Azienda Ospedaliera Ospedali Riuniti di Bergamo, Italy

Funding: This study was supported by grants from the Bio & Medical Technology Development Program of the National Research Foundation (NRF) funded by the Korean government (2010-0020258) and from the IRICT, Seoul National University Hospital (A062260), sponsored by the Ministry of Health and Welfare, Republic of Korea. The funders had no role in study design, data collection and analysis, decision to publish, or preparation of the manuscript.

Competing Interests: The authors have declared that no competing interests exist.

* Email: hyosoo@snu.ac.kr

⊙ These authors contributed equally to this work.

Introduction

Contrast-induced acute kidney injury (CIAKI) is a well-recognized complication of coronary angiography (CAG) with iodinated contrast medium and is the third leading cause of hospital-acquired acute renal failure. CIAKI has been known to be associated with prolonged hospitalization, increased costs, and increased short and long-term morbidity and mortality. [1] The incidence of CIAKI varies widely depending on the patient's underlying co-morbidities, definition criteria, and preventive strategies. But, certain subgroup of coronary heart disease patients, especially with acute coronary syndrome or chronic kidney disease, showed higher risk for the CIAKI. [2,3] Investigators have examined several strategies to prevent CIAKI, such as fenolopam, mannitol, theophylline, iloprost, furosemide, dopamine, hemofiltration, ascorbic acid, and N-acetylcystein (NAC). [4] However, none of the agents were proved to be effective in preventing CIAKI. [4,5] Currently, recommendations of the

European Society of Cardiology/European Association for Cardio-Thoracic Surgery (ESC/EACTS) or the ACCF/AHA/SCAI guideline are limited to the prophylactic intravenous hydration, use of iso- or low-osmolar contrast agents, and reduced dosages of contrast agents to prevent occurrence of CIAKI. [6,7] Since a few observational studies suggested that 3-hydroxyl-3-methylglutaryl coenzyme A reductase inhibitors (statins) may reduce CIAKI incidence, several RCTs have evaluated the potential benefit of statin in prevention of CIAKI. [8,9]Statin's postulated mechanism of kidney protection was through its pleotropic effects, i.e. antioxidant, anti-inflammatory, and anti-thrombotic actions. However, these previous RCTs and meta-analysis of high-dose statin pre-treatment showed disappointing results. [10–12] Recently, three RCTs with relatively large sample size (NAPLES II, PRATO-ACS, TRACK-D trial) have reported promising results favoring prophylactic efficacy of high-dose statin in prevention of CIAKI. [13–15] Considering insufficient evidences regarding efficacy of high-dose statin pre-treatment and prognostic importance of CIAKI, we therefore performed a systematic review and comprehensive meta-analysis of all published randomized control trials, in order to evaluate the efficacy of high-dose statin pre-treatment to reduce the incidence of CIAKI in various clinical situations including overall population, chronic kidney disease, or acute coronary syndrome.

Methods

Data Sources and Searches

Relevant published or unpublished studies were independently searched in PubMed, Cochrane Central Register of Controlled Trials, EMBASE, the United States National Institutes of Health registry of clinical trials (www.clinicaltrials.gov), and relevant websites (www.crtonline.org, www.clinicaltrialresults.com, www.tctmd.com, www.cardiosource.com, and www.pcronline.com) were also searched. Detailed search strategy was presented in the Method S1. The electronic search strategy was complemented by manual review of reference lists of included articles. References of recent reviews, editorials, and meta-analyses were also examined. No restrictions were imposed on language, study period, or sample size.

Study Selection

We included RCTs assessing preventive strategies for CIAKI that met following criteria. First, we selected studies which enrolled adult patients undergoing CAG with or without percutaneous coronary intervention (PCI). Second, the intervention was high-dose statin (defined as a daily dose of at least 40 mg of Atorvastatin or equivalent dose of available statins including Simvastatin, Pitavastatin, Fluvastatin, Lovastatin, Pravastatin, or Rosuvastatin), compared with low-dose statin (defined as a daily dose of less than 40 mg of Atorvastatin or equivalent dose of available statins), placebo or none of medication pre-treatment. In cases where a concomitant prophylactic measures were used (for example, NAC, sodium bicarbonate, or other preventive medications), both arms must have shared the same concomitant prophylactic measures, with only a difference in statin protocol. Finally, the incidences of post-procedural CIAKI were reported in both arms, regardless of its definition or the timing of data collection. We excluded RCTs conducted on pediatric patients (including neonates and preterm infants) and randomized crossover trials that assigned patients to both high-dose and low-dose or placebo arms.

Data Extraction and Quality Assessment

Data extraction and quality assessment was performed as previously described. [16] Summarized data as reported in the published manuscripts were used in the analysis. A standardized form was used to extract characteristics of trials, study design (including randomization sequence generation, allocation concealment, crossover between assigned groups, number of post-randomization withdrawals or follow-up loss), number of study patients, age, eligibility criteria of each trials, definition of CIAKI in each trials, baseline serum creatinine and estimated glomerular filtration rates (eGFR), mean change of serum creatinine after procedure, total cumulative dose of statin before procedure, protocols for statin treatment, hydration protocols, type or mean dosage of radio-contrast agents, the proportion of diabetes mellitus, hypertension, chronic kidney disease, timing of data collection, length of follow-up, adverse events data associated with statin treatment reported on an intention-to-treat basis. We primarily focused our analysis on the effect of prophylactic treatment with high-dose statin on the incidence of CIAKI, not on the surrogate markers of inflammation or oxidative stress. The quality of eligible RCTs was assessed using the Cochrane Collaboration's tool for assessing the risk of bias for RCTs (Table S1 in File S1). Because most previous meta-analyses have reported the methodological quality of each trial using the Jadad score, we also provided this score, as well as the Cochran Collaboration's tool, for each RCT. [17] Two investigators (JML and JP) independently performed screening of titles and abstracts, identified duplicates, reviewed full articles, and determined their eligibility. Disagreements were resolved by discussions. The last search was performed in February 2014.

Outcomes and Definitions

The primary outcome was the incidence of post-procedural CIAKI within 2–5 days after index procedure. Secondary outcomes included the incidence of post-procedural CIAKI, stratified according to the various subgroups for example, type of contrast agents (iso-osmolar or low-osmolar) used, mean age of the study patients, presence of underlying chronic kidney disease, patients with acute coronary syndrome, NAC usage, or placebo control. All of the patients and outcomes were analyzed according to the originally assigned group.

Data Synthesis and Analysis

Data synthesis and analsysis was performed as described in detail previously [16], The primary outcome was analyzed by both a random effects model and a fixed effects model. Relative risks (RR) with 95% confidence interval (CI) were presented as summary statistics. The pooled RR was calculated with the DerSimonian and Laird method for random effects model, as well as the Mantel–Haenszel method for fixed effects model. [18] To evaluate the effect of progressive chronological change in study design, such as study population, protocol of statin pre-treatment, hydration protocols or concomitant prophylactic medications including NAC or sodium bicarbonate, we evaluated the impact of publication date on the overall effect of pooled RRs for incidence of CIAKI by a cumulative meta-analysis. Stratified subgroup analyses were performed to assess treatment effects according to the control group (low-dose statin, placebo, or no medication), type of contrast agent, mean age of the patients, underlying chronic kidney disease, acute coronary syndrome, and usage of NAC along with tests for interaction derived from random effects meta-regression. Statistical heterogeneity was assessed by Cochran's Q via a $\chi 2$ test and was quantified with the I^2 test. [19] Publication bias was assessed by funnel plot asymmetry, along with Egger's and Begg's test. The κ statistic was used to assess agreement between investigators for study selection. Results were considered statistically significant at 2-sided p<0.05. Statistical analysis was performed with the use of STATA/SE 12.0 (Stata Corp LP, College Station, Texas, USA). The present study was performed in compliance with the Preferred Reporting Items for Systematic Reviews and Meta-Analyses (PRISMA) guidelines and the review protocol has not been registered (Checklist S1). [20]

Results

Search Results

We identified 465 citations from searches as previously described. Among these, 24 studies were retrieved for detailed evaluation, of which 13 RCTs met inclusion criteria (Figure 1). [11–15,21–28] These 13 RCTs included a total of 5,825 adult patients, 2,889 (49.6%) of which were allocated to the high-dose statin group and 2,936 (50.4%) of which were allocated to the control group (low-dose statin or placebo group). The characteristics of 11 excluded studies after full article review are summarized in the Method S2. The inter-observer agreement for study selection was high (κ = 0.92).

Trial Characteristics

The main characteristics of the individual studies are summarized in Table 1 and 2. All trials reported the incidence of CIAKI within 2-5days from index procedure using contrast agents. Four trials exclusively enrolled the patients with chronic kidney disease, which was defined as eGFR of less than 60 ml/min/1.73 m^2 in

PROMISS, Toso et al, and NAPLES II trial, and eGFR of between 30–90 ml/min/1.73 m^2 in TRACK-D trial. [11–14] Only one trial (TRACK-D) exclusively enrolled type 2 diabetes mellitus patients, whereas the others enrolled the patients regardless of diabetes mellitus. [14] Among the 13 trials, 4 trials compared high-dose statin versus low-dose statin pre-treatment. [21,22,25,27] Majority of trials used Atorvastin, whereas 2 trials [11,21] used Simvastatin, and 2 trials [14,15] used Rosuvastatin. Total cumulative dose of statin in high-dose statin group ranged from 40 mg to 560 mg of Atorvastatin equivalent dose from 1 to 7 days before CAG. The detailed medication protocols in each included trials are summarized in Table 1. The definition of CIAKI slightly differed across trials. Ten trials [11,14,15,21, 22,24–28] used an increase in serum creatinine of ≥0.5mg/dL or ≥25% from baseline within 48–72 hours after radiocontrast exposure, whereas 2 trials [12,23] regarded an absolute increase in serum creatinine of ≥0.5 mg/dL within 5 days as their primary definition of CIAKI. One trial (NAPLES II) used an increase in serum cystatin C ≥10% from baseline, which was used in this analysis, although they reported the incidence of CIAKI on the base of the change in serum creatinine as secondary outcomes. [13] All trials evaluated patients with coronary artery disease undergoing CAG with or without percutaneous coronary intervention. Among the trials, 5 studies [15,21,26–28] exclusively enrolled the patients with acute coronary syndrome including unstable angina and non ST-segment elevation myocardial infarction, and 2 of these 5 studies [21,28] further included the patients with ST-segment elevation myocardial infarction. Four trials [12,13,15,24] used NAC (600 mg or 1200 mg twice daily) as additional preventive measure of CIAKI in both arms, and 1 trial

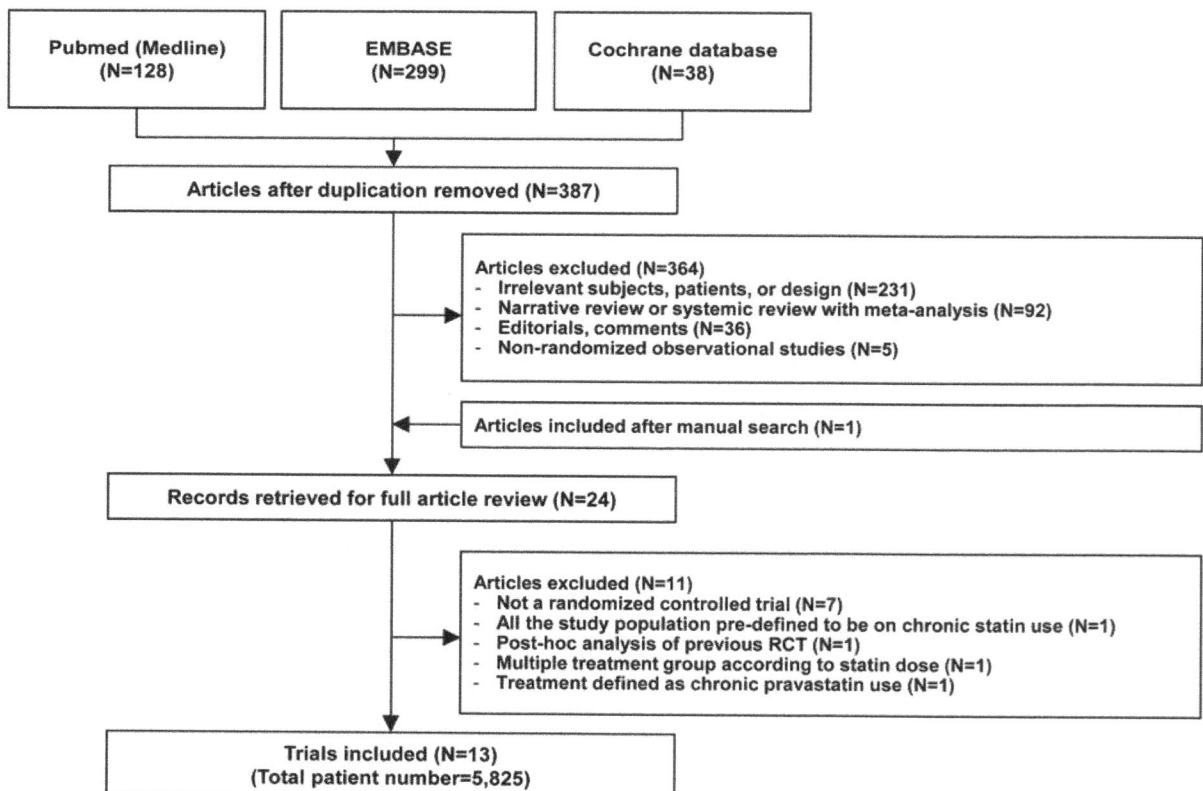

Figure 1. Flow diagram of trial selection. Abbreviations: RCT, randomized controlled trial.

Table 1. Characteristics of the study, trial characteristics and protocols.

Trial (Year)	Patients number Statin (N=2889)	Patients number Control (N=2936)	Inclusion criteria	Definition of CIN	Medication Protocols Statin	Medication Protocols Control	Contrast agent	Contrast volumes (mean), ml Statin	Contrast volumes (mean), ml Control	Hydration protocols
PROMISS (2008)	118	118	CKD patients undergoing CAG or PCI, CrCl≤60 mL/min or SCr≥ 1.1 mg/dL	Increase of SCr≥ 0.5 mg/dL or ≥25% at 48 hours	Simvastatin 40 mg bid, 1 day pre-procedure and 1 day post-procedure	Placebo	Visipaque (iodixanol)	173.3	190.9	NS 1 mg/kg/h for 12 h before and 12 h after procedure
Toso et al. (2009)	152	152	CKD patients undergoing CAG or PCI, CrCl<60 mL/min	Increase of SCr≥ 0.5 mg/dl within 5 days.	Atorvastatin 80 mg/day 2 days pre-procedure and 2 days post-procedure, NAC 1200 mg bid from 1 day before to 1 day post-procedure	Placebo + NAC 1200 mg bid from 1day before to 1 day post-procedure	Visipaque (iodixanol)	151.0	164.0	NS 1 ml/kg/h for 12 h before and after the procedure
Xinwei et al. (2009)	113	115	ACS (UA/NSTEMI) including STEMI patients undergoing PCI	Increase of SCr≥ 0.5 mg/dL or ≥25% at 48 hours	Simvastatin 80 mg/day from admission to the day before, 20 mg/day after procedure	Simvastatin, 20 mg/day from admission to the end	Visipaque (iodixanol) for CKD, Omnipaque (iohexol) for non-CKD	227.0	240.0	NS 1 ml/kg/h for 6 to 12 h before and 12 h after procedure
Zhou Xia et al. (2009)	50	50	Patients undergoing CAG or PCI	Increase of SCr≥ 0.5 mg/dL or ≥ 25% at 72 hours	Atorvastatin 80 mg/ day before for 1day,10 mg/day for 6days after procedure	Atorvastatin 10 mg/day for 7 days	Iopamidol 370 mg/ml	118.7	112.9	NS 1000 mL infusion, for 12 h before and 12 h after intervention
Acikel et al. (2010)	80	80	Patients undergoing elective CAG or PCI (excluding ACS), LDL≥ 70 mg/dl, eGFR≥60 ml/min/ 1.73 m²	Increase of SCr≥ 0.5 mg/dL at 48 hours	Atorvastatin 40 mg/ day 3 days pre-procedure and 2 days post-procedure	None	Omnipaque(iohexol)	105.0	103.0	NS 1 ml/kg/h starting 4 h before and continuing until 24 h after procedure
Ozhan et al. (2010)	60	70	Patients undergoing CAG or PCI, eGFR≥70 ml/min/1.73 m² or SCr≤1.5 mg/dL	Increase of SCr≥ 0.5 mg/dL or ≥25% at 48 hours	Atorvastatin 80 mg 1 day pre-procedure and 2 days post-procedure, NAC 600 mg bid pre-procedure	No statin pre-procedure, NAC 600 mg bid pre-procedure	Iopamidol	97.0	93.0	NS 1000 ml infusion during 6 h after procedure
Hua et al. (2010)	76	97	Patients undergoing CAG or PCI	Increase of SCr≥ 0.5 mg/dL or ≥25% at 72 hours	Atorvastatin 80 mg/day pre-procedure	Atorvastatin 20 mg/day pre-procedure	Iopromide	173.0	177.0	NR
ARMYDA-CIN (2011)	120	121	ACS (UA/NSTEMI) Patients undergoing CAG or PCI (excluding high-risk NSTEMI requiring emergency PCI), SCr≤3 mg/dl	Increase of SCr≥ 0.5 mg/dL or ≥25% at 48 hours	Atorvastatin 80 mg (12 h before) → 40 mg (2 h before), 40 mg for 2days after procedure	Placebo before procedure → Atorvastatin 40 mg for 2days after procedure	Xenetix (iobitridol)	209.0	213.0	For patients CrCl < 60 ml/min, NS 1 ml/ kg/h for 12 h before and 24 h after intervention

Table 1. Cont.

Trial (Year)	Patients number		Inclusion criteria	Definition of CIN	Medication Protocols		Contrast agent	Contrast volumes (mean), ml		Hydration protocols
	Statin (N=2889)	Control (N=2936)			Statin	Control		Statin	Control	
Wei Li et al. (2012)	78	83	STEMI patients undergoing emergency PCI within 12 hours of symptom onset	Increase of SCr≥ 0.5 mg/dL or ≥25% at 72 hours	Atorvastatin 80 mg loading pre-procedure, long-term 40 mg/day after procedure	Placebo 801mg loading pre-procedure, long-term 40 mg/day after procedure	Ultravist 370 (iopromide)	100.0	103.6	NS 1 ml/kg/h before the procedure and for 12 h after the procedure
NAPLES II (2012)	202	208	CKD patients undergoing CAG or PCI, eGFR<60 ml/min/1.73 m²	Increase of Serum Cystatin C concentration ≥10% at 24 hours	Atorvastatin 80 mg before procedure, NAC 1200 mg bid the day before and the day of procedure	No statin pre-procedure, NAC 1200 mg bid the day before and the day of procedure	Visipaque (iodixanol)	177.0	184.0	Sodium bicarbonate solution (154 mEq/ L), initial bolus of 3 mL/kg/h for 1 h before procedure, 1 mL/kg/h during and for 6 h after the procedure
CAO et al. (2012)	90	90	Patients undergoing CAG or PCI	Increase of SCr≥ 0.5 mg/dL or ≥25% at 72 hours	Atorvastatin 40 mg/day from 3days before procedure, 20 mg/day after procedure	Atorvastatin 20 mg/day from 3days before procedure, 20 mg/day after procedure	NR	162.3	158.9	NR
PRATO-ACS (2014)	252	252	ACS (UA/NSTEMI) patients undergoing CAG or PCI (excluding STEMI and high-risk NSTEMI requiring emergency PCI), SCr≤ 3 mg/dl	Increase of SCr≥ 0.5 mg/dL or ≥25% at 72 hours	Rosuvastatin 40 mg loading → 20 mg/day before procedure, Rosuvastatin 20 mg/day continued after procedure, NAC 1200 mg bid the day before and the day of procedure	No statin pre-procedure, Atorvastatin 40 mg/day after procedure, NAC 1200 mg bid the day before and the day of pro cedure	Visipaque (iodixanol)	149.7	138.2	NS 1 ml/kg/h for 12 h both before and after the procedure. Hydration rate was reduced to 0.5 ml/ kg/h in both arms for patients with LVEF <40%
TRACK-D (2014)	1498	1500	Stage 2 or 3 CKD and type II DM patients undergoing CAG or PCI, eGFR ≥30 ml/min/1.73 m² and < 90 ml/min/1.73 m² (excluded stage 0,1,4,5 CKD patients)	Increase of SCr≥ 0.5 mg/dL or ≥25% at 72 hours	Rosuvastatin 10 mg/day from 2 days before to 3 days after procedure → continued after procedure	No statin pre-procedure, Rosuvastatin 10 mg. day 3 days after procedure	Visipaque (iodixanol)	120.0	110.0	NS 1 ml/kg/h started 12 h before and continued for 24 h after procedure

Abbreviations: ACS, acute coronary syndrome; CAG, coronary angiography; CIN, contrast induced nephropathy; CKD, chronic kidney disease; CrCl, creatinine clearance; DM, diabetes mellitus; eGFR, estimated glomerular filtration rate; LDL, low-density lipoprotein; LVEF, left ventricular ejection fraction; NAC, N-acetylcystein; NS, normal saline (isotonic saline, 0.9%); NR, not reported; NS, normal saline (isotonic saline, 0.9%); NSTEMI, non ST-segment elevation myocardial infarction; PCI, percutaneous coronary intervention; SCr, serum creatinine; STEMI, ST-segment elevation myocardial infarction; UA, unstable angina.

Table 2. Characteristics of the study, baseline characteristics.

Trial (Year)	Mean age, year		Mean baseline SCr (mg/dL)		Mean baseline eGFR (ml/min)		Male proportion	Diabetes Mellitus proportion	Hypertension proportion	Additional measures
	Statin	Control	Statin	Control	Statin	Control				
PROMISS (2008)	65	66	1.29	1.25	53.46	55.40	72.5%	25.9%	63.2%	None
Toso et al. (2009)	75	76	1.20	1.18	46.00	46.00	64.5%	21.1%	60.5%	NAC
Xinwei et al. (2009)	65	66	0.82	0.83	86.50	93.60	36.0%	20.6%	63.6%	None
Zhou Xia et al. (2009)	60	61	1.04	1.08	76.88	70.54	59.0%	20.0%	75.0%	None
Acikel et al. (2010)	59	61	0.84	0.85	97.70	97.00	63.8%	24.4%	58.1%	None
Ozhan et al. (2010)	54	55	0.88	0.88	92.00	89.00	59.2%	16.2%	22.3%	NAC
Hua et al. (2010)	65	65	1.34	1.40	68.20	66.70	67.1%	26.6%	74.6%	None
ARMYDA-CIN (2011)	65	66	1.04	1.04	79.80	77.00	77.6%	28.2%	75.1%	None
Wei Li et al. (2012)	66	65	0.93	0.93	NR	NR	75.8%	28.0%	80.7%	None
NAPLES II (2012)	70	70	1.32	1.29	42.00	43.00	54.4%	41.2%	86.3%	NAC, bicarbonate
CAO et al. (2012)	63	63	0.85	0.83	109.60	106.80	57.2%	21.7%	37.2%	None
PRATO-ACS (2014)	66	66	0.95	0.96	69.90	69.30	65.7%	21.2%	55.8%	NAC
TRACK-D (2014)	62	61	1.08	1.07	74.16	74.43	65.2%	100.0%	71.9%	None

Abbreviations: ACS, acute coronary syndrome; CAG, coronary angiography; CIN, contrast induced nephropathy; CKD, chronic kidney disease; CrCl, creatinine clearance; DM, diabetes mellitus; eGFR, estimated glomerular filtration rate; LDL, low-density lipoprotein; LVEF, left ventricular ejection fraction; NAC, N-acetylcystein; NR, not reported; NS, normal saline (isotonic saline, 0.9%); NSTEMI, non ST-segment elevation myocardial infarction; PCI, percutaneous coronary intervention; SCr, serum creatinine; STEMI, ST-segment elevation myocardial infarction; UA, unstable angina.

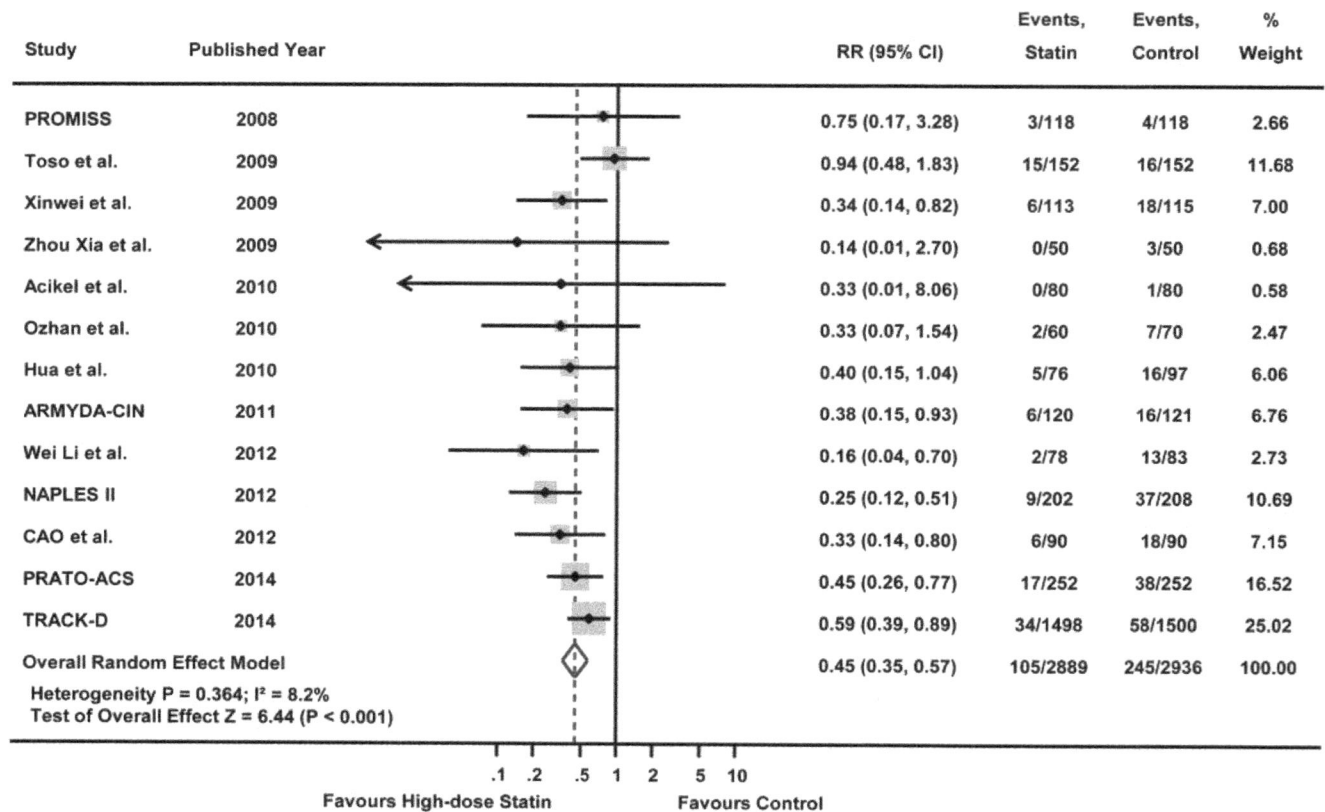

Study	Published Year	RR (95% CI)	Events, Statin	Events, Control	% Weight
PROMISS	2008	0.75 (0.17, 3.28)	3/118	4/118	2.66
Toso et al.	2009	0.94 (0.48, 1.83)	15/152	16/152	11.68
Xinwei et al.	2009	0.34 (0.14, 0.82)	6/113	18/115	7.00
Zhou Xia et al.	2009	0.14 (0.01, 2.70)	0/50	3/50	0.68
Acikel et al.	2010	0.33 (0.01, 8.06)	0/80	1/80	0.58
Ozhan et al.	2010	0.33 (0.07, 1.54)	2/60	7/70	2.47
Hua et al.	2010	0.40 (0.15, 1.04)	5/76	16/97	6.06
ARMYDA-CIN	2011	0.38 (0.15, 0.93)	6/120	16/121	6.76
Wei Li et al.	2012	0.16 (0.04, 0.70)	2/78	13/83	2.73
NAPLES II	2012	0.25 (0.12, 0.51)	9/202	37/208	10.69
CAO et al.	2012	0.33 (0.14, 0.80)	6/90	18/90	7.15
PRATO-ACS	2014	0.45 (0.26, 0.77)	17/252	38/252	16.52
TRACK-D	2014	0.59 (0.39, 0.89)	34/1498	58/1500	25.02
Overall Random Effect Model		0.45 (0.35, 0.57)	105/2889	245/2936	100.00
Heterogeneity P = 0.364; I² = 8.2%					
Test of Overall Effect Z = 6.44 (P < 0.001)					

Figure 2. The effect of high-dose statin on the incidence of contrast-induced acute kidney injury by random effects model. Forest plot with relative risks for the incidence of contrast-induced acute kidney injury associated with high-dose statin pre-treatment, compared with control group (low-dose statin or placebo) for individual trials and the pooled population. Abbreviations: CI, confidence intervals; RR, relative risks.

[13] used sodium bicarbonate solution as primary hydration protocol.

Risk of Bias within Trials

Figure S1 in File S1 shows the risk of bias graph illustrating the proportion of studies with each of the judgments ('Yes', 'No', 'Unclear') for each entry in the Cochrane Collaboration's tool. A full description of the summary of risk of bias judgments of each study is available in Figure S2 and Table S1 in File S1. All of the included trials were RCTs and no substantial risk of bias was observed in random sequence generation. The included trials showed relatively high methodological quality. Among the 13 RCTs, 5 trials [11,12,15,26,28] had double-blinded design, whereas others were open-label or non-blinded trials. However, all trials used objective findings (serum creatinine or cystatin C) to define the primary endpoint (the incidence of CIAKI), the authors, therefore, judged that the outcomes were not likely to be influenced by lack of blinding.

Effect of Statin on the Incidence of Contrast-Induced Acute Kidney Injury

As shown in Figure 1, this meta-analysis included 13 RCTs [11–15,21–28], all of which provided the incidence of CIAKI. Figure 2 illustrates the RRs of individual study and pooled RR in regards to the incidence of CIAKI, the primary outcome. The overall incidence of CIAKI in the intention-to-treat population was 3.6% (105/2889) in high-dose statin group and 8.3% (245/2936) in control group, respectively. In pooled analysis using random effects model, patients receiving high-dose statin pre-treatment had 55% less risk of CIAKI compared with the control group (RR 0.45, 95% CI 0.35–0.57, p<0.001) (Figure 2). A fixed effects model yielded a similar result (RR 0.44, 95% CI 0.35–0.55, p<0.001) (Figure S3 in File S1). The number needed to treat (NNT) of high-dose statin was 16 in random effects model which means that treatment of 16 patients with high-dose statin will reduce 1 event of CIAKI. There was no significant heterogeneity in either the random effects or the fixed effects model (I² = 8.2%, heterogeneity p = 0.364 for both random and fixed effects model). Since 4 trials compared high-dose versus low-dose statin group and 9 trials compared high-dose versus placebo or no treatment, we performed stratified analysis according to the type of treatment (Figure 3). High-dose statin significantly reduced the risk of CIAKI by 53% (RR 0.47, 95% CI 0.34–0.65, p<0.001, I² = 28.4%, heterogeneity p = 0.192) or 66% (RR 0.34, 95% CI 0.21–0.58, p< 0.001, I² = 0.0%, heterogeneity p = 0.931), when compared with placebo or low-dose statin group, respectively.

Visual estimation of the funnel plot indicated no apparent publication or small study effect bias with the support of the Egger's test (p = 0.128) and Begg's test (p = 0.625) (Figure S4 in File S1). No individual study unduly influenced the pooled estimate of high-dose statin for the incidence of CIAKI (Figure S5 in File S1). Cumulative meta-analysis, which sorts trials chronologically, showed no apparent progressive shift of pooled estimate of high-dose statin from a negative to a positive effect, despite of differences in practice patterns or patient populations from 2008 to 2014 (Figure S6 in File S1). Along with the

Study	Published Year	RR (95% CI)	Events, Statin	Events, Control	% Weight
(A) High-dose Statin versus Control					
PROMISS	2008	0.75 (0.17, 3.28)	3/118	4/118	2.66
Toso et al.	2009	0.94 (0.48, 1.83)	15/152	16/152	11.68
Acikel et al.	2010	0.33 (0.01, 8.06)	0/80	1/80	0.58
Ozhan et al.	2010	0.33 (0.07, 1.54)	2/60	7/70	2.47
ARMYDA-CIN	2011	0.38 (0.15, 0.93)	6/120	16/121	6.76
Wei Li et al.	2012	0.16 (0.04, 0.70)	2/78	13/83	2.73
NAPLES II	2012	0.25 (0.12, 0.51)	9/202	37/208	10.69
PRATO-ACS	2014	0.45 (0.26, 0.77)	17/252	38/252	16.52
TRACK-D	2014	0.59 (0.39, 0.89)	34/1498	58/1500	25.02
Subtotal Effect (Z = 4.52, P < 0.001) Heterogeneity (P = 0.192 , I² = 28.4%)		0.47 (0.34, 0.65)	88/2560	190/2584	79.10
(B) High-dose Statin versus Low-dose Statin					
Xinwei et al.	2009	0.34 (0.14, 0.82)	6/113	18/115	7.00
Zhou Xia et al.	2009	0.14 (0.01, 2.70)	0/50	3/50	0.68
Hua et al.	2010	0.40 (0.15, 1.04)	5/76	16/97	6.06
CAO et al.	2012	0.33 (0.14, 0.80)	6/90	18/90	7.15
Subtotal Effect (Z = 4.06, P < 0.001) Heterogeneity (P = 0.931 , I² = 0.0%)		0.34 (0.21, 0.58)	17/329	55/352	20.90
Overall Random Effect Model Heterogeneity P = 0.364; I² = 8.2% Test of Overall Effect Z = 6.44 (P < 0.001)		0.45 (0.35, 0.57)	105/2889	245/2936	100.00

.1 .2 .5 1 2 5 10

Favours High-dose Statin   Favours Control

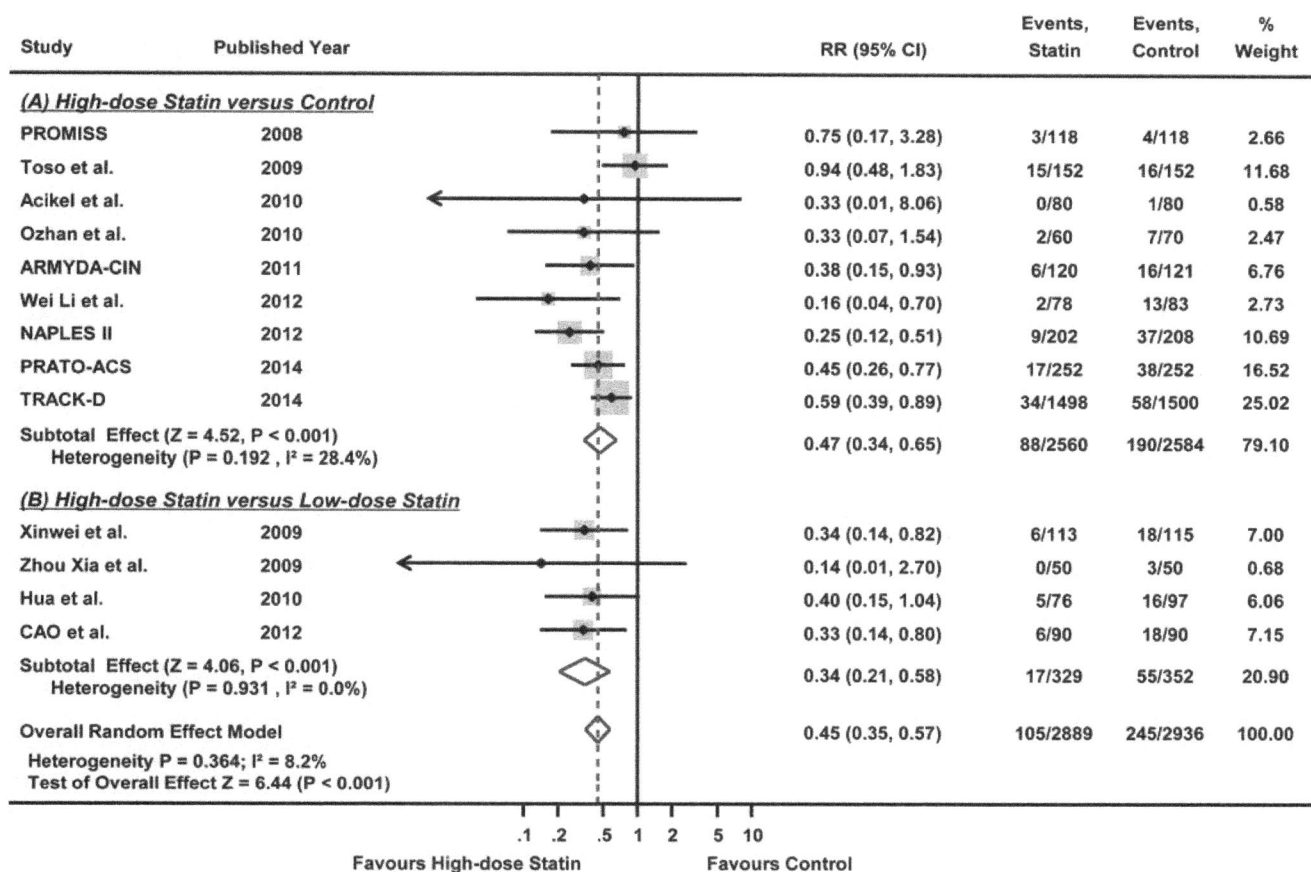

Figure 3. The effect of high-dose statin on the incidence of contrast-induced acute kidney injury, stratified according to the high-dose versus low-dose statin or high-dose versus placebo. Forest plot with relative risks for the incidence of contrast-induced acute kidney injury associated with (A) high-dose statin versus low-dose statin or (B) high-dose statin versus placebo for individual trials and the pooled population. Abbreviations: CI, confidence intervals; RR, relative risks.

significantly reduced incidence of CIAKI in high-dose statin group, mean change of post-procedural serum creatinine was also significantly lower in the high-dose statin group, compared with control group (SMD −0.37, 95% CI −0.59 to −0.15, p = 0.001) (Figure S7 in File S1).

Subgroup Analysis

The results of subgroup analysis are presented in Figure 4. The beneficial effect of high-dose statin pre-treatment was consistent across all the subgroups, except the subgroup of age less than 60 years old. The high-dose statin showed significantly less development of CIAKI in the patients with old age (≥60 years old), underlying chronic kidney disease, or acute coronary syndrome. When the high-risk subgroup was defined with the patients with chronic kidney disease or acute coronary syndrome, the high-dose statin showed also significant beneficial effect in reducing CIAKI in both high-risk and low-risk subgroup. In addition, the protective effect of high-dose statin was also significant regardless of the osmolality of the contrast agents (iso- or low-osmolar) or concomitant treatment of NAC. Lastly, high-dose statin significantly reduced the incidence of CIAKI compared with placebo or low-dose statin. The NNT of high-dose statin ranged from 12 to 26 (Figure 4). Detailed results of pooled analysis in each subgroup are summarized in the Figure S8-S12 in File S1.

Discussion

The results of this meta-analysis indicate that high-dose statin pre-treatment in patients undergoing CAG with or without PCI significantly reduced the incidence of CIAKI, compared with control (placebo or low-dose statin). The beneficial effect of high-dose statin was obvious in various subgroups of patients including underlying chronic kidney disease, acute coronary syndrome, or old age (≥60 years). The effect of high-dose statin was also clear regardless of type of contrast agent or concomitant treatment of NAC.

This study is the most up-to-date comprehensive meta-analysis with improved statistical power to address the effect of statin for CIAKI prevention in CAG. [10,29–33] The inconclusive results of previous meta-analyses regarding the efficacy of statin pre-treatment, might mainly originate from the limited sample size of included trials. [29–31] Some of these studies included both randomized and non-randomized clinical trials, which might have led to potential bias. [10,32] In the most recent meta-analysis by Li et al. [33], the authors showed significant benefit of statin pre-treatment in reducing the incidence of CIAKI. However, they argued that statin pre-treatment had no protective effect in the patients with underlying chronic kidney disease (RR 0.79, 95% CI 0.47–1.32, p = 0.37), however, the included studies in this subgroup analysis were only 3 studies with total sample size of

	No. of Trials	No. of Patients	Relative Risks (95% CI) for CIN	NNT	I² (heterogeneity P)	Interaction P
Statistical Model						
Fixed effects	13	5825	0.44 (0.35-0.55)	22	8.2% (0.364)	
Radom Effects	13	5825	0.45 (0.35-0.57)	16	8.2% (0.364)	
Type of Intervention						0.356
High-dose Statin versus Control	9	5144	0.47 (0.34-0.65)	19	28.4% (0.192)	
High-dose Statin versus Low-dose Statin	4	681	0.34 (0.21-0.58)	16	0.0% (0.931)	
Type of Contrast agent						0.156
Iso-osmolar, non-ionic contrast	5	4452	0.52 (0.34-0.79)	21	50.2% (0.090)	
Low-osmolar, non-ionic contrast	7	1193	0.33 (0.21-0.52)	14	0.0% (0.962)	
Mean Age of the Population						0.718
≥ 60 years old	11	5535	0.44 (0.34-0.58)	14	22.3% (0.231)	
< 60 years old	2	290	0.33 (0.08-1.33)	31	0.0% (1.000)	
Chronic Kidney Disease						0.144
Exclusively enrolled CKD patients	4	3948	0.55 (0.31-0.96)	26	60.5% (0.055)	
Others	9	1877	0.37 (0.27-0.51)	13	0.0% (0.973)	
Acute coronary syndrome						0.265
Exclusively enrolled ACS patients	5	1314	0.37 (0.26-0.53)	10	0.0% (0.776)	
Others	8	4511	0.50 (0.34-0.73)	24	24.2% (0.236)	
N-acetylcystein was administered						0.710
Yes	4	1348	0.46 (0.25-0.83)	13	59.9% (0.058)	
No	9	4477	0.45 (0.34-0.60)	18	0.0% (0.695)	
Placebo controlled or Not						0.047
Placebo controlled	5	3940	0.56 (0.36-0.88)	28	32.5% (0.205)	
No	8	1885	0.35 (0.26-0.49)	12	0.0% (0.953)	
Risk of CIAKI						
High-risk (CKD or ACS patient)	9	5262	0.45 (0.33-0.61)	14	34.1% (0.145)	0.583
Low-risk (Others)	4	563	0.35 (0.16-0.75)	19	0.0% (0.932)	

0.1   1   10

Favours High-dose Statin   Favours Control

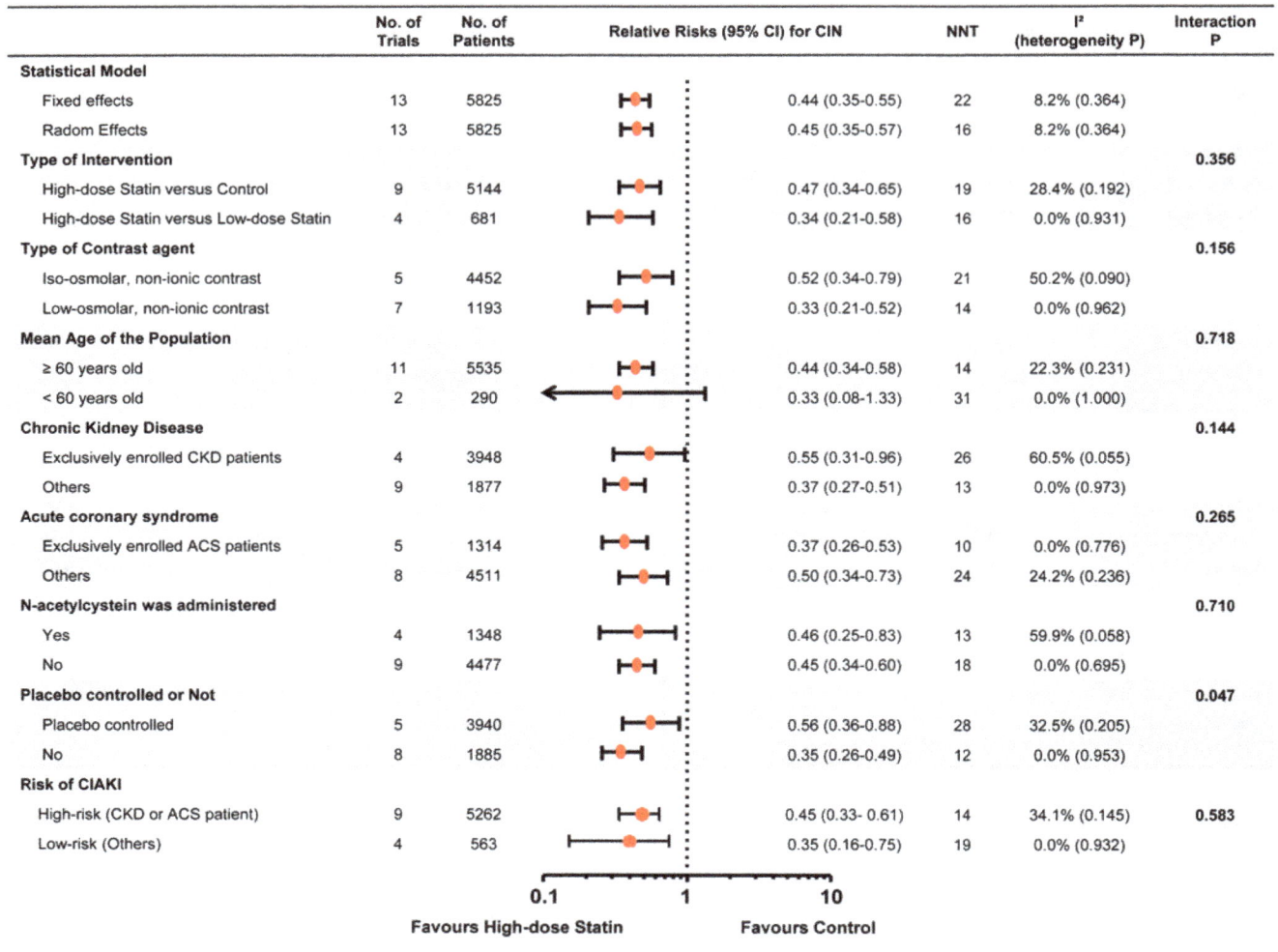

Figure 4. Subgroup analyses according to the study protocols. The forest plot shows relative risks (by random effects model) for the incidence of contrast-induced acute kidney injury associated with high-dose statin pre-treatment, compared with control group (low-dose statin or placebo), stratified according to (1) type of intervention, (2) type of contrast agent, (3) mean age of the patients, (4) underlying chronic kidney disease, (5) acute coronary syndrome, (6) N-acetylcystein as concomitant prophylactic measure, and (7) placebo controlled trial or not. Abbreviations: ACS, acute coronary syndrome; CI, confidence intervals; CKD, chronic kidney disease; RR, relative risks.

390 in high-dose statin versus 391 in control group. [33] In the present meta-analysis we evaluated over 5,800 patients from 13 RCTs, the benefit of high-dose statin was consistently observed in both overall population and various subgroups including patients with chronic kidney disease (RR 0.55, 95% CI 0.31–0.96, p = 0.036). The limited sample size of the pooled analysis and larger chance of type II error would explain the negative result of Li et al.

Previous studies have suggested that statin protects CIAKI through its pleotropic effect rather than its lipid lowering effect. The pleotropic effect includes enhancement of nitric oxide production, anti-inflammatory, and antioxidative effect. [34,35] These pleotropic effects could decrease renal cell injury after iodinated contrast exposure. In the NAPLES II trial, high-dose atorvastatin reduced contrast-induced JNK activation and p53 phosphorylation which is the key steps of oxidative stress induced intrinsic apoptosis. [13] Also, statin may modulate the kidney hypoperfusion after radio-contrast exposure by down-regulation of angiotensin receptors and by decrease of endothelin-1 synthesis.

[36] Lastly, anti-inflammatory effect of statin may prevent renal cell damage through decrease of pro-inflammatory cytokines which induce tissue factor expression by macrophage and activate nuclear factor-kappa B [37].

Although high-dose statin showed clear beneficial effect in preventing CIAKI, the risk of high-dose statin should be considered. Among the 13 RCTs, only 2 trials reported adverse events related with high-dose statin treatment. [14,28] Wei Li et al. reported that the rates of hepatotoxicity (defined as>3 times of upper normal limits of alanine aminotransferase within 1 month of the procedure) were 3.85% in high-dose statin group and 1.20% in control group (p = 0.57). In TRACK-D trial, they described that the rates of muscle pain, liver function abnormality, gastrointestinal disorders, edema or rash were not statistically different between high-dose statin and control group without presentation of actual numbers of the complications. Since limited data of adverse events in the included trials, the hazard of high-dose statin pre-treatment could not be evaluated in this meta-analysis. Previous meta-analysis of 35 RCTs comparing statin versus placebo, which was not a meta-analysis for CIAKI, reported that the absolute risk differences (RD) of most frequent adverse drug reactions were as follows; transaminase elevation (RD 4.2%, 95% CI 1.5 to 6.9%), myalgia (RD 2.7%, 95% CI −3.2 to 8.7%), rhabdomyolysis (RD 0.4%, 95% CI −0.1 to 0.9%), and discontinuation due to any adverse drug reaction (RD −0.5%, 95% CI −4.3 to 3.3%). [38] According to this report, the number needed to harm of statin treatment regarding adverse drug reaction are from 24 (hepatotoxicity) to 250 (rhabdomyolysis, defined as creatinine kinase elevations ≥10 times upper normal limit). Considering substantially lower NNT of 16 in this meta-analysis for reducing CIAKI and the clinical importance of CIAKI, high-dose statin pre-treatment before CAG with or without PCI could be considered as an effective prophylactic measure to prevent CIAKI.

Limitations

Several important limitations of the study should not be ignored. First, this meta-analysis included clinically- and methodologically-diverse studies. Although we included only RCTs to the final analysis and assured statistically insignificant heterogeneity, there were some differences in the enrollment criteria (some studies exclusively enrolled patients with chronic kidney disease or diabetes mellitus), definition of the CIAKI, medication or hydration protocols. Also, basically this meta-analysis comprising 13 RCTs inherently shares the limitations of each trial. Second, variations in the type, dose, and duration of statin pretreatment among the included trials might have potential effects to our results, since all statins may not be equivalent to each other in their pleotropic and nephroprotective effects. Finally, as this study was a study-level meta-analysis, individual patient data were not included in the analysis, and therefore, we could not adjust for patient-level confounders.

Conclusion

High-dose statin pre-treatment significantly reduced the incidence of CIAKI in patients undergoing CAG. Considering prognostic importance of CIAKI and clear beneficial effect of statin in this meta-analysis, high-dose statin pre-treatment may be more actively employed as an effective prophylactic measure to prevent CIAKI.

Supporting Information

Checklist S1 PRISMA checklist.

File S1 Supporting information files. Method S1, Search Strategy on Medline, EMBASE and Cochran Central. Method S2, Characteristics of the Excluded Study. Table S1, The Cochrane Collaboration's tool for assessing risk of bias. Figure S1, Risk of bias assessment graph. Risk of bias of each included trial was assessed with the Cochrane Collaboration's tool. This 'risk of bias graph' illustrates the proportion of studies with each of the judgments for each entry in the tool. Green represents 'Yes (low risk of bias)'; yellow, 'Unclear'; red, 'No (high risk of bias)'. Figure S2, Risk of bias assessment summary. Risk of bias of each included trial was assessed with the Cochrane Collaboration's tool. This 'risk of bias summary' figure presents all of the judgments in a cross-tabulation of study by entry. Green represents 'Yes (low risk of bias)'; yellow, 'Unclear'; red, 'No (high risk of bias)'. Figure S3,

The effect of High-dose statin on the incidence of contrast-induced nephropathy by fixed effects model. Forest plot with relative risks for the incidence of contrast-induced nephropathy associated with high-dose statin versus low-dose statin or placebo for individual trials and the pooled population. The squares and the horizontal lines indicate the relative risks (by fixed effects model) and the 95% confidence intervals (CI) for each trial included; the size of each square is proportional to the statistical weight of a trial in the frequentist meta-analysis; diamond indicates the effect estimate derived from meta-analysis, with the center indicating the point estimate and the left and the right ends the 95% CI. Abbreviations: CI, confidence intervals; RR, relative risks. Figure S4, The effect of High-dose statin on mean change of post-procedural serum creatinine. Forest plot with standardized mean difference (SMD) for the mean change of post-procedural serum creatinine from the baseline value associated with high-dose statin versus low-dose statin or placebo for individual trials and the pooled population. The squares and the horizontal lines indicate the SMD (by random effects model) and the 95% confidence intervals (CI) for each trial included; the size of each square is proportional to the statistical weight of a trial in the frequentist meta-analysis; diamond indicates the effect estimate derived from meta-analysis, with the center indicating the point estimate and the left and the right ends the 95% CI. Abbreviations: CI, confidence intervals; SD, standard deviation; SMD, standardized mean difference. Figure S5, Funnel plot for evaluation of publication and small study bias. Figure S6, Influence of individual studies Abbreviations: CI, confidence intervals; RR, relative risks. Figure S7, Cumulative Meta-analysis of high-dose statin on the incidence of contrast-induced nephropathy. The first row shows the effect of one study, the second row shows the cumulative pooled estimates based on the two studies, and so on. The squares and the horizontal lines indicate the cumulative relative risks (by random effects model) and the 95% confidence intervals (CI) for each trial included. Abbreviations: CI, confidence intervals; RR, relative risks. Figure S8, The effect of High-dose statin on the incidence of contrast-induced nephropathy, stratified according to the type of contrast. The squares and the horizontal lines indicate the relative risks (by random effects model) and the 95% confidence intervals (CI) for each trial included; the size of each square is proportional to the statistical weight of a trial in the meta-analysis; diamond indicates the effect estimate derived from meta-analysis, with the center indicating the point estimate and the left and the right ends the 95% CI. Abbreviations: CI, confidence intervals; RR, relative risks. Figure S9, The effect of High-dose statin on the incidence of contrast-induced nephropathy, stratified according to the mean age of the patients. The squares and the horizontal lines indicate the relative risks (by random effects model) and the 95% confidence intervals (CI) for each trial included; the size of each square is proportional to the statistical weight of a trial in the meta-analysis; diamond indicates the effect estimate derived from meta-analysis, with the center indicating the point estimate and the left and the right ends the 95% CI. Abbreviations: CI, confidence intervals; RR, relative risks. Figure S10, The effect of High-dose statin on the incidence of contrast-induced nephropathy, stratified according to the underlying chronic kidney disease. The squares and the horizontal lines indicate the relative risks (by random effects model) and the 95% confidence intervals (CI) for each trial included; the size of each square is proportional to the statistical weight of a trial in the meta-analysis; diamond indicates the effect estimate derived from meta-analysis, with the center indicating the point estimate and the left and the right ends the 95% CI. Abbreviations: CI, confidence intervals; CKD, chronic kidney disease; eGFR, estimated glomerular filtration rates; RR, relative risks. Figure S11, The effect of High-dose statin on the incidence of contrast-induced nephropathy, stratified according to the acute coronary syndrome. The squares and the horizontal lines indicate the relative risks (by random effects model) and the 95% confidence intervals (CI) for each trial included; the size of each square is proportional to the statistical weight of a trial in the meta-analysis; diamond indicates the effect estimate derived from meta-analysis, with the center indicating the point estimate and the left and the right ends the 95% CI. Abbreviations: CI, confidence intervals; RR, relative risks. Figure S12, The effect of High-dose statin on the incidence of contrast-induced nephropathy, stratified according to the concomitant treatment of N-acetylcystein. The squares and the

horizontal lines indicate the relative risks (by random effects model) and the 95% confidence intervals (CI) for each trial included; the size of each square is proportional to the statistical weight of a trial in the meta-analysis; diamond indicates the effect estimate derived from meta-analysis, with the center indicating the point estimate and the left and the right ends the 95% CI. Abbreviations: CI, confidence intervals; RR, relative risks.

Author Contributions

Conceived and designed the experiments: JML JP HSK. Analyzed the data: JML JP KHJ JHJ SEL JKH HLK HMY KWP HJK BKK SHJ HSK. Contributed reagents/materials/analysis tools: JHJ SEL JKH HLK HMY KWP HJK BKK SHJ. Wrote the paper: JML JP.

References

1. McCullough PA (2008) Contrast-induced acute kidney injury. J Am Coll Cardiol 51: 1419–1428.
2. McCullough PA, Adam A, Becker CR, Davidson C, Lameire N, et al. (2006) Epidemiology and prognostic implications of contrast-induced nephropathy. Am J Cardiol 98: 5K–13K.
3. Klein LW, Sheldon MW, Brinker J, Mixon TA, Skelding K, et al. (2009) The use of radiographic contrast media during PCI: a focused review: a position statement of the Society of Cardiovascular Angiography and Interventions. Catheter Cardiovasc Interv 74: 728–746.
4. Kelly AM, Dwamena B, Cronin P, Bernstein SJ, Carlos RC (2008) Meta-analysis: effectiveness of drugs for preventing contrast-induced nephropathy. Ann Intern Med 148: 284–294.
5. Kitzler TM, Jaberi A, Sendlhofer G, Rehak P, Binder C, et al. (2012) Efficacy of vitamin E and N-acetylcysteine in the prevention of contrast induced kidney injury in patients with chronic kidney disease: a double blind, randomized controlled trial. Wien Klin Wochenschr 124: 312–319.
6. O'Gara PT, Kushner FG, Ascheim DD, Casey DE Jr, Chung MK, et al. (2013) 2013 ACCF/AHA guideline for the management of ST-elevation myocardial infarction: executive summary: a report of the American College of Cardiology Foundation/American Heart Association Task Force on Practice Guidelines: developed in collaboration with the American College of Emergency Physicians and Society for Cardiovascular Angiography and Interventions. Catheter Cardiovasc Interv 82: E1–27.
7. Task Force on Myocardial Revascularization of the European Society of C, the European Association for Cardio-Thoracic S, European Association for Percutaneous Cardiovascular I, Wijns W, Kolh P, et al. (2010) Guidelines on myocardial revascularization. Eur Heart J 31: 2501–2555.
8. Attallah N, Yassine L, Musial J, Yee J, Fisher K (2004) The potential role of statins in contrast nephropathy. Clin Nephrol 62: 273–278.
9. Khanal S, Attallah N, Smith DE, Kline-Rogers E, Share D, et al. (2005) Statin therapy reduces contrast-induced nephropathy: an analysis of contemporary percutaneous interventions. Am J Med 118: 843–849.
10. Pappy R, Stavrakis S, Hennebry TA, Abu-Fadel MS (2011) Effect of statin therapy on contrast-induced nephropathy after coronary angiography: a meta-analysis. Int J Cardiol 151: 348–353.
11. Jo SH, Koo BK, Park JS, Kang HJ, Cho YS, et al. (2008) Prevention of radiocontrast medium-induced nephropathy using short-term high-dose simvastatin in patients with renal insufficiency undergoing coronary angiography (PROMISS) trial—a randomized controlled study. Am Heart J 155: 499 e491–498.
12. Toso A, Maioli M, Leoncini M, Gallopin M, Tedeschi D, et al. (2010) Usefulness of atorvastatin (80 mg) in prevention of contrast-induced nephropathy in patients with chronic renal disease. Am J Cardiol 105: 288–292.
13. Quintavalle C, Fiore D, De Micco F, Visconti G, Focaccio A, et al. (2012) Impact of a high loading dose of atorvastatin on contrast-induced acute kidney injury. Circulation 126: 3008–3016.
14. Han Y, Zhu G, Han L, Hou F, Huang W, et al. (2014) Short-term rosuvastatin therapy for prevention of contrast-induced acute kidney injury in patients with diabetes and chronic kidney disease. J Am Coll Cardiol 63: 62–70.
15. Leoncini M, Toso A, Maioli M, Tropeano F, Villani S, et al. (2014) Early high-dose rosuvastatin for contrast-induced nephropathy prevention in acute coronary syndrome: Results from the PRATO-ACS Study (Protective Effect of Rosuvastatin and Antiplatelet Therapy On contrast-induced acute kidney injury and myocardial damage in patients with Acute Coronary Syndrome). J Am Coll Cardiol 63: 71–79.
16. Lee JM, Bae W, Lee YJ, Cho YJ (2014) The efficacy and safety of prone positional ventilation in acute respiratory distress syndrome: updated study-level meta-analysis of 11 randomized controlled trials. Crit Care Med 42: 1252–1262.
17. Jadad AR, Moore RA, Carroll D, Jenkinson C, Reynolds DJ, et al. (1996) Assessing the quality of reports of randomized clinical trials: is blinding necessary? Control Clin Trials 17: 1–12.
18. DerSimonian R, Laird N (1986) Meta-analysis in clinical trials. Control Clin Trials 7: 177–188.
19. Higgins JP, Thompson SG, Deeks JJ, Altman DG (2003) Measuring inconsistency in meta-analyses. BMJ 327: 557–560.
20. Moher D, Liberati A, Tetzlaff J, Altman DG (2009) Preferred reporting items for systematic reviews and meta-analyses: the PRISMA statement. Ann Intern Med 151: 264–269, W264.
21. Xinwei J, Xianghua F, Jing Z, Xinshun G, Ling X, et al. (2009) Comparison of usefulness of simvastatin 20 mg versus 80 mg in preventing contrast-induced nephropathy in patients with acute coronary syndrome undergoing percutaneous coronary intervention. Am J Cardiol 104: 519–524.
22. Zhou X, Jin YZ, Wang Q, Min R, Zhang XY (2009) [Efficacy of high dose atorvastatin on preventing contrast induced nephropathy in patients underwent coronary angiography]. Zhonghua Xin Xue Guan Bing Za Zhi 37: 394–396.
23. Acikel S, Muderrisoglu H, Yildirir A, Aydinalp A, Sade E, et al. (2010) Prevention of contrast-induced impairment of renal function by short-term or long-term statin therapy in patients undergoing elective coronary angiography. Blood Coagul Fibrinolysis 21: 750–757.
24. Ozhan H, Erden I, Ordu S, Aydin M, Caglar O, et al. (2010) Efficacy of short-term high-dose atorvastatin for prevention of contrast-induced nephropathy in patients undergoing coronary angiography. Angiology 61: 711–714.
25. X-p H, R-x W, Y Y, Zheng C, Bin C (2010) Prevention of contrast-induced nephropathy using high-dose atorvastatin in patients with coronary heart disease undergoing elective percutaneous coronary intervention] [in Chinese. Milit Med J South China 24: 448–451.
26. Patti G, Ricottini E, Nusca A, Colonna G, Pasceri V, et al. (2011) Short-term, high-dose Atorvastatin pretreatment to prevent contrast-induced nephropathy in patients with acute coronary syndromes undergoing percutaneous coronary intervention (from the ARMYDA-CIN [atorvastatin for reduction of myocardial damage during angioplasty—contrast-induced nephropathy] trial. Am J Cardiol 108: 1–7.
27. Cao S, Wang P, Cui K, Zhang L, Hou Y (2012) [Atorvastatin prevents contrast agent-induced renal injury in patients undergoing coronary angiography by inhibiting oxidative stress]. Nan Fang Yi Ke Da Xue Xue Bao 32: 1600–1602.
28. Li W, Fu X, Wang Y, Li X, Yang Z, et al. (2012) Beneficial effects of high-dose atorvastatin pretreatment on renal function in patients with acute ST-segment elevation myocardial infarction undergoing emergency percutaneous coronary intervention. Cardiology 122: 195–202.
29. Takagi H, Umemoto T (2011) A meta-analysis of randomized trials for effects of periprocedural atorvastatin on contrast-induced nephropathy. Int J Cardiol 153: 323–325.
30. Zhang BC, Li WM, Xu YW (2011) High-dose statin pretreatment for the prevention of contrast-induced nephropathy: a meta-analysis. Can J Cardiol 27: 851–858.
31. Zhang L, Zhang L, Lu Y, Wu B, Zhang S, et al. (2011) Efficacy of statin pretreatment for the prevention of contrast-induced nephropathy: a meta-analysis of randomised controlled trials. Int J Clin Pract 65: 624–630.
32. Zhang T, Shen LH, Hu LH, He B (2011) Statins for the prevention of contrast-induced nephropathy: a systematic review and meta-analysis. Am J Nephrol 33: 344–351.
33. Li Y, Liu Y, Fu L, Mei C, Dai B (2012) Efficacy of short-term high-dose statin in preventing contrast-induced nephropathy: a meta-analysis of seven randomized controlled trials. PLoS One 7: e34450.
34. John S, Schneider MP, Delles C, Jacobi J, Schmieder RE (2005) Lipid-independent effects of statins on endothelial function and bioavailability of nitric oxide in hypercholesterolemic patients. Am Heart J 149: 473.

35. Ridker PM, Rifai N, Clearfield M, Downs JR, Weis SE, et al. (2001) Measurement of C-reactive protein for the targeting of statin therapy in the primary prevention of acute coronary events. N Engl J Med 344: 1959–1965.

36. Ichiki T, Takeda K, Tokunou T, Iino N, Egashira K, et al. (2001) Downregulation of angiotensin II type 1 receptor by hydrophobic 3-hydroxy-3-methylglutaryl coenzyme A reductase inhibitors in vascular smooth muscle cells. Arterioscler Thromb Vasc Biol 21: 1896–1901.

37. Bonetti PO, Lerman LO, Napoli C, Lerman A (2003) Statin effects beyond lipid lowering—are they clinically relevant? Eur Heart J 24: 225–248.

38. Kashani A, Phillips CO, Foody JM, Wang Y, Mangalmurti S, et al. (2006) Risks associated with statin therapy: a systematic overview of randomized clinical trials. Circulation 114: 2788–2797.

28

Association of Versican Turnover with All-Cause Mortality in Patients on Haemodialysis

Federica Genovese[1]*, **Morten A. Karsdal**[1], **Diana J. Leeming**[1], **Alexandra Scholze**[2], **Martin Tepel**[2]

1 Nordic Bioscience, Fibrosis Biology and Biomarkers, Herlev, Denmark, **2** Odense University Hospital, Department of Nephrology, Institute for Molecular Medicine, Cardiovascular and Renal Research, Institute of Clinical Research, University of Southern Denmark, Odense, Denmark

Abstract

Objective: Cardiovascular diseases are among the most common causes of mortality in renal failure patients undergoing haemodialysis. A high turnover rate of the proteoglycan versican, represented by the increased presence of its fragmentation products in plasma, has previously been associated with cardiovascular diseases. The objective of the study was to investigate the association of versican turnover assessed in plasma with survival in haemodialysis patients.

Methods: A specific matrix metalloproteinase-generated neo-epitope fragment of versican (VCANM) was measured in plasma of 364 haemodialysis patients with a 5-years follow-up, using a robust competitive enzyme-linked immunosorbent assays. Association between VCANM plasma concentration and survival was assessed by Kaplan-Meier analysis and adjusted Cox model.

Results: Haemodialysis patients with plasma VCANM concentrations in the lowest quartile had increased risk of death (odds ratio, as compared to the highest quartile: 7.1, $p<0.001$), with a reduced survival of 152 days compared to 1295 days for patients with plasma VCANM in the highest quartile. Multivariate analysis showed that low VCANM ($p<0.001$) and older age ($p<0.001$) predicted death in haemodialysis patients.

Conclusions: Low concentrations of the versican fragment VCANM in plasma were associated with higher risk of death among haemodialysis patients. A possible protective role for the examined versican fragment is suggested.

Editor: Konradin Metze, University of Campinas, Brazil

Funding: The authors acknowledge the Danish Research Fund (Den Danske Forskningfond) for providing the funding for this research. FG, DJL, and MAK are full-time employees at Nordic Bioscience. Nordic Bioscience provided support in the form of salaries for authors FG, DJL, and MAK, but did not have any additional role in the study design, data collection and analysis, decision to publish, or preparation of the manuscript. The specific roles of these authors are articulated in the 'author contributions' section.

Competing Interests: Federica Genovese has read the journal's policy and the authors of this manuscript have the following competing interests: FG, DJL, and MAK are full-time employees at Nordic Bioscience. All other authors have no competing financial interests.

* Email: fge@nordicbioscience.com

Introduction

Patients with renal failure who undergo haemodialysis have an increased mortality compared to the general population [1,2]. Cardiovascular diseases are frequently a co-morbidity affecting end stage kidney disease (ESKD) patients [3,4], and they are the major cause of death in patients on dialysis [5]. A dysregulated equilibrium between extracellular matrix (ECM) formation and degradation characterizes fibrotic disorders, neoplasia and cardiovascular diseases [6]. Renal fibrosis is the pathological process underlying kidney failure, and most of the co-morbidities affecting ESKD patients can be related to the altered matrix turnover [7]. Thus, novel non-invasive biomarkers able to describe the rate of ECM turnover have the potential to be useful instruments to identify patients with a worse prognosis [8].

Versican is a large extracellular matrix proteoglycan whose role in chronic kidney disease (CKD) has only been described to a certain extent [9]. Versican belongs to the family of the large aggregating proteoglycans, and it has been localized in the ECM

of many organs, including kidneys [9,10]. It has a modular structure constituted by a G1 domain at the N-terminal, a glycosaminoglycan (GAG) domain for the attachment of the chondroitin sulphate chains that constitute its carbohydrate fraction, and a G3 domain at the C-terminal end. The G3 domain is further organized in a modular structure containing two EGF-like repeats, a lectin-like subdomain and a complement binding protein (CBP)-like subdomain, which are dedicated to the binding with different ECM components and cytokines [11]. The main protein associated with versican is hyaluronan [12], which interacts with the G1 domain of versican. Moreover versican binds and interacts with elastic fibers, collagen type I, fibronectin and integrins [11]. Versican turnover can be estimated by the amount of fragmentation products released into circulation. A novel neo-epitope specific enzyme-linked immunosorbent assays (ELISA) has been developed to detect a unique fragmentation product generated by the cleavage of matrix metalloproteinases. This fragment of versican variant V0 measurable in plasma (VCANM), has previously been associated with different cardiovascular manifestations [13].

In the present study we tested the hypothesis that versican turnover may be associated with mortality in haemodialysis patients, by measuring plasma levels of VCANM.

Subjects and Methods

Participants

We performed an observational cohort study of 364 haemodialysis patients. The study was approved by the local ethics committee (Ethikkommission Free University Berlin, Reference numbers: ek.211-19, ek.Te2.02) and adhered to the declaration of Helsinki. Inclusion criteria were haemodialysis treatment due to end-stage renal disease and written informed consent.

All patients were routinely dialyzed for four to five hours three times weekly using biocompatible membranes with no dialyser reuse. Blood flow rates were 250 to 300 mL/min, dialysate flow rates were 500 mL/min, dialysate conductivity was 135 mS. Blood pressure was measured pre-dialysis in patients in a recumbent position. Pre-dialysis blood samples were taken at study entry.

Blood was collected immediately before the start of the haemodialysis session. Clinical and laboratory data included age, gender, medication (use of angiotensin-converting-enzyme inhibitors, ß-blockers, calcium channel blockers, and erythropoietin), body mass index (calculated as weight in kilograms divided by height in meters squared), systolic and diastolic blood pressure, serum urea, serum calcium, serum potassium, and serum phosphorus. 179 patients (49%) died during the 5-years follow up. The causes of death were classified as cardiovascular, infection, cancer, or unknown. Controls consisted of nineteen age- and sex-matched CKD patients not undergoing dialysis. Among these, two patients had stage two CKD (glomerular filtration rate, GFR, according to MDRD: 90–60 mL/min), and seventeen patients had stage three CKD (GFR according to MDRD: 60–30 mL/min).

Procedures

The neo-epitope peptide generated by matrix metalloproteinase (MMP) degradation of versican (VCANM) was measured in plasma of haemodialysis patients and controls by means of a robust competitive enzyme-linked immunosorbent assays (ELISA) using a specific monoclonal antibody (mAb). The protocols and

Table 1. Baseline clinical and biochemical characteristics of haemodialysis patients stratified by plasma VCANM quartiles (Q1, Q2, Q3, Q4).

Characteristic	Q1	Q2	Q3	Q 4	P-value[a]
Number of patients	92	90	92	90	–
VCANM (range; ng/ml)	0.50 (0.20–0.59)	0.70 (0.60–0.79)	0.80 (0.80–0.99)	1.10 (1.00–1.50)	<0.001
Age (years)	68.0 (60.5–76)	64.2 (56–75)	64.3 (52–76)	64.5 (57–72)	0.12
Gender (% Male)	68%	72%	66%	56%	0.06
Dialysis vintage (months)	25.4 (1.0–35.3)	27.8 (1.0–51.7)	26.5 (1.6–43.0)	23.4 (1.0–30.4)	0.88
Diabetes mellitus (%)	50%	31%	62%	60%	0.30
Weight (kg)	71 (60–80)	74 (63–81)	73 (62–79)	75 (64–83)	0.33
Body mass index[b] (kg/m^2)	24.4 (21–27.7)	25.3 (22–27.8)	24.6 (21.6–26)	25.6 (22.4–29)	0.13
Systolic blood pressure (mmHg)	131 (114–149)	135 (117–153)	134 (114–150)	134 (117–150)	0.73
Diastolic blood pressure (mmHg)	68 (57–80)	71 (59–80)	70 (58–80)	71 (60–82)	0.35
Hemoglobin (mg/dL)	9.9 (8.7–10.8)	10.0 (9.1–11.4)	10.6 (9.3–11.8)	10.6 (9.3–11.9)	0.02
Leukocytes (10^9/L)	10.0 (6.6–12.6)	10.0 (6.5–12.8)	8.4 (6.2–9.7)	7.9 (5.7–9.5)	0.002
Platelets (10^9/L)	243 (173–305)	232 (176–256)	227 (165–271)	248 (187–300)	0.43
Albumin (g/dL)	3.2 (2.6–3.4)	3.2 (2.8–3.6)	3.4 (3.1–3.7)	3.5 (3.1–3.8)	<0.001
High sensitive CRP (mg/dL)	6.7 (2.3–8.0)	4.2 (1.2–4.5)	3.0 (0.75–4.1)	3.8 (0.9–4.7)	<0.001
Urea (mg/dL)	34 (20–36)	33 (20–41)	26 (16–31)	27 (17–35)	0.02
Serum potassium (mmol/L)	4.7 (4.1–5.2)	4.8 (4–5.5)	4.8 (4.3–5.2)	4.8 (4.2–5.4)	0.80
Serum calcium (mmol/L)	2.2 (2–2.4)	2.3 (2.1–2.4)	2.2 (2.1–2.4)	2.2 (2.1–2.4)	0.34
Serum phosphorus (mg/dL)	1.6 (1.2–1.9)	1.7 (1.2–2.1)	1.7 (1.2–2)	1.6 (1.1–2.1)	0.69
Parathyroid hormone (ng/mL)	164 (39–197)	213 (45–272)	199 (43–213)	212 (42–278)	0.96
Serum cholesterol (mg/dL)	142 (108–178)	162 (124–201)	156 (135–181)	166 (137–189)	0.06
LDL-cholesterol (mg/dl)	92 (66–114)	101 (70–129)	98 (79–116)	100 (79–123)	0.55
Dialysis dose (kt/V)	1.2 (1.0–1.3)	1.2 (1.1–1.3)	1.2 (1.0–1.3)	1.2 (1.0–1.3)	0.67
ACE inhibitors (%)	24%	20%	33%	28%	0.23
ß-Blockers (%)	59%	62%	55%	62%	0.87
Calcium channel blockers (%)	23%	29%	38%	29%	0.20
Erythropoietin therapy (%)	48%	42%	62%	45%	0.57

Continuous variables are given as medians (IQR).
[a]Comparisons between groups were made using Kruskal-Wallis test for continuous variables and Chi-square test for categorical variables.
[b]Body mass index was calculated as weight in kilograms divided by height in meters squared.

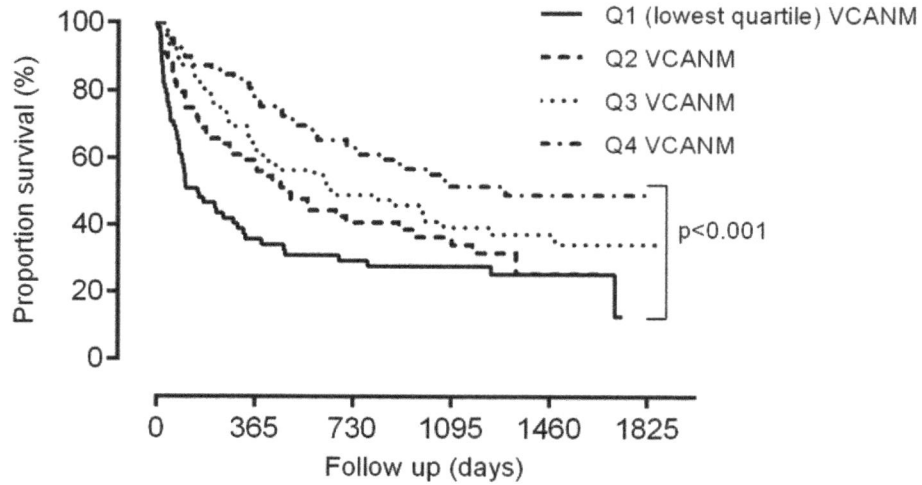

Figure 1. Kaplan-Meier survival curves for haemodialysis patients stratified in quartiles according to plasma VCANM levels.

technical specifications of the assay have already been described [13]. The VCANM mAb was raised against the sequence KTFGKMKPRY, a neo-epitope generated by *in vitro* proteolytic cleavage at the position 3306 by MMP-12. The antibody was selected to recognize specifically the neo-epitope generated after MMP cleavage, and not the total protein.

Statistical analysis

Continuous variables were expressed as median with interquartile range and compared with Kruskal-Wallis test and Dunn's multiple comparison post-hoc test. Time-to-event analyses were performed using the Kaplan-Meier method. Comparison of survival curves was performed using the log-rank (Mantel-Cox) test. 46 patients (12%) underwent kidney transplantation during the follow up. These patients were censored on the day of

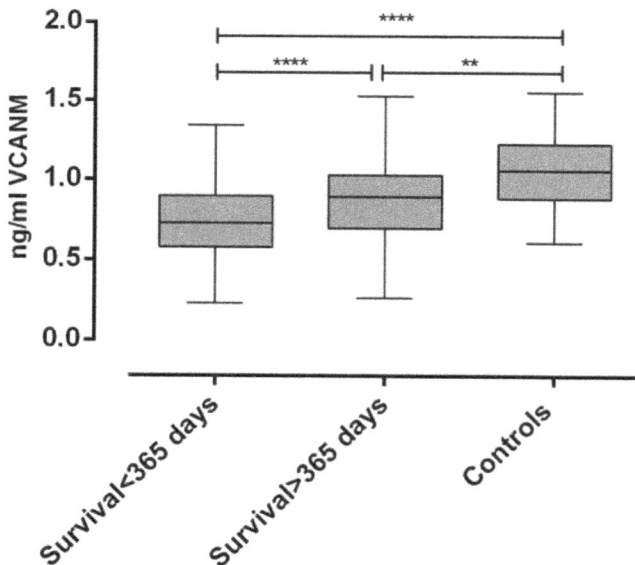

Figure 2. Plasma VCANM levels in haemodialysis patients with survival <365 days and survival >365 days and in the control group. Horizontal line: median; hashed box = IQR; error bars: range of non-outlying values. Significance levels (calculated with one-way ANOVA test, multiple comparison): ** = p<0.01; **** = p<0.001.

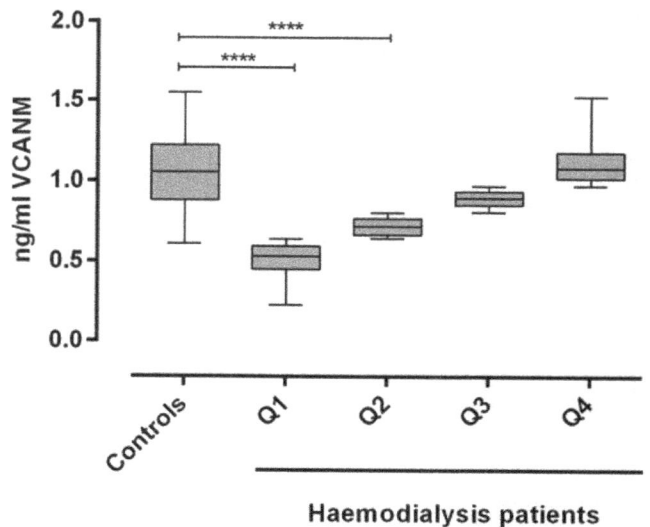

Figure 3. Plasma VCANM levels divided into quartiles in haemodialysis patients and in CKD stage two and three patients (controls). Horizontal line: median; hashed box = IQR; error bars: range of non-outlying values. Significance levels (calculated with Kruskal Wallis test and one-way ANOVA test, multiple comparison): **** = p<0.001.

Table 2. Univariate and multivariate Cox regression showing the odds for death in haemodialysis patients.

	Univariate Odds Ratio (95% CI)	P-value	Multivariate Odds Ratio (95% CI)	P-value
VCANM	0.23 (0.12–0.42)	<0.001	0.23 (0.13–0.42)	<0.001
Age	1.06 (1.05–1.08)	<0.001	1.06 (1.05–1.07)	<0.001
Gender (Ref=male)	0.89 (0.66–1.43)	0.31		
High sensitive CRP	1.69 (1.25–2.28)	<0.001		
Albumin	0.67 (0.52–0.86)	0.002		

transplantation. Univariate and multivariate survival analyses were performed using the proportional hazards regression model. The multivariate model was constructed with backward variable selection, using P<0.05 for variable retention. Statistical analyses were conducted using GraphPad Prism 5.0 (GraphPad Software, San Diego, CA), SPSS for windows (version 15; SPSS, Chicago, IL) and MedCalc (version 12.3.0.0, MedCalc software bvba for Windows).

Results

Characteristics of cohort at baseline

A total of 364 haemodialysis patients (240 men and 124 women) with a median age of 67 years (IQR, 56 to 75 years), a median time since initiation of dialysis of 247 days (IQR, 31 to 1142 days), and a median dialysis dose (kt/V) of 1.2 (IQR, 1.0 to 1.3) entered into the study. The primary diseases leading to end stage kidney disease were hypertensive nephrosclerosis in 122 cases (34%), diabetic nephropathy in 118 cases (32%), chronic glomerular nephritis in 30 cases (8%), polycystic kidney disease in 10 cases (3%) and other/unknown in 84 cases (23%). Median plasma VCANM concentration was 0.81 ng/mL (IQR, 0.64 to 0.97 ng/mL). Quartiles of plasma VCANM were used for the survival analysis. Table 1 describes the quartiles and summarizes clinical and laboratory variables stratified according to plasma VCANM quartiles.

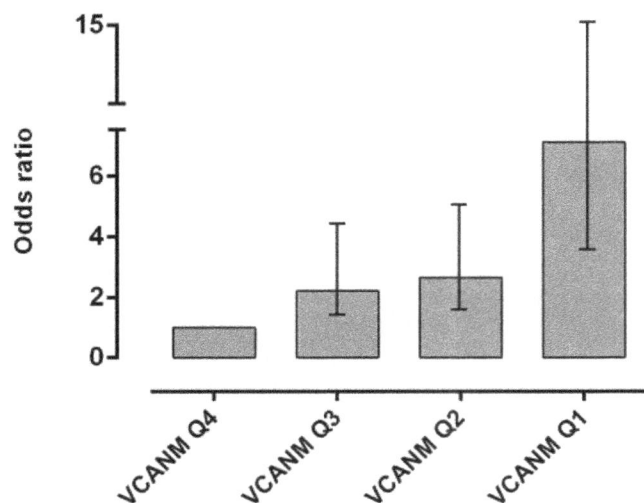

Figure 4. Odds ratio calculated for a cut-off of 365 days in the different VCANM quartiles. Bars: 95% CI.

Plasma VCANM levels are related to mortality

179 patients (49%) died during the 5 year follow up. Death occurred at a median of 201 days (IQR, 63 to 477 days) after study entry. The causes of death were cardiovascular diseases (including sudden death, fatal myocardial infarction, or fatal stroke) in 111 patients (62%), infectious disease (including septicemia) in 35 patients (20%), cancer (any type) in 22 patients (12%), and others/unknown in 11 patients (6%).

When patients were stratified according to quartiles of plasma VCANM, the survival rate differed significantly between the different groups (p<0.001). Patients belonging to the lowest VCANM quartile had a survival of 152 days compared to 1295 days for patients with plasma VCNAM in the highest quartile (Figure 1). VCANM was associated to all-cause mortality, and could not distinguish between cardiovascular disease-driven mortality and other mortality causes (data not shown).

The differences in survival rate among the different groups appeared to be evident already at early time points, such as 365 days. Therefore a survival time of 365 days was chosen as cut-off and the haemodialysis patients were divided into two groups: one including patients with survival time below 365 days and the other including patients that survived longer than 365 days. The levels of the analyzed marker in these two groups were compared to those of our control group constituted of patients with chronic kidney disease stage two and three (Figure 2). Plasma VCANM levels were highest in the control group, and lowest in the group of patients with short survival. Figure 3 illustrates the concentration levels in the different quartiles in the haemodialysis patient population and in the controls. VCANM levels were the same in controls and in Q4 and decreased significantly in Q3, Q2 and in the lowest quartile Q1.

The univariate Cox regression analysis showed a significant association of VCANM, age, high sensitive CRP and albumin with survival (Table 2). VCANM and age were retained in the model obtained with a multivariate analysis, showing independency from one another. CRP levels were significantly different in the VCANM quartile groups, decreasing with increasing VCANM concentrations (Table 1).

From the Cox regression analysis it was possible to calculate the odds ratio for an increase of ten years in age (odds = 1.87) and a decrease of 0.5 ng/ml of plasma VCANM (odds = 2.1).

The odds ratio for the different VCANM quartiles was calculated for death at 365 days as outcome (figure 4). VCANM Q1 showed an odds ratio of 7.1 (using as reference the fourth quartile).

Discussion

In the present study we have identified a novel marker of mortality in haemodialysis patients.

This marker represents a fragmentation product of versican, an ECM proteoglycans implicated in vascular remodeling [14], and it was previously associated with cardiovascular diseases caused by dysregulated ECM turnover [13]. The VCANM assay measures a pool of fragments of versican long up to 90 aminoacids, which have a common N-terminal end generated by proteolytic cleavage mediated by matrix metalloproteinases. This fragment is localized in the proximity of the protein C-terminal, in the G3 domain, and belongs to the complement binding protein (CBP)-like motif.

Haemodialysis patients with higher VCANM levels showed better outcome. This finding was strengthened by the observation of higher plasma VCANM levels in CKD patients stage two and three (controls) than in haemodialysis patients with shorter survival. Plasma VCANM concentration and age were retained in a multivariate regression model and were independent from each other. Furthermore, a decrease in plasma VCANM levels of 0.5 ng/ml, which corresponded to the median difference between the lowest and the highest plasma VCANM quartile, described a higher risk of death when compared to an increase of ten years of age. The separation between the different survival curves was maximal at early time points. For this reason we chose a cut-off time point of 365 days to calculate the odds ratio. The odds ratio for mortality for patients in the lowest plasma VCANM quartile was seven times higher compared to that for patients in the highest quartile. Interestingly, levels of VCANM were not exclusively associated to cardiovascular mortality, despite the previous findings that versican fragmentation was increased in cardiovascular diseases such as acute myocardial infarction and coronary calcification [13]. This suggests that in ESKD patients VCANM is not a marker for cardiovascular morbidity. The association of lower plasma levels of this specific fragment with a worse outcome might have different possible explanations: an increased fragmentation of versican in patients with a better prognosis may facilitate its clearance. An upregulated versican mRNA expression in the kidney was associated with the degree of histological damage [15], and histological accumulation of versican was observed in the tubulointerstitium of patients with proteinuric nephropathy [9], and in cellular crescents and periglomerular areas of patients with human crescentic glomerulonephritis [16]; therefore the ability to degrade the accumulated proteoglycan might be a factor that ameliorates the disease burden. Versican has been shown to be produced by stromal cells and leukocytes [17]: the correlation between number of leukocytes and VCANM quartiles (as shown in table 1) suggests that versican formation is more elevated than versican degradation during sustained inflammation. It has been demonstrated that complexes of versican and hyaluronan (HA) promote leukocytes adhesion and that a failed incorporation of versican into the ECM blocks monocyte adhesion and reduces the inflammatory response [17]. Therefore when versican is degraded (hence VCANM presence in plasma increases), the formation of the complex versican-hyaluronan is impaired and inflammation is reduced. This hypothesis is further confirmed by the inverse correlation between serum CRP levels and VCANM levels (table 1). Furthermore, as lower levels of VCANM are associated with higher mortality risk, it can be hypothesized that this fragment may have a protective role in end stage kidney disease patients. Such protective functions have been previously observed for other ECM protein fragments, such as endostatin and tumstatin [18,19]. The paracrine and endocrine functions of the ECM proteins are more and more object of investigation, and the proteins belonging to the matrix are not considered anymore as structural components only. Beside ECM proteins in their native conformation having signaling roles, there are evidences suggesting that ECM proteins that normally don't exert matricellular functions, gain powerful signaling potential after protease cleavage [6,20]. As of today, versican has only been seen as a therapeutic target [21], but the finding that high levels of its degradation product VCANM are associated with longer survival introduces the novel concept of its potential as therapeutic *per se*, which, however, needs to be carefully examined. Further investigations are needed to confirm whether VCANM is not only a fragment generated by proteolytic cleavage of versican, but has also paracrine or endocrine functions.

Acknowledgments

We acknowledge the Danish Research Fund (Den Danske Forskningfond) for providing the funding for this research.

Author Contributions

Conceived and designed the experiments: FG MAK DJL AS MT. Performed the experiments: FG AS MT. Analyzed the data: FG DJL MT. Contributed reagents/materials/analysis tools: MT AS MAK. Contributed to the writing of the manuscript: FG MT DJL MAK.

References

1. Hallan SI, Matsushita K, Sang Y, Mahmoodi BK, Black C, et al. (2012) Age and association of kidney measures with mortality and end-stage renal disease. JAMA 308: 2349–2360.

2. de Jager DJ, Grootendorst DC, Jager KJ, van Dijk PC, Tomas LM, et al. (2009) Cardiovascular and noncardiovascular mortality among patients starting dialysis. JAMA 302: 1782–1789.

3. Raggi P, Boulay A, Chasan-Taber S, Amin N, Dillon M, et al. (2002) Cardiac calcification in adult hemodialysis patients. A link between end-stage renal disease and cardiovascular disease? J Am Coll Cardiol 39: 695–701.

4. Goodman WG, Goldin J, Kuizon BD, Yoon C, Gales B, et al. (2000) Coronary-artery calcification in young adults with end-stage renal disease who are undergoing dialysis. N Engl J Med 342: 1478–1483.

5. Al-Dadah A, Omran J, Nusair MB, Dellsperger KC (2012) Cardiovascular mortality in dialysis patients. Adv Perit Dial 28: 56–59.

6. Karsdal MA, Nielsen MJ, Sand JM, Henriksen K, Genovese F, et al. (2013) Extracellular matrix remodeling: the common denominator in connective tissue diseases. Possibilities for evaluation and current understanding of the matrix as more than a passive architecture, but a key player in tissue failure. Assay Drug Dev Technol 11: 70–92.

7. Gross ML, Ritz E (2008) Hypertrophy and fibrosis in the cardiomyopathy of uremia–beyond coronary heart disease. Semin Dial 21: 308–318.

8. Genovese F, Manresa AA, Leeming DJ, Karsdal MA, Boor P (2014) The extracellular matrix in the kidney: a source of novel non-invasive biomarkers of kidney fibrosis? Fibrogenesis Tissue Repair 7: 4.

9. Rudnicki M, Perco P, Neuwirt H, Noppert SJ, Leierer J, et al. (2012) Increased renal versican expression is associated with progression of chronic kidney disease. PLoS One 7: e44891.

10. Bode-Lesniewska B, Dours-Zimmermann MT, Odermatt BF, Briner J, Heitz PU, et al. (1996) Distribution of the large aggregating proteoglycan versican in adult human tissues. J Histochem Cytochem 44: 303–312.

11. Wu YJ, La Pierre DP, Wu J, Yee AJ, Yang BB (2005) The interaction of versican with its binding partners. Cell Res 15: 483–494.

12. Selbi W, de la Motte CA, Hascall VC, Day AJ, Bowen T, et al. (2006) Characterization of hyaluronan cable structure and function in renal proximal tubular epithelial cells. Kidney Int 70: 1287–1295.

13. Barascuk N, Genovese F, Larsen L, Byrjalsen I, Zheng Q, et al. (2013) A MMP derived versican neo-epitope is elevated in plasma from patients with atherosclerotic heart disease. Int J Clin Exp Med 6: 174–184.

14. Wight TN, Merrilees MJ (2004) Proteoglycans in atherosclerosis and restenosis: key roles for versican. Circ Res 94: 1158–1167.

15. Melk A, Mansfield ES, Hsieh SC, Hernandez-Boussard T, Grimm P, et al. (2005) Transcriptional analysis of the molecular basis of human kidney aging using cDNA microarray profiling. Kidney Int 68: 2667–2679.

16. Stokes MB, Hudkins KL, Zaharia V, Taneda S, Alpers CE (2001) Up-regulation of extracellular matrix proteoglycans and collagen type I in human crescentic glomerulonephritis. Kidney Int 59: 532–542.

17. Wight TN, Kang I, Merrilees MJ (2014) Versican and the control of inflammation. Matrix Biol 35: 152–161.

18. Yamaguchi Y, Takihara T, Chambers RA, Veraldi KL, Larregina AT, et al. (2012) A peptide derived from endostatin ameliorates organ fibrosis. Sci Transl Med 4: 136ra71.

19. Yamamoto Y, Maeshima Y, Kitayama H, Kitamura S, Takazawa Y, et al. (2004) Tumstatin peptide, an inhibitor of angiogenesis, prevents glomerular hypertrophy in the early stage of diabetic nephropathy. Diabetes 53: 1831–1840.

20. Karsdal MA, Henriksen K, Leeming DJ, Woodworth T, Vassiliadis E, et al. (2010) Novel combinations of Post-Translational Modification (PTM) neo-epitopes provide tissue-specific biochemical markers–are they the cause or the consequence of the disease? Clin Biochem 43: 793–804.

21. Merrilees MJ, Wight TN (2012) Targeting the matrix: potential benefits for versican therapeutics. Elsevier Current Opinion doi:10.1016/j.ceb.2013.01.001.

29

Triglyceride Levels Are Closely Associated with Mild Declines in Estimated Glomerular Filtration Rates in Middle-Aged and Elderly Chinese with Normal Serum Lipid Levels

Xinguo Hou[1][9], Chuan Wang[1][9], Xiuping Zhang[2], Xiangmin Zhao[2], Yulian Wang[3], Chengqiao Li[3], Mei Li[3], Shaoyuan Wang[4], Weifang Yang[4], Zeqiang Ma[5], Aixia Ma[1], Huizhen Zheng[1], Jiahui Wu[1], Yu Sun[1], Jun Song[1], Peng Lin[1], Kai Liang[1], Lei Gong[1], Meijian Wang[1], Fuqiang Liu[1], Wenjuan Li[1], Juan Xiao[1], Fei Yan[1], Junpeng Yang[1], Lingshu Wang[1], Meng Tian[1], Jidong Liu[1], Ruxing Zhao[1], Shihong Chen[6]*, Li Chen[1]*

1 Department of Endocrinology of Qilu Hospital and Institute of Endocrinology and Metabolism, Shandong University, Jinan, Shandong, China, 2 Shantui Community Health Center, Jining, Shandong, China, 3 Department of Endocrinology, Second People's Hospital of Jining, Jining, Shandong, China, 4 Lukang Hospital of Jining, Jining, Shandong, China, 5 China National Heavy Duty Truck Group Corporation Hospital, Jinan, Shandong, China, 6 Department of Endocrinology, the Second Hospital of Shandong University, Jinan, Shandong, China

Abstract

Objective: To investigate the relationship between lipid profiles [including total cholesterol (TC), triglyceride (TG), low-density lipoprotein cholesterol (LDL-C) and high-density lipoprotein cholesterol (HDL-C)] and a mild decline in the estimated glomerular filtration rate (eGFR) in subjects with normal serum lipid levels.

Design and Methods: In this study, we included 2647 participants who were $\geq$40 years old and had normal serum lipid levels. The Chronic Kidney Disease Epidemiology Collaboration (CKD-EPI) equation was used to estimate the GFR. A mildly reduced eGFR was defined as 60–90 mL/min/1.73 m^2. First, multiple linear regression analysis was used to estimate the association of lipid profiles with the eGFR. Then, the levels of each lipid component were divided into four groups, using the 25th, 50th and 75th percentiles as cut-off points. Finally, multiple logistic regression analysis was used to investigate the association of different lipid components with the risk of mildly reduced eGFR.

Results: In the group with a mildly reduced eGFR, TG and LDL-C levels were significantly increased, but HDL-C levels were significantly decreased. After adjusting for age, gender, body mass index (BMI), systolic blood pressure (SBP), glycated hemoglobin (HbA$_{1c}$), smoking and drinking, only TC and TG were independently related to the eGFR. Additionally, only TG showed a linear relationship with an increased risk of a mildly reduced eGFR, with the highest quartile group (TG: 108–150 mg/dl [1.22–1.70 mmol/L]) having a significantly increased risk after adjusting for the above factors.

Conclusions: Triglyceride levels are closely associated with a mildly reduced eGFR in subjects with normal serum lipid levels. Dyslipidemia with lower TG levels could be used as new diagnostic criteria for subjects with mildly reduced renal function.

Editor: Yanqiao Zhang, Northeast Ohio Medical University, United States of America

Funding: This study was supported by grants from the Chinese Society of Endocrinology, the National Natural Science Foundation of China (No. 81100617), the Medical and Health Science and Technology Development Projects of Shandong Province (2011HD005), the National Science and Technology Support Plan (2009BAI80B04), the Natural Science Foundation of Shandong Province (ZR2012HM014), the International Science and Technology Projects of Shandong Province (2012GGE27126), the Business Plan of Jinan Students Studying Abroad (20110407), and the special scientific research fund of clinical medicine of Chinese Medical Association (12030420342). The funders had no role in study design, data collection and analysis, decision to publish, or preparation of the manuscript.

Competing Interests: The authors have declared that no competing interests exist.

* Email: 515751512@qq.com (SC); wangchuansdu.edu@163.com (LC)

[9] These authors contributed equally to this work.

Introduction

Chronic kidney disease (CKD), characterized by albuminuria or reduced kidney function, is a worldwide public health problem [1,2] that increases the risk of cardiovascular events and mortality [3,4]. Even mild renal insufficiency increases the risk of cardiovascular events [5,6] and is predictive of the progression of kidney disease [7]. Therefore, screening for risk factors is critical during the early stage of CKD, which is characterized by a mildly reduced eGFR.

Dyslipidemia is often detected in patients with CKD and has been shown to mediate atherosclerotic disease. Therefore, statin treatment has been recommended for patients with CKD according to the lipid management guidelines developed by Kidney Disease: Improving Global Outcomes (KDIGO) [8]. However, the specific target range of serum lipid levels remains to be determined. Additionally, most previous studies of the relationship between serum lipid levels and CKD have focused on dyslipidemia and severe kidney disease where the eGFR was less than 60 mL/min/1.73 m^2 [9]. Few studies have been conducted to determine the association of normal serum lipid levels, as defined by current criteria, with a mildly reduced eGFR. Whether the current criteria for normal serum lipid levels are appropriate for patients with mild renal insufficiency remains to be clarified. Here, to explain this issue, we explored the relationship between lipid profiles and a mildly reduced eGFR in subjects with normal serum lipid levels.

Materials and Methods

Ethics Statement

This cross-sectional study is part of the REACTION study [10,11] and was approved by the Ruijin Hospital Ethics Committee of the Shanghai Jiao Tong University School of Medicine. Written informed consent was obtained from all participants in this study.

Study population

The present study recruited 10,028 subjects who were ≥40 years old in Shandong province from January to April 2012. We excluded subjects with (1) missing data for calculation of the eGFR; (2) an eGFR <60 mL/min/1.73 m^2; (3) dyslipidemia (see below); (4) previously diagnosed kidney disease, including autoimmune or drug-induced kidney disease, nephritis, renal fibrosis or renal failure, or subjects who had a kidney transplant and were receiving dialysis treatment; (5) previously diagnosed hepatic disease, including fatty liver, liver cirrhosis and autoimmune hepatitis; and (6) any malignant disease. Finally, 2647 subjects (1734 women) were eligible for the analysis.

Data collection

Demographic characteristics, lifestyle information and previous medical history were obtained by trained investigators through a standard questionnaire. BMI was calculated as weight (kg) divided by height squared (m^2). Blood pressure (BP) was measured 3 times consecutively (OMRON Model HEM-752 FUZZY, Omron Company, Dalian, China), and the average reading was used for analysis. After an overnight fasting, venous blood samples were collected between 07:00 and 09:00 for measurement of fasting blood glucose (FBG), creatinine and lipid profiles (TC, TG, LDL-C and HDL-C). Postprandial blood glucose (PBG) was measured after subjects had completed a 75-g OGTT. HbA$_{1c}$ was measured by high-performance liquid chromatography (VARIANT II and D-10 Systems, BIO-RAD, USA).

The estimated GFR (eGFR) was calculated from creatinine levels using the CKD-EPI formula [12].

Definition

Normal eGFR was defined as ≥90 mL/min/1.73 m^2; mildly reduced eGFR was defined as 60–90 mL/min/1.73 m^2.

Diabetes was defined by the 1999 World Health Organization (WHO) criteria [13]: FBG ≥126 mg/dl (7.0 mmol/L) and/or PBG ≥200 mg/dl (11.1 mmol/L) or a history of diabetes.

Dyslipidemia was defined by the 2007 Guidelines for Prevention and Treatment of Dyslipidemia in Adults in China [14]: (1) TC ≥ 200 mg/dl (5.18 mmol/L); (2) TG ≥150 mg/dl (1.70 mmol/L);

(3) LDL-C ≥130 mg/dl (3.37 mmol/L); (4) HDL-C <40 mg/dl (1.04 mmol/L); or (5) the patient was undergoing treatment for any of these conditions.

Statistical analysis

The continuous variables in this study, which contained a large cohort of patients, exhibited normal distribution or approximately normal distribution and are presented as the means ± SD, and the categorical variables are presented as numbers (%). Differences between groups were analyzed using Student's t test for continuous data and the chi-square test for categorical data. After verifying the assumption of a linear relationship between the dependent and independent variables that were introduced into the linear regression model (assessed using a histogram of the residuals, together with a scatter plot of the standardized residuals to the standardized predicted values in different models, as described below), multiple linear regression analysis was used to estimate the association of lipid profiles with the eGFR. Three models were constructed for each component of lipid profiles: the first model was not adjusted; the second model was adjusted for age and gender; and the third model was adjusted for age, gender, BMI, systolic blood pressure (SBP), HbA$_{1c}$, smoking and drinking. The levels of each lipid component were divided into four groups, using the 25th, 50th and 75th percentiles as cut-off points: 163.10, 177.02 and 189.00 mg/dl (4.22, 4.58 and 4.89 mmol/L) for TC; 65.49, 84.08 and 108.00 mg/dl (0.74, 0.95 and 1.22 mmol/L) for TG; 85.97, 98.30 and 109.87 mg/dl (2.23, 2.55 and 2.85 mmol/L) for LDL-C; and 50.44, 57.37 and 65.84 mg/dl (1.31, 1.49 and 1.71 mmol/L) for HDL-C. Then, the associations of the different lipid components (we introduced the ordinal independent variables as quartiles of TC, TG, LDL-C and HDL-C as dummy variables) with the risk of a mildly reduced eGFR were estimated using multiple logistic regression analysis in the same three models mentioned above. P-values for the trends were calculated by Spearman correlation analysis of categorical variables and odds ratios for the different groups, scored 0, 1, 2 and 3, respectively. $P<0.05$ was considered statistically significant. All statistical analyses were performed using SPSS 16.0 (SPSS Inc., Chicago, IL, USA).

Results

Characteristics of study participants

We included 2647 subjects (1734 women) who were divided into two groups according to the eGFR, using 90 mL/min/1.73 m^2 as the cut-off value. As shown in Table 1, almost all characteristics were different between the two groups, except for TC. In the group with a mildly reduced eGFR, age, BMI, SBP, DBP, FBG, PBG, HbA$_{1c}$, TG, LDL-C, the percentages of males and diabetics and smoking and drinking statuses among the patients were significantly increased, while the HDL-C level was significantly decreased (all $P<0.001$).

Multiple linear regression analysis

As shown in Table 2, we constructed three models to analyze the association of each lipid component with the eGFR (the 4 lipid components were analyzed separately due to colinearity). The assumption of a linear relationship between each lipid component and the eGFR was assessed using a histogram of the residuals, together with a scatter plot of the standardized residuals to the standardized predicted value in the different models, showing an approximately linear relationship, especially in models 2 and 3. In model 1, the TC, TG, LDL-C and HDL-C levels were independently related to the eGFR. However, after adjusting for

Table 1. Characteristics of the study participants.

Characteristics	eGFR (mL/min/1.73 m^2)		P-value
	≥90 (n = 1665)	(60–90) (n = 982)	
Female (%)	77.60%	45.01%	<0.001
Age (years)	51.09±7.73	63.08±9.38	<0.001
BMI (kg/m^2)	25.26±3.52	26.00±3.48	<0.001
SBP (mmHg)	131.60±19.31	141.92±20.49	<0.001
DBP (mmHg)	77.55±10.93	80.29±11.40	<0.001
FBG (mg/dl)	99.72±22.22	111.49±32.14	<0.001
PBG (mg/dl)	113.05±53.69	136.03±71.38	<0.001
HbA$_{1c}$ (%)	5.81±0.84	6.20±1.21	<0.001
Diabetes (%)	6.79%	18.13%	<0.001
TC (mg/dl)	173.87±17.92	175.27±14.85	0.051
TG (mg/dl)	85.22±27.65	91.97±26.94	<0.001
LDL-C (mg/dl)	95.21±17.46	99.15±17.68	<0.001
HDL-C (mg/dl)	60.21±11.05	56.21±10.53	<0.001
Smoking (%)	8.89%	23.73%	<0.001
Drinking (%)	14.23%	35.13%	<0.001
eGFR (mL/min/1.73 m^2)	102.29±6.69	78.47±7.86	<0.001

Data are the means ± SD or numbers (%). BMI, body mass index; SBP, systolic blood pressure; DBP, diastolic blood pressure; FBG, fasting blood glucose; PBG, postprandial blood glucose; TC, total cholesterol; TG, triglyceride; LDL-C, low-density lipoprotein cholesterol; HDL-C, high-density lipoprotein cholesterol; eGFR, estimated glomerular filtration rate.

age and gender, HDL-C levels were no longer related to the eGFR in model 2. Finally, in model 3, only TC and TG were chosen as independent variables in subjects with normal serum lipid levels.

Multiple logistic regression analysis

As shown in Table 3, we analyzed the association of increased lipid profiles with the risk of a mildly reduced eGFR in three models. In model 1, both TG and LDL-C levels were positively related, but HDL-C levels were negatively related, to an increased

Table 2. The association of lipid profiles with the eGFR.

Models	Independent variable	β Coefficient	95% CI	P-value
Model 1				
Model 1a	TC, mg/dl	−0.061	−0.090 to −0.033	**<0.001**
Model 1b	TG, mg/dl	−0.074	−0.093 to −0.056	**<0.001**
Model 1c	LDL-C, mg/dl	−0.105	−0.134 to −0.076	**<0.001**
Model 1d	HDL-C, mg/dl	0.227	0.181 to 0.273	**<0.001**
Model 2				
Model 2a	TC, mg/dl	−0.029	−0.045 to −0.014	**<0.001**
Model 2b	TG, mg/dl	−0.024	−0.034 to −0.014	**<0.001**
Model 2c	LDL-C, mg/dl	−0.025	−0.040 to −0.009	**0.002**
Model 2d	HDL-C, mg/dl	0.017	−0.008 to 0.043	0.179
Model 3				
Model 3a	TC, mg/dl	−0.028	−0.044 to −0.013	**<0.001**
Model 3b	TG, mg/dl	−0.017	−0.027 to −0.006	**<0.001**
Model 3c	LDL-C, mg/dl	−0.012	−0.028 to 0.003	0.125
Model 3d	HDL-C, mg/dl	−0.012	−0.038 to 0.014	0.356

Model 1: not adjusted.
Model 2: adjusted for age and gender.
Model 3: adjusted for age, gender, BMI, SBP, HbA$_{1c}$, smoking and drinking.

risk of a mildly reduced eGFR. In contrast, there was no linear relationship between TC levels and an increased risk of a mildly reduced eGFR, though the highest quartile group of TC levels had a significantly increased risk ($P = 0.035$). However, after adjusting for age and gender (model 2) or further adjusting for BMI, SBP, HbA_{1c}, smoking and drinking (model 3), only TG showed a linear relationship with an increased risk of a mildly reduced eGFR, with the highest quartile group (TG: 108–150 mg/dl [1.22–1.70 mmol/L]) significantly increasing the risk.

Discussion

A recent study revealed that patients with CKD have cardiovascular mortality rates at least 10 times higher than those of the general population [15] and that dyslipidemia may play an important role in mediating cardiovascular disease and many other complications of CKD [16]. Therefore, an increasing number of experts suggest lipid-lowering therapies in patients with CKD [8,17,18]. Additionally, more and more studies have indicated that lipid-lowering therapy clearly affects the incidence of cardiovascular disease, total mortality, stroke, and myocardial infarction in patients with CKD [19,20]. However, the specific target range of serum lipid levels remains to be determined.

Aside from advanced CKD, a mild reduction of the eGFR was also observed to increase the risk of cardiovascular events, such as arterial stiffness, coronary artery calcium, higher rates of stress-induced ischemia, myocardial hypertrophy, and even mortality [5,6,21,22,23]. Moreover, two cross-sectional studies performed in China found that the percentage of dyslipidemia was significantly higher in patients with a mildly reduced eGFR than in subjects with a normal eGFR [24,25], suggesting that dyslipidemia might also be closely associated with a mildly reduced eGFR. Therefore, it is important to identify a specific range of normal serum lipid levels for subjects with a mildly reduced eGFR. However, the association of normal serum lipid levels, as defined by the current criteria, with a mildly reduced eGFR remains unclear; if they are closely associated, new criteria for dyslipidemia might need to be determined.

In the present study, we found that TG and LDL-C levels were significantly increased but HDL-C levels were significantly decreased in the group with a mildly reduced eGFR in middle-aged and elderly Chinese subjects with normal serum lipid levels. The traditional risk factors for CKD include age, gender, overweight, hypertension, diabetes, smoking and drinking [2,26,27,28]. Therefore, we adjusted for age, gender, BMI, SBP, HbA1c, smoking and drinking to analyze the association of lipid profiles with the eGFR and the risk of a mildly reduced eGFR, and

Table 3. The association of lipid profiles with the risk of a mildly reduced eGFR.

Independent variable	Model 1 Odds ratio (95% CI)	P-value	Model 2 Odds ratio (95% CI)	P-value	Model 3 Odds ratio (95% CI)	P-value
TC						
Q1	1		1		1	
Q2	1.05 (0.84–1.32)	0.664	0.93 (0.65–1.32)	0.665	0.97 (0.67–1.39)	0.855
Q3	1.00 (0.80–1.25)	0.973	0.90 (0.63–1.28)	0.558	0.91 (0.64–1.30)	0.608
Q4	1.27 (1.02–1.59)	**0.035**	1.21 (0.86–1.70)	0.276	1.23 (0.87–1.74)	0.237
P for trend	1.00		0.80		0.80	
TG						
Q1	1		1		1	
Q2	1.41 (1.11–1.78)	**0.004**	1.33 (0.92–1.92)	0.129	1.25 (0.86–1.81)	0.245
Q3	1.82 (1.44–2.30)	**<0.001**	1.43 (1.00–2.06)	0.052	1.31 (0.90–1.91)	0.154
Q4	1.98 (1.57–2.49)	**<0.001**	1.78 (1.25–2.53)	**0.001**	1.61 (1.12–2.32)	**0.011**
P for trend	**<0.01**		**<0.01**		**<0.01**	
LDL-C						
Q1	1		1		1	
Q2	1.03 (0.82–1.30)	0.803	0.89 (0.62–1.28)	0.523	0.92 (0.64–1.33)	0.655
Q3	1.47 (1.18–1.84)	**0.001**	1.25 (0.89–1.76)	0.204	1.21 (0.85–1.71)	0.295
Q4	1.76 (1.41–2.20)	**<0.001**	1.29 (0.92–1.81)	0.141	1.19 (0.84–1.68)	0.334
P for trend	**<0.01**		0.20		0.20	
HDL-C						
Q1	1		1		1	
Q2	0.69 (0.55–0.85)	**0.001**	0.92 (0.66–1.27)	0.604	0.96 (0.69–1.34)	0.818
Q3	0.47 (0.37–0.59)	**<0.001**	0.81 (0.58–1.13)	0.207	0.85 (0.60–1.20)	0.344
Q4	0.38 (0.31–0.48)	**<0.001**	0.85 (0.60–1.20)	0.341	1.02 (0.71–1.46)	0.936
P for trend	**<0.01**		0.20		0.80	

Model 1: not adjusted.
Model 2: adjusted for age and gender.
Model 3: adjusted for age, gender, BMI, SBP, HbA_{1c}, smoking and drinking.

we found that TC and TG levels were significantly associated with a decreased eGFR, independently of the above risk factors. Moreover, only TG showed a linear relationship with an increased risk of a mildly reduced eGFR, with the highest quartile group (TG: 108–150 mg/dl [1.22–1.70 mmol/L]), significantly increasing the risk after adjusting for the factors mentioned above. All of the results suggest that even within a normal range of serum lipid levels, as defined by the current criteria, TG significantly increased the risk of a mildly reduced eGFR, indicating that we should pay more attention to controlling TG levels to prevent the progression of CKD. Additionally, new criteria for dyslipidemia might need to be determined in subjects with mildly reduced eGFR.

Creatinine-based equations for estimating the GFR include the Cockcroft-Gault equation proposed in 1976 [29], the Modification of Diet in Renal Disease (MDRD) study equation proposed in 1999 [30] and the CKD-EPI equation proposed in 2009 [11]. Currently, the Cockcroft-Gault equation has been supplanted by the MDRD study equation and the CKD-EPI equation [31]. A recent study performed in South Asians, aged 40 years or older as in the present study, demonstrated that the CKD-EPI equation was more accurate and precise in estimating the GFR than the MDRD study equation [32]. Therefore, we selected the CKD-EPI equation to calculate the eGFR.

Of course, our study has some limitations. First, a cross-sectional study cannot infer causality between lipid profiles and a mildly reduced eGFR, so whether the decline in the eGFR produces the high levels of TG and cholesterol, or the inverse, where the high levels of TG and cholesterol lead to a decline in the eGFR, remains unknown. Second, we could not provide sufficient evidence to change the current dyslipidemia criteria. Though a dose-dependent effect was observed between TG and a reduced eGFR in this study (the higher the TG levels, the higher the risk for a reduced eGFR, Table 3), the causality between lipid profiles and a mildly reduced eGFR remains unclear. Moreover, there was not good evidence that pharmacological treatment effects of high triglycerides on cardiovascular outcomes differed between those with and without lower baseline eGFR[33]. Therefore, more

randomized controlled trials are needed to clarify the specific range of normal serum lipid levels for patients with a mildly reduced eGFR at baseline to prevent the progression of CKD and related cardiovascular complications. Third, the risk was not very high for the highest quartile of TG (OR = 1.61), further adjustments for other unknown risk factors may drop the risk to 1, as was observed with TC, LDL-C and HDL-C when adjusted for the risk factors considered in this study. Therefore, as new risk factors are found, the association of TG with a mildly reduced eGFR may need to be reassessed. Fourth, our study contained only middle-aged and elderly Chinese subjects; the present results may not be appropriate for subjects of different ages or ethnicities. Finally, the GFR based on creatinine and estimated by the CKD-EPI equation may not accurately reflect kidney function, which may have influenced the outcomes of this study. However, the gold standard method for measuring the GFR (isotope clearance measurement) is very expensive and time-consuming, so the use of creatinine-based equations to estimate the GFR is logical for large epidemiological studies. The CKD-EPI equation was more accurate and precise than the MDRD study equation and the Cockcroft-Gault equation and, therefore, may be the best choice for estimating the GFR.

In conclusion, we found that TG levels were closely associated with a mildly reduced eGFR in subjects with normal serum lipid levels. Though the evidence is not sufficient, new criteria for dyslipidemia may be needed for middle-aged and elderly Chinese subjects with a mildly reduced eGFR. Longitudinal studies are needed to explore how much the TG value should be controlled in clinical practice to have a beneficial effect on CKD.

Author Contributions

Conceived and designed the experiments: XH CW. Performed the experiments: XH CW X. Zhang X. Zhao YW CL ML SW WY ZM AM HZ JW YS JS PL KL LG MW FL WL JX FY JY LW MT JL RZ SC LC. Analyzed the data: XH CW. Wrote the paper: XH CW SC LC.

References

1. Tomonaga Y, Risch L, Szucs TD, Ambuehl PM (2013) The prevalence of chronic kidney disease in a primary care setting: a Swiss cross-sectional study. PLoS One 8: e67848.
2. Zhang L, Wang F, Wang L, Wang W, Liu B, et al. (2012) Prevalence of chronic kidney disease in China: a cross-sectional survey. Lancet 379: 815–822.
3. Chen YC, Su YC, Lee CC, Huang YS, Hwang SJ (2012) Chronic kidney disease itself is a causal risk factor for stroke beyond traditional cardiovascular risk factors: a nationwide cohort study in Taiwan. PLoS One 7: e36332.
4. Hallan SI, Matsushita K, Sang Y, Mahmoodi BK, Black C, et al. (2012) Age and association of kidney measures with mortality and end-stage renal disease. JAMA 308: 2349–2360.
5. Hermans MM, Henry R, Dekker JM, Kooman JP, Kostense PJ, et al. (2007) Estimated glomerular filtration rate and urinary albumin excretion are independently associated with greater arterial stiffness: the Hoorn Study. J Am Soc Nephrol 18: 1942–1952.
6. Henry RM, Kostense PJ, Bos G, Dekker JM, Nijpels G, et al. (2002) Mild renal insufficiency is associated with increased cardiovascular mortality: The Hoorn Study. Kidney Int 62: 1402–1407.
7. Fox CS, Larson MG, Leip EP, Culleton B, Wilson PW, et al. (2004) Predictors of new-onset kidney disease in a community-based population. JAMA 291: 844–850.
8. Tonelli M, Wanner C (2013) Lipid Management in Chronic Kidney Disease: Synopsis of the Kidney Disease: Improving Global Outcomes 2013 Clinical Practice Guideline. Ann Intern Med.
9. Iseki K (2014) Epidemiology of dyslipidemia in chronic kidney disease. Clin Exp Nephrol.
10. Ning G (2012) Risk Evaluation of cAncers in Chinese diabeTic Individuals: a lONgitudinal (REACTION) study. J Diabetes 4: 172–173.
11. Bi Y, Lu J, Wang W, Mu Y, Zhao J, et al. (2014) Cohort profile: Risk evaluation of cancers in Chinese diabetic individuals: a longitudinal (REACTION) study. J Diabetes 6: 147–157.
12. Levey AS, Stevens LA, Schmid CH, Zhang YL, Castro AF, 3rd, et al. (2009) A new equation to estimate glomerular filtration rate. Ann Intern Med 150: 604–612.
13. Alberti KG, Zimmet PZ (1998) Definition, diagnosis and classification of diabetes mellitus and its complications. Part 1: diagnosis and classification of diabetes mellitus provisional report of a WHO consultation. Diabet Med 15: 539–553.
14. Dyslipidemia TACoPaTo (2007) [Chinese guidelines on prevention and treatment of dyslipidemia in adults]. Zhonghua Xin Xue Guan Bing Za Zhi 35: 390–419.
15. Gansevoort RT, Correa-Rotter R, Hemmelgarn BR, Jafar TH, Heerspink HJ, et al. (2013) Chronic kidney disease and cardiovascular risk: epidemiology, mechanisms, and prevention. Lancet 382: 339–352.
16. Vaziri ND, Norris K (2011) Lipid disorders and their relevance to outcomes in chronic kidney disease. Blood Purif 31: 189–196.
17. Barsoum RS (2006) Chronic kidney disease in the developing world. N Engl J Med 354: 997–999.
18. Zhang L, Zhang P, Wang F, Zuo L, Zhou Y, et al. (2008) Prevalence and factors associated with CKD: a population study from Beijing. Am J Kidney Dis 51: 373–384.
19. Upadhyay A, Earley A, Lamont JL, Haynes S, Wanner C, et al. (2012) Lipid-lowering therapy in persons with chronic kidney disease: a systematic review and meta-analysis. Ann Intern Med 157: 251–262.
20. Zhang X, Xiang C, Zhou YH, Jiang A, Qin YY, et al. (2014) Effect of statins on cardiovascular events in patients with mild to moderate chronic kidney disease: a systematic review and meta-analysis of randomized clinical trials. BMC Cardiovasc Disord 14: 19.
21. Roy SK, Cespedes A, Li D, Choi TY, Budoff MJ (2011) Mild and moderate pre-dialysis chronic kidney disease is associated with increased coronary artery calcium. Vasc Health Risk Manag 7: 719–724.

Triglyceride Levels Are Closely Associated with Mild Declines in Estimated Glomerular Filtration Rates...

253

22. Natali A, Boldrini B, Baldi S, Rossi M, Landi P, et al. (2013) Impact of mild to moderate reductions of glomerular filtration rate on coronary artery disease severity. Nutr Metab Cardiovasc Dis.

23. Campbell NG, Varagunam M, Sawhney V, Ahuja KR, Salahuddin N, et al. (2012) Mild chronic kidney disease is an independent predictor of long-term mortality after emergency angiography and primary percutaneous intervention in patients with ST-elevation myocardial infarction. Heart 98: 42–47.

24. Wang F, Ye P, Luo L, Xiao W, Wu H (2010) Association of risk factors for cardiovascular disease and glomerular filtration rate: a community-based study of 4,925 adults in Beijing. Nephrol Dial Transplant 25: 3924–3931.

25. Ji B, Zhang S, Gong L, Wang Z, Ren W, et al. (2013) The risk factors of mild decline in estimated glomerular filtration rate in a community-based population. Clin Biochem 46: 750–754.

26. Chen W, Wang H, Dong X, Liu Q, Mao H, et al. (2009) Prevalence and risk factors associated with chronic kidney disease in an adult population from southern China. Nephrol Dial Transplant 24: 1205–1212.

27. Noborisaka Y (2013) Smoking and chronic kidney disease in healthy populations. Nephrourol Mon 5: 655–667.

28. Shankar A, Klein R, Klein BE (2006) The association among smoking, heavy drinking, and chronic kidney disease. Am J Epidemiol 164: 263–271.

29. Cockcroft DW, Gault MH (1976) Prediction of creatinine clearance from serum creatinine. Nephron 16: 31–41.

30. Levey AS, Bosch JP, Lewis JB, Greene T, Rogers N, et al. (1999) A more accurate method to estimate glomerular filtration rate from serum creatinine: a new prediction equation. Modification of Diet in Renal Disease Study Group. Ann Intern Med 130: 461–470.

31. Delanaye P, Mariat C (2013) The applicability of eGFR equations to different populations. Nat Rev Nephrol 9: 513–522.

32. Jessani S, Levey AS, Bux R, Inker LA, Islam M, et al. (2014) Estimation of GFR in South Asians: a study from the general population in Pakistan. Am J Kidney Dis 63: 49–58.

33. Wanner C, Tonelli M, Cass A, Garg AX, Holdaas H, et al. (2014) KDIGO Clinical Practice Guideline for Lipid Management in CKD: summary of recommendation statements and clinical approach to the patient. Kidney Int.

30

Triglycerides in the Human Kidney Cortex: Relationship with Body Size

Ion Alexandru Bobulescu[1]*, Yair Lotan[2], Jianning Zhang[3], Tara R. Rosenthal[3], John T. Rogers[3], Beverley Adams-Huet[4], Khashayar Sakhaee[1], Orson W. Moe[5]

1 Department of Internal Medicine and the Charles and Jane Pak Center for Mineral Metabolism and Clinical Research, University of Texas Southwestern Medical Center, Dallas, Texas, United States of America, **2** Department of Urology, University of Texas Southwestern Medical Center, Dallas, Texas, United States of America, **3** Department of Internal Medicine, University of Texas Southwestern Medical Center, Dallas, Texas, United States of America, **4** Department of Clinical Sciences and the Charles and Jane Pak Center for Mineral Metabolism and Clinical Research, University of Texas Southwestern Medical Center, Dallas, Texas, United States of America, **5** Departments of Internal Medicine, Physiology, and the Charles and Jane Pak Center for Mineral Metabolism and Clinical Research, University of Texas Southwestern Medical Center, Dallas, Texas, United States of America

Abstract

Obesity is associated with increased risk for kidney disease and uric acid nephrolithiasis, but the pathophysiological mechanisms underpinning these associations are incompletely understood. Animal experiments have suggested that renal lipid accumulation and lipotoxicity may play a role, but whether lipid accumulation occurs in humans with increasing body mass index (BMI) is unknown. The association between obesity and abnormal triglyceride accumulation in non-adipose tissues (steatosis) has been described in the liver, heart, skeletal muscle and pancreas, but not in the human kidney. We used a quantitative biochemical assay to quantify triglyceride in normal kidney cortex samples from 54 patients undergoing nephrectomy for localized renal cell carcinoma. In subsets of the study population we evaluated the localization of lipid droplets by Oil Red O staining and measured 16 common ceramide species by mass spectrometry. There was a positive correlation between kidney cortex trigyceride content and BMI (Spearman $R = 0.27$, $P = 0.04$). Lipid droplets detectable by optical microscopy had a sporadic distribution but were generally more prevalent in individuals with higher BMI, with predominant localization in proximal tubule cells and to a lesser extent in glomeruli. Total ceramide content was inversely correlated with triglycerides. We postulate that obesity is associated with abnormal triglyceride accumulation (steatosis) in the human kidney. In turn, steatosis and lipotoxicity may contribute to the pathogenesis of obesity-associated kidney disease and nephrolithiasis.

Editor: Giuseppe Danilo Norata, University of Milan, Italy

Funding: This work was supported by the United States National Institutes of Health (NIH) grants K01-DK090282 (to IAB) and R01-DK081423 (to KS). OWM was supported by NIH grants R01-DK041612 and R01-DK091392, the Simmons Family Foundation, and the Charles and Jane Pak Foundation. The authors also acknowledge support from the research cores of the UT Southwestern O'Brien Kidney Research Center, supported by NIH grant P30DK-07938. The funders had no role in study design, data collection and analysis, decision to publish, or preparation of the manuscript.

Competing Interests: The authors have declared that no competing interests exist.

* Email: Alexandru.Bobulescu@UTSouthwestern.edu

Introduction

The prevalence of obesity (body mass index ≥ 30) among adults in the European Union ranges from 8% in Romania to 24% in the United Kingdom [1], exceeds 35% in the United States [2], and is approximately 11% worldwide [3]. Although body mass index (BMI) is not an ideal measure of body adiposity and associated health risk [4], multiple studies have shown that increased BMI is an independent risk factor for chronic kidney disease (CKD) and end-stage renal disease (ESRD), even after adjustment for obesity-related conditions such as hypertension and type 2 diabetes [5–7]. The mechanisms by which obesity can directly contribute to increased CKD and ESRD risk, independent of its association with hypertension and type 2 diabetes, are incompletely understood. Various non-mutually exclusive and partly overlapping mechanisms have been proposed, including inflammation, hyperfiltration, podocyte stress, oxidative stress, changes in various hormones or signaling molecules such as leptin and adiponectin, as well as renal lipid accumulation and lipotoxicity [8–11].

In addition to its association with CKD and ESRD, obesity has been linked with increased risk for kidney stones in general [12,13], and uric acid stones in particular [14,15]. While the pathophysiology of uric acid nephrolithiasis is likely multifactorial [16], animal and cell culture experiments have shown that lipid accumulation in proximal tubule cells may contribute to the urinary biochemical abnormalities that underpin uric acid stone risk [17–19].

Lipid accumulation in other organs, including skeletal muscle, myocardium, pancreas and liver, has been associated with obesity in humans [20–23], and has been implicated in cell and organ dysfunction [24–27]. Lipid accumulation in the kidney has been described in a number of animal models, but very little human data are available [8,9]. In particular, establishing whether renal lipid accumulation occurs in humans with increased BMI, thus potentially contributing to obesity-related CKD, ESRD and nephrolithiasis risk, is of fundamental importance, and there is no database on this topic. To address this knowledge gap, we measured renal triglycerides and defined their localization in normal kidney surgical specimens obtained from patients undergoing nephrectomy, with a wide range of BMI. In addition, we measured tissue levels of 16 common ceramide species in representative samples.

Methods

Ethics Statement

The human study was approved by the University of Texas Southwestern Medical Center Institutional Review Board, was conducted in strict accordance with the Helsinki Declaration of 1975, as revised in 2000, and all study participants provided written informed consent prior to nephrectomy. The animal study protocol was approved by the Institutional Animal Care and Use Committee (IACUC) at University of Texas Southwestern Medical Center, and all animal work was performed in strict accordance with institutional guidelines and with the National Academy of Sciences Guide for the Care and Use of Laboratory Animals.

Study participants and tissue collection protocol

We studied surgical specimens obtained from patients undergoing total nephrectomy at the University of Texas Southwestern Medical Center and affiliated hospitals between 2007 and 2012. Included in the study were patients older than 21 years, of either gender and of any race/ethnicity, undergoing nephrectomy as first-line therapy for unilateral renal cell carcinoma. Race/ethnicity was self-reported. Exclusion criteria were serum creatinine ≥ 1.5 mg/dL, proteinuria, treatment with insulin or thiazolidinediones, genetic diseases of the kidney, inborn defects of lipid metabolism, and a history of recurrent urinary tract infections. None of the study participants were alcohol abusers. After nephrectomy, an experienced surgical pathologist dissected 1–3 separate, 0.1–1 cm^3 normal kidney cortex samples from each kidney, away from the tumor. Patients with no normal kidney cortex upon pathological examination of the surgical specimen were excluded from the study. Tissue samples were immediately frozen in liquid nitrogen and stored at $-80°C$ for biochemical measurement of triglycerides. For 29 subjects from which 2 or more samples were available, one sample was fixed in 4% paraformaldehyde, cryosectioned and stained for lipids using Oil Red O on the same day.

Lipid measurements and tissue lipid staining

Biochemical measurement of kidney cortex triglycerides and Oil Red O lipid staining were performed as previously described [17]. Briefly, frozen tissue samples were homogenized using a Polytron (Brinkmann Instruments, Westbury, NY) in 300 mM mannitol, 18 mM HEPES and 5 mM EGTA (pH 7.5), and lipids were extracted by the method of Folch et al. [28]. Total triglyceride content was quantified using a triglyceride colorimetric assay kit (Sigma, St. Louis, MO) according to the method of Danno et al. [29]. Measurements from each tissue sample were performed in triplicate, with mean triglyceride values for each subject included in further analyses.

For lipid staining, 4 µm tissue sections were rinsed with distilled deionized water, rinsed briefly with 60% isopropanol, stained with Oil Red O for 1 hour, and then subjected to standard hematoxylin staining and mounted on glass slides. Quantitative assessment of Oil Red O staining was performed in a blinded fashion by two independent investigators using the color deconvolution method of Ruifrock and Johnston [30] and the National Institutes of Health ImageJ software [31].

Tissue ceramides were measured in frozen tissue samples by the Mouse Metabolic Phenotyping Core at UT Southwestern Medical Center using high performance liquid chromatography-electrospray ionization-tandem mass spectrometry (HPLC-ESI-MS/MS), on a Shimadzu Prominence HPLC system coupled to an API 5000 LC-MS/MS mass spectrometer (ABSCIEX, Framingham, MA) equipped with a Turbo VTM electrospray ionization source operated in positive mode. Quantitative analysis of ceramides was achieved using selective reaction monitoring scan mode, with the concentration of each analyte determined according to calibration curves using peak-area ratio of analyte vs. corresponding internal standard. Calibration curves were generated using serial dilutions of ceramide standards (Avanti Polar Lipids, Alabaster, AL).

Animals

Nine Zucker ZDF (fa/fa) rats, 7–10 months of age, and eight age-matched lean wild-type (+/+) rats, were a gift from Dr. Roger Unger (Touchstone Center for Diabetes Research, UT Southwestern Medical Center). Rats were fed standard chow (Harlan Teklad, Madison, WI) ad libitum and had free access to water. Euthanasia was performed by exsanguination under anesthesia with ketamine-xylazine-acepromazine (100, 10, and 1 mg/kg intraperitoneally). Kidneys were dissected on ice, and cortical samples were frozen in liquid nitrogen and stored at $-80°C$ for lipid measurements.

Statistical analysis

For continuous variables, one-way analysis of variance with orthogonal linear contrasts was used to assess the trend over the kidney cortex triglyceride content tertiles. Adjustments for potential confounding variables were made with analysis of covariance models. Categorical variables were analyzed with the Cochran-Armitage trend test. Correlations were evaluated with Spearman rank-order correlation coefficients. A two-sided P value<0.05 was considered statistically significant. Analyses were performed with SAS v9.3 (SAS Institute, Cary, NC).

Results

Kidney cortex triglyceride content and characteristics of the study population

Triglyceride content was measured biochemically in non-cancerous kidney cortex samples obtained from 54 patients undergoing total nephrectomy. Selected demographic characteristics of the study population are presented in **Table 1**, with further stratification by tertiles of cortical triglyceride content. Body mass index (BMI) increased across tertiles of increasing kidney cortex triglyceride, and there was a significant positive correlation between triglycerides and BMI analyzed as continuous variables (**Figure 1**). Patients with higher renal cortical triglyceride content tended to be younger in the unadjusted analysis, but only BMI was a significant predictor of kidney triglyceride content (P = 0.003) in a multivariable analysis including age and BMI as covariates. There were also no statistically significant differences in tertile distribution by gender or race/ethnicity, though women and minorities were numerically over-represented in the highest tertile (**Table 1**).

Serum creatinine, estimated glomerular filtration rate (eGFR), serum lipids (with and without adjustment for the use of antidyslipidemic medications) and diagnosed hypertension were not different across tertiles of kidney cortex triglyceride content (**Table 2**). We noted a borderline significant association between higher renal cortical triglyceride content and documented type 2

Table 1. Demographic and anthropometric characteristics.

	Overall cohort (N = 54)	Tertile 1 (N = 18)	Tertile 2 (N = 19)	Tertile 3 (N = 17)	P_{trend}	P for tertile 1 vs. 3
Body mass index, * kg/m^2	27.8 (24.9, 32.2)	26.7 (24.2, 29.1)	27.2 (24.8, 32.8)	30.0 (26.5, 33.7)	0.06	0.04
Age	65 (56, 71)	66 (60, 71)	66 (58, 74)	59 (50, 64)	0.07	0.06
Gender					0.41	0.41
Female	19 (35.2%)	6 (33.3%)	5 (26.3%)	8 (47.1%)		
Male	35 (64.8%)	12 (66.7%)	14 (73.7%)	9 (52.9%)		
Race/ethnicity†					0.61	0.63
Black	4 (7.4%)	1 (5.6%)	0	3 (17.6%)		
Hispanic	3 (5.6%)	1 (5.6%)	1 (5.3%)	1 (5.9%)		
Native American	1 (1.9%)	0	0	1 (5.9%)		
White	43 (79.6%)	14 (77.8%)	17 (89.5%)	12 (70.6%)		
Unknown	3 (5.6%)	2 (11.1%)	1 (5.3%)	0		

Data are presented as median (25th, 75th percentiles) or number of subjects (percentage) for the overall study population, as well as stratified by tertiles of renal cortical triglyceride content.
* Adjusted for body mass index.
†Because of rounding, not all percentages for race/ethnicity add up to exactly 100%.

diabetes in unadjusted analyses, but statistical significance was not upheld after adjustment for BMI.

Localization of triglyceride droplets

Triglyceride localization within kidney structures was examined in a blinded fashion by two investigators using Oil Red O staining of lipid droplets followed by computerized color deconvolution, in a subset of 29 subjects for which fixed tissue was available. Of these, 19 subjects had detectable Oil Red O staining. In spite of inter-individual variability, generally more lipid droplets were detected in samples from individuals with higher BMI (**Figure 2A**). Lipid droplets were predominantly localized in tubular cells, mostly in proximal tubules, and to a lesser extent within glomeruli and in the interstitium (**Figures 2B and 2C**). Of note, even in samples with high triglyceride content by biochemistry, lipid droplets detectable by Oil Red O staining and optical microscopy had a relatively sparse distribution, likely because only larger droplets can be visualized using this technique [32].

Kidney cortex ceramide content

Kidney cortex ceramide content was measured retrospectively in samples from a subset of 14 patients with available tissue stored at $-80°C$. The abundance of 16 common ceramide species in individual study subjects is shown in **Figure 3A**. We noted an inverse correlation trend between tissue triglycerides and several ceramides, with ceramide 16:0 reaching statistical significance ($R = -0.61$, $P = 0.02$). As shown in **Figure 3B**, within-sample molar sums of all measured ceramides were significantly and inversely correlated with triglyceride content. In spite of the positive correlation between triglycerides and BMI in the overall study population, there was no detectable relationship between BMI and individual ceramides or total ceramide content in the subset of subjects with measured renal ceramide content.

In an effort to further explore the significance of ceramides in relationship with renal lipid accumulation, we also measured ceramide content in obese Zucker diabetic fatty (ZDF) rats and lean age-matched controls. In spite of much higher triglyceride content in the kidney cortex of ZDF versus lean rats, there was no difference in total ceramides between groups (**Figure 3C**), and no relationship between total ceramides and triglyceride content.

Discussion

Key findings and interpretation

There are several key findings from this study of normal kidney surgical specimens obtained from 54 patients undergoing nephrectomy. There was a modest but statistically robust correlation between body mass index and total kidney cortex triglyceride content, suggesting that renal lipid accumulation occurs in humans with increasing body size. Lipid droplets detectable by conventional staining were primarily localized within epithelial cells of the proximal tubule, and to a lesser extent within glomeruli, suggesting that lipid accumulation and lipotoxicity may interfere with the normal physiology of these structures. Finally, evaluation of kidney ceramides in humans and rodents suggested that lipid accumula-

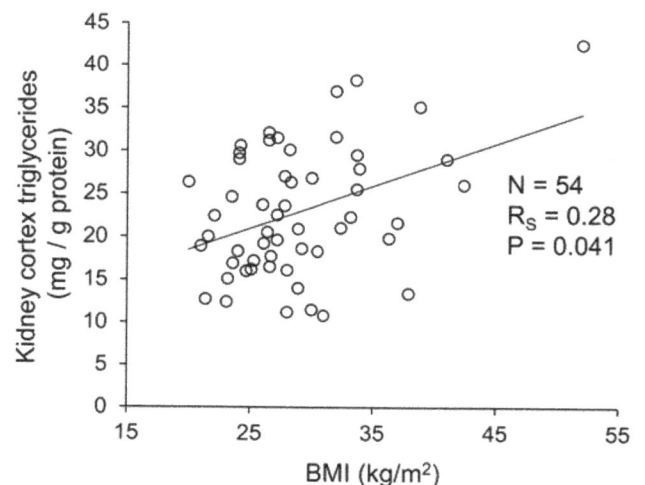

Figure 1. Kidney cortex triglyceride content and relationship with body mass index (BMI). Nephrectomy cortex samples were obtained from 54 patients with serum creatinine <1.5 mg/dL and no proteinuria. All surgical specimens were dissected by experienced clinical pathologists and confirmed to be healthy, away from the tumor. R_S, Spearman rank-order correlation coefficient.

Table 2. Biochemical and clinical characteristics.

	Overall cohort	Tertile 1	Tertile 2	Tertile 3	P$_{trend}$	P for tertile 1 vs. 3
Creatinine (mg/dL)	1.0 (0.8, 1.2)	1.0 (0.8, 1.2)	1.0 (0.9, 1.1)	0.9 (0.7, 1.3)	0.62	0.82
eGFR* (ml/min/1.73 m^2)	79 (62, 92)	74 (61, 98)	81 (67, 90)	75 (61, 88)	0.64	0.85
Triglycerides (mg/dL)[†]	132 (96, 195)	132 (95, 150)	154 (93, 232)	125 (101, 234)	0.47	0.52
Total Cholesterol (mg/dL)[†]	171 (137, 200)	190 (144, 194)	180 (135, 214)	153 (135, 179)	0.35	0.26
HDL-Cholesterol (mg/dL)[†]	39 (34, 49)	44 (34, 51)	36 (31, 45)	39 (35, 47)	0.61	0.56
LDL-Cholesterol (mg/dL)[†]	95 (76, 117)	106 (90, 119)	97 (79, 128)	85 (65, 96)	0.15 (0.58[§])	0.10 (0.24[§])
Antidyslipidemic medications[‡]	13 (31.7%)	2 (18.2%)	6 (35.3%)	5 (29.4%)	0.30	0.28
Diabetes[‖]	12 (22.2%)	1 (5.6%)	6 (31.6%)	5 (29.4%)	0.09 (0.24[#])	0.06 (0.12[#])
Hypertension	35 (64.8%)	14 (77.8%)	11 (57.9%)	10 (58.8%)	0.24	0.23

Data are presented as median (25th, 75th percentiles) or number of subjects (percentage) for the overall study population, as well as stratified by tertiles of renal cortical triglyceride content.
* eGFR was calculated using the CKD-EPI formula, http://www.kidney.org/professionals/kdoqi/gfr_calculator.cfm.
[†]Lipid values were available for 34 of the 54 study participants (13, 10 and 11 respectively in the 3 tertiles).
[‡]Antidyslipidemic medications included statins in 11 patients, statin combined with cholesterol absorption inhibitor in 1 patient, and fibrate in 1 patient.
[§]Adjusted for the use of antidyslipidemic medications.
[‖]All type 2 diabetes.
Of these, 4 were taking metformin, 3 sulfonylurea (glipizide or glyburide), one metformin+glimepiride, and 4 were managed with lifestyle intervention alone.
[#]Adjusted for body mass index.

tion in the kidney may not associate with lipotoxicity via the ceramide pathway.

Obesity and triglyceride accumulation in non-adipose tissues

Lipid accumulation with increasing BMI has been described in multiple non-adipose tissues, including the liver [21,23], pancreas [22], myocardium [23] and skeletal muscle [20]. With some exceptions, such as the "athlete's paradox" of high intramuscular lipid associated with marked insulin sensitivity in endurance-trained athletes [33], lipid accumulation has been associated with lipotoxicity and organ dysfunction [24–27].

In the human kidney, various patterns of lipid accumulation have been described in patients with genetic defects of lipid metabolism, including familial dysbetalipoproteinemia [34], lecithin-cholesterol acyltransferase deficiency [35], lipoprotein glomerulopathy [36] and alpha-galactosidase A deficiency (Fabry's disease) [37], as well as in patients with acquired conditions such as hypertensive nephrosclerosis [38], focal segmental glomerulosclerosis [39], minimal change disease with massive proteinuria [40] and hepatorenal syndrome [41]. However, whether lipid accumulation occurs with increasing BMI was not known prior to the present study.

As the general definition of steatosis is "any abnormal accumulation of triglycerides within parenchymal cells" [42], our data suggest that obesity may be associated with renal steatosis, although absolute triglyceride levels in the steatotic kidney are much lower than in the steatotic liver [43].

Localization of lipid droplets and pathophysiological implications

A large number of animal studies using genetic, pharmacologic or dietary manipulations have shown that renal lipid accumulation can occur both in glomeruli and in tubule cells, primarily in proximal tubules, with some variations between genetic strains and experimental models (reviewed in [9]). Lipid accumulation in glomeruli as well as in tubule cells has been postulated to contribute to the pathogenesis of kidney disease in animal models

of progressive renal injury [8,9]. In addition, prior *in vivo* and *in vitro* studies from our group have proposed a causal relationship between lipid accumulation in the proximal tubule and altered renal acidification, which can increase uric acid stone risk [17,18]. It is absolutely imperative to determine whether these studies are relevant for human pathophysiology. One *sine qua non* condition is detectability of lipid accumulation within the respective renal structures in at-risk individuals. Our findings that kidney cortex triglycerides are localized in both tubule cells and in glomeruli, and track with increasing BMI, suggest that renal lipid accumulation could play a role in obesity-related kidney disease and nephrolithiasis risk.

Lipid droplets, lipotoxicity and the role of ceramides

Intracellular lipid droplets are not static fat depots, but dynamic and highly regulated organelles with important normal functions in cellular energy storage and metabolism [44]. When net delivery of fatty acids to non-adipose cells exceeds cellular energy needs or beta-oxidative capacity, one key mechanism of defense against lipotoxicity is the storage of excess fatty acids as triglycerides in lipid droplets. It is thus important to note that triglyceride accumulation is not considered harmful *per se*, but is instead a quantifiable marker of a disturbed balance between fatty acid supply and utilization [8,9,45]. Excess fatty acids that are not beta-oxidized or incorporated in triglycerides enter alternative metabolic pathways, resulting in increased cellular content of potentially lipotoxic metabolites, with ceramides as a much touted candidate [8,9,45]. This model is compatible with the negative correlation between renal triglyceride and ceramide levels in a subset of samples from our study, suggesting that effective incorporation of excess fatty acids into triglycerides may protect against ceramide-induced renal lipotoxicity.

Importantly, there was no detectable relationship between ceramide levels and BMI in our dataset. We postulate that our data on triglycerides reflect a general state of obesity-associated renal fatty acid oversupply, while our data on ceramides reflect inter-individual differences in the metabolic fates of excess fatty acids in the kidney due to factors unrelated to BMI. These differences could potentially contribute to clinical variability, with

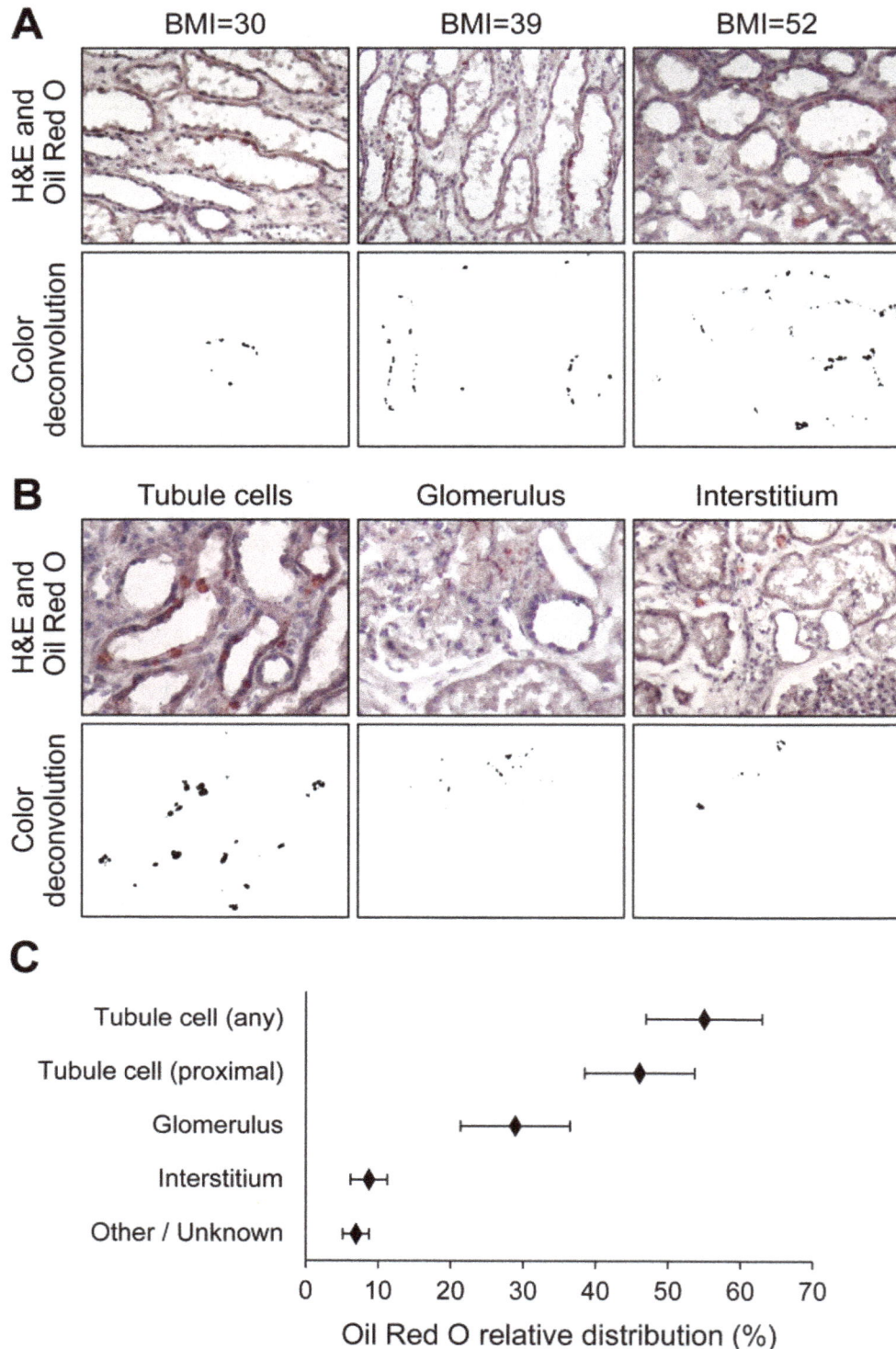

Figure 2. Lipid staining. Kidney cortex sections were stained with Oil Red O and standard hematoxylin to visualize lipid localization within renal structures. After image acquisition, a computer-based color deconvolution and thresholding algorithm was used to separately visualize and quantify Oil Red O staining, with the original image serving as reference for the manual assignment of lipid staining to discrete structures (i.e. tubule cells, glomeruli, interstitium, other). A. Oil Red O staining was noted predominantly in proximal tubule cells, and generally increased with increasing body mass index (BMI). B. Examples of the localization of lipids within tubule cells, glomeruli and interstitium. C. Relative distribution of lipids within kidney structures based on Oil Red O staining quantified by color deconvolution in 29 study participants with available fixed tissue. Whiskers represent 95% confidence intervals.

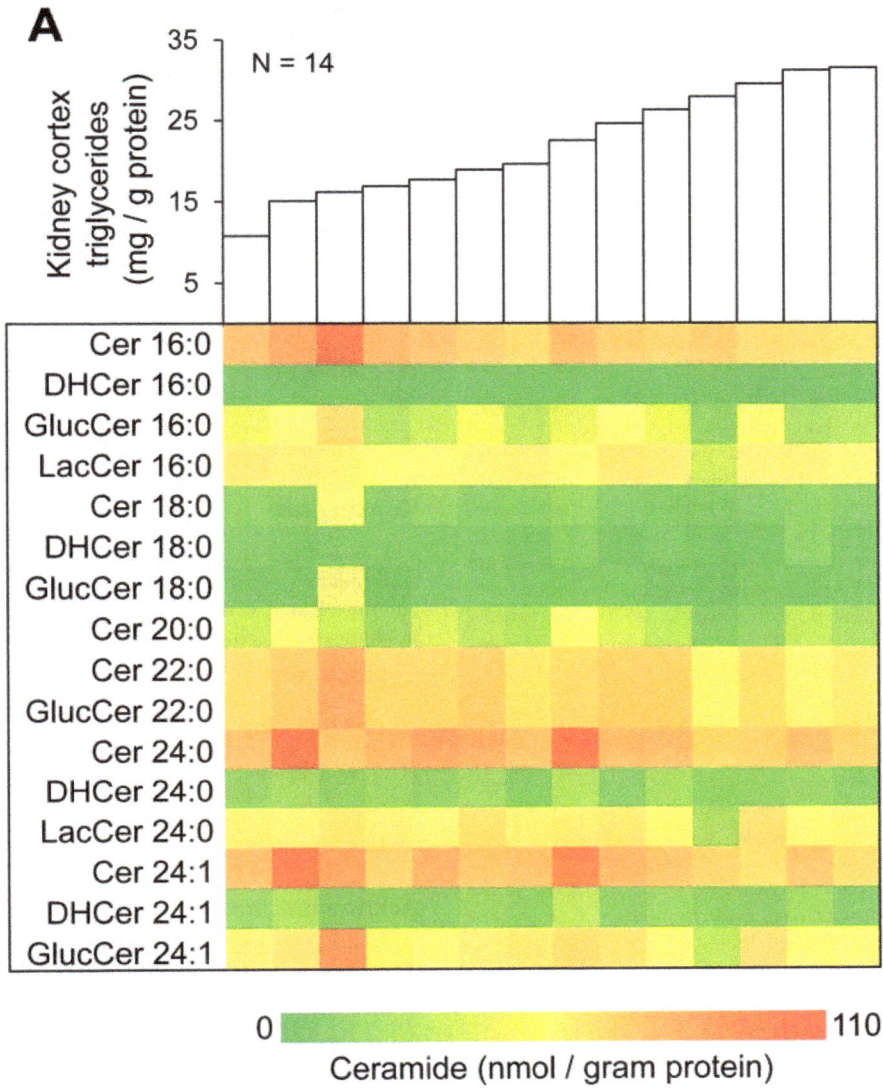

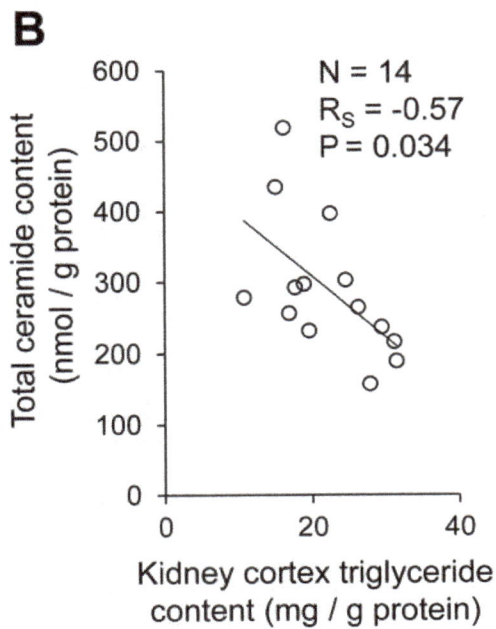

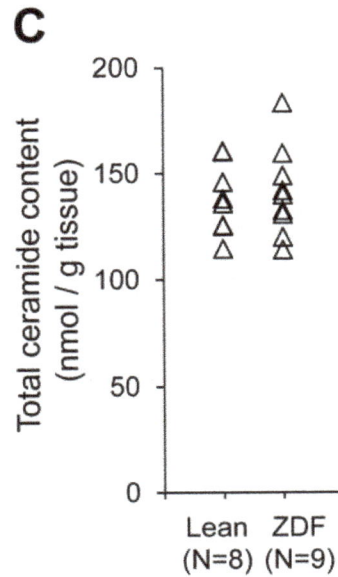

Figure 3. Kidney cortex ceramide content and relationship with triglycerides. Sixteen common ceramide species (Cer, ceramide; GlucCer, glucosylceramide; LacCer, lactosylceramide; DHCer, dihydroceramide) were measured by high performance liquid chromatography-electrospray ionization-tandem mass spectrometry (HPLC-ESI-MS/MS) in kidney cortex samples previously frozen at $-80°C$. A. The abundance of each ceramide species in human kidney cortex samples with increasing triglyceride content. B. Relationship between total ceramide content (molar sum of all measured ceramides) and triglyceride content in human kidney cortex samples. R_S, Spearman rank-order correlation coefficient. C. Total ceramide content in kidney cortex samples from Zucker diabetic fatty (ZDF) and lean control rats.

obesity-related kidney disease and nephrolithiasis risk not uniformly manifested in the general population. However, while ceramides have been implicated in lipotoxicity in other organs, little is known about their role in the kidney, and the potential contribution of other lipid metabolites to renal lipotoxicity is also unclear [8,24,46,47].

Renal ceramides in Zucker diabetic fatty rats

To further explore the potential role of ceramides in renal pathophysiology, while controlling for the genetic and environmental heterogeneity inherent in human subject research, we studied a rodent model in which renal triglyceride accumulation has been linked with surrogate functional markers of uric acid stone risk, including data showing that reduction of triglyceride accumulation with a PPARγ agonist reversed the functional defects [18,19]. There were no differences in total kidney cortex ceramide content between ZDF rats and lean control rats, suggesting that renal dysfunction in ZDF rats is not attributable to ceramide-induced lipotoxicity. Other lipid metabolites may contribute to renal lipotoxicity in this animal model [8,24,46,47].

Strengths and Limitations

Key strengths of the present study include the quantitation of triglycerides by a combination of direct biochemical and histological methods and the assessment of a relatively large number of samples from patients with a wide range of BMI. While most recent studies in humans have evaluated triglyceride content in various tissues indirectly by ^{1}H magnetic resonance spectroscopy (MRS) [20–23], direct biochemical quantitation of triglycerides, as used in the present study, remains the gold-standard [48]. Despite widespread use in the heart, skeletal muscle, liver and pancreas [49], MRS-based measurement of triglycerides in the kidney has only recently been reported by Hammer *et al.* [50]. However, the technique does not have adequate reliability in our hands. We and our collaborators have performed careful measurements including respiratory motion compensation, but these yielded borderline signal-to-noise ratios and unacceptable intra-assay variation (unpublished data). This is largely attributable to the much lower fat content in the kidney, even in pathologic states, compared with other tissues in which this technique is established. The study of Hammer *et al.* found mean triglyceride-to-water peak ratios in the renal parenchyma less than 0.5%, with a reported intra-assay coefficient of variation (CV) of 27% in optimal conditions [50]. For comparison, triglyceride peak ratios

as high as 40% have been reported in steatotic liver, with $CV = 8.5\%$ [51].

The study also has important limitations. Our cohort of patients undergoing nephrectomy for renal tumors is not representative of the general population. Measures of adiposity other than BMI, such as waist circumference, waist to hip ratio, or truncal fat content determined by dual energy X-ray absorptiometry, were not available. Finally, because of limited tissue availability, we could only perform Oil Red O staining and ceramide measurements in subsets of the study population.

Conclusions

This is the first demonstration of obesity-related triglyceride accumulation (steatosis) in the human kidney. Even though the amount of lipid is not large and the distribution is sporadic, the predominant localization of lipid droplets appears to be within proximal tubule cells, and to a lesser extent within glomeruli. Triglyceride accumulation in individuals with high BMI is likely a marker of renal fatty acid oversupply, as well as a cellular defense mechanism against the accumulation of potentially toxic metabolites, as suggested by our quantitation of 16 common ceramide species. This study supports the potential association between renal lipid accumulation and obesity-related kidney disease and nephrolithiasis risk.

Acknowledgments

The authors are grateful for the skilled assistance of Carolyn Griffith, RN, Elaine Isaminger, RN (clinical research coordinators), Adrien Jump, Anthony Nguyen, Hillary Thompson, Sun Park (technical staff), John Poindexter (database manager) and to the many staff members in the Departments of Urology and Pathology at UT Southwestern and affiliated hospitals who facilitated the timely transfer of surgical specimens for this study. Special thanks go to Dr. Roger Unger and Dr. Connie Hsia for generously providing ZDF and control rats, to Dr. Lili Wu and Dr. Priya Ravikumar for help with animal experiments, to Dr. Ruth Gordillo for help with the quantitation of ceramides by LC-ESI-MS/MS, and to Dr. Philipp Scherer for helpful discussions.

Author Contributions

Conceived and designed the experiments: IAB KS OWM. Performed the experiments: IAB JZ TRR. Analyzed the data: IAB YL JZ TRR JTR BA KS OWM. Wrote the paper: IAB. Revised the article for important intellectual content: IAB YL JZ TRR JTR BA KS OWM. Approved the final version: IAB YL JZ TRR JTR BA KS OWM.

References

1. European Commission's European Statistics (Eurostat) website: Overweight and obesity - BMI statistics - Statistics Explained. Available: http://epp.eurostat.ec. europa.eu/statistics_explained/index.php/Overweight_and_obesity_-_BMI_ statistics# Accessed 2014 June 7.

2. Ogden CL, Carroll MD, Kit BK, Flegal KM (2012) Prevalence of obesity in the United States, 2009–2010. NCHS data brief, no 82. Hyattsville, MD: NationalCenter for Health Statistics. Available on the Centers for Disease Control and Prevention website: http://www.cdc.gov/nchs/data/databriefs/db82.pdf Accessed 2014 June 7.

3. World Health Organization website: Fact sheet N°311 - Obesity and overweight. Available: http://www.who.int/mediacentre/factsheets/fs311/en/ Accessed 2014 June 7.

4. Janssen I, Katzmarzyk PT, Ross R (2004) Waist circumference and not body mass index explains obesity-related health risk. Am J Clin Nutr 79: 379–384.

5. Fox CS, Larson MG, Leip EP, Culleton B, Wilson PW, et al. (2004) Predictors of new-onset kidney disease in a community-based population. JAMA 291: 844–850.

6. Vivante A, Golan E, Tzur D, Leiba A, Tirosh A, et al. (2012) Body mass index in 1.2 million adolescents and risk for end-stage renal disease. Arch Intern Med 172: 1644–1650.

7. Hsu CY, McCulloch CE, Iribarren C, Darbinian J, Go AS (2006) Body mass index and risk for end-stage renal disease. Ann Intern Med 144: 21–28.

8. Weinberg JM (2006) Lipotoxicity. Kidney Int 70: 1560–1566.

9. Bobulescu IA (2010) Renal lipid metabolism and lipotoxicity. Curr Opin Nephrol Hypertens 19: 393–402.

10. Zoccali C, Mallamaci F (2011) Adiponectin and leptin in chronic kidney disease: causal factors or mere risk markers? J Ren Nutr 21: 87–91.

11. Wickman C, Kramer H (2013) Obesity and kidney disease: potential mechanisms. Semin Nephrol 33: 14–22.

12. Taylor EN, Stampfer MJ, Curhan GC (2005) Obesity, weight gain, and the risk of kidney stones. JAMA 293: 455–462.

13. Scales CD, Jr., Smith AC, Hanley JM, Saigal CS, Urologic Diseases in America P(2012) Prevalence of kidney stones in the United States. Eur Urol 62: 160–165.

14. Daudon M, Lacour B, Jungers P (2006) Influence of body size on urinary stone composition in men and women. Urol Res 34: 193–199.

15. Maalouf NM, Sakhaee K, Parks JH, Coe FL, Adams-Huet B, et al. (2004) Association of urinary pH with body weight in nephrolithiasis. Kidney Int 65: 1422–1425.

16. Sakhaee K, Maalouf NM (2008) Metabolic syndrome and uric acid nephrolithiasis. Semin Nephrol 28: 174–180.

17. Bobulescu IA, Dubree M, Zhang J, McLeroy P, Moe OW (2008) Effect of renal lipid accumulation on proximal tubule Na+/H+ exchange and ammonium secretion. Am J Physiol Renal Physiol 294: F1315–1322.

18. Bobulescu IA, Dubree M, Zhang J, McLeroy P, Moe OW (2009) Reduction of renal triglyceride accumulation: effects on proximal tubule Na+/H+ exchange and urinary acidification. Am J Physiol Renal Physiol 297: F1419–1426.

19. Bobulescu IA, Dubree M, Zhang J, Moe OW (2007) Effect of lipid accumulation on renal proximal tubule Na+/H+ exchange and NH4+ secretion. Am J Physiol Renal Physiol: submitted.

20. Sinha R, Dufour S, Petersen KF, LeBon V, Enoksson S, et al. (2002) Assessment of skeletal muscle triglyceride content by (1)H nuclear magnetic resonance spectroscopy in lean and obese adolescents: relationships to insulin sensitivity, total body fat, and central adiposity. Diabetes 51: 1022–1027.

21. Thomas EL, Hamilton G, Patel N, O'Dwyer R, Dore CJ, et al. (2005) Hepatic triglyceride content and its relation to body adiposity: a magnetic resonance imaging and proton magnetic resonance spectroscopy study. Gut 54: 122–127.

22. Lingvay I, Esser V, Legendre JL, Price AL, Wertz KM, et al. (2009) Noninvasive quantification of pancreatic fat in humans. J Clin Endocrinol Metab 94: 4070–4076.

23. Graner M, Siren R, Nyman K, Lundbom J, Hakkarainen A, et al. (2013) Cardiac steatosis associates with visceral obesity in nondiabetic obese men. J Clin Endocrinol Metab 98: 1189–1197.

24. Unger RH, Clark GO, Scherer PE, Orci L (2010) Lipid homeostasis, lipotoxicity and the metabolic syndrome. Biochim Biophys Acta 1801: 209–214.

25. Wende AR, Abel ED (2010) Lipotoxicity in the heart. Biochim Biophys Acta 1801: 311–319.

26. Muoio DM (2010) Intramuscular triacylglycerol and insulin resistance: Guilty as charged or wrongly accused? Biochim Biophys Acta 1801: 281–288.

27. Suganami T, Tanaka M, Ogawa Y (2012) Adipose tissue inflammation and ectopic lipid accumulation. Endocr J 59: 849–857.

28. Folch J, Lees M, Sloane Stanley GH (1957) A simple method for the isolation and purification of total lipides from animal tissues. J Biol Chem 226: 497–509.

29. Danno H, Jincho Y, Budiyanto S, Furukawa Y, Kimura S (1992) A simple enzymatic quantitative analysis of triglycerides in tissues. J Nutr Sci Vitaminol (Tokyo) 38: 517–521.

30. Ruifrok AC, Johnston DA (2001) Quantification of histochemical staining by color deconvolution. Anal Quant Cytol Histol 23: 291–299.

31. Rasband WS (1997–2007) ImageJ, U. S. National Institutes of Health, Bethesda, Maryland, USA. Available: http://rsb.info.nih.gov/ij/ Accessed 2014 June 7.

32. Olofsson SO, Bostrom P, Andersson L, Rutberg M, Perman J, et al. (2009) Lipid droplets as dynamic organelles connecting storage and efflux of lipids. Biochim Biophys Acta 1791: 448–458.

33. Goodpaster BH, He J, Watkins S, Kelley DE (2001) Skeletal muscle lipid content and insulin resistance: evidence for a paradox in endurance-trained athletes. J Clin Endocrinol Metab 86: 5755–5761.

34. Balson KR, Niall JF, Best JD (1996) Glomerular lipid deposition and proteinuria in a patient with familial dysbetalipoproteinaemia. J Intern Med 240: 157–159.

35. Gjone E (1981) Familial lecithin:cholesterol acyltransferase deficiency - a new metabolic disease with renal involvement. Adv Nephrol Necker Hosp 10: 167–185.

36. Sam R, Wu H, Yue L, Mazzone T, Schwartz MM, et al. (2006) Lipoprotein glomerulopathy: a new apolipoprotein E mutation with enhanced glomerular binding. Am J Kidney Dis 47: 539–548.

37. Gubler MC, Lenoir G, Grunfeld JP, Ulmann A, Droz D, et al. (1978) Early renal changes in hemizygous and heterozygous patients with Fabry's disease. Kidney Int 13: 223–235.

38. Druilhet RE, Overturf ML, Kirkendall WM (1978) Cortical and medullary lipids of normal and nephrosclerotic human kidney. Int J Biochem 9: 729–734.

39. Magil AB, Cohen AH (1989) Monocytes and focal glomerulosclerosis. Lab Invest 61: 404–409.

40. Jennette JC, Falk RJ (1990) Adult minimal change glomerulopathy with acute renal failure. Am J Kidney Dis 16: 432–437.

41. Hovig T, Blomhoff JP, Holme R, Flatmark A, Gjone E (1978) Plasma lipoprotein alterations and morphologic changes with lipid deposition in the kidney of patients with hepatorenal syndrome. Lab Invest 38: 540–549.

42. Kumar V, Abbas AK, Aster JC (2012) Robbins Basic Pathology. Philadelphia, PA: Elsevier Saunders.

43. Reddy JK, Rao MS (2006) Lipid metabolism and liver inflammation. II. Fatty liver disease and fatty acid oxidation. Am J Physiol Gastrointest Liver Physiol 290: G852–858.

44. Greenberg AS, Coleman RA, Kraemer FB, McManaman JL, Obin MS, et al. (2011) The role of lipid droplets in metabolic disease in rodents and humans. J Clin Invest 121: 2102–2110.

45. Listenberger LL, Han X, Lewis SE, Cases S, Farese RV, Jr., et al. (2003) Triglyceride accumulation protects against fatty acid-induced lipotoxicity. Proc Natl Acad Sci U S A 100: 3077–3082.

46. Unger RH (2002) Lipotoxic diseases. Annu Rev Med 53: 319–336.

47. Samuel VT, Shulman GI (2012) Mechanisms for insulin resistance: common threads and missing links. Cell 148: 852–871.

48. Szczepaniak LS, Babcock EE, Schick F, Dobbins RL, Garg A, et al. (1999) Measurement of intracellular triglyceride stores by H spectroscopy: validation in vivo. Am J Physiol 276: E977–989.

49. Thomas EL, Fitzpatrick JA, Malik SJ, Taylor-Robinson SD, Bell JD (2013) Whole body fat: Content and distribution. Prog Nucl Magn Reson Spectrosc 73: 56–80.

50. Hammer S, de Vries AP, de Heer P, Bizino MB, Wolterbeek R, et al. (2013) Metabolic imaging of human kidney triglyceride content: reproducibility of proton magnetic resonance spectroscopy. PLoS One 8: e62209.

51. Szczepaniak LS, Nurenberg P, Leonard D, Browning JD, Reingold JS, et al. (2005) Magnetic resonance spectroscopy to measure hepatic triglyceride content: prevalence of hepatic steatosis in the general population. Am J Physiol Endocrinol Metab 288: E462–468.

Permissions

The contributors of this book come from diverse backgrounds, making this book a truly international effort. This book will bring forth new frontiers with its revolutionizing research information and detailed analysis of the nascent developments around the world.

We would like to thank all the contributing authors for lending their expertise to make the book truly unique. They have played a crucial role in the development of this book. Without their invaluable contributions this book wouldn't have been possible. They have made vital efforts to compile up to date information on the varied aspects of this subject to make this book a valuable addition to the collection of many professionals and students.

This book was conceptualized with the vision of imparting up-to-date information and advanced data in this field. To ensure the same, a matchless editorial board was set up. Every individual on the board went through rigorous rounds of assessment to prove their worth. After which they invested a large part of their time researching and compiling the most relevant data for our readers.

The editorial board has been involved in producing this book since its inception. They have spent rigorous hours researching and exploring the diverse topics which have resulted in the successful publishing of this book. They have passed on their knowledge of decades through this book. To expedite this challenging task, the publisher supported the team at every step. A small team of assistant editors was also appointed to further simplify the editing procedure and attain best results for the readers.

Apart from the editorial board, the designing team has also invested a significant amount of their time in understanding the subject and creating the most relevant covers. They scrutinized every image to scout for the most suitable representation of the subject and create an appropriate cover for the book.

The publishing team has been an ardent support to the editorial, designing and production team. Their endless efforts to recruit the best for this project, has resulted in the accomplishment of this book. They are a veteran in the field of academics and their pool of knowledge is as vast as their experience in printing. Their expertise and guidance has proved useful at every step. Their uncompromising quality standards have made this book an exceptional effort. Their encouragement from time to time has been an inspiration for everyone.

The publisher and the editorial board hope that this book will prove to be a valuable piece of knowledge for researchers, students, practitioners and scholars across the globe.

List of Contributors

Bauke Schievink, Hiddo Lambers Heerspink and Dick De Zeeuw
Department of Clinical Pharmacy and Pharmacology, University of Groningen, University Medical Center Groningen, Groningen, The Netherlands

Jarno Hoekman
Utrecht Institute for Pharmaceutical Sciences, Division of Pharmacoepidemiology and Clinical Pharmacology, Utrecht University, Utrecht, The Netherlands

Hubert Leufkens
Utrecht Institute for Pharmaceutical Sciences, Division of Pharmacoepidemiology and Clinical Pharmacology, Utrecht University, Utrecht, The Netherlands
Medicines Evaluation Board, Utrecht, The Netherlands

Fatemeh Saheb Sharif-Askari, Syed Azhar Syed Sulaiman and Narjes Saheb Sharif-Askari
School of Pharmacy, Universiti Sains Malaysia, Penang, Malaysia

Ali Al Sayed Hussain
Pharmacy Department, Dubai Health Authority, Dubai, United Arab Emirates,

Mohammad Jaffar Railey
Nephrology Unit, Dubai Hospital, Dubai, United Arab Emirates

Xinguo Hou, Chuan Wang, Aixia Ma, Huizhen Zheng, Jiahui Wu, Yu Sun, Jun Song, Peng Lin, Kai Liang, Lei Gong, Meijian Wang, Fuqiang Liu, Wenjuan Li, Juan Xiao, Fei Yan, Junpeng Yang, Lingshu Wang, Meng Tia, Jidong Liu, Ruxing Zhao and Li Chen
Department of Endocrinology of Qilu Hospital and Institute of Endocrinology and Metabolism, Shandong University, Jinan, Shandong, China

Xiuping Zhang and Xiangmin Zhao
Shantui Community Health Center, Jining, Shandong, China

Yulian Wang, Chengqiao Li and Mei Li
Department of Endocrinology, Second People's Hospital of Jining, Jining, Shandong, China

Shaoyuan Wang and Weifang Yang
Lukang Hospital of Jining, Jining, Shandong, China

Zeqiang Ma
China National Heavy Duty Truck Group Corporation Hospital, Jinan, Shandong, China

Shihong Chen
Department of Endocrinology, the Second Hospital of Shandong University, Jinan, Shandong, China

Christine A. Murakami, Gregory M. Lucas, Michelle M. Estrella, Derek M. Fine and Mohamed G. Atta
Department of Medicine, Johns Hopkins University School of Medicine, Baltimore, Maryland, United States of America

Doaa Attia
Faculty of Medicine, Alexandria, Egypt

Naima Carter-Monroe
Department of Pathology, Johns Hopkins University School of Medicine, Baltimore, Maryland, United States of America

Shuo-Meng Wang
Department of Urology, National Taiwan University Hospital, Taipei, Taiwan
Institute of Occupational Medicine and Industrial Hygiene, College of Public Health, National Taiwan University, Taipei, Taiwan

Ming-Nan Lai
Department of Statistics, Feng Chia University, Taichung, Taiwan

Alan Wei
School of Medicine, Stony Brook University, Stony Brook, New York, United States of America

Yeong-Shiau Pu
Department of Urology, National Taiwan University Hospital, Taipei, Taiwan

Pau-Chung Chen
Institute of Occupational Medicine and Industrial Hygiene, College of Public Health, National Taiwan University, Taipei, Taiwan

Jung-Der Wang
Department of Public Health, National Cheng Kung University Medical College, Tainan City, Taiwan
Departments of Internal Medicine and Occupational and Environmental Medicine, National Cheng Kung University Hospital, Tainan City, Taiwan
Ya-Yin Chen
Department of Urology, National Taiwan University Hospital, Taipei, Taiwan
Department of Statistics, Feng Chia University, Taichung, Taiwan

Yi-Chun Tsai and Mei-Chuan Kuo
Graduate Institute of Clinical Medicine, Kaohsiung Medical University, Kaohsiung, Taiwan
Division of Nephrology, Department of Internal Medicine, Kaohsiung Medical University Hospital, Kaohsiung, Taiwan
Faculty of Renal Care, College of Medicine, Kaohsiung Medical University, Kaohsiung, Taiwan

Su-Chu Lee
Division of Nephrology, Department of Internal Medicine, Kaohsiung Medical University Hospital, Kaohsiung, Taiwan

Ming-Yen Lin
Faculty of Renal Care, College of Medicine, Kaohsiung Medical University, Kaohsiung, Taiwan

Yi-Wen Chiu, Jer-Chia Tsai, Hung-Tien Kuo, Chi-Chih Hung and Hung-Chun Chen
Division of Nephrology, Department of Internal Medicine, Kaohsiung Medical University Hospital, Kaohsiung, Taiwan
Faculty of Renal Care, College of Medicine, Kaohsiung Medical University, Kaohsiung, Taiwan

Shang-Jyh Hwang
Graduate Institute of Clinical Medicine, Kaohsiung Medical University, Kaohsiung, Taiwan
Division of Nephrology, Department of Internal Medicine, Kaohsiung Medical University Hospital, Kaohsiung, Taiwan
Faculty of Renal Care, College of Medicine, Kaohsiung Medical University, Kaohsiung, Taiwan
Institute of Population Sciences, National Health Research Institutes, Miaoli, Taiwan

Janaína Garcia Gonçalves, Ana Carolina de Bragança, Daniele Canale, Maria Heloisa Massola Shimizu, Talita Rojas Sanches, Rosa Maria Affonso Moysés, Lúcia Andrade, Antonio Carlos Seguro and Rildo Aparecido Volpini
Nephrology Department, University of São Paulo School of Medicine, São Paulo, Brazil

Shinichi Saito, Shaniya Abudureyimu and Yelixiati Adelibieke
Department of Advanced Medicine for Uremia, Nagoya University Graduate School of Medicine, Nagoya, Japan

Fuyuhiko Nishijima
Biomedical Research Laboratories, Kureha Co., Tokyo, Japan

Kyosuke Takeshita and Toyoaki Murohara
Department of Cardiology, Nagoya University Graduate School of Medicine, Nagoya, Japan

Maimaiti Yisireyili
Department of Advanced Medicine for Uremia, Nagoya University Graduate School of Medicine, Nagoya, Japan
Department of Cardiology, Nagoya University Graduate School of Medicine, Nagoya, Japan

Hwee-Yeong Ng
Division of Nephrology, Department of Internal Medicine, Kaohsiung Chang Gung Memorial Hospital and Chang Gung University College of Medicine, Kaohsiung, Taiwan

Toshimitsu Niwa
Department of Advanced Medicine for Uremia, Nagoya University Graduate School of Medicine, Nagoya, Japan
Faculty of Health and Nutrition, Shubun University, Aichi, Japan

Dov Shiffman, Judy Z. Louie, Charles M. Rowland and James J. Devlin
Celera, Alameda, CA, United States of America

Guillaume Pare and Matthew J. McQueen
Population Health Research Institute, Hamilton Health Sciences and McMaster University, Hamilton, Ontario, Canada

Rainer Oberbauer
Department of Nephrology, KH Elisabethinen, Linz, Austria and Department of Nephrology, Medical University of Vienna, Vienna, Austria

Johannes F. Mann
Department of Nephrology and Hypertension, Friedrich Alexander University, Erlangen, Germany

Ping Wen, Hong Ye, Xiaochun Wu, Lei Jiang, Bing Tang, Yang Zhou, Li Fang, Hongdi Cao, Weichun He, Chunsun Dai and Junwei Yang
Center for Kidney Disease, Second Affiliated Hospital, Nanjing Medical University, Nanjing, China

Yafang Yang
Department of Radiology, Second Affiliated Hospital, Nanjing Medical University, Nanjing, China

Dan Song
Department of Nephrology, Affiliated Wuxi Hospital, Nanjing Medical University, Wuxi, China

Luis E. Morales-Buenrostro, Omar I. Salas-Nolasco, Gustavo Casas-Aparicio and Sergio Irizar-Santana
Department of Nephrology Nefrología y Metabolismo Mineral, Instituto Nacional de Ciencias Médicas y Nutrición Salvador Zubirán, México City, México

Jonatan Barrera-Chimal, Rosalba Pérez-Villalva and Norma A. Bobadilla
Department of Nephrology Nefrología y Metabolismo Mineral, Instituto Nacional de Ciencias Médicas y Nutrición Salvador Zubirán, México City, México
Unidad de Fisiología Molecular, Instituto de Investigaciones Biomídicas, Universidad Nacional Autónoma de México, México City, México

Wai H. Lim
University of Western Australia School of Medicine and Pharmacology, Sir Charles Gairdner Hospital Unit, Perth, Australia
Department of Renal Medicine, Sir Charles Gairdner Hospital, Perth, Australia

Joshua R. Lewis and Richard L. Prince
University of Western Australia School of Medicine and Pharmacology, Sir Charles Gairdner Hospital Unit, Perth, Australia
Department of Endocrinology and Diabetes, Sir Charles Gairdner Hospital, Perth, Australia

Germaine Wong
Centre for Kidney Research, Children's Hospital at Westmead, Sydney, Australia
School of Public Health, Sydney Medical School, The University of Sydney, Sydney, Australia

Robin M. Turner
School of Public Health, The University of New South Wales, Sydney, Australia

Ee M. Lim
Department of Renal Medicine, Sir Charles Gairdner Hospital, Perth, Australia
PathWest, Sir Charles Gairdner Hospital, Perth, Australia

Peter L. Thompson
Department of Cardiovascular Medicine, Sir Charles Gairdner Hospital, Perth, Australia

Jeonghwan Lee
Department of Internal Medicine, Hallym University Hangang Sacred Heart Hospital, Seoul, Korea
Clinical Research Center for End Stage Renal Disease (CRC for ESRD), Daegu, Korea

Jung Nam An
Department of Internal Medicine, Seoul National University Boramae Medical Center, Seoul, Korea

Jin Ho Hwang
Department of Internal Medicine, Chung-Ang University Medical Center, Seoul, Korea

Yong-Lim Kim
Clinical Research Center for End Stage Renal Disease (CRC for ESRD), Daegu, Korea
Department of Internal Medicine, Kyungpook National University School of Medicine, Daegu, Korea

Shin-Wook Kang
Clinical Research Center for End Stage Renal Disease (CRC for ESRD), Daegu, Korea
Department of Internal Medicine, Yonsei University College of Medicine, Seoul, Korea

Chul Woo Yang
Clinical Research Center for End Stage Renal Disease (CRC for ESRD), Daegu, Korea
Department of Internal Medicine, The Catholic University of Korea College of Medicine, Seoul, Korea

Nam-Ho Kim
Clinical Research Center for End Stage Renal Disease (CRC for ESRD), Daegu, Korea
Department of Internal Medicine, Chonnam National University Medical School, Gwangju, Korea

Yun Kyu Oh, Chun Soo Lim and Jung Pyo Lee
Clinical Research Center for End Stage Renal Disease (CRC for ESRD), Daegu, Korea
Department of Internal Medicine, Seoul National University Boramae Medical Center, Seoul, Korea

Yon Su Kim
Clinical Research Center for End Stage Renal Disease (CRC for ESRD), Daegu, Korea
Department of Internal Medicine, Seoul National University Hospital, Seoul National University College of Medicine, Seoul, Korea

Minako Wakasugi
Center for Inter-organ Communication Research, Niigata University Graduate School of Medical and Dental Sciences, Niigata, Japan

Junichiro James Kazama
Department of Clinical Nephrology and Rheumatology, Niigata University Graduate School of Medical and Dental Sciences, Niigata, Japan

Ichiei Narita, Kunitoshi Iseki, Toshiki Moriyama, Kunihiro Yamagata, Shouichi Fujimoto, Kazuhiko Tsuruya, Koichi Asahi, Tsuneo Konta, Kenjiro Kimura, Masahide Kondo and Tsuyoshi Watanabe
Steering Committee for "Design of the comprehensive health care system for chronic kidney disease (CKD) based on the individual risk assessment by Specific Health Checkups," Fukushima, Japan

Issei Kurahashi
iAnalysis LLC, Tokyo, Japan

Yasuo Ohashi
Department of Integrated Science and Engineering for Sustainable Society, Chuo University, Tokyo, Japan

Zhuo Liang and Yu-tang Wang
Department of Geriatric Cardiology, Chinese PLA General Hospital, Beijing, China

Li-feng Liu, Xin-pei Chen, Xiang-min Shi, Hong-yang Guo, Kun Lin, Jian-ping Guo and Zhao-liang Shan
Department of Cardiology, Chinese PLA General Hospital, Beijing, China

Xuehong Dong, Dingting Wu, Chengfang Jia, Yu Ruan, Xiaocheng Feng, Guoxing Wang, Jun Liu and Hong Li
Departments of Endocrinology and Metabolism, Sir Run Run Shaw Hospital, School of Medicine, Zhejiang University, Hangzhou, P. R. China

Yi Shen
Department of Epidemiology and Health Statistics School of Public Health, Zhejiang University, Hangzhou, P. R. China

Lianxi Li
Department of Endocrinology and Metabolism, Shanghai Jiao Tong University Affiliated Sixth People's Hospital, Shanghai, P. R. China

Yu-Jen Yu, I-Wen Wu, Chin-Chan Lee, Chio-Yin Sun and Heng-Jung Hsu
Department of Nephrology, Chang Gung Memorial Hospital, Keelung, Taiwan
College of Medicine, Chang Gung University, Tao-Yuan, Taiwan

Chun-Yu Huang and Kuang-Hung Hsu
Laboratory for Epidemiology, Department of Health Care Management, Chang Gung University, Tao-Yuan, Taiwan

Mai-Szu Wu
Department of Nephrology, Chang Gung Memorial Hospital, Keelung, Taiwan
Division of Nephrology, Taipei Medical University Hospital, Taipei, Taiwan
School of Medicine, Taipei Medical University, Taipei, Taiwan

Xinguo Hou, Chuan Wang, Yu Sun, Jun Song, Peng Lin, Kai Liang, Lei Gong, Meijian Wang, Fuqiang

Liu, Wenjuan Li, Fei Yan, Junpeng Yang, Lingshu Wang, Meng Tian, Jidong Liu, Ruxing Zhao
Department of Endocrinology of Qilu Hospital, Shandong University, Jinan, Shandong, China

Shaoyuan Wang and Weifang Yang
Lukang Hospital of Jining, Jining, Shandong, China

Zeqiang Ma
China National Heavy Duty Truck Group Corporation Hospital, Jinan, Shandong, China

Yulian Wang, Chengqiao Li and Mei Li
Department of Endocrinology, Second People's Hospital of Jining, Jining, Shandong, China

Xiuping Zhang and Xiangmin Zhao
Shantui Community Health Center, Jining, Shandong, China

Shihong Chen
Department of Endocrinology, the Second Hospital of Shandong University, Jinan, Shandong, China

Dongsheng Cheng, Yang Fei, Yumei Liu, Junhui Li, Yuqiang Chen, Xiaoxia Wang and Niansong Wang
Department of Nephrology and Rheumatology, Shanghai Jiaotong University Affiliated Sixth People's Hospital, Shanghai, P.R. China

Marc Froissart
CESP, Centre for Epidemiology and Population Health, INSERM Unit 1018, Villejuif, France

Elena Tynkevich, Marie Metzger, Bénédicte Stengel and on behalf of the NephroTest Study Group
CESP, Centre for Epidemiology and Population Health, INSERM Unit 1018, Villejuif, France
University Paris-Sud 11, UMRS 1018, Villejuif, France

Martin Flamant
AP-HP, Hôpital Bichat, Department of Physiology, Paris, France

Jean-Philippe Haymann
AP-HP, Hôpital Tenon, Department of Physiology, Paris, France
INSERM UNIT 702, Paris, France
University Pierre et Marie Curie-Paris 6, UMRS 702, Paris, France

Eric Thervet
AP-HP, Hôpital Européen Georges Pompidou, Department of Nephrology, Paris, France
AP-HP, Hôpital Européen Georges Pompidou, DHU Common and Rare Arterial Diseases, Paris, France

Jean-Jacques Boffa
INSERM UNIT 702, Paris, France
University Pierre et Marie Curie-Paris 6, UMRS 702, Paris, France
AP-HP, Hôpital Tenon, Department of Nephrology, Paris, France

François Vrtovsnik
AP-HP, Hôpital Bichat, Department of Nephrology, Paris, France

Pascal Houillier
University Paris Descartes-Paris 5, UMRS 775, Paris, France
AP-HP, Hôpital Européen Georges Pompidou, Department of Physiology, Paris, France

Yi-Chun Tsai and Mei-Chuan Kuo
Graduate Institute of Clinical Medicine, Kaohsiung Medical University, Kaohsiung, Taiwan
Division of Nephrology, Kaohsiung Medical University Hospital, Kaohsiung, Taiwan
Faculty of Renal Care, Kaohsiung Medical University, Kaohsiung, Taiwan

Yi-Wen Chiu, Hung-Tien Kuo and Hung-Chun Chen
Division of Nephrology, Kaohsiung Medical University Hospital, Kaohsiung, Taiwan
Faculty of Renal Care, Kaohsiung Medical University, Kaohsiung, Taiwan

Szu-Chia Chen
Faculty of Renal Care, Kaohsiung Medical University, Kaohsiung, Taiwan
Department of Internal Medicine, Kaohsiung Municipal Hsiao-Kang Hospital, Kaohsiung, Taiwan

Shang-Jyh Hwang
Graduate Institute of Clinical Medicine, Kaohsiung Medical University, Kaohsiung, Taiwan
Division of Nephrology, Kaohsiung Medical University Hospital, Kaohsiung, Taiwan
Faculty of Renal Care, Kaohsiung Medical University, Kaohsiung, Taiwan
Institute of Population Sciences, National Health Research Institutes, Miaoli, Taiwan

Tzu-Hui Chen
Department of Nursing, Kaohsiung Medical University Hospital, Kaohsiung, Taiwan

Xingqiang Lai, Guodong Chen, Jiang Qiu, Changxi Wang and Lizhong Chen
Organ Transplant Center, The First Affiliated Hospital, Sun Yat-sen University, Guangzhou, China

Ingo Flamme
Cardiology/Hematology, Acute Care Research, Global Drug Discovery, Bayer Pharma AG, Wuppertal, Germany

Felix Oehme
Biotech Development, Global Biologics, Bayer Pharma AG, Wuppertal, Germany

Peter Ellinghaus
Clinical Science, Global Biomarkers, Bayer Pharma AG, Wuppertal, Germany

Mario Jeske
Global Chemical Product Development, Bayer Pharma AG, Wuppertal, Germany

Jörg Keldenich and Uwe Thuss
Drug Metabolism and Pharmacokinetics, Global Early Development, Bayer Pharma AG, Wuppertal, Germany

Michiya Ohno, Kumiko Izumi, Hirotoshi Ishigaki and Hiroshige Ohashi
Division of Nephrology, Murakami Memorial Hospital, Asahi University School of Dentistry, Gifu City, Gifu, Japan

Fumiko Deguchi and Takao Kojima
Division of Health Center, Murakami Memorial Hospital, Asahi University School of Dentistry, Gifu City, Gifu, Japan

Hiroshi Sarui and Akihiko Sasaki
Division of Diabetes and Endocrinology, Murakami Memorial Hospital, Asahi University School of Dentistry, Gifu City, Gifu, Japan

Tomonori Segawa and Takahiko Yamaki
Division of Cardiology, Murakami Memorial Hospital, Asahi University School of Dentistry, Gifu City, Gifu, Japan

Tae Ik Chang, Sug Kyun Shin and Ea Wha Kang
Department of Internal Medicine, NHIS Medical Center, Ilsan Hospital, Goyangshi, Gyeonggi–do, Republic of Korea

Yung Ly Kim, Hyungwoo Kim, Geun Woo Ryu, Jung Tak Park, Tae-Hyun Yoo, Kyu Hun Choi, Dae Suk Han and Seung Hyeok Han
Department of Internal Medicine, College of Medicine, Yonsei University, Seoul, Republic of Korea

Shin-Wook Kang
Department of Internal Medicine, College of Medicine, Yonsei University, Seoul, Republic of Korea

Brain Korea 21 for Medical Science, Severance Biomedical Science Institute, Yonsei University, Seoul, Republic of Korea

Serena M. Bagnasco, Srinivas Gottipati, Lorraine C. Racusen and Lois J. Arend
Department of Pathology, Johns Hopkins University, Baltimore, Maryland, United States of America

Edward Kraus and Nada Alachkar
Department of Medicine, Johns Hopkins University, Baltimore, Maryland, United States of America

Robert A. Montgomery
Department of Surgery, Johns Hopkins University, Baltimore, Maryland, United States of America

Ikechi G. Okpechi, Thandiwe A. L. Dlamini, Brian L. Rayner and Charles R. Swanepoel
Division of Nephrology and Hypertension, Groote Schuur Hospital and University of Cape Town, South Africa

Maureen Duffield
Division of Anatomical Pathology, National Health and Laboratory Services (NHLS), University of Cape Town, South Africa

George Moturi
Department of Medicine, Aga Khan University Hospital, Nairobi, Kenya

Joo Myung Lee, Jonghanne Park, Ki-Hyun Jeon, Ji-hyun Jung, Sang Eun Lee, Jung-Kyu Han, Han-Mo Yang, Kyung Woo Park, Hyun-Jae Kang and Bon-Kwon Koo
Department of Internal Medicine and Cardiovascular Center, Seoul National University Hospital, Seoul, Korea

Hack-Lyoung Kim
Cardiovascular Center, Seoul National University, Boramae Medical Center, Seoul, Korea

Sang-Ho Jo
Division of Cardiology, Department of Internal Medicine, Hallym University Sacred Heart Hospital, Anyang-si, Gyeonggi-do, Korea,

Hyo-Soo Kim
Department of Internal Medicine and Cardiovascular Center, Seoul National University Hospital, Seoul, Korea

Department of Molecular Medicine and Biopharmaceutical Sciences, Graduate School of Convergence Science and Technology, Seoul National University, Seoul, Korea

Federica Genovese, Morten A. Karsdal and Diana J. Leeming
Nordic Bioscience, Fibrosis Biology and Biomarkers, Herlev, Denmark

Alexandra Scholze and Martin Tepel
Odense University Hospital, Department of Nephrology, Institute for Molecular Medicine, Cardiovascular and Renal Research, Institute of Clinical Research, University of Southern Denmark, Odense, Denmark

Terri R. Fried
Clinical Epidemiology Research Center, VA Connecticut Healthcare System, West Haven, Connecticut, United States of America
Department of Medicine, Yale School of Medicine, New Haven, Connecticut, United States of America

Ion Alexandru Bobulescu and Khashayar Sakhaee
Department of Internal Medicine and the Charles and Jane Pak Center for Mineral Metabolism and Clinical Research, University of Texas Southwestern Medical Center, Dallas, Texas, United States of America

Yair Lotan
Department of Urology, University of Texas Southwestern Medical Center, Dallas, Texas, United States of America

Jianning Zhang, Tara R. Rosenthal and John T. Rogers
3 Department of Internal Medicine, University of Texas Southwestern Medical Center, Dallas, Texas, United States of America

Beverley Adams-Huet
Department of Clinical Sciences and the Charles and Jane Pak Center for Mineral Metabolism and Clinical Research, University of Texas Southwestern Medical Center, Dallas, Texas, United States of America

Orson W. Moe
Departments of Internal Medicine, Physiology, and the Charles and Jane Pak Center for Mineral Metabolism and Clinical Research, University of Texas Southwestern Medical Center, Dallas, Texas, United States of America

Index

www.ingramcontent.com/pod-product-compliance
Lightning Source LLC
Chambersburg PA
CBHW080455200326
41458CB00012B/3983